D1666160

Osteoarthritis: From Molecular Pathways to Therapeutic Advances

Osteoarthritis: From Molecular Pathways to Therapeutic Advances

Editor

Nicola Veronese

MDPI • Basel • Beijing • Wuhan • Barcelona • Belgrade • Manchester • Tokyo • Cluj • Tianjin

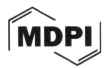

Editor
Nicola Veronese
Medicine
University of Palermo
Palermo
Italy

Editorial Office
MDPI
St. Alban-Anlage 66
4052 Basel, Switzerland

This is a reprint of articles from the Special Issue published online in the open access journal *International Journal of Molecular Sciences* (ISSN 1422-0067) (available at: www.mdpi.com/journal/ijms/special_issues/Osteoarthritis_2020).

For citation purposes, cite each article independently as indicated on the article page online and as indicated below:

LastName, A.A.; LastName, B.B.; LastName, C.C. Article Title. *Journal Name* **Year**, *Volume Number*, Page Range.

ISBN 978-3-0365-3464-0 (Hbk)
ISBN 978-3-0365-3463-3 (PDF)

Contents

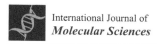
International Journal of
Molecular Sciences

Review

Nutraceutical Approach to Chronic Osteoarthritis: From Molecular Research to Clinical Evidence

Alessandro Colletti [1,2] **and Arrigo F. G. Cicero** [2,3,*]

1   Department of Science and Drug Technology, University of Turin, 10125 Turin, Italy;
    alessandro.colletti@unito.it
2   Italian Nutraceutical Society (SINut), 40138 Bologna, Italy
3   IRCCS AOU Policlinico S. Orsola-Malpighi, Medical and Surgical Sciences Department, University of
    Bologna, 40138 Bologna, Italy
*   Correspondence: arrigo.cicero@unibo.it

Abstract: Osteoarthritis (OA) is a degenerative inflammatory condition of the joint cartilage that currently affects approximately 58 million adults in the world. It is characterized by pain, stiffness, and a reduced range of motion with regard to the arthritic joints. These symptoms can cause in the long term a greater risk of overweight/obesity, diabetes mellitus, and falls and fractures. Although the current guidelines for the treatment of OA suggest, as the gold standard for this condition, pharmacological treatment characterized by non-steroidal anti-inflammatory drugs (NSAID), opioids, and cyclooxygenase (COX)-2-specific drugs, a great interest has been applied to nutraceutical supplements, which include a heterogeneous class of molecules with great potential to reduce inflammation, oxidative stress, pain, and joint stiffness and improve cartilage formation. The purpose of this review is to describe the potential application of nutraceuticals in OA, highlighting its molecular mechanisms of actions and data of efficacy and safety (when available).

Keywords: osteoarthritis; nutraceuticals; glucosamine; chondroitin; collagen; methylsulfonylmethane; vitamin C; vitamin D; hyaluronic acid

Citation: Colletti, A.; Cicero, A.F.G. Nutraceutical Approach to Chronic Osteoarthritis: From Molecular Research to Clinical Evidence. *Int. J. Mol. Sci.* **2021**, *22*, 12920. https://doi.org/10.3390/ijms222312920

Academic Editor: Yousef Abu-Amer

Received: 5 November 2021
Accepted: 27 November 2021
Published: 29 November 2021

1. Introduction

Osteoarthritis (OA) is a degenerative inflammatory condition of the joint cartilage that currently affects approximately 58 million adults, with an estimated increase to 78.4 million by 2040 [1]. It represents the principal reason for joint pain and functional impairment in the world [2].

This inflammation is characterized by pain, stiffness, and a reduced range of motion with regard to the arthritic joints. These symptoms can cause a greater risk of overweight/obesity, diabetes mellitus, and falls and fractures in the long term [3]. Factors predisposing to OA could be classified as local biochemical factors, including joint injury, joint space, and physical activities, and general factors, such as sex, age, comorbidities like obesity, and nutrition disorders [4].

Current guidelines for the treatment of OA suggest three types of approaches, which can be also combined if necessary. The first approach includes pharmacological treatment, which is characterized by non-steroidal anti-inflammatory drugs (NSAIDs), opioids, and cyclooxygenase (COX)-2-specific drugs. However, it has only a "palliative" role by reducing symptoms but not considering the essential problem of the cartilage disorder. In addition, the conventional therapies can cause (especially for long period of consumption) possible side effects, which can reduce the compliance for the appearance of gastrointestinal problems, cardiovascular effects, and others [5]. The second approach regards lifestyle change, a non-pharmacological approach characterized by rehabilitation to facilitate healthy body composition, physical activity, and the optimization of an appropriate nutrition plan and a nutraceutical treatment [6]. In this context, a chronic nutritional intervention associated with conventional therapies demonstrated to improve OA condition (joint of knee, hip, and hand) compared with only pharmacological treatments [7]. If lifestyle changes and medications are not enough, the third approach is surgery. Nevertheless, in recent years, a great interest has been applied to nutraceutical supplements, which include a hetero-geneous class of molecules with great potential to reduce inflammation, oxidative stress, pain, and joint stiffness and improve cartilage formation [8]. The use of nutraceuticals might be particularly interesting for the action on pain, which is typically chronic in OA and represents the main cause of disability for this condition. In this regard, for evaluation of OA pain intensity, the most common criteria include the visual analog scale (VAS) or numerical rating scale (NRS), the pain subscale of the Western Ontario and McMaster Universities Arthritis Index (WOMAC), and the Knee injury and Osteoarthritis Outcome Score (KOOS) [9]. In particular, the WOMAC index is widely used in the evaluation of hip and knee osteoarthritis based on a self-administered questionnaire consisting of items regarding pain, stiffness, and physical function. In this regard, a recent meta-analysis of 42 random clinical trials (RCTs) utilizing nutraceuticals (such as chondroitin sulphate, glucosamine sulphate, collagen, and hyaluronic acid) found improvements across all OA measurement parameters expressed through the total WOMAC index, WOMAC pain and WOMAC stiffness subscales,and VAS [10]. Among the most used nutraceuticals in OA, chondroitin sulphate, glucosamine sulphate, collagen, hyaluronic acid, and methylsulfonyl-methane were shown to be impressive in the improvement of clinical symptoms and in decreasing inflammatory indices in subjects with OA [11]. Confirming this, 69% of patients with OA receive various forms of nutraceuticals for their problem [12]. However, although numerous studies have detailed the benefits of nutraceutical usage in OA, inconsistent reports of the side effects and results of little statistical significance have kept them from mainstream medical usage as described in further sections.

The purpose of this narrative review is to describe the molecular mechanisms of action of the most used and clinically tested chondroprotective nutraceuticals.

2. Methods

As a first step, we focused our literature search on the search for the most clinically studied dietary supplements using as key words on PubMed "Osteoarthritis", "Nutraceuti-cals", "Dietary supplements", "Randomized", and "Clinical trials". Then, we searched for studies investigating the mechanism of action of the selected nutraceuticals and critically described it.

A summary of the discussed nutraceuticals and their proposed mechanisms of actions is reported in Table 1.

Table 1. Nutraceuticals useful in OA diseases: dosages of administration, molecular mechanism of actions, and effect on OA-related behavior and biomarkers.

Nutraceutical	Tested Daily Dose	Molecular Mechanism of Actions	Effect on OA and Related Behavior	Ref.
Anthocyanins from pomegranate juice	300–600 mg	IL-1β, TNF-α, CCR2, NF-κB, JNK-MAPK, ROS, NO, COX-2, PGE2	↓ VAS pain, WOMAC pain	[13]
Avocado/soybean unsaponifiables	300 mg	IL-1, IL-6, IL-8, and PGE2	↓ VAS pain, WOMAC pain, ↓ Analgesic and NSAIDs use	[14]
Acetyl-keto-β-boswellic acid (AKBA) (from *Boswellia serrata*)	150–250 mg (AKBA)	iNOS, NF-κB, COX, LOX	↓ VAS pain, WOMAC pain	[15]
Capsaicin (from Chili pepper)	10 mg	TRPV1 agonist	↓ VAS pain, WOMAC pain	[16]

Table 1. *Cont.*

Nutraceutical	Tested Daily Dose	Molecular Mechanism of Actions	Effect on OA and Related Behavior	Ref.
Chondroitin	500–1500 mg	IL-1, IL-6, TNF-α, IL-1β, TGF-β MMPs,NF-κB, ROS formation, improve of proteoglycans, type II collagen and GAGs expression	↓ VAS pain, WOMAC pain, stiffness, function and total, ↓ Analgesic and NSAIDs use	[17–19]
Collagen	4000–10000 mg	Cartilage regeneration by increasing the synthesis of macromolecules in the extracellular matrix, CTXII, MMP-13, T regulatory (Treg) modulation	↓ VAS pain, WOMAC pain, stiffness, function and total	[20]
Curcumin (from *Curcuma longa*)	1000–3000 mg	IL-1β, TNF-α, NF-κB, COX-2, PGE2	↓ VAS pain, WOMAC pain, stiffness, function and total, ↓ Analgesic and NSAIDs use	[21]
Epigallocatechin 3-gallate (from green tea)	400–1000 mg	IL-1β, TNF-α, CCR2, NF-κB, JNK-MAPK, ROS, NO, COX-2, PGE2	↓ VAS pain, WOMAC pain	[22]
Gingerols (from ginger)	250–400 mg ginger (5% gingerols)	iNOS, NF-κB, TRPV1 agonist	↓ VAS pain, WOMAC pain	[23,24]
Glucosamine	500–1500 mg	IL-1, IL-6, TNF-α, IL-1β, TGF-β MMPs,NF-κB, ROS formation, improve of proteoglycans, type II collagen and GAGs expression	↓ VAS pain, WOMAC pain, ↓ Analgesic and NSAIDs use	[17–19]
Hyaluronic acid	80–200 mg	CD44 receptors, IL-1β, -6, -9, MMPs, PGE2, TNFα, RHAMM, TLR4, ICAM-1, Nf-kB	↓ VAS pain, WOMAC pain, stiffness, function and total	[25]
Methylsulfonylmethane	500–1500 mg	NF-Kb, IL-1, IL-6, IL-1β, TNF-α ROS, COX	↓ VAS pain, WOMAC pain, stiffness, function and total, ↑ SF-36 quality of life all eight domains including pain, ↑ Global patient and physician assessments of disease status	[26]
Omega-3 (EPA and DHA)	500–4500 mg (EPA + DHA)	NF-κB, COX	↓ Mean WOMAC scores for pain, stiffness, and function, ↓ Analgesic and NSAIDs use, ↓ OA symptoms including morning stiffness, pain in hips and knees	[27,28]
Pycnogenol	100–200 mg	MMPs, COX-1, -2, NF-κB, ROS	↓ VAS pain, WOMAC pain	[29]
Vitamin C	500–2000 mg	MMPs, ROS	↓ VAS pain	[30]
Vitamin D	2000–60000 UI	Bone formation and mineralization, MMPs, osteoclast and osteoblast activity, VEGF	Unclear	[31,32]

CCR2 = C-C chemokine receptor type 2, CD44 = Cluster of differentiation 44, COX = Cyclooxygenase, IL = Interleukin, GAGs = glycosaminoglycans, ICAM-1 = Intercellular adhesion molecule, MMPs = Matrix metalloproteinases, LOX = Lipoxygenase, NF-kB = Nuclear factor-kappa B, NO = Nitric oxide, NSAIDs = Non-steroidal anti-inflammatory drug, OA = Osteoarthritis, PGE2 = Prostaglandin E2, RHAMM = receptor for hyaluronan mediated motility, ROS = Reactive oxygen species, SF-36 = 36-Item short form survey, TGF = Tumor grown factor, TLR4 = Toll like receptor 4, TNF = Tumor necrosis factor, VAS = Visual analogue scale, VEGF = Vascular endothelial growth factor, WOMAC = Western Ontario and McMaster University, ↓ = reduction, ↑ = improvement.

3. Nutraceuticals Used for the Prevention of Worsening and Management of OA

3.1. Glucosamine and Chondroitin

Chondroitin and glucosamine are nutraceuticals commonly used in clinical practice for OA patients for its analgesic and chondroprotective effects [33]. Glucosamine is a water-soluble amino monosaccharide available in two forms (glucosamine sulphate and glucosamine hydrochloride), which is a normal constituent of glycosaminoglycans (GAGs) in cartilage matrix and in the synovial fluid and consequently present in high quantities in articular cartilage. It is a constituent of keratan sulphate. Chondroitin is a major component of the extracellular matrix of articular cartilage, which played an important role in creating considerable osmotic pressure. In this way, it could provide cartilage with resistance and elasticity to resist tensile stresses during loading conditions [34].

3.1.1. Mechanisms of Action

Glucosamine and chondroitin act first as anti-inflammatory agents. A study conducted in rats treated with different dosages of glucosamine (20, 40, 80, or 160 mg/kg/day) showed, by the 6th day, the capability of this substance to reduce the levels of proinflammatory cytokines interleukin (IL)-1, IL-6, and tumor necrosis factor (TNF)-α, also preventing the increase in plasma nitrite levels [35]. Similar results were obtained by Li et al., and Waly et al., on mice with monosodium iodoacetate-induced OA in which glucosamine was shown to downregulate serum pro-inflammatory cytokines (IL-1β, IL-6, and TNF-α) and C-reactive protein levels and upregulate the anti-inflammatory cytokines IL-2 and IL-10 levels [17,18]. Oral glucosamine administration is able to suppress the early increase in tumor grown factor (TGF)-β levels in monosodium iodoacetate-induced OA rats [17]. Nevertheless, the precise role of TGF-β in different stages of OA is still unclear as well as the effects of glucosamine on this function required further confirmations [17]. Glucosamine appears to also have immune-modulatory activity by inhibiting the expression and/or activity of catabolic enzymes, such as phospholipase A2, MMPs, or aggrecanases [36].

Both chondroitin and glucosamine sulphate were demonstrated to reduce the activation of the nuclear factor κB (NF-κB) and p38 mitogen-activated protein kinase (MAPK) pathway, which represent a pathway of inflammation in OA [37]. In addition, further studies showed that these molecules prevent the cytokine-induced IL-1β expression by suppressing the demethylation of the IL-1β promoter region [36], inhibiting the lipopolysaccharide (LPS)-induced reactive oxygen species (ROS) generation, nucleotide-binding oligomerization domain-like receptor containing pyrin domain 3 (NLRP3) inflammasome activation and caspase-1 activation, and upregulation and release of IL-1β [38].

Another important activity of both chondroitin and glucosamine concerns its antioxidant properties, which have been reported in several in vitro models [21]. Even though glucosamine hydrochloride and glucosamine sulphate possess antioxidant activity, glucosamine sulphate shows greater antioxidant and radical scavenging activities compared with glucosamine hydrochloride [39].

The reduction of ROS produced during the early OA stage by mechanical stress, trauma, or chemicals is important in order to reduce the cellular damage on the adjacent cartilage and collagen degradation [40]. Glucosamine was shown to bind directly with malondialdehyde (MDA) and block the subsequent formation of MDA adducts and protein cross-linkages and thus prevent lipoprotein oxidation and inhibit MDA adduct formation in the articular chondrocyte cell matrix [41]. Other in vitro studies reported the ability of these molecules to inhibit hydrogen peroxide (H2O2)-mediated membrane lipid peroxidation, protein and DNA oxidation, as well as the intracellular ROS level in chondrocytes, with the upregulation of glutathione (GSH) and other antioxidant enzymes, including superoxide dismutase (SOD), catalase (CAT), and glutathione peroxidase (GPx) in chondrocytes [42]. However, direct evidence of the antioxidant activity of both glucosamine and chondroitin in OA animal models is limited. In a study conducted in the formalin-induced osteoarthritic rat knee joint, the association of glucosamine hydrochloride, chondroitin sulphate, methylsulfonylmethane, *Harpagophytum procumbens* root extract, and bromelain administered orally for 30 days resulted in a significant reduction in MDA, NO, and 8-hydroxyguanine levels and an increased total GSH level was observed. These reductions were higher in the combination group (with plants) if compared with the administration of glucosamine or chondroitin alone, probably due to the additional analgesic effects [43].

Glucosamine and chondroitin are also known to improve tissue regeneration as demonstrated by different in vivo studies. In New Zealand rabbits with surgical-induced knee joint cartilage damage, treatment with glucosamine sulphate remarkably improved hyaline cartilage regeneration on autologous chondrocyte implantation repair sites, with upregulation of proteoglycans, type II collagen, and GAGs expression compared with autologous chondrocyte implantation alone [19]. In addition, these nutraceuticals simultaneously suppressed the osteoclastic cell differentiation in MC3T3-E1 osteoblasts, downregulating the receptor activator of NF-κB ligand (RANKL) expression [44] and blocked IL-1β-mediated downregulation of type II collagen and aggrecan gene expression and inhibited the MMP-13 gene expression in both normal and OA chondrocytes [45].

3.1.2. Efficacy and Safety

Chondroitin and glucosamine were tested in several clinical trials of OA. However, the results remain at least in part contrasting. A recent meta-analysis of 30 randomized clinical trials including 7127 patients showed that chondroitin could alleviate pain symptoms (-0.071, 95%CI: -0.228 to 0.085) and improve physical function (-0.090, 95%CI: -0.242 to 0.061) compared with the placebo [46]. Similar results were shown in a previous meta-analysis in which treatments with glucosamine and chondroitin were found to significantly reduce pain in VAS [weighted mean difference (WMD) -7.41 mm, 95%CI–14.31, -0.51, $p = 0.04$ and WMD–8.35 mm, 95% CI–11.84, -4.85, $p < 0.001$, respectively] [47]. Even the meta-analysis by Ogata et al., including 18 RCTs, demonstrated glucosamine's potential to alleviate knee OA pain [48]. Moreover, Zhu et al., reported the superiority of the combination of glucosamine and chondroitin for pain reduction and joint stiffness in comparison with acetaminophen, even if celecoxib was most likely the best option for knee or hip OA [49]. In a large meta-analysis of 54 randomized clinical trials including 16,427 patients, the effects of glucosamine and chondroitin were compared with conventional treatments. Although, even in this case, celecoxib was considered the best option for pain reduction, only glucosamine plus chondroitin showed a clinically significant improvement from baseline function. In terms of the structure-modifying effect, both glucosamine alone and chondroitin alone achieved a statistically significant reduction in joint space narrowing [50].

However, other studies reported no significant improvement of the OA condition after both glucosamine and chondroitin supplementation. Kwoh et al., did not observe any significant changes in the joint structure in people with chronic knee pain treated with glucosamine 1500 mg/day [51]. In addition, supplementation with chondroitin or glucosamine (1500 mg/day) for 2 years also did not cause remarkable changes in the joint structure of OA patients (aged 45–75 years) [52]. Similar conclusions were obtained from a study regarding 59 people with temporomandibular OA randomly receiving glucosamine sulphate 1200 mg/day or placebo. At the end of the study (six weeks), no significant differences in all signs and symptoms of OA were observed in both groups [53]. In accordance with this data, in a meta-analysis of 17 clinical studies, only seven showed a statistically significant reduction in pain (-0.35, 95%CI = -0.54 to -0.16) and four studies met the review criteria for joint space narrowing (SMD= -0.10, 95%CI = -0.23 to +0.04) [54]. Moreover, several smaller dosages throughout the day of glucosamine seem to be better in pain reduction effects if compared with a single daily large dose (1500 mg) [38].

Both glucosamine and chondroitin were also demonstrated to reduce joint inflammation and oxidative stress. In an RCT including elderly people with temporomandibular joint OA, treatment with an intra-articular hyaluronic acid injection in combination with glucosamine hydrochloride (oral 720 mg for 3 months) was shown to be greatly beneficial by further reducing the IL-6, IL-1β, and TGF-β levels if compared with people treated with only hyaluronic acid injection [55]. Glucosamine sulphate (1500 mg/day) in addition with celecoxib (200 mg/day) supplemented in patients with knee OA for 8 weeks showed a better redox status expressed as higher serum SOD activity and lower serum MDA levels compared with the control group (celecoxib alone) [56].

In conclusion, data indicates that both glucosamine and chondroitin may have a small to moderate effect in reducing OA-related pain and joint inflammation but little effect on joint-space narrowing. The discrepancies in the effectiveness of chondroitin and glucosamine on osteoarthritis between different studies should be further examined.

The supplementation of both chondroitin and glucosamine in the medium term is considered safe and well tolerated. Different studies reported some mild and transitory effects, such as diarrhea, abdominal pain, nausea, and headache. However, there was no significant difference in the comparison between any options (glucosamine alone, chondroitin alone, glucosamine + chondroitin) versus placebo.

3.2. Methylsulfonylmethane

Methylsulfonylmethane (MSM) is a supplement containing organic sulphur suggested for relieving joint/muscle pain, thanks to its anti-inflammatory properties and it has also been reported to slow anatomical joint progressivity in the knee OA. It is a natural member of the methyl-S-methane compounds, but it can also be obtained through the oxidation of dimethylsophoxide with H_2O_2 [42].

3.2.1. Mechanism of Action

In vitro studies showed the ability of MSM to act as an anti-inflammatory agent through the inhibition of the nuclear factor kappa-light-chain-enhancer of activated B cells (NF-κB) [57] as well as p65-S536 phosphorylation [58], reducing the expression of interleukins (IL-1, IL-6, IL-1β) and TNF-α [59,60]. MSM downregulates NF-κB production of the leucine-rich repeat family pyrin domain-containing 3 (NLRP3) inflammasome transcript and/or it blocks the activation signal in the form of mitochondrial-generated ROS, negatively affecting the expression of the NLRP3 inflammasome [44]. In addition, MSM reduces the expression of cyclooxygenase-2 and nitric oxide synthase, reducing the formation of superoxide radical (O_2^-) and nitric oxide (NO) [61]. MSM influences the balance of ROS and antioxidant enzymes by mediating at least four types of transcription factors including NF-κB, signal transducers and activators of transcription (STAT), p53, and nuclear factor (erythroid-derived 2)-like 2 (Nrf2) [45]. Other pleiotropic effects of MSM include the improvement of osteoblast differentiation acting through the Jak2/STAT5b pathway [62] and the upregulation of the master gene RUNX2, which transactivates its downstream partner SP7 (Osterix) and thus the expression of osteogenic genes (e.g., COL1A1 and COL1A2 (collagen type I), BGLAP (osteocalcin), SPARC (osteonectin), and SSP1 (osteopontin)) [63]. The osteogenic differentiation operated by MSM is also stimulated by the induction of BMP2 or transglutaminase-2 (TG2) [64].

3.2.2. Efficacy and Safety

Although the MSM anti-arthritic data of in vitro and in animal models are numerous and promising [58,65], human studies are for the most part conducted on small samples of people and in combination with other molecules, such as chondroitin and glucosamine.

RCTs suggest MSM is effective in reducing pain, as indicated by the WOMAC pain subscale [66,67], the 36-Item Short Form Survey (SF36) pain subscale [26], the VAS pain scale, and the Lequesne Index [68]. Significant improvements were also observed in swelling [55] and stiffness [53].

Other RCTs utilizing MSM in combination with other therapies report similar results. In this regard, the study conducted by Usha et al., reported an improvement in pain, pain intensity, and swelling after supplementation with MSM and glucosamine, in people with OA [55]. In another double-blind RCT including 147 people with knee OA, Kellgren–Lawrence grade I-II, patients were randomized to receive 1500 mg of glucosamine +

1200 mg of chondroitin sulphate or 1500 mg of glucosamine + 1200 mg of chondroitin sulphate + 500 mg of MSM or placebo for 3 months. At the end of the treatments, the MSM treatment group was found to have a statistically significant WOMAC score ($p = 0.01$) and VAS score ($p < 0.001$) compared with the control and the glucosamine and chondroitin group (WOMAC score ($p = 0.03$) and VAS score ($p = 0.004$) [69]. The combination of glucosamine, chondroitin, and MSM has also been demonstrated to improve functional ability and joint mobility [70]. However, these positive observations were not confirmed in the trial by Magrans-Courtney et al. [71]. Further larger and long-term clinical trials are needed to quantify its efficacy, especially when compared to chondroitin and glucosamine.

MSM appears to be well-tolerated and safe as reported by the Food and Drug Administration (FDA) GRAS notification, at dosages under 4845.6 mg/day [72].

3.3. Collagen

Collagen is an extracellular matrix protein localized in the skin, tendons, cartilage, and bone, which is usually contained in foods, such as fish and meat [73]. It is characterized by a triple-helix configuration with a repeating amino acid sequence, (Gly-X-Y)n, where X and Y are typically proline and hydroxyproline, respectively. Type II collagen is the major component (90–95% of total collagen content) of the articular cartilage, forming the fibrils that give cartilage its tensile strength [74]. It is also generally commercialized as a nutritional supplement obtained by the action of proteases, which hydrolyze the gelatine [75]. In fact, the bioavailability of undenatured collagen is very low because it is not hydrolyzed and thus physiologically available for enteric absorption [76]. However, it has been demonstrated that bioactive di- or tripeptides containing proline and hydroxyproline could be absorbed into the blood circulation and exert anti-OA activities [77].

3.3.1. Mechanism of Action

The site of interaction of collagen and its subfractions on cartilage has not yet been fully clarified. Several in vitro studies have investigated the potential molecular mechanisms regarding the protection of articular cartilage [78]. Firstly, collagen is well known to be an extracellular matrix molecule used by cells for structural integrity [79]. Hydrolyzed collagen may induce cartilage regeneration by increasing the synthesis of macromolecules in the extracellular matrix [80]. After a single administration with labeled collagen peptide, a significant improvement in the levels of collagen detected in the skin and cartilage was shown, indicating an accumulation of these peptides in the connective tissue [81].

Collagen is able to modulate the humoral and cellular immune response. In fact, it activates the immune cells (it takes place in the gut-associated lymphoid tissue (GALT)) and regulates the oral tolerance, which is an immune process that the body uses to distinguish between innocuous molecules, such as dietary proteins or intestinal bacteria, from potentially harmful foreign invaders [82]. In this regard, the transformation of naive T cells into T regulatory (Treg) cells permits the secretion of anti-inflammatory mediators, including the transforming growth factor-beta (TGF-β), interleukin 4 (IL-4), and interleukin 10 (IL-10), which help in the reduction of joint inflammation and promotion of cartilage repair [83,84].

Proline and hydroxyproline are considered to be the biologically active substances of collagen, inducing hyaluronic acid synthesis as reported by in-cultured synovial cells [85] and suppressing the hypertrophic differentiation of chondrocytes, which is well known to be involved in the pathogenesis of OA [86]. Furthermore, these amino acids stimulate glycosaminoglycan synthesis by chondrocytes [79]. In a rat experimental osteoarthritis (OA) model, collagen peptides administration was demonstrated to reduce the CTX-II (type II collagen degradation) levels and suppress the Mankin score ($p < 0.05$ for both). In addition, type II collagen reduced inflammation expressed as MMP-13 levels [87].

Based on these findings, oral administration of hydrolyzed collagen has anti-inflammatory and chondroprotective actions, which could represent the basis of the protection of OA initiation/progression. Further in vitro studies investigating the components of collagen peptides are required to elucidate the detailed mechanism behind the beneficial effect of these peptides on joint health.

3.3.2. Efficacy and Safety

Different clinical studies have investigated the protective effects of collagen on joints [88,89]. It has been suggested that supplementation with 4.5–10 g/day of collagen peptides, at least for 2 months, relieves knee and hip joint pain in people with OA [90]. In a RCT involving 147 athletes, 10 g collagen/day for 24 weeks reduced activity-related joint pain [91]. In another RCT including 30 subjects with knee OA, supplementation of 5 g/day of collagen for 13 weeks showed a significant improvement of all the score levels of WOMAC, VAS, and quality of life ($p < 0.01$ compared with placebo). In accordance with these results, in a meta-analysis of five RCTs, collagen treatment showed a significant reduction in the total WOMAC index score (WMD–8.00; 95% CI–13.04, –2.95; $p = 0.002$) and in the VAS score (WMD–16.57; 95% CI–26.24, –6.89; $p < 0.001$). Subgroup analysis of the WOMAC subscores also revealed a significant decrease in the stiffness subscore (WMD–0.41; 95% CI–0.74, –0.08; $p = 0.01$) [20]. Based on the available data, it is estimated that collagen peptides are effective at dosages of 0.166 g/kg body weight/day (10 g/60 kg/day) in treating joint pain in humans [92]. In the multicenter RCT by Trc et al., supplementation for 90 days of hydrolyzed collagen at a dosage of 10 g/day was demonstrated to be superior to glucosamine sulphate 1.5 g/day in improving the WOMAC and VAS score (reduction of the WOMAC and VAS index observed in the collagen group: 80.8% of the study population vs. 46.6% observed in the glucosamine sulphate group) [93]. The pain reduction after collagen supplementation in patients with OA indirectly indicates an improvement in joint conditions. In fact, as discussed below, the initiation of the repair process by the accumulation of collagen peptide in cartilage tissue helps to maintain the structure and function of cartilage, resulting in joint comfort, subsequent improvement in pain, and a reduction in the progression of degradation of articular cartilage tissue.

Collagen supplementation is generally safe with no reported adverse events. Further studies are needed to elucidate medical use in OA disease and to determine the optimal dosing regimens as well as the period of treatments.

3.4. Hyaluronic Acid

Hyaluronic acid (HA) is a mucopolysaccharide constituted by repeated monomers of β-1,4-D-glucuronic acid and β-1,3-N-acetylglucosamine. This molecule is particularly present in the synovial fluid with excellent viscoelasticity, high moisture retention capacity, high biocompatibility, and hygroscopic properties, thus acting as a lubricant, shock absorber, joint structure stabilizer, and water balance and flow resistance regulator [94]. HA is considered the treatment of choice for people with knee/hip OA, working slowly if compared with steroid treatments, but its effect may last considerably longer [95]. Although HA injection has shown great advantages in improving the clinical symptoms of OA patients, it must be administered repeatedly into the joint cavity [96]. The need for multiple injections of HA is a major drawback of the therapy because of the proportional increase of side effects with the repeated injections and the discomfort of repeated clinic visits. For these reasons, considering the disadvantages of HA injection, it is more favorable for the symptoms of OA to be relieved by oral administration [97].

3.4.1. Mechanism of Action

The first proposed HA mechanism of action regards chondroprotection. HA has been shown to reduce chondrocyte apoptosis, while increasing chondrocyte proliferation [98]. This phenomenon is possible through HA binding to cluster of differentiation 44 (CD44) receptors that cause inhibition of interleukin (IL)-1β expression and a decline in matrix metalloproteinase (MMP)−1, 2, 3, 9, and 13 production [99]. HA also binds to the receptor for hyaluronan-mediated motility (RHAMM), which is thought to aid in chondroprotection in addition to CD44 binding [92]. In addition, it may affect the subchondral bone by the suppression of MMP-13 and IL-6 via CD44 binding [100]. The suppression of MMP-13 expression has been suggested to be a critical factor in the effect on OA subchondral bone [93].

Although human studies demonstrated that oral supplementation with HA can reach the blood and be distributed to the skin and joints [101], the therapeutic effects of this molecule on OA may not necessarily require its absorption. HA could in fact bind to toll-like receptor 4 (TLR4) in the intestine and exert its biological activities, increasing the secretion of suppressor of cytokine signaling 3 (SOCS3), which leads to the suppression of pro-inflammatory cytokine expression [102]. In this regard, the suppression of pro-inflammatory mediators IL-8, IL-6, PGE2, and TNFα has been observed with HA [103]. In addition, the binding of HA to TLR4 also suppresses the expression of pleiotrophin, a pro-inflammatory molecule [102]. HA also binds to the intercellular adhesion molecule (ICAM-1), downregulating NF-kB, which in turn decreases the production of IL-6 [104].

Another possible mechanism of action regards the N-acetyl glucosamine, which is the monosaccharide that comprises HA together with D-glucuronic acid. N-acetyl glucosamine is converted into glucosamine in the cells by the actions of lysosomal enzymes, which permit the chondroprotective and anti-inflammatory activities of glucosamine described in the dedicated paragraph [105]. HA treatment stimulated proteoglycan synthesis (such as aggrecan), reducing the progression of OA [106].

HA has a mechanical effect, which contributes to the lubrification of the joint capsule, preventing degeneration through decreased friction. HA provides cushioning to absorb pressure and vibration, avoiding the degradation of chondrocyte tissue [107].

HA possesses analgesic effects, probably by decreasing the mechanical sensitivity of stretch-activated ion channels, which effectively blocks the pain response. Moreover, HA reduces the action of joint-sensitized nociceptors, which are affected by the HA concentration, reducing the pain response exhibited by these terminals [108].

3.4.2. Efficacy and Safety

The results of animal experiments using radiolabeled HA clearly demonstrated that oral HA would indeed be absorbed and distributed to the skin, bone, and synovial joints and would be retained in those tissues for prolonged periods [109]. In agreement with these findings, RCTs in humans showed that oral supplementation with this molecule can reach the blood and can be distributed to the skin and joints, preserving its biological activities [101].

Several studies have suggested that oral supplementation with HA could alleviate the symptoms of knee OA [110,111]. Sato et al., demonstrated that treatment with 240 mg/day of HA for 12 weeks was associated with an improvement of the Japanese Knee Osteoarthritis Measure (JKOM) score and the Japan Orthopaedic Association (JOA) score improved significantly compared with baseline values [112]. Supplementation with 200 mg/day of HA in OA people for 8 weeks was also shown to improve the WOMAC scores compared with the placebo group [108]. Similar results were described by Iwaso et al., who highlighted an improvement of both WOMAC and JKOM scores after 200 mg of HA supplementation for 8 weeks [113].

In a one-year RCT, 60 osteoarthritic subjects (Kellgren-Lawrence grade 2 or 3) were randomly assigned to receive HA (200 mg/day) or placebo. At the end of treatment, the improvement was most evident in the subscale for "pain and stiffness", and it was more obvious in patients who performed therapeutic exercises in combination with HA therapy [114].

Although different studies report positive effects of oral HA supplementation on OA, several limitations should be described before arriving at any conclusion. In fact, the lack of appropriate controls, shortness of study periods, small sample size, as well as the different forms of supplemented hyaluronic acid (in many cases, this was not described in the studies) may influence the results. To clarify these issues, new long-term RCTs with standardized HA are urgently required and desirable to recommend such a nutraceutical in clinical practice.

It was confirmed that oral supplementation of HA is safe in humans at dosages up to 200 mg/day ingested for periods up to 12 months [109]. Several safety studies were conducted with medium-term (3–6 months) supplementation periods, and safety was confirmed [115].

3.5. Vitamin C

Vitamin C or ascorbic acid was first isolated in 1923 by Szent-Gyorgyi and synthesized by Howarth and Hirst. It is especially found in citrus fruits, red and green peppers, tomatoes, strawberries, broccoli, Brussels sprouts, turnips, and other leafy vegetables. It is a water-soluble molecule with highly effective antioxidant properties due to its reactivity with numerous aqueous-free radicals and ROS [116]. A deficiency of this molecule can be associated with a higher risk of various diseases including scurvy, anemia, capillary hemorrhage, muscle degeneration, infections, bleeding gums, poor wound healing, atherosclerotic plaques, and neurotic disturbances. In addition, dietary intake of vitamin C seems to be associated with a decreased risk of cartilage loss and OA in humans, probably by the reduction of oxidative stress, as highlighted by different studies [117,118]. However, although vitamin C has an approved claim by the EFSA (European Food Safety Authority) regarding its role on the normal formation of collagen, it is still unknown whether this supplement has additional effects on the prevention of OA progression.

3.5.1. Mechanism of Action

Vitamin C acts prevalently as an antioxidant and antiradical supplement. In fact, it exists in both reduced (ascorbate) and oxidized forms as dehydroascorbic acid, which are easily inter-convertible and biologically active, thus it acts as an important antioxidant. In this regard, ascorbic acid reacts directly with free radicals undergoing single-electron oxidation to produce a relatively poor reactive intermediate, the ascorbyl radical, which disproportionates to ascorbate and dehydroascorbate. In this sense, ascorbic acid has the ability to reduce toxic ROS superoxide anion ($O^2\bullet$), and hydroxyl radical ($OH\bullet$), as well as organic (RO^2) and nitrogen ($NO^2\bullet$) oxy radicals. In addition, this molecule could also act indirectly, by protecting the oxidation of other vitamins, such as vitamin A and E. In this context, damage caused by ROS has long been thought to be pathogenic and it has an important role in the progression of OA, causing cytotoxicity and cellular damage [8]. Although OA is classified as a 'non-inflammatory arthropathy', growing evidence highlights the key role of pro-inflammatory mediators in the pathogenesis of OA [119]. Vitamin C also plays an important role as an electron donor in the synthesis of type II collagen [120] and a sulphate carrier in glycosaminoglycan synthesis [121]. Moreover, ascorbic acid is a co-factor for the hydroxylation and activity of mono-oxygenase enzymes in the synthesis of collagen, carnitine, and neurotransmitters, maintaining the active center of metal ions in a reduced state for optimal activity of the enzymes hydroxylase and oxygenase [109]. The depletion of sulphated proteoglycans' extracellular matrix of the articular cartilage is considered one of the most relevant expressions of OA, often associated with cartilage degeneration [117]. Vitamin C deficiency could therefore be considered a risk factor for OA development and thus, its supplementation in primary prevention may represent a possible solution for OA, especially in combination with conventional or unconventional therapies.

3.5.2. Efficacy and Safety

Vitamin C possesses multiple abilities for the prevention of OA progress, including the modulation of apoptosis processes (via procaspase-3 and procaspase-9 and Bax expression) and the expression of pro-inflammatory cytokines and MMPs, in addition to the well-known antioxidation. In an in vitro chondrosarcoma cell line (SW1353), treatment with 100 μM of vitamin C was shown to prevent oxidative stress, apoptosis, and proteoglycan loss induced by the treatment with 5 µM of monosodium iodoacetate (MIA). Moreover, the expression levels of the pro-inflammatory cytokines IL-6, IL-17A, and TNF-α and MMP-1, MMP-3, and MMP-13 were also prevented [122]. Similar results were obtained in in vivo monosodium iodoacetate (MIA)-induced OA rats (vitamin C supplemented: 100 mg/kg) [118]. Many in vivo studies indicated that increased intake of vitamin C may decrease the risk of OA progression and cartilage loss in humans, a causal association with its capacity against oxidative stress [113,117]. However, some studies indicated a non-correlation between circulating vitamin C levels and incident radiographic knee OA [123]. In a prospective cohort study including 1023 people, individuals without baseline knee OA who self-reported vitamin C supplement usage were 11% less likely to develop knee OA than those individuals who self-reported no vitamin C supplement usage (risk ratio (RR)=0.89, 95% CI 0.85, 0.93). In addition, among those participants with radiographic knee OA at baseline, after controlling for confounding variables, vitamin C supplementation was demonstrated to be potentially useful in preventing incident knee OA [124]. In a cross-sectional analysis (4685 participants) regarding the associations between the intake of dietary antioxidants (carotenoid, vitamin C, E, and selenium) and radiographic knee OA, radiographic knee OA was not significantly associated with dietary carotenoids, vitamin E, and selenium but significantly associated with vitamin C intake [117]. Moreover, the use of vitamin C significantly decreased the lipoperoxides ($p < 0.05$ compared with the placebo group) linked with hip bone loss [125]. Vitamin C may also reduce the use of painkillers and improve quality of life, probably acting as a cofactor for the enzyme peptidyl glycine α-amidating mono-oxygenase (PAM), which is involved in the synthesis of the endomorphin-1 [30,126].

Given the massive economic burden of OA, the use of a simple, inexpensive, and widely available supplement to potentially reduce the impact of this disease merits further consideration. However, long-term RCTs are urgently required before making any final consideration.

Overall, vitamin C appears to be a safe and effective adjunctive therapy for acute and chronic pain relief in specific patient groups [125]. Nevertheless, future studies are needed in order to measure the vitamin C concentrations at baseline and following intervention to determine if specific patient groups respond, determination of the optimal route of administration, the optimal dose and frequency of administration, and the potential mechanisms of action of this molecule in OA disease.

3.6. Vitamin D

Vitamin D is well known to be a lipophilic molecule, which was recommended by the Institute of Medicine (IOM) in 2011for bone health, in order to improve the calcium absorption, bone mineral density, and vitamin D deficiency rickets/osteomalacia [127]. Although it can be obtained both through foods, such as mushrooms fatty fish, and vitamin D-fortified products, and through the cutaneous synthesis in response to ultraviolet-B exposure, vitamin D deficiency occurs in <20% of the population in northern Europe; in 30–60% in western, southern, and eastern Europe; and up to 80% in Middle East countries. Severe deficiency (serum 25(OH)D < 30 nmol/L or 12 ng/mL) is found in >10% of Europeans [128].

Several studies have investigated the possible role of vitamin D on the initiation and progression of OA. In this regard, the expression of vitamin D receptors (VDRs) in the articular cartilage of OA people, but not in that of healthy volunteers, may indicate the direct influence of this hormone on the potential damage of articular cartilage [129,130]. In addition, vitamin D may also act on OA indirectly through the endocrine system.

3.6.1. Mechanism of Action

Vitamin D is an important immunoregulator of inflammation, influencing the response of white cells (macrophages, dendritic cells, T and B lymphocytes) [131]. In particular, the activation of VDR localized on white cell membranes also promotes the blocking of cytokine genes' transcription, such as NF-AT (nuclear factor of activated T cells) and NF-κB, reducing the production of TNF-α and IL-1, which are considered inflammatory pathways for the deterioration of cartilage [129]. In addition, several studies have shown that VDRs are upregulated on damaged cartilage. An in vitro study reported the hyperexpression of VDR in the areas of erosion of late-stage rheumatoid arthritis cells [129]. This result was confirmed in humans by the same research group [131] and by Orfanidou et al. [132]. The upregulation of VDR seems to stimulate a signaling cascade that enhances the production of MMPs 1, 3, and 9 from chondrocytes, which induces the degradation of both cartilage and bone [133].

Vitamin D acts also with the VDRs expressed on osteoblasts. A study by Corrado et al. [134] found that OA osteoblasts expressed a significantly lower receptor activator of NF-κ B ligand (RANKL)/osteoprotegerin (OPG) ratio compared to healthy and osteoporotic cells. RANKL and its decoy receptor OPG are regulators of osteoclastogenesis and thus bone resorption. Moreover, OPG expression in OA osteoblasts was significantly higher than in controls and in osteoporosis patients. Nevertheless, these results contrasted with those obtained by Giner et al., who found OPG secretions to be higher in osteoporotic osteoblasts compared to OA [135].

Vitamin D may regulate the angiogenesis process, which is an important pathway in the pathophysiology of OA. In fact, the expression of vascular endothelial growth factor (VEGF) is regulated in part by 1α,25(OH)2D3 as demonstrated by studies in vitro, including osteoarthritic osteoblasts [136]. This supports the idea that osteoblasts could regulate angiogenesis in subchondral bone and may link vitamin D with the development and progression of OA.

Limited evidence suggests that vitamin D acts indirectly on osteoclasts through the activation of the abovementioned RANKL signaling, increasing bone resorption [137].

Lastly, vitamin D may also regulate the transforming growth factor-beta (TGF-β)/SMAD pathway that is involved in OA [133]. In healthy joints, TGF-β protects the joint, repressing MMP13 expression [138]. In this regard, the blockage of TGF-β, the expression of which decreases with age, results in alteration of the repairing responses in the joint and cartilage damage [139]. However, in contrast with these results, TGF-β seems to aggravate OA in OA joints. The inhibition of TGF-β signaling was shown to attenuate OA in the mesenchymal stem cells of subchondral bone [140]. These observations indicate that TGF-β may protect healthy joints from OA, even if it may aggravate the condition of joints with existing OA. Nevertheless, vitamin D should be recommended, especially in OA elderly with low plasmatic levels of this hormone (<30 ng/mL) associated with comorbidities, such as cardiovascular diseases and disorders related to bone health. In fact, it was demonstrated to reduce oxidative protein damage, decrease pain (VAS), improve quality of life, and improve grip strength and physical performance in these patients [141].

3.6.2. Efficacy and Safety

Whether vitamin D deficiency increases the risk of developing OA is still unclear and results are contrasting. Several observational studies have shown no relationship between relatively high (≥50 nmol/L) vitamin D status and OA initiation expressed as pain, radiologic OA, and cartilage volume loss [142–145]. In a study in Ireland including rheumatology outpatients, 26% were found to be severely deficient (<12 ng/mL) and 70% vitamin D deficient (<21 ng/mL) [146]. In this regard, 62% of OA patients suffered from hypovitaminosis D and a low vitamin D status has also been associated with radiographic hip OA [147]. Similar conclusions were obtained by the osteoporotic fractures in a study of men in which vitamin D insufficiency or deficiency status were associated with a doubled risk of hip OA [148]. Even in Egypt [149] and in Iran [150], people with lower serum 25(OH)D3 had a major risk of developing knee OA. A systematic review by Cao and colleagues [151], including 15 studies, showed strong evidence for an association between 25(OH)D3 and cartilage loss in knee joints and moderate evidence to support a positive association between low levels of vitamin D and radiographic knee OA. In accordance with this observation, the Tasmanian Older Adult Cohort Study found an inverse correlation between time of sunlight exposure and knee cartilage loss [143].

In contrast with these results, the research group of Konstari and colleagues showed no correlation between vitamin D status and the risk of developing knee OA in Scandinavian people [152,153]. Felson et al., found no association between low vitamin D and structural worsening of affected joints (cartilage loss by magnetic resonance imaging and joint space narrowing by radiography) in two longitudinal studies (1203 people) [145].

People with deficiencies of plasma vitamin D (12.5–25 nmol/L) at baseline predicted a five-year change in knee pain and hip pain [154]. However, although elevated vitamin D status may attenuate joint pain and possibly radiologic OA in subjects with hypovitaminosis D [155,156], studies regarding the potential relationship between vitamin D status and the initiation of radiologic OA or cartilage volume loss in people with 'suboptimal' 25(OH)D are still lacking or contrasting. In a 2-year RCT, supplementation of cholecalciferol in patients with symptomatic knee OA showed no difference in the WOMAC knee pain scores or cartilage loss compared with the placebo group [156]. In partial accordance with this result, 787 members of the Hertfordshire Cohort Study (enrolled in a cross-sectional study) showed no association between vitamin D status and radiographic knee OA, even if there was a significant correlation between vitamin D and knee pain [157]. Furthermore, an RCT including 103 knee OA people treated with vitamin D oral supplements (60,000 IU/day for 10 days followed by 60,000 IU/month for 12 months) showed a small but significant correlation between the supplementation and the severity of pain and the functional scores (in comparison with the placebo group) [32].

In people undergoing total hip replacement, vitamin D levels have been shown to predict the OA outcomes, also suggesting a positive correlation of both preoperative and postoperative Harris hip scores and plasma 25(OH)D3 levels [158].

In conclusion, the research presented to date is conflicting as to the effects low vitamin D levels have on the functional aspects of knee OA. Although it appears that vitamin D has negative effects on OA cartilage health, as reported by the studies in vitro, which investigated the molecular mechanisms of action of this hormone, other human studies reported a possible role in prevention of pain, radiologic OA, and cartilage volume loss. In this context, to fully determine the relationship between vitamin D supplementation and the progression or development of OA, large scale longitudinal and multicentric studies including individuals with various skin pigmentations and different nationalities and ethnicities are urgent. In addition to this, large scale meta-analyses will yield more powerful interpretations of the existing findings and help to elucidate any associations low vitamin D has with OA.

Vitamin D supplementation is in general safe and well tolerated. The upper limit of vitamin D dose safety could differ depending on several factors, such as the vitamin D plasmatic levels, dose of administration and regimen, outcomes, as well as sex and age, which may play a role. However, the prevention or correction of vitamin D deficiency/insufficiency with 1000–2000 IU/daily of vitamin D is considered safe [159].

3.7. Other Promising Nutraceuticals

Avocado/soybean unsaponifiables have been shown to be effective in pain reduction as highlighted by human RCTs. In a 3-month RCT, daily intake of avocado/soybean unsaponifiables was demonstrated to significantly reduce the NSAID intake and the Lesquesne pain score [14]. Similar results were observed using the combination of avocado/soybean unsaponifiables with chondroitin sulphate (50% decrease in WOMAC scores) [160].

Boswellia serrata is well known to be rich in anti-inflammatory boswellic acids (3-O-acetyl-11-keto-beta-boswellic acid (AKBA), as the major potential active ingredient), which were shown to decrease pain (VAS, WOMAC pain), increase knee/hip flexion and walking distance (function and stiffness), as well as affecting the frequency of swelling if administered in patients with OA [5,161,162]. Similar results were observed in patients who took N-acetylglucosamine, ginger (5% gingerols at 250 mg/tablet), and *B. serrata* (65% boswellic acids at 180 mg/tablet), who reported a significant improvement in pain-free walking distance [15].

Another anti-inflammatory molecule is capsaicin, which is an agonist that binds to transient receptor potential V1 (TRPV1) channels in sensory nerve endings. This molecule extracted from the chili pepper is responsible for producing the sensation of heat or piquancy, which was shown to reduce mean WOMAC pain, stiffness, and functional scores compared with placebo in people with OA [16].

Curcumin, the most important curcuminoid in turmeric (*Curcuma longa*), has been well studied in OA disease, showing chondroprotective, antioxidative, and anti-inflammatory effects. In a 6-week trial including people with OA, the analgesic effect of oral curcumin (2 g/day) was comparable to ibuprofen (800 mg/day), improving the time spent walking 100 m and going up and down stairs [163]. The same conclusion was reported in another study in which curcumin (1500 mg/day) administered for 4 weeks resulted in a reduction in pain comparable to that with ibuprofen at 1200 mg per day [21]. In addition, it decreases inflammatory markers in the serum including IL-1β, IL-6, soluble CD40 ligand, sVCAM-1, and Coll2-1, a biomarker of type II collagen degradation [164].

Even ginger powder (titrated in gingerols) supplementation (1 g/day) can reduce inflammatory markers in patients with OA in addition to decreasing pain on standing, pain after walking, and WOMAC stiffness scores [23,24].

Polyphenols from pomegranate juice, pine bark, and green tea have demonstrated anti-inflammatory and antioxidative efficacy in relieving OA pain in human trials [13]. In particular, epigallocatechin 3-gallate (EGCG) from green tea reported a lower VAS pain score, as well as the total WOMAC score and physical function subscore after 4 weeks of administration in people with OA, compared with diclofenac 100 mg [22]. Similar results were observed with 150/200 mg/day of pycnogenol [29] and anthocyanins from pomegranate juice [13].

Lastly, omega-3 fatty acids (EPA and DHA) were reported to improve WOMAC pain, stiffness, and physical function scores and reduce NSAID use after 3 months of treatment [27]. These actions were confirmed even in association with the co-administration of 500 mg/day of glucosamine sulphate and other nutraceutical supplements like *Urtica dioica*, zinc, and vitamin E [165].

4. Discussion

Nutraceuticals supplementation has been shown to be a significant adjuvant strategy in the management of OA as reported by extensive evidence collected in cellular OA models, animals, and human RCTs.

From a molecular point of view, the abovementioned nutraceuticals act predominantly in the signaling pathways underlying OA pathogenesis, inflammation, and oxidative stress, with the former triggering the latter and vice versa [166].

Although complete knowledge of all the molecular effects in OA management is still lacking, a summary of the latter is shown in Table 1. As reported by different in vitro and in vivo studies, the advantage of most of the nutraceutical molecules is they exert pleiotropic effects, acting through different but complementary pathways of action regarding the reduction of inflammation and oxidative stress. For this reason, the synergistic integration of nutraceuticals with conventional therapy could eventually reduce the dosages and/or the number of administrations of drugs and thus the side effects [167].

An important point with regard to the nutritional supplements is the low bioavailability of the more promising compounds, which inevitably reduces the final effectiveness of the treatments. In this context, it is important to underline how the success of a nutraceutical supplementation does not depend exclusively on the correct choice of the active ingredient and the dosage of administration, but also on the correct bionutraceutical formulations [164]. This aspect may explain in part the great heterogeneity of results from clinical studies, which depend on the principles of clinical research, including the careful selection

Int. J. Mol. Sci. **2021**, 22, 12920

and stratification of the patients with inclusion and exclusion criteria, power analyses, and avoidance of confounding variables, in order to avoid inconsistent results.

However, one of the most relevant limits in the use of anti-OA nutraceuticals regards the high costs involved in obtaining titrated and standardized extracts. In general, the conventional techniques that are naturally available and used by industries do not always allow the production of inexpensive quality extracts and thus low-cost strategies to prevent or treat OA disease. The problem of cheap but poor-quality nutraceutical extracts is a serious, underestimated, and potentially dangerous problem for people's health, not only because of the absence of specific active ingredients or the low quality of un-titrated extracts, but above all due to the presence of contaminants [168]. An important challenge for the future is to develop a food-compatible method for the extraction of specific phytochemicals and thus produce qualitatively effective and safe nutraceutical extracts with anti-OA properties. In this context, unconventional techniques, such as ultrasound or microwave-assisted extraction associated with hydroalcoholic solvents, may potentially improve the quality of the extracts and ensure good yields [169]. Nevertheless, although the unconventional processes used for extracting value-added products are well established in the laboratory, industrial-scale production with specific cost-effective analyses is still a challenge.

Finally, another important goal in OA management is the reduction of pain, which remains a major source of distress and disability, and the improvement of quality of life. In fact, current pharmacological analgesics have limited efficacy, in addition to being potentially correlated with important adverse events, especially for chronic administrations. In this regard, the abovementioned nutraceuticals could be associated with other extracts of both botanical and animal origin in order to act comprehensively on the clinical picture of the patient with OA. While the specific molecular mechanism underlying the effect of these nutraceuticals on OA pain is at least in part unknown and not well understood, growing evidence suggests it may be attributable to their anti-inflammatory actions [11].

5. Conclusions

In conclusion, nutraceuticals may represent a valid strategy in OA management in association with conventional therapies. However, larger and longer studies are urgently required to definitively consider this unconventional approach in clinical practice, in order to focus the attention on the molecular mechanisms of nutraceuticals in mitigating OA processes and pain, the potential combination of anti-OA molecules with pain relief nutraceuticals, as well as both the efficacy and the safety of these treatments in long-term periods.

Author Contributions: Conceptualization, A.F.G.C.; methodology, A.F.G.C. and A.C.; data curation, A.C.; writing—original draft preparation, A.C.; writing—review and editing, A.C.; and A.F.G.C. All authors have read and agreed to the published version of the manuscript.

Funding: This research received no external funding.

Institutional Review Board Statement: Not applicable.

Informed Consent Statement: Not applicable.

Acknowledgments: We are grateful to Elisa Grandi for help in paper revision.

Conflicts of Interest: The authors declare no conflict of interest.

References

1. Hootman, J.M.; Helmick, C.G.; Barbour, K.E.; Theis, K.A.; Boring, M.A. Updated projected prevalence of self-reported doctor-diagnosed arthritis and arthritis-attributable activity limitation among us adults, 2015–2040. *Arthritis Rheumatol.* **2016**, *68*, 1582–1587. [CrossRef] [PubMed]
2. Szychlinska, M.A.; Trovato, F.M.; Di Rosa, M.; Malaguarnera, L.; Puzzo, L.; Leonardi, R.; Castrogiovanni, P.; Musumeci, G. Co-expression and co-localization of cartilage glycoproteins CHI3L1 and lubricin in osteoarthritic cartilage: Morphological, immunohistochemical and gene expression profiles. *Int. J. Mol. Sci.* **2016**, *17*, 359. [CrossRef] [PubMed]

3. Aiello, F.C.; Trovato, F.M.; Szychlinska, M.A.; Imbesi, R.; Castrogiovanni, P.; Loreto, C.; Musumeci, G. Molecular links between diabetes and osteoarthritis: The role of physical activity. *Curr. Diabetes Rev.* **2017**, *13*, 50–58. [CrossRef] [PubMed]

4. Fajardo, M.; Di Cesare, P.E. Disease-modifying therapies for osteoarthritis. *Drugs Aging* **2005**, *22*, 141–161. [CrossRef]

5. Sengupta, K.; Alluri, K.V.; Satish, A.R.; Mishra, S.; Golakoti, T.; Sarma, K.V.; Dey, D.; Raychaudhuri, S.P. A double blind, randomized, placebo controlled study of the efficacy and safety of 5-Loxin for treatment of osteoarthritis of the knee. *Arthritis Res. Ther.* **2008**, *10*, R85. [CrossRef] [PubMed]

6. Szychlinska, M.A.; Castrogiovanni, P.; Trovato, F.M.; Nsir, H.; Zarrouk, M.; Lo Firno, D.; Di Rosa, M.; Imbesi, R.; Musumeci, G. Physical activity and Mediterranean diet based on olive tree phenolic compounds from two different geographical areas have protective effects on early osteoarthritis, muscle atrophy and hepatic steatosis. *Eur. J. Nutr.* **2019**, *58*, 565–581. [CrossRef]

7. Toopchizadeh, V.; Dolatkhah, N.; Aghamohammadi, D.; Rasouli, M.; Hashemian, M. Dietary inflammatory index is associated with pain intensity and some components of quality of life in patients with knee osteoarthritis. *BMC Res. Not.* **2020**, *13*, 1–7. [CrossRef]

8. Ameye, L.G.; Chee, W.S. Osteoarthritis and nutrition. From nutraceuticals to functional foods: A systematic review of the scientific evidence. *Arthritis Res. Ther.* **2006**, *8*, 127. [CrossRef]

9. Neogi, T. The epidemiology and impact of pain in osteoarthritis. *Osteoarthr. Cartil.* **2013**, *21*, 1145–1153. [CrossRef]

10. Aghamohammadi, D.; Dolatkhah, N.; Bakhtiari, F.; Eslamian, F.; Hashemian, M. Nutraceutical supplements in management of pain and disability in osteoarthritis: A systematic review and meta-analysis of randomized clinical trials. *Sci. Rep.* **2020**, *10*, 20892. [CrossRef]

11. Castrogiovanni, P.; Trovato, F.M.; Loreto, C.; Nsir, H.; Szychlinska, M.A.; Musumeci, G. Nutraceutical supplements in the management and prevention of osteoarthritis. *Int. J. Mol. Sci.* **2016**, *17*, 2042. [CrossRef]

12. Shen, C.L.; Smith, B.J.; Lo, D.F.; Chyu, M.C.; Dunn, D.M.; Chen, C.H.; Kwun, I.S. Dietary polyphenols and mechanisms of osteoarthritis. *J. Nutr. Biochem.* **2012**, *23*, 1367–1377. [CrossRef]

13. Ghoochani, N.; Karandish, M.; Mowla, K.; Haghighizadeh, M.H.; Jalali, M.T. The effect of pomegranate juice on clinical signs, matrix metalloproteinases and antioxidant status in patients with knee osteoarthritis. *J. Sci. Food Agric.* **2016**, *96*, 4377–4381. [CrossRef]

14. Appelboom, T.; Schuermans, J.; Verbruggen, G.; Henrotin, Y.; Reginster, J.Y. Symptoms modifying effect of avocado/soybean unsaponifiables (ASU) in knee osteoarthritis. A double blind, prospective, placebo-controlled study. *Scand. J. Rheumatol.* **2001**, *30*, 242–247. [PubMed]

15. Belcaro, G.; Dugall, M.; Luzzi, R.; Ledda, A.; Pellegrini, L.; Cesarone, M.R.; Hosoi, M.; Errichi, M.; Francis, S.; Cornelli, U. FlexiQule (Boswellia extract) in the supplementary management of osteoarthritis: A supplement registry. *Minerva Med.* **2014**, *105*, 9–16.

16. Schnitzer, T.J.; Pelletier, J.P.; Haselwood, D.M.; Ellison, W.T.; Ervin, J.E.; Gordon, R.D.; Lissie, J.R.; Archambault, W.T.; Sampson, A.R.; Fezatte, H.B.; et al. Civamide cream 0.075% in patients with osteoarthritis of the knee: A 12-week randomized controlled clinical trial with a longterm extension. *J. Rheumatol.* **2012**, *39*, 610–620. [CrossRef] [PubMed]

17. Li, Y.; Chen, L.; Liu, Y.; Zhang, Y.; Liang, Y.; Mei, Y. Anti-inflammatory effects in a mouse osteoarthritis model of a mixture of glucosamine and chitooligosaccharides produced by bi-enzyme single-step hydrolysis. *Sci. Rep.* **2018**, *8*, 5624. [CrossRef]

18. Waly, N.E.; Refaiy, A.; Aborehab, N.M. IL-10 and TGF-beta: Roles in chondroprotective effects of Glucosamine in experimental Osteoarthritis? *Pathophysiology* **2017**, *24*, 45–49. [CrossRef]

19. Kamarul, T.; Ab-Rahim, S.; Tumin, M.; Selvaratnam, L.; Ahmad, T.S. A preliminary study of the effects of glucosamine sulphate and chondroitin sulphate on surgically treated and untreated focal cartilage damage. *Eur. Cells Mater.* **2011**, *21*, 259–271, discussion 270–51. [CrossRef]

20. García-Coronado, J.M.; Martínez-Olvera, L.; Elizondo-Omaña, R.E.; Acosta-Olivo, C.A.; Vilchez-Cavazos, F.; Simental-Mendía, L.E.; Simental-Mendía, M. Effect of collagen supplementation on osteoarthritis symptoms: A meta-analysis of randomized placebo-controlled trials. *Int. Orthop.* **2019**, *43*, 531–538. [CrossRef] [PubMed]

21. Kuptniratsaikul, V.; Dajpratham, P.; Taechaarpornkul, W.; Buntragulpoontawee, M.; Lukkanapichonchut, P.; Chootip, C.; Saengsuwan, J.; Tantayakom, K.; Laongpech, S. Efficacy and safety of Curcuma domestica extracts compared with ibuprofen in patients with knee osteoarthritis: A multicenter study. *Clin. Interv. Aging* **2014**, *9*, 451–458. [CrossRef]

22. Hashempur, M.H.; Sadrneshin, S.; Mosavat, S.H.; Ashraf, A. Green tea (Camellia sinensis) for patients with knee osteoarthritis: A randomized open-label activecontrolled clinical trial. *Clinical Nutrition* **2018**, *37*, 85–90. [CrossRef] [PubMed]

23. Altman, R.D.; Marcussen, K.C. Effects of a ginger extract on knee pain in patients with osteoarthritis. *Arthr. Rheum.* **2001**, *44*, 2531–2538. [CrossRef]

24. Rondanelli, M.; Riva, A.; Morazzoni, P.; Allegrini, P.; Faliva, M.A.; Naso, M.; Miccono, A.; Peroni, G.; Degli Agosti, I.; Perna, S. The effect and safety of highly standardized Ginger (Zingiber officinale) and Echinacea (Echinacea angustifolia) extract supplementation on inflammation and chronic pain in NSAIDs poor responders. A pilot study in subjects with knee arthrosis. *Nat. Prod. Res.* **2017**, *31*, 1309–1313. [CrossRef]

25. Altman, R.D.; Manjoo, A.; Fierlinger, A.; Niazi, F.; Nicholls, M. The mechanism of action for hyaluronic acid treatment in the osteoarthritic knee: A systematic review. *BMC Musculoskelet Disord* **2015**, *16*, 321. [CrossRef] [PubMed]

26. Pagonis, T.A.; Givissis, P.A.; Kritis, A.C.; Christodoulou, A.C. The effect of methylsulfonylmethane on osteoarthritic large joints and mobility. *Int. J. Orthop.* **2014**, *1*, 19–24. [CrossRef]

27. Jacquet, A.; Girodet, P.O.; Pariente, A.; Forest, K.; Mallet, L.; Moore, N. Phytalgic, a food supplement, vs placebo in patients with osteoarthritis of the knee or hip: A randomised double-blind placebo-controlled clinical trial. *Arthritis Res. Ther.* **2009**, *11*, R192. [CrossRef] [PubMed]

28. Hill, C.L.; March, L.M.; Aitken, D.; Lester, S.E.; Battersby, R.; Hynes, K.; Jones, G. Fish oil in knee osteoarthritis: A randomised clinical trial of low dose versus high dose. *Ann. Rheum. Dis.* **2016**, *75*, 23–29. [CrossRef]

29. Cisar, P.; Jany, R.; Waczulikova, I.; Sumegova, K.; Muchova, J.; Vojtassak, J.; Duraćková, Z.; Lisý, M.; Rohdewald, P. Effect of pine bark extract (Pycnogenol) on symptoms of knee osteoarthritis. *Phytother Res* **2008**, *22*, 1087–1092. [CrossRef]

30. Carr, A.C.; McCall, C. The role of vitamin C in the treatment of pain: New insights. *J. Transl. Med.* **2017**, *15*, 77. [CrossRef]

31. Arden, N.K.; Cro, S.; Sheard, S.; Doré, C.J.; Bara, A.; Tebbs, S.A.; Hunter, D.J.; James, S. The effect of vitamin D supplementation on knee osteoarthritis, the VIDEO study: A randomised controlled trial. *Osteoarthr. Cartil.* **2016**, *24*, 1858–1866. [CrossRef] [PubMed]

32. Sanghi, D.; Mishra, A.; Sharma, A.C.; Singh, A.; Natu, S.M.; Agarwal, S.; Srivastava, R.N. Does vitamin D improve osteoarthritis of the knee: A randomized controlled pilot trial. *Clin. Orthop. Relat. Res.* **2013**, *471*, 3556–3562. [CrossRef]

33. DiNubile, N.A. Glucosamine and chondroitin sulfate in the management of osteoarthritis. *Postgrad. Med.* **2009**, *121*, 48–50. [CrossRef] [PubMed]

34. Jomphe, C.; Gabriac, M.; Hale, T.M.; Héroux, L.; Trudeau, L.-R.; Deblois, D.; Montell, E.; Vergés, J.; du Souich, P. Chondroitin sulfate inhibits the nuclear translocation of nuclear factor-kappaB in interleukin-1beta-stimulated chondrocytes. *Basic Clin. Pharmacol. Toxicol.* **2008**, *102*, 59–65. [CrossRef] [PubMed]

35. Aghazadeh-Habashi, A.; Kohan, M.H.; Asghar, W.; Jamali, F. Glucosamine dose/concentration-effect correlation in the rat with adjuvant arthritis. *J. Pharm. Sci.* **2014**, *103*, 760–767. [CrossRef] [PubMed]

36. Imagawa, K.; de Andrés, M.C.; Hashimoto, K.; Pitt, D.; Itoi, E.; Goldring, M.B.; Roach, H.I.; Oreffo, R.O. The epigenetic effect of glucosamine and a nuclear factor-kappa B (NF-kB) inhibitor on primary human chondrocytes—implications for osteoarthritis. *Biochem. Biophys. Res. Commun.* **2011**, *405*, 362–367. [CrossRef]

37. Wen, Z.H.; Tang, C.C.; Chang, Y.C.; Huang, S.Y.; Hsieh, S.P.; Lee, C.H.; Huang, G.S.; Ng, H.F.; Neoh, C.A.; Hsieh, C.S.; et al. Glucosamine sulfate reduces experimental osteoarthritis and nociception in rats: Association with changes of mitogen-activated protein kinase in chondrocytes. *Osteoarthr. Cartil.* **2010**, *18*, 1192–1202. [CrossRef]

38. Chiu, H.W.; Li, L.H.; Hsieh, C.Y.; Rao, Y.K.; Chen, F.H.; Chen, A.; Ka, S.M.; Hua, K.F. Glucosamine inhibits IL-1beta expression by preserving mitochondrial integrity and disrupting assembly of the NLRP3 inflammasome. *Sci. Rep.* **2019**, *9*, 5603. [CrossRef] [PubMed]

39. Mendis, E.; Kim, M.M.; Rajapakse, N.; Kim, S.K. Sulfated glucosamine inhibits oxidation of biomolecules in cells via a mechanism involving intracellular free radical scavenging. *Eur. J. Pharmacol.* **2008**, *579*, 74–85. [CrossRef]

40. Panasyuk, A.; Frati, E.; Ribault, D.; Mitrovic, D. Effect of reactive oxygen species on the biosynthesis and structure of newly synthesized proteoglycans. *Free Radic. Biol. Med.* **1994**, *16*, 157–167. [CrossRef]

41. Tiku, M.L.; Narla, H.; Jain, M.; Yalamanchili, P. Glucosamine prevents in vitro collagen degradation in chondrocytes by inhibiting advanced lipoxidation reactions and protein oxidation. *Arthritis. Res. Ther.* **2007**, *9*, R76. [CrossRef]

42. Wu, S.; Dai, X.; Shilong, F.; Zhu, M.; Shen, X.; Zhang, K.; Li, S. Antimicrobial and antioxidant capacity of glucosamine-zinc(II) complex via non-enzymatic browning reaction. *Food Sci. Biotechnol.* **2018**, *27*, 1–7. [CrossRef] [PubMed]

43. Ucuncu, Y.; Celik, N.; Ozturk, C.; Turkoglu, M.; Cetin, N.; Kockara, N.; Sener, E.; Dundar, C.; Arslan, A.; Dogan, H.; et al. Chondroprotective effects of a new glucosamine combination in rats: Gene expression, biochemical and histopathological evaluation. *Life Sci.* **2015**, *130*, 31–37. [CrossRef] [PubMed]

44. Igarashi, M.; Sakamoto, K.; Nagaoka, I. Effect of glucosamine, a therapeutic agent for osteoarthritis, on osteoblastic cell differentiation. *Int. J. Mol. Med.* **2011**, *28*, 373–379. [CrossRef]

45. Derfoul, A.; Miyoshi, A.D.; Freeman, D.E.; Tuan, R.S. Glucosamine promotes chondrogenic phenotype in both chondrocytes and mesenchymal stem cells and inhibits MMP-13 expression and matrix degradation. *Osteoarthr. Cartil.* **2007**, *15*, 646–655. [CrossRef] [PubMed]

46. Zhu, X.; Sang, L.; Wu, D.; Rong, J.; Jiang, L. Effectiveness and safety of glucosamine and chondroitin for the treatment of osteoarthritis: A meta-analysis of randomized controlled trials. *J. Orthop. Surg. Res.* **2018**, *13*, 170. [CrossRef]

47. Simental-Mendía, M.; Sánchez-García, A.; Vilchez-Cavazos, F.; Acosta-Olivo, C.A.; Peña-Martínez, V.M.; Simental-Mendía, L.E. Effect of glucosamine and chondroitin sulfate in symptomatic knee osteoarthritis: A systematic review and meta-analysis of randomized placebo-controlled trials. *Rheumatol. Int.* **2018**, *38*, 1413–1428. [CrossRef]

48. Ogata, T.; Ideno, Y.; Akai, M.; Seichi, A.; Hagino, H.; Iwaya, T.; Doim, T.; Yamadam, K.; Chen, A.Z.; Li, Y.; et al. Effects of glucosamine in patients with osteoarthritis of the knee: A systematic review and meta-analysis. *Clin. Rheumatol.* **2018**, *37*, 2479–2487. [CrossRef]

49. Zhu, X.; Wu, D.; Sang, L.; Wang, Y.; Shen, Y.; Zhuang, X.; Chu, M.; Jiang, L. Comparative effectiveness of glucosamine, chondroitin, acetaminophen or celecoxib for the treatment of knee and/or hip osteoarthritis: A network meta-analysis. *Clin. Exp. Rheumatol.* **2018**, *36*, 595–602. [PubMed]

50. Zeng, C.; Wei, J.; Li, H.; Wang, Y.L.; Xie, D.X.; Yang, T.; Gao, S.G.; Li, Y.S.; Luo, W.; Lei, G.H. Effectiveness and safety of Glucosamine, chondroitin, the two in combination, or celecoxib in the treatment of osteoarthritis of the knee. *Sci. Rep.* **2015**, *5*, 16827. [CrossRef] [PubMed]

51. Kwoh, C.K.; Roemer, F.W.; Hannon, M.J.; Moore, C.E.; Jakicic, J.M.; Guermazi, A.; Green, S.M.; Evans, R.W.; Boudreau, R. Effect of oral glucosamine on joint structure in individuals with chronic knee pain: A randomized, placebo-controlled clinical trial. *Arthritis Rheumatol.* **2014**, *66*, 930–939. [CrossRef]

52. Fransen, M.; Agaliotis, M.; Nairn, L.; Votrubec, M.; Bridgett, L.; Su, S.; Jan, S.; March, L.; Edmonds, J.; Norton, R.; et al. LEGS study collaborative group. Glucosamine and chondroitin for knee osteoarthritis: A double-blind randomised placebocontrolled clinical trial evaluating single and combination regimens. *Ann. Rheum. Dis.* **2015**, *74*, 851–858. [CrossRef]

53. Cahlin, B.J.; Dahlstrom, L. No effect of glucosamine sulfate on osteoarthritis in the temporomandibular joints–A randomized, controlled, short-term study. *Oral Surg. Oral Med. Oral Pathol. Oral Radiol. Endod.* **2011**, *112*, 760–766. [CrossRef]

54. Knapik, J.J.; Pope, R.; Hoedebecke, S.S.; Schram, B.; Orr, R.; Lieberman, H.R. Effects of Oral Glucosamine Sulfate on Osteoarthritis-Related Pain and Joint-Space Changes: Systematic Review and Meta-Analysis. *J. Spec. Oper. Med.* **2018**, *18*, 139–147.

55. Cen, X.; Liu, Y.; Wang, S.; Yang, X.; Shi, Z.; Liang, X. Glucosamine oral administration as an adjunct to hyaluronic acid injection in treating temporomandibular joint osteoarthritis. *Oral Dis.* **2018**, *24*, 404–411. [CrossRef]

56. Gang, D.; Xiaguang, C.; Kanghua, Y.; Aiping, W.; Guangxuan, Z. Combined effect of celecoxib and glucosamine sulfate on inflammatory factors and oxidative stress indicators in patients with knee osteoarthritis. *Trop. J. Pharm. Res.* **2019**, *18*, 397–402. [CrossRef]

57. Joung, Y.H.; Darvin, P.; Kang, D.Y.; Sp, N.; Byun, H.J.; Lee, C.-H.; Lee, H.K.; Yang, Y.M. Methylsulfonylmethane inhibits RANKL-induced osteoclastogenesis in BMMs by suppressing NF-κB and STAT3 activities. *PLoS ONE* **2016**, *11*, e0159891. [CrossRef]

58. Kloesch, B.; Liszt, M.; Broell, J.; Steiner, G. Dimethyl sulphoxide and dimethyl sulphone are potent inhibitors of IL-6 and IL-8 expression in the human chondrocyte cell line C-28/I2. *Life Sci.* **2011**, *89*, 473–478. [CrossRef] [PubMed]

59. Cheleschi, S.; Fioravanti, A.; De Palma, A.; Corallo, C.; Franci, D.; Volpi, N.; Bedogni, G.; Giannotti, S.; Giordano, N. Methylsulfonylmethane and mobilee prevent negative effect of IL-1β in human chondrocyte cultures via NF-κB signaling pathway. *Int. Immunopharmacol.* **2018**, *65*, 129–139. [CrossRef] [PubMed]

60. Ahn, H.; Kim, J.; Lee, M.-J.; Kim, Y.J.; Cho, Y.-W.; Lee, G.-S. Methylsulfonylmethane inhibits NLRP3 inflammasome activation. *Cytokine* **2015**, *71*, 223–231. [CrossRef]

61. Butawan, M.; Benjamin, R.L.; Bloomer, R.J. Methylsulfonylmethane: Applications and safety of a novel dietary supplement. *Nutrients* **2017**, *9*, 290. [CrossRef]

62. Joung, Y.H.; Lim, E.J.; Darvin, P.; Chung, S.C.; Jang, J.W.; Do Park, K.; Lee, H.K.; Kim, H.S.; Park, T.; Yang, Y.M. MSM enhances GH signaling via the Jak2/STAT5b pathway in osteoblast-like cells and osteoblast differentiation through the activation of STAT5b in MSCs. *PLoS ONE* **2012**, *7*, e47477. [CrossRef] [PubMed]

63. Dalle Carbonare, L.; Bertacco, J.; Marchetto, G.; Cheri, S.; Deiana, M.; Minoia, A.; Tiso, N.; Mottes, M.; Valenti, M.T. Methylsulfonylmethane enhances MSC chondrogenic commitment and promotes pre-osteoblasts formation. *Stem Cell Res. Ther.* **2021**, *12*, 326. [CrossRef]

64. Aljohani, H.; Senbanjo, L.T.; Chellaiah, M.A. Methylsulfonylmethane increases osteogenesis and regulates the mineralization of the matrix by transglutaminase 2 in SHED cells. *PLoS ONE* **2019**, *14*, e0225598. [CrossRef] [PubMed]

65. Oshima, Y.; Amiel, D.; Theodosakis, J. The effect of distilled methylsulfonylmethane (msm) on human chondrocytes in vitro. *Osteoarthr. Cartil.* **2007**, *15*, C123. [CrossRef]

66. Debbi, E.M.; Agar, G.; Fichman, G.; Ziv, Y.B.; Kardosh, R.; Halperin, N.; Elbaz, A.; Beer, Y.; Debi, R. Efficacy of methylsulfonylmethane supplementation on osteoarthritis of the knee: A randomized controlled study. *BMC Complement. Altern. Med.* **2011**, *11*, 50. [CrossRef] [PubMed]

67. Debi, R.; Fichman, G.; Ziv, Y.B.; Kardosh, R.; Debbi, E.; Halperin, N.; Agar, G. The role of msm in knee osteoarthritis: A double blind, randomized, prospective study. *Osteoarthr. Cartil.* **2007**, *15*, C231. [CrossRef]

68. Usha, P.; Naidu, M. Randomised, double-blind, parallel, placebo-controlled study of oral glucosamine, methylsulfonylmethane and their combination in osteoarthritis. *Clin. Drug Investig.* **2004**, *24*, 353–363. [CrossRef]

69. Lubis, A.M.T.; Siagian, C.; Wonggokusuma, E.; Marsetyo, A.F.; Setyohadi, B. Comparison of Glucosamine-Chondroitin Sulfate with and without Methylsulfonylmethane in Grade I-II Knee Osteoarthritis: A Double Blind Randomized Controlled Trial. *Acta Med. Indones.* **2017**, *49*, 105–111.

70. Vidyasagar, S.; Mukhyaprana, P.; Shashikiran, U.; Sachidananda, A.; Rao, S.; Bairy, K.L.; Adiga, S.; Jayaprakash, B. Efficacy and tolerability of glucosamine chondroitin sulphate-methyl sulfonyl methane (MSM) in osteoarthritis of knee in indian patients. *Iran J. Pharmacol. Ther.* **2004**, *3*, 61–65.

71. Magrans-Courtney, T.; Wilborn, C.; Rasmussen, C.; Ferreira, M.; Greenwood, L.; Campbell, B.; Kerksick, C.M.; Nassar, E.; Li, R.; Iosia, M. Effects of diet type and supplementation of glucosamine, chondroitin, and msm on body composition, functional status, and markers of health in women with knee osteoarthritis initiating a resistance-based exercise and weight loss program. *J. Int. Soc. Sports Nutr.* **2011**, *8*, 8. [CrossRef]

72. Borzelleca, J.F.; Sipes, I.G.; Wallace, K.B. *Dossier in Support of the Generally Recognized as Safe (GRAS) Status of Optimsm (Methylsulfonylmethane MSM) as a Food Ingredient*; Food and Drug Administration: Vero Beach, FL, USA, 2007.

73. Kawaguchi, T.; Nanbu, P.N.; Kurokawa, M. Distribution of prolylhydroxyproline and its metabolites after oral administration in rats. *Biol. Pharm. Bull.* **2012**, *35*, 422–427. [CrossRef]

74. Garnero, P.; Rousseau, J.C.; Delmas, P.D. Molecular basis and clinical use of biochemical markers of bone, cartilage, and synovium in joint diseases. *Arthritis Rheum.* **2000**, *43*, 953–968. [CrossRef]
75. Bos, K.J.; Rucklidge, G.J.; Dunbar, B.; Robins, S.P. Primary structure of the helical domain of porcine collagen X. *Matrix Biol.* **1999**, *18*, 149–153. [CrossRef]
76. Sibilla, S.; Godfrey, M.; Brewer, S.; Budh-Raja, A.; Genovese, L. An overview of the beneficial effects of hydrolysed collagen as a nutraceutical on skin properties: Scientific background and clinical studies. *Open Nutraceuticals J.* **2015**, *8*, 29–42. [CrossRef]
77. Ohara, H.; Matsumoto, H.; Ito, K.; Iwai, K.; Sato, K. Comparison of quantity and structures of hydroxyproline-containing peptides in human blood after oral ingestion of gelatin hydrolysates from different sources. *J. Agric. Food Chem.* **2007**, *55*, 1532–1535. [CrossRef] [PubMed]
78. Bourdon, B.; Contentin, R.; Cassé, F.; Maspimby, C.; Oddoux, S.; Noël, A.; Legendre, F.; Gruchy, N.; Galéra, P. Marine Collagen Hydrolysates Downregulate the Synthesis of Pro-Catabolic and Pro-Inflammatory Markers of Osteoarthritis and Favor Collagen Production and Metabolic Activity in Equine Articular Chondrocyte Organoids. *Int. J. Mol. Sci.* **2021**, *22*, 580. [CrossRef]
79. Gordon, M.K.; Hahn, R.A. Collagens. *Cell Tissue Res.* **2010**, *339*, 247–257. [CrossRef]
80. Henrotin, Y.; Sanchez, C.; Balligand, M. Pharmaceutical and nutraceutical management of canine osteoarthritis: Present and future perspectives. *Vet. J.* **2005**, *170*, 113–123. [CrossRef]
81. Oesser, S.; Adam, M.; Babel, W.; Seifert, J. Oral Administration of 14C Labeled Gelatin Hydrolysate Leads to an Accumulation of Radioactivity in Cartilage of Mice (C57/BL). *J. Nutr.* **1999**, *129*, 1891–1895. [CrossRef]
82. Bagchi, D.; Misner, B.; Bagchi, M.; Kothari, S.C.; Downs, B.W.; Fafard, R.D.; Preuss, H.G. Effects of orally administered undenatured type II collagen against arthritic inflammatory diseases: A mechanistic exploration. *Int. J. Clin. Pharmacol. Res.* **2002**, *22*, 101–110.
83. Tong, T.; Zhao, W.; Wu, Y.-Q.; Chang, Y.; Wang, Q.-T.; Zhang, L.-L.; Wei, W. Chicken type II collagen induced immune balance of main subtype of helper T cells in mesenteric lymph node lymphocytes in rats with collagen-induced arthritis. *Inflamm. Res. Off. J. Eur. Histamine Res. Soc.* **2010**, *59*, 369–377. [CrossRef]
84. D'Altilio, M.; Peal, A.; Alvey, M.; Simms, C.; Curtsinger, A.; Gupta, R.C.; Canerdy, T.D.; Goad, J.T.; Bagchi, M.; Bagchi, D. Therapeutic efficacy and safety of undenatured type II collagen singly or in combination with glucosamine and chondroitin in arthritic dogs. *Toxicol. Mech. Methods* **2007**, *17*, 189–196. [CrossRef]
85. Ohara, H.; Iida, H.; Ito, K.; Takeuchi, Y.; Nomura, Y. Effects of Pro-Hyp, a collagen hydrolysate-derived peptide, on hyaluronic acid synthesis using in vitro cultured synovium cells and oral ingestion of collagen hydrolysates in a guinea pig model of osteoarthritis. *Biosci. Biotechnol. Biochem.* **2010**, *74*, 2096–2099. [CrossRef]
86. Nakatani, S.; Mano, H.; Sampei, C.; Shimizu, J.; Wada, M. Chondroprotective effect of the bioactive peptide prolyl-hydroxyproline in mouse articular cartilage in vitro and in vivo. *Osteoarthr. Cartil.* **2009**, *17*, 1620–1627. [CrossRef] [PubMed]
87. Isaka, S.; Someya, A.; Nakamura, S.; Naito, K.; Nozawa, M.; Inoue, N.; Sugihara, F.; Nagaoka, I.; Kaneko, K. Evaluation of the effect of oral administration of collagen peptides on an experimental rat osteoarthritis model. *Exp. Ther. Med.* **2017**, *13*, 2699–2706. [CrossRef]
88. Kumar, S.; Sugihara, F.; Suzuki, K.; Inoue, N.; Venkateswarathirukumara, S. A double-blind, placebo-controlled, randomised, clinical study on the effectiveness of collagen peptide on osteoarthritis. *J. Sci. Food Agric.* **2015**, *95*, 702–707. [CrossRef] [PubMed]
89. Lugo, J.P.; Saiyed, Z.M.; Lane, N.E. Efficacy and tolerability of an undenatured type II collagen supplement in modulating knee osteoarthritis symptoms: A multicenter randomized, double-blind, placebo-controlled study. *Nutr. J.* **2016**, *15*, 14. [CrossRef]
90. Moskowitz, R.W. Role of collagen hydrolysate in bone and joint disease. *Semin. Arthritis Rheum.* **2000**, *30*, 87–99. [CrossRef] [PubMed]
91. Clark, K.L.; Sebastianelli, W.; Flechsenhar, K.R.; Aukermann, D.F.; Meza, F.; Millard, R.L.; Deitch, J.R.; Sherbondy, P.S.; Albert, A. 24-Week study on the use of collagen hydrolysate as a dietary supplement in athletes with activity-related joint pain. *Curr. Med. Res. Opin.* **2008**, *24*, 1485–1496. [CrossRef]
92. Wu, J.; Fujioka, M.; Sugimoto, K.; Mu, G.; Ishimi, Y. Assessment of effectiveness of oral administration of collagen peptide on bone metabolism in growing and mature rats. *J. Bone Miner Metab.* **2004**, *22*, 547–553. [CrossRef] [PubMed]
93. Trc, T.; Bohmova, J. Efficacy and tolerance of enzymatic hydrolysed collagen (EHC) vs. Glucosamine sulphate (GS) in the treatment of knee osteoarthritis (KOA). *Int. Orthop.* **2011**, *35*, 341–348. [CrossRef]
94. Necas, J.; Bartosicova, L.; Brauner, P.; Kolar, J. Hyaluronic acid. (hyaluronan): A review. *Vet. Med.* **2008**, *8*, 397–411. [CrossRef]
95. Bowman, S.; Awad, M.E.; Hamrick, M.W.; Hunter, M.; Fulzele, S. Recent advances in hyaluronic acid based therapy for osteoarthritis. *Clin. Transl. Med.* **2018**, *7*, 6. [CrossRef]
96. Day, R.; Brooks, P.; Conaghan, P.G.; Petersen, M. A double blind, randomized, multicenter, parallel group study of the effectiveness and tolerance of intraarticular hyaluronan in osteoarthritis of the knee. *J. Rheumatol.* **2004**, *31*, 775–782. [CrossRef]
97. Adams, M.E.; Lussier, A.J.; Peyron, J.G. A risk-benefit assessment of injections of hyaluronan and its derivatives in the treatment of osteoarthritis of the knee. *Drug Saf.* **2000**, *23*, 115–130. [CrossRef] [PubMed]
98. Brun, P.; Panfilo, S.; Daga Gordini, D.; Cortivo, R.; Abatangelo, G. The effect of hyaluronan on CD44-mediated survival of normal and hydroxyl radical-damaged chondrocytes. *Osteoarthr. Cartil.* **2003**, *11*, 208–216. [CrossRef]
99. Karna, E.; Miltyk, W.; Surazynski, A.; Palka, J.A. Protective effect of hyaluronic acid on interleukin-1-induced deregulation of beta1-integrin and insulin-like growth factor-I receptor signaling and collagen biosynthesis in cultured human chondrocytes. *Mol. Cell Biochem.* **2008**, *308*, 57–64. [CrossRef]

100. Hiraoka, N.; Takahashi, Y.; Arai, K.; Honjo, S.; Nakawaga, S.; Tsuchida, S.; Sakao, K.; Kubo, T. Hyaluronan and intermittent hydrostatic pressure synergistically suppressed MMP-13 and Il-6 expressions in osteoblasts from OA subchondral bone. *Osteoarthr. Cartil.* 2009, *17*, S97. [CrossRef]
101. Kajimoto, O.; Odanaka, Y.; Sakamoto, W.; Yoshida, K.; Takahashi, T. Clinical effects of dietary hyaluronic acid on dry skin. *J. New Remedies* 2001, *50*, 548–560.
102. Asari, A.; Kanemitsu, T.; Kurihara, H. Oral administration of high molecular weight hyaluronan (900 kDa) controls immune system via toll-like receptor 4 in the intestinal epithelium. *J. Biol. Chem.* 2010, *285*, 24751–24758. [CrossRef]
103. Chang, C.C.; Hsieh, M.S.; Liao, S.T.; Chen, Y.H.; Cheng, C.W.; Huang, P.T.; Lin, J.-F.; Chen, C.-H. Hyaluronan regulates PPARgamma and inflammatory responses in IL-1beta-stimulated human chondrosarcoma cells, a model for osteoarthritis. *Carbohydr. Polym.* 2012, *90*, 1168–1175. [CrossRef]
104. Yasuda, T. Hyaluronan inhibits Akt, leading to nuclear factor-kappaB down-regulation in lipopolysaccharide-stimulated U937 macrophages. *J. Pharmacol. Sci.* 2011, *115*, 509–515. [CrossRef]
105. Meikle, P.J.; Whittle, A.M.; Hopwood, J.J. Human acetyl-coenzyme A: α-glucosaminide N-acetyltransferase: Kinetic characterization and mechanistic interpretation. *Biochem. J.* 1995, *308*, 327–333. [CrossRef]
106. Han, F.; Ishiguro, N.; Ito, T.; Sakai, T.; Iwata, H. Effects of sodium hyaluronate on experimental osteoarthritis in rabbit knee joints. *Nagoya Med. Sci.* 1999, *62*, 115–126.
107. Forsey, R.; Fisher, J.; Thompson, J.; Stone, M.; Bell, C.; Ingham, E. The effect of hyaluronic acid and phospholipid based lubricants on friction within a human cartilage damage model. *Biomaterials* 2006, *27*, 4581–4590. [CrossRef] [PubMed]
108. Gomis, A.; Miralles, A.; Schmidt, R.F.; Belmonte, C. Intra-articular injections of hyaluronan solutions of different elastoviscosity reduce nociceptive nerve activity in a model of osteoarthritic knee joint of the guinea pig. *Osteoarthr. Cartil.* 2009, *17*, 798–804. [CrossRef] [PubMed]
109. Balogh, L.; Polyak, A.; Mathe, D.; Kiraly, R.; Thuroczy, J.; Terez, M.; Janoki, G.; Ting, Y.; Bucci, L.R.; Schauss, A.G. Absorption, uptake and tissue affinity of high-molecular-weight hyaluronan after oral administration in rats and dogs. *J. Agric. Food. Chem.* 2008, *56*, 10582–10593. [CrossRef] [PubMed]
110. Sato, T.; Iwaso, H. An effectiveness study of hyaluronic acid (Hyabest J) in the treatment of osteoarthritis of the knee. *J. New Rem. Clin.* 2008, *57*, 260–269.
111. Nagaoka, I.; Nabeshima, K.; Murakami, S.; Yamamoto, T.; Watanabe, K.; Tomonaga, A.; Yamaguchi, H. Evaluation of the effects of a supplementary diet containing chicken comb extract on symptoms and cartilage metabolism in patients with knee osteoarthritis. *Exp. Ther. Med.* 2010, *1*, 817–827. [CrossRef]
112. Sato, T.; Iwaso, H. An effectiveness study of hyaluronic acid (Hyabest J) in the treatment of osteoarthritis of the knee on the patint in the United States. *J. New Rem. Clin.* 2009, *58*, 551–558.
113. Iwaso, H.; Sato, T. Examination of the efficacy and safety of oral administration of Hyabest J, highly pure hyaluronic acid, for knee joint pain. *J. Jap. Soc. Clin. Sports Med.* 2009, *17*, 566–572.
114. Tashiro, T.; Seino, S.; Sato, T.; Matsuoka, R.; Masuda, Y.; Fukui, N. Oral administration of polymer hyaluronic acid alleviates symptoms of knee osteoarthritis: A double-blind, placebo-controlled study over a 12-month period. *Sci. World J.* 2012, *2012*, 167928. [CrossRef] [PubMed]
115. Oe, M.; Sakai, S.; Yoshida, H.; Okado, N.; Kaneda, H.; Masuda, Y.; Urushibata, O. Oral hyaluronan relieves wrinkles: A double-blinded, placebo-controlled study over a 12-week period. *Clin. Cosmet. Investig. Dermatol.* 2017, *10*, 267–273. [CrossRef]
116. Padayatty, S.J.; Katz, A.; Wang, Y.; Eck, P.; Kwon, O.; Lee, J.H.; Chen, S.; Corpe, C.; Dutta, A.; Dutta, S.K.; et al. Vitamin C as an antioxidant: Evaluation of its role in disease prevention. *J. Am. Coll. Nutr.* 2003, *22*, 18–35. [CrossRef] [PubMed]
117. Li, H.; Zeng, C.; Wei, J.; Yang, T.; Gao, S.G.; Li, Y.S.; Lei, G.H. Associations between dietary antioxidants intake and radiographic knee osteoarthritis. *Clin. Rheumatol.* 2016, *35*, 1585–1592. [CrossRef]
118. Chang, Z.; Huo, L.; Li, P.; Wu, Y.; Zhang, P. Ascorbic acid provides protection for human chondrocytes against oxidative stress. *Mol. Med. Rep.* 2015, *12*, 7086–7092. [CrossRef] [PubMed]
119. Pinto, S.; Rao, A.V.; Rao, A. Lipid peroxidation, erythrocyte antioxidants and plasma antioxidants in osteoarthritis before and after homeopathic treatment. *Homeopathy* 2008, *97*, 185–189. [CrossRef] [PubMed]
120. Kurz, B.; Jost, B.; Schünke, M. Dietary vitamins and selenium diminish the development of mechanically induced osteoarthritis and increase the expression of antioxidative enzymes in the knee joint of STR/1N mice. *Osteoarth. Cartil.* 2002, *10*, 119–126. [CrossRef]
121. Sowers, M.; Lachance, L. Vitamins and arthritis—the roles of vitamins A, C, D, and E. *Rheum. Dis. Clin. N. Am.* 1999, *25*, 315–332. [CrossRef]
122. Chiu, P.R.; Hu, Y.C.; Huang, T.C.; Hsieh, B.-S.; Yeh, J.-P.; Cheng, H.-L.; Huang, L.-W.; Chang, K.-L. Vitamin C Protects Chondrocytes against Monosodium Iodoacetate-Induced Osteoarthritis by Multiple Pathways. *Int. J. Mol. Sci.* 2016, *18*, 38. [CrossRef] [PubMed]
123. Chaganti, R.K.; Tolstykh, I.; Javaid, M.K.; Neogi, T.; Torner, J.; Curtis, J.; Jacques, P.; Felson, D.; Lane, N.E.; Nevitt, M.C. Multicenter Osteoarthritis Study Group (MOST). High plasma levels of vitamin C and E are associated with incident radiographic knee osteoarthritis. *Osteoarthr. Cartil. OARS Osteoarthr. Res. Soc.* 2014, *22*, 190–196. [CrossRef] [PubMed]
124. Peregoy, J.; Wilder, F.V. The effects of vitamin C supplementation on incident and progressive knee osteoarthritis: A longitudinal study. *Public Health Nutr.* 2011, *14*, 709–715. [CrossRef]

125. Iolascon, G.; Gimigliano, R.; Bianco, M.; De Sire, A.; Moretti, A.; Giusti, A.; Malavolta, N.; Migliaccio, S.; Migliore, A.; Napoli, N.; et al. Are Dietary Supplements and Nutraceuticals Effective for Musculoskeletal Health and Cognitive Function? A Scoping Review. *J. Nutr. Health Aging.* **2017**, *21*, 527–538. [CrossRef] [PubMed]
126. Carr, A.C.; Vissers, M.C.; Cook, J.S. The effect of intravenous vitamin C on cancer- and chemotherapy-related fatigue and quality of life. *Front Oncol.* **2014**, *4*, 283. [CrossRef]
127. IOM. *Dietary Refence Intakes for Calcium and Vitamin D*; The National Academies Press: Washington, DC, USA, 2011.
128. Lips, P.; Cashman, K.D.; Lamberg-Allardt, C.; Bischoff-Ferrari, H.A.; Obermayer-Pietsch, B.; Bianchi, M.L.; Stepan, J.; El-Hajj Fuleihan, G.; Bouillon, R. Current vitamin D status in European and Middle East countries and strategies to prevent vitamin D deficiency: A position statement of the European Calcified Tissue Society. *Eur. J. Endocrinol.* **2019**, *180*, P23–P54. [CrossRef]
129. Tetlow, L.C.; Woolley, D.E. Expression of vitamin D receptors and matrix metalloproteinases in osteoarthritic cartilage and human articular chondrocytes in vitro. *Osteoarthr. Cartil.* **2001**, *9*, 423–431. [CrossRef]
130. Fairney, A.; Straffen, A.M.; May, C.; Seifert, M.H. Vitamin D metabolites in synovial fluid. *Ann. Rheum. Dis.* **1987**, *46*, 370–374. [CrossRef] [PubMed]
131. Guillot, X.; Semerano, L.; Saidenberg-Kermanac'h, N.; Falgarone, G.; Boissier, M. Vitamin D and inflammation. *Jt. Bone Spine* **2010**, *77*, 552–557. [CrossRef]
132. Orfanidou, T.; Malizos, K.N.; Varitimidis, S.; Tsezou, A. 1,25-Dihydroxyvitamin D(3) and extracellular inorganic phosphate activate mitogen-activated protein kinase pathway through fibroblast growth factor 23 contributing to hypertrophy and mineralization in osteoarthritic chondrocytes. *Exp. Biol. Med.* **2012**, *237*, 241–253. [CrossRef]
133. Mabey, T.; Honsawek, S. Role of vitamin D in osteoarthritis: Molecular, cellular, and clinical perspectives. *Int. J. Endocrinol.* **2015**, *2015*, 383918. [CrossRef] [PubMed]
134. Corrado, A.; Neve, A.; Macchiarola, A.; Gaudio, A.; Marucci, A.; Cantatore, F.P. RANKL/OPG ratio and DKK-1 expression in primary osteoblastic cultures from osteoarthritic and osteoporotic subjects. *J. Rheumatol.* **2013**, *40*, 684–694. [CrossRef] [PubMed]
135. Giner, M.; Rios, M.J.; Montoya, M.J.; Vázquez, M.A.; Naji, L.; Pérez-Cano, R. RANKL/OPG in primary cultures of osteoblasts from post-menopausal women. Differences between osteoporotic hip fractures and osteoarthritis. *J. Steroid Biochem. Molec. Biol.* **2009**, *113*, 46–51. [CrossRef]
136. Neve, A.; Cantatore, F.P.; Corrado, A.; Gaudio, A.; Ruggieri, S.; Ribatti, D. In vitro and in vivo angiogenic activity of osteoarthritic and osteoporotic osteoblasts is modulated by VEGF and vitamin D3 treatment. *Regul. Pep.* **2013**, *184*, 81–84. [CrossRef] [PubMed]
137. Rossini, M.; Adami, S.; Viapiana, O.; Fracassi, E.; Idolazzi, L.; Povino, M.R.; Gatti, D. Dose-dependent short-term effects of single high doses of oral vitamin D3 on bone turnover markers. *Calcif. Tissue Intern.* **2012**, *91*, 365–369. [CrossRef] [PubMed]
138. Uitterlinden, A.G.; Fang, Y.; Bergink, A.P.; Van Meurs, J.B.J.; Van Leeuwen, H.P.T.M.; Pols, H.A.P. The role of vitamin D receptor gene polymorphisms in bone biology. *Mol. Cell Endocr.* **2002**, *197*, 15–21. [CrossRef]
139. Keen, R.W.; Hart, D.J.; Lanchbury, J.S.; Spector, T.D. Association of early, osteoarthritis of the knee with a Taq I polymorphism of the vitamin D receptor gene. *Arth. Rheum.* **1997**, *40*, 1444–1449. [CrossRef]
140. Kerkhof, H.J.M.; Lories, R.J.; Meulenbelt, I.; Jonsdottir, I.; Valdes, A.M.; Arp, P.; Ingvarsson, T.; Jhamai, M.; Jonsson, H.; Stolk, L.; et al. A genome-wide association study identifies an osteoarthritis susceptibility locus on chromosome 7q22. *Arthritis Rheum.* **2010**, *62*, 499–510. [CrossRef]
141. Manoy, P.; Yuktanandana, P.; Tanavalee, A.; Anomasiri, W.; Ngarmukos, S.; Tanpowpong, T.; Honsawek, S. Vitamin D Supplementation Improves Quality of Life and Physical Performance in Osteoarthritis Patients. *Nutrients* **2017**, *9*, 799. [CrossRef]
142. Hunter, D.J.; Hart, D.; Snieder, H.; Bettica, P.; Swaminathan, R.; Spector, T.D. Evidence of altered bone turnover, vitamin D and calcium regulation with knee osteoarthritis in female twins. *Rheumatology* **2003**, *42*, 1311–1316. [CrossRef]
143. Ding, C. Serum levels of vitamin D, sunlight exposure, and knee cartilage loss in older adults: The Tasmanian older adult cohort study. *Arthritis Rheum.* **2009**, *60*, 1381–1389. [CrossRef] [PubMed]
144. Bergink, A.P.; Uitterlinden, A.G.; Van Leeuwen, J.P.; Buurman, C.J.; Hofman, A.; Verhaar, J.A.; Pols, H.A. Vitamin D status, bone mineral density, and the development of radiographic osteoarthritis of the knee: The Rotterdam Study. *J. Clin. Rheumatol.* **2009**, *15*, 230–237. [CrossRef]
145. Felson, D.T.; Niu, J.; Clancy, M.; Aliabadi, P.; Sack, B.; Guermazi, A.; Hunter, D.J.; Amin, S.; Rogers, G.; Booth, S.L. Low levels of vitamin D and worsening of knee osteoarthritis: Results of two longitudinal studies. *Arthritis Rheum.* **2007**, *56*, 129–136. [CrossRef]
146. Haroon, M.; Bond, U.; Quillinan, N.; Phelan, M.J.; Regan, M.J. The prevalence of vitamin D deficiency in consecutive new patients seen over a 6-month period in general rheumatology clinics. *Clin. Rheum.* **2011**, *30*, 789–794. [CrossRef] [PubMed]
147. Lane, N.E.; Gore, L.R.; Cummings, S.R.; Hochberg, M.C.; Scott, J.C.; Williams, E.N.; Nevitt, M.C. Serum vitamin D levels and incident changes of radiographic hip osteoarthritis: A longitudinal study. Study of osteoporotic fractures research group. *Arthritis Rheum.* **1999**, *42*, 854–860. [CrossRef]
148. Chaganti, R.K.; Parimi, N.; Cawthon, P.; Dam, T.L.; Nevitt, M.C.; Lane, N.E. Association of 25-hydroxyvitamin D with prevalent osteoarthritis of the hip in elderly men: The osteoporotic fractures in men study. *Arthritis Rheum.* **2010**, *62*, 511–514. [CrossRef]
149. Abu El Maaty, M.A.; Hanafi, R.S.; Badawy, S.E.; Gad, M.Z. Association of suboptimal 25-hydroxyvitamin D levels with knee osteoarthritis incidence in post-menopausal Egyptian women. *Rheum Intern.* **2013**, *33*, 2903–2907. [CrossRef]
150. Heidari, B.; Heidari, P.; Hajian-Tilaki, K. Association between serum vitamin D deficiency and knee osteoarthritis. *Intern. Orthop.* **2011**, *35*, 1627–1631. [CrossRef]

151. Cao, Y.; Winzenberg, T.; Nguo, K.; Lin, J.; Jones, G.; Ding, C. Association between serum levels of 25-hydroxyvitamin D and osteoarthritis: A systematic review. *Rheumatology* **2013**, *52*, 1323–1334. [CrossRef]
152. Konstari, S.; Paananen, M.; Heliövaara, M.; Knekt, P.; Marniemi, P.; Impivaara, O.; Arokoski, J.; Karppinen, J. Association of 25-hydroxyvitamin D with the incidence of knee and hip osteoarthritis: A 22-year follow-up study. *Scand. J. Rheumatol.* **2012**, *41*, 124–131. [CrossRef] [PubMed]
153. Konstari, S.; Kaila-Kangas, L.; Jaaskelainen, T.; Heliövaara, M.; Rissanen, H.; Marniemi, J.; Knekt, P.; Arokoski, K.; Karppinen, J. Serum 25-hydroxyvitamin D and the risk of knee and hip osteoarthritis leading to hospitalization: A cohort study of 5274 Finns. *Rheumatology* **2014**, *53*, 1778–1782. [CrossRef]
154. Laslett, L.L.; Quinn, S.; Burgess, J.R.; Parameswaran, V.; Winzenberg, T.M.; Jones, G.; Ding, C. Moderate vitamin D deficiency is associated with changes in knee and hip pain in older adults: A 5-year longitudinal study. *Ann. Rheum. Dis.* **2014**, *73*, 697–703. [CrossRef]
155. Wang, X.; Cicuttini, F.; Jin, X.; Wluka, A.E.; Han, W.; Zhu, Z.; Blizzard, L.; Antony, B.; Winzenberg, T.; Jones, G.; et al. Knee effusion-synovitis volume measurement and effects of vitamin D supplementation in patients with knee osteoarthritis. *Osteoarthr. Cartil.* **2017**, *25*, 1304–1312. [CrossRef] [PubMed]
156. McAlindon, T.; LaValley, M.; Schneider, E.; Nuite, M.; Lee, J.Y.; Price, L.L.; Lo, G.; Dawson-Hughes, B. Effect of vitamin D supplementation on progression of knee pain and cartilage volume loss in patients with symptomatic osteoarthritis: A randomized controlled trial. *J. Am. Med. Ass.* **2013**, *309*, 155–162. [CrossRef]
157. Muraki, S.; Dennison, E.; Jameson, K.; Boucher, B.J.; Akune, T.; Yoshimura, N.; Judge, A.; Arden, N.K.; Javaid, K.; Cooper, C. Association of vitamin D status with knee pain and radiographic knee osteoarthritis. *Osteoarthr. Cartil.* **2011**, *19*, 1301–1306. [CrossRef]
158. Nawabi, D.H.; Chin, K.F.; Keen, R.W.; Haddad, F.S. Vitamin D deficiency in patients with osteoarthritis undergoing total hip replacement: A cause for concern? *J. Bone Jt. Surg. Br.* **2010**, *92*, 496–499. [CrossRef]
159. Rizzoli, R. Vitamin D supplementation: Upper limit for safety revisited? *Aging Clin. Exp. Res.* **2021**, *33*, 19–24. [CrossRef] [PubMed]
160. Pavelka, K.; Coste, P.; Geher, P.; Krejci, G. Efficacy and safety of piascledine 300 versus chondroitin sulfate in a 6 months treatment plus 2 months observation in patients with osteoarthritis of the knee. *Clin. Rheumatol.* **2010**, *29*, 659–670. [CrossRef]
161. Kimmatkar, N.; Thawani, V.; Hingorani, L.; Khiyani, R. Efficacy and tolerability of Boswellia serrata extract in treatment of osteoarthritis of knee–A randomized double blind placebo controlled trial. *Phytomedicine* **2003**, *10*, 3–7. [CrossRef] [PubMed]
162. Sengupta, K.; Krishnaraju, A.V.; Vishal, A.A.; Mishra, A.; Trimurtulu, G.; Sarma, K.V.; Raychaudhuri, S.P. Comparative efficacy and tolerability of 5-Loxin and Aflapin against osteoarthritis of the knee: A double blind, randomized, placebo controlled clinical study. *Int. J. Med. Sci.* **2010**, *7*, 366–377. [CrossRef]
163. Kuptniratsaikul, V.; Thanakhumtorn, S.; Chinswangwatanakul, P.; Wattanamongkonsil, L.; Thamlikitkul, V. Efficacy and safety of Curcuma domestica extracts in patients with knee osteoarthritis. *J. Altern. Complement. Med.* **2009**, *15*, 891–897. [CrossRef] [PubMed]
164. Belcaro, G.; Cesarone, M.R.; Dugall, M.; Pellegrini, L.; Ledda, A.; Grossi, M.G.; Togni, S.; Appendino, G. Efficacy and safety of Meriva(R), a curcumin-phosphatidylcholine complex, during extended administration in osteoarthritis patients. *Altern. Med. Rev.* **2010**, *15*, 337–344.
165. Gruenwald, J.; Petzold, E.; Busch, R.; Petzold, H.P.; Graubaum, H.J. Effect of glucosamine sulfate with or without omega-3 fatty acids in patients with osteoarthritis. *Adv. Ther.* **2009**, *26*, 858–871. [CrossRef]
166. D'Adamo, S.; Cetrullo, S.; Panichi, V.; Mariani, E.; Flamigni, F.; Borzì, R.M. Nutraceutical Activity in Osteoarthritis Biology: A Focus on the Nutrigenomic Role. *Cells* **2020**, *9*, 1232. [CrossRef] [PubMed]
167. Davidson, R.K.; Green, J.; Gardner, S.; Bao, Y.; Cassidy, A.; Clark, I.M. Identifying chondroprotective diet-derived bioactives and investigating their synergism. *Sci. Rep.* **2018**, *8*, 17173. [CrossRef]
168. Siddiqui, R.A.; Moghadasian, M.H. Nutraceuticals and Nutrition Supplements: Challenges and Opportunities. *Nutrients* **2020**, *12*, 1593. [CrossRef]
169. Zhang, Q.W.; Lin, L.G.; Ye, W.C. Techniques for extraction and isolation of natural products: A comprehensive review. *Chin. Med.* **2018**, *13*, 20. [CrossRef] [PubMed]

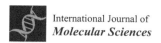

International Journal of

Molecular Sciences

MDPI

Article

Pleiotropic Roles of NOTCH1 Signaling in the Loss of Maturational Arrest of Human Osteoarthritic Chondrocytes

Manuela Minguzzi [1,†], Veronica Panichi [2,†], Stefania D'Adamo [1], Silvia Cetrullo [2], Luca Cattini [3], Flavio Flamigni [2], Erminia Mariani [1,3] and Rosa Maria Borzì [3,*]

1   Dipartimento di Scienze Mediche e Chirurgiche, Università di Bologna, 40138 Bologna, Italy; manuela.minguzzi@gmail.com (M.M.); stefania.dadamo2@unibo.it (S.D.); erminia.mariani@ior.it (E.M.)
2   Dipartimento di Scienze Biomediche e Neuromotorie, Università di Bologna, 40138 Bologna, Italy; veronica.panichi2@unibo.it (V.P.); silvia.cetrullo@unibo.it (S.C.); flavio.flamigni@unibo.it (F.F.)
3   Laboratorio di Immunoreumatologia e Rigenerazione Tissutale, IRCCS Istituto Ortopedico Rizzoli, 40136 Bologna, Italy; luca.cattini@ior.it
*   Correspondence: rosamaria.borzi@ior.it
†   These authors contributed equally to this work.

Abstract: Notch signaling has been identified as a critical regulator of cartilage development and homeostasis. Its pivotal role was established by both several joint specific Notch signaling loss of function mouse models and transient or sustained overexpression. NOTCH1 is the most abundantly expressed NOTCH receptors in normal cartilage and its expression increases in osteoarthritis (OA), when chondrocytes exit from their healthy "maturation arrested state" and resume their natural route of proliferation, hypertrophy, and terminal differentiation. The latter are hallmarks of OA that are easily evaluated in vitro in 2-D or 3-D culture models. The aim of our study was to investigate the effect of NOTCH1 knockdown on proliferation (cell count and Picogreen mediated DNA quantification), cell cycle (flow cytometry), hypertrophy (gene and protein expression of key markers such as RUNX2 and MMP-13), and terminal differentiation (viability measured in 3-D cultures by luminescence assay) of human OA chondrocytes. NOTCH1 silencing of OA chondrocytes yielded a healthier phenotype in both 2-D (reduced proliferation) and 3-D with evidence of decreased hypertrophy (reduced expression of RUNX2 and MMP-13) and terminal differentiation (increased viability). This demonstrates that NOTCH1 is a convenient therapeutic target to attenuate OA progression.

Keywords: osteoarthritis; chondrocytes; hypertrophy; remodeling; angiogenesis

Citation: Minguzzi, M.; Panichi, V.; D'Adamo, S.; Cetrullo, S.; Cattini, L.; Flamigni, F.; Mariani, E.; Borzì, R.M. Pleiotropic Roles of NOTCH1 Signaling in the Loss of Maturational Arrest of Human Osteoarthritic Chondrocytes. *Int. J. Mol. Sci.* **2021**, *22*, 12012. https://doi.org/10.3390/ijms222112012

Academic Editor: Alfonso Baldi

Received: 14 July 2021
Accepted: 30 October 2021
Published: 5 November 2021

Publisher's Note: MDPI stays neutral with regard to jurisdictional claims in published maps and institutional affiliations.

1. Introduction

Osteoarthritis (OA) is the leading cause of chronic disability in the elderly, with worldwide estimates showing that 9.6% of men and 18.0% of women over 60 years old suffer for symptomatic OA [1]. Therefore, OA represents a huge problem for the quality of life of millions of individuals and for the national healthcare systems. Established OA is associated with the progressive derangement of articular cartilage structure and function and is maintained by positive feedback loops with the involvement of subchondral bone and synovial tissue [2]. However, at its onset most often OA is an articular cartilage disease caused by the failure of the homeostatic mechanisms that actively maintain chondrocytes in a differentiation arrested state [3]. Indeed, chondrocytes are post-mitotic cells that in healthy cartilage do not proliferate and are only in charge of a very limited turnover of extracellular matrix (ECM) [4]. It has become increasingly evident that degeneration of articular cartilage is sustained by multiple inflammatory loops that can be targeted in order to restore the functionality of the tissue or at least to delay OA progression [5].

Notch signaling has been identified as a critical regulator of cartilage development and homeostasis with an on/off expression in the different phases of chondrogenesis as resumed in the growth plate [6]. As detailed elsewhere, the activation of this pathway occurs after triggering the receptor with a ligand [7]. The pathway requires proteolytic cleavages of the internal portion of the transmembrane receptor, which translocates to the nucleus to act as a transcription coactivator on target genes, thereby being renamed as Notch intracellular domain (NICD). NICD binds to RBPJ (recombination signal-binding protein for Ig region) and Maml (mastermind-like) in order to start transcription [7]. Although there is occurrence of multiple crosstalks with other pathways as detailed in [8], Notch activation directly leads to the induction of several target genes, among which HES1 (hairy and enhancer of split-1) has been recognized as relevant in OA pathogenesis [9].

Expression of members of the Notch pathway occurs in early differentiation phases of skeletal development, such as mesenchymal progenitor condensation [10]. Likewise, functional genomic studies carried out in mice indicated that proper functioning of the pathway in postnatal chondrocytes is required for the correct cartilage differentiation as well as for the expression of ECM genes (col2, aggrecan), transcription factors (Sox9), and ECM degrading enzymes (adamts 4, adamts 5, and mmp-13) [11]. Later on, a subsequent time specific expression of Notch1 and Notch2 drives the progression from the proliferating to the pre-hypertrophic and hypertrophic chondrocyte phenotype in the context of endochondral ossification in the growth plate [6].

Although transient (growth plate) and stable (articular) cartilages are different tissues from an anatomical and morphogenetic point of view, steps occurring in the former have represented a reference to understand OA pathogenesis. This represents the so-called EVO-DEVO approach [4], i.e., a pathogenetic model whereby functional changes occurring in OA in adulthood in many species (EVO) are interpreted as an attempt to recapitulate developmental programs (DEVO) to contrast structural changes. The expression of NOTCH receptors and ligands in healthy articular cartilage has been reported several years ago [12] as well as changes due to OA. Both NOTCH1 and NOTCH2 were found expressed in human cartilage particularly in the superficial zone, but major changes in OA are related to NOTCH1, whose increased expression in OA cartilage, particularly in the so-called "clusters", suggests its involvement in the abnormal cell activation and differentiation process of OA chondrocytes [13,14]. Indeed, NOTCH1 and NOTCH2 move to the nucleus in chondrocytes of developing growth plate cartilage and drive endochondral ossification via RPBJ signaling and are also found increased in murine and human OA [15]. Karlsson et al. showed the dramatic increase of the cells positive for NOTCH1, Jagged, and HES in OA compared to healthy cartilage [16]. A more recent study reported an increase in NOTCH1, Jagged-1, HES1, and NICD1 in human OA, a pattern also reproduced in a murine OA model [17]: the destabilization of the medial meniscus (DMM), the method of choice for surgically induced OA in mice that reproduces the slow onset and progression of human OA [18,19]. Interestingly, Jagged-1, the pivotal trigger of NOTCH1 activation is a NF-κB target gene [20] and resulted upregulated at early (2 weeks) stages of DMM [19] as shown in a matched comparison of nine microarrays carried out in similar conditions [21]. This suggests an early and pivotal involvement of the NOTCH pathway in OA development as well as occurrence of crosstalks with other master signaling pathways in OA.

Gain of function mouse models for the Notch pathway have shown an OA-like phenotype [15,22,23]. On the other hand, a chondroprotective role of "housekeeping" NOTCH levels is consistent with worsening of the disease following Notch1 inactivation in surgical mouse OA models [17,24]. Therefore, in human articular cartilage, the NOTCH pathway might have a dual role both in cartilage homeostasis maintenance and OA development. NOTCH1 and its target genes are overexpressed in OA compared to healthy articular cartilage [14]. Conversely, the prevention of pathway activation by γ-secretase inhibitors leads to reduced expression of ECM catabolic factors in in vitro cultured chondrocytes [15,22,25].

A recent report has shed light on the signaling network that links NOTCH1 with chondrocyte proliferation, differentiation, and MMP-13 expression via RUNX2 [26] and modulation with γ secretase inhibition (via *N*-[*N*-(3,5-Difluorophenacetyl)-L-alanyl]-S-phenylglycine t-butyl ester or DAPT) or Jagged induction.

Despite the large amount of information reported above, further investigation is needed to shed light on the role of NOTCH1 role in human OA. In particular, no literature data are available about the effects of NOTCH inactivation on human primary OA chondrocytes. As described above, the pathway is overexpressed in OA compared to healthy chondrocytes, and a nonspecific DAPT-dependent NOTCH pathway inactivation exerts chondroprotective and anabolic effects in human OA cartilage explants [27]. Therefore, tuning NOTCH signaling down to a homeostatic level may represent one of the constraints that prevent progression of the differentiation of articular chondrocytes toward hypertrophy.

The aim of our work has been to characterize the effects of NOTCH1 silencing on major features of OA chondrocytes (increased proliferation and loss of maturational arrest driven by increased extracellular remodeling) in suitable culture models. Given the pleiotropic effects of NOTCH that are peculiar to the differentiation stage of the cells, we undertook the present study to characterize the effects of its silencing on proliferation and differentiation in vitro, exploiting both 2-D and 3-D culture models, established with primary human OA chondrocytes, in the perspective of elaborating a potential therapeutic strategy for OA management. Some preliminary findings presented in this manuscript have been already presented at an OARSI Congress in 2018 [28].

2. Results

2.1. NOTCH1 Expression Is Higher in 2-D Compared to 3-D Chondrocyte Culture

Figure 1a shows that the level of NOTCH1 (as assessed by evaluating the intensity of the NICD1 band at 105–110 kDa) was higher in 2-D (monolayer) compared to 3-D (micromass) chondrocyte cultures ($p < 0.05$, $n = 3$), the latter representing a culture model where chondrocytes stop proliferation and recover their differentiated status, with progression to hypertrophy and terminal differentiation over time [29]. On the other hand, monolayer chondrocyte cultures maintain a small fraction of proliferating cells, although its percentage is further reduced at high density [30]. Thus, the different NOTCH1 level may be related to the proliferative status. The relationship between NOTCH1 expression level and the percentage of cells in mitosis is further highlighted in Figure 1b and Supplementary Figures S2 and S3: NOTCH1 expression is much higher in the immortalized chondrocyte cell line C28/I2 compared to primary chondrocytes, with the former showing about 40% cells in the S-G_2M cell cycle phases [31] and the latter about 5% [30].

The level of cleaved NOTCH1 (Val1744) was also investigated in both primary chondrocytes and C28/I2 cells upon stimulation with EDTA [32] or IL-1 [9]. Supplementary Figure S4 shows that the level of this antigen is almost undetectable in primary chondrocytes.

With regard to NOTCH1 proteolytic processing, it is well known that NOTCH1 cleaved at the level of Val1744 is the result of sequential cleavages of the membrane bound NOTCH1 [8]: (1) S1: furin mediated cleavage to obtain a 120 kDa peptide, (2) S2: ADAM10 or 17 mediated cleavage to obtain a 115 kDa, and (3) S3: γ-secretase mediated cleavage to obtain the 110 kDa NICD1 peptide that exposes Val1744 epitope [32].

The NICD1 band presented in our Western blot has a molecular weight of 105–110, therefore, it likely corresponds to the NICD1 fragment, that possibly becomes suddenly post-translational modified with masking/degradation of the epitope, so that the signal of anti-cleaved (Val1744) NOTCH1 is hardly detectable at least in primary chondrocytes (Supplementary Figure S4).

Despite the marked difference in band intensity, a similar pattern of anti-cleaved (Val1744) NOTCH1 is observable in both C28/I2 and primary chondrocytes, with a fraction of the signal under 1 h EDTA treatment showing higher molecular weight in both cell types. This possibly indicates a fraction of the molecules that undergo marked phosphorylation with a massive apparent shift (5–10 kDa) [33] in molecular weight. Phosphorylation, the "fulcrum of NOTCH1 signaling [34]", then increases activity of NICD1, that is however immediately degraded. Taken together, the findings presented in Figure 1b and Supplementary Figure S4, we can conclude that there is much less active NOTCH1 in primary chondrocytes, i.e., cleaved NICD1 able to enter the nucleus and regulate NOTCH1 target genes in a canonical (RBPJ dependent) way. In addition, the protease rich cellular environment of chondrocytes may concur to rapidly terminate the pathway.

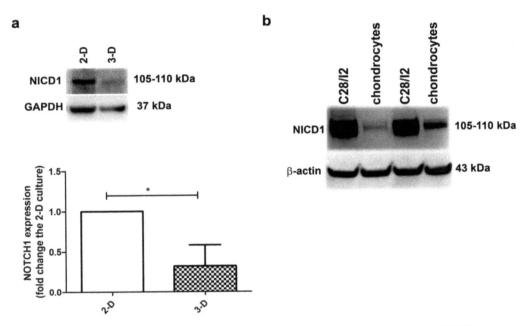

Figure 1. Higher NOTCH1 expression is evident in proliferating chondrocyte cultures. (**a**) To assess NOTCH1 expression and modulation in human chondrocyte cultures, the active form of the receptor was evaluated in monolayer culture and in micromasses at 1 week maturation. GAPDH was used as a loading control. A representative example and a cumulative evaluation performed with samples from three different patients. * $p < 0.05$. (**b**) Western blot analysis of NOTCH1 expression in C28/I2 cells compared to primary chondrocytes, with β-actin as a loading control.

2.2. NOTCH1 Transient Silencing Is Efficient at Both Protein and RNA Level

The siRNA-mediated NOTCH1 silencing of the primary chondrocyte cultures was quite efficient, as determined by both Western blot and real time RT-PCR. At the protein level, assessment in Western blot of the intensity of the NOTCH1 intracellular and transcriptionally active domain (NICD1 fragment of about 110 kDa) pointed at a 58 ± 20 (mean ± SD, $n = 4$) percentage reduction in NOTCH1 KD cells (N1) compared to the level in the control siRNA (NC) chondrocytes (Figure 2, left image). At the RNA level, assessment in real time RT-PCR of NOTCH1 expression in NOTCH1 KD chondrocytes at 48 h post transfection pointed at a 82 ± 14 ($p = 0.0023$, mean ± SD, $n = 5$) percentage reduction compared to the level in the control siRNA cells (Figure 2, right image). The difference was statistically significant.

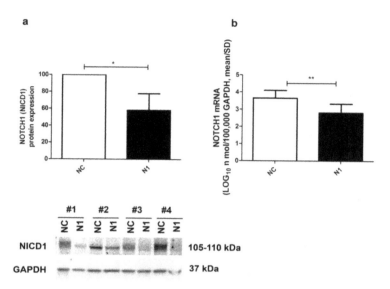

Figure 2. Efficiency of NOTCH1 silencing. (**a**) Cumulative Western blot evaluation of NOTCH1 KD in four different samples (Western blot shown below) as evaluated by assessment of the 110 kDa NICD1 active form at 48 h after transfection (mean ± SD, $n = 4$) with GAPDH used as a loading control; * $p < 0.05$. (**b**) NOTCH1 KD in five different samples assessed by real time RT-PCR (mean ± SD, $n = 5$). NC—control; N1—NOTCH1 silenced chondrocytes; ** $p < 0.01$.

The earlier effects of the siRNA on NOTCH1 transcripts are consistent with the higher knockdown efficiency as assessed by mRNA compared to the protein quantification. This is possibly because in the case of abundantly expressed proteins such as NOTCH1 the cells need time to get rid of it according to the physiological turnover of the siRNA target. On the other hand, the downstream experimental design of our work relied on the stability of the silencing effects. For this purpose, it has been reported that rather than on intracellular siRNA half-life, the duration of gene silencing is mostly dependent on dilution effects due to cell division, with differences according to the type of cells: rapidly dividing or slowly dividing (such as chondrocytes), with a duration of at least 3 weeks in the latter [35].

2.3. NOTCH1 KD Determines Biphasic Effects on Cell Proliferation

Compared to the effects on NOTCH1 RNA, the delayed kinetic of NOTCH1 protein reduction was also reflected in the different proliferative behavior of cells after NOTCH1 silencing at early or late time points.

At 48 h post transfection (Figure 3a), NOTCH1 silencing gave an advantage in cell proliferation. Cell count of different primary chondrocyte cultures indicated a higher recovery of NOTCH1 KD cells ($p = 0.033$, $n = 7$), in keeping with a significantly lower percentage of cells in the G1 phase and higher percentage of cells in the S-G$_2$M phase ($p = 0.0331$, $n = 4$).

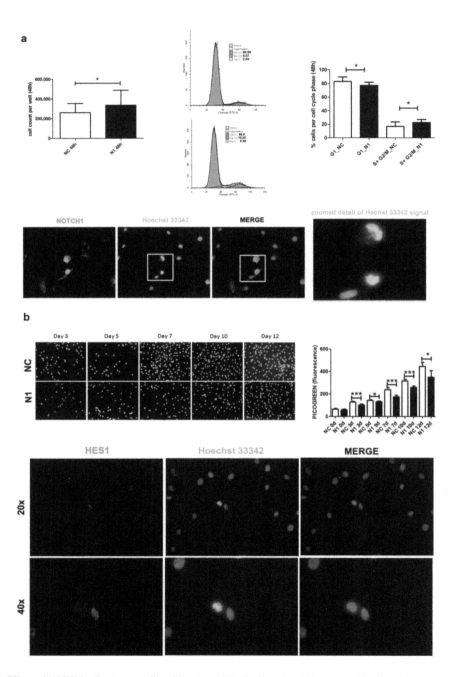

Figure 3. Effects of NOTCH1 silencing on cell proliferation. (**a**) Early effects (at 48 h) of increased cell proliferation in different NOTCH1 KD primary chondrocyte cultures (*n* = 7) in keeping with statistically significant increased percentage of cells in the S-G_2M fraction as shown by one representative sample and cumulative data (*n* = 4); * *p* < 0.05. Immunofluorescence indicates the close NOTCH1/DNA interaction during mitosis. Bottom: NOTCH1 immunofluorescence in chondrocytes at

72 h post control siRNA transfection. NOTCH1 staining (red), nuclei (blue), and merged images obtained with a NIKON Eclipse 90i fluorescence microscope equipped with 20 × objective lens. The white square indicates a detail that has been further zoomed and represented in the right image to indicate that the cells with strong NOTCH1 signal are caught during mitosis based on condensed chromatin. (**b**) Late effects (plating the cells recovered at 48 h post-transfection and assessment at days 0, 3, 5, 7, 10, 12) of delayed cell proliferation in NOTCH1 KD chondrocytes. Upper image shows the signal of the highly specific Picogreen staining of the nuclei of control cells (upper row) or NOTCH1 silenced cells (lower row). The right graph represents the mean ± SD of the fluorescence intensity obtained by scanning the bottom of the quintuplicate wells; * $p < 0.05$, *** $p < 0.001$. Bottom: HES1 immunofluorescence in chondrocytes at 72 h post control siRNA transfection. HES1 staining (red), nuclei (blue), and merged images obtained with a NIKON Eclipse 90i fluorescence microscope equipped with either 20× objective lens (with gain 1.2×, upper row) or 40x (with gain 1.2×, lower row).

Immunofluorescence indicated a stronger and mainly nuclear NOTCH1 staining in the cells during mitosis, suggesting a close interaction of NOTCH1 with DNA compared to those in interphase (Figure 3a).

Possibly because of its involvement in DNA replication [36], at a later analysis, NOTCH1 silencing showed opposite consequences in cell proliferation, as shown in Figure 3b that presents Picogreen (i.e., a specific dye for dsDNA) staining relative to one out of three different experiments performed, along with the quantitative assessment of fluorescence performed in quintuplicate that shows decreased cell proliferation of NOTCH1 KD cells. The right graph shows the cumulative data represented as mean ± standard deviation. The reason for the impaired cell proliferation may correspond to a reduced expression of HES1, the main NOTCH target gene. HES1 localizes in actively dividing cells suggesting an active role in controlling cell cycle progression, namely G_1/S transition as also reported in other cell types [37] and in the output of the research for pathways in the Reactome pathway analyzer, (https://reactome.org/PathwayBrowser/#/DTAB=AN&ANALYSIS=MjAyMTA2MTUxNDQ2NTJfMTU%3D&FLG=HES1, accessed on 25 march 2021).

2.4. NOTCH1 KD Determines a Delayed Differentiation in 3-D Culture

2.4.1. Reduced Transcription of Differentiation Related Genes

The data provided above about the delayed but persistent clearance of the protein were confirmed in the evaluation of the effects of NOTCH1 silencing in differentiation recapitulated in 3-D cultures [38], as a model whereby evaluating correlated phenomena in differentiation progression from hypertrophy to terminal differentiation, including hypertrophy, catabolic markers, and chondrocyte viability. The 3-D cultures were established at 48 h after transfection with either control or NOTCH1 silenced chondrocytes, so that the amounts of siRNA in the cells were not diluted because of division [35] and collected at 1, 2, and 3 weeks. Data shown in Supplementary Figure S6 show the persistence of NOTCH1 silencing over time. To analyze the effects on transcription we focused on micromasses at 1 week maturation. We selected this time point in order to avoid biases connected with the reduced viability at later time points due to recapitulation of terminal differentiation in these 3-D cultures [29].

At first, we checked and confirmed the maintenance of NOTCH1 knockdown (Figure 4 upper left graph, showing that the level of knockdown remained high: 73 ± 30 (mean ± SD, $p = 0.0134$, $n = 5$).

Then, we assessed the effects on signaling intermediates and NOTCH1 targets. As expected, we found that HES1 was significantly reduced in NOTCH1 silenced micromasses. We also confirmed significantly reduced levels of CHUK (i.e., IKKα, one of the NF-κB upstream activating kinases and a NOTCH target gene [39]) and a reduction of NFKB1, i.e., NF-κB p105, one member of the family of NF-κB monomers recognized among the NF-κB target genes [40].

We then moved to assess expression of genes connected with progressed differentiation from resting to hypertrophic and terminal differentiated chondrocytes, in keeping with [3,4].

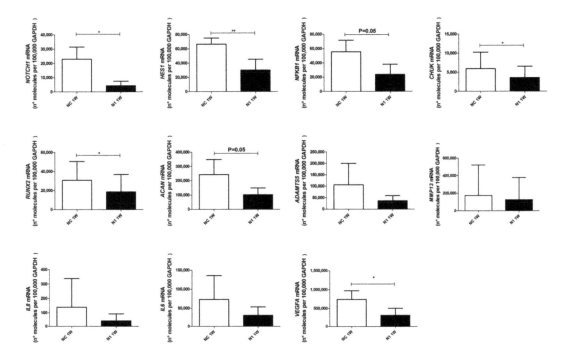

Figure 4. Effects of NOTCH1 silencing at the level of transcription of key genes in osteoarthritis. Total RNA was extracted from 1 week micromasses established with control (NC) or NOTCH1 silenced chondrocytes (N1). mRNA levels were calculated for each target gene and normalized using the reference housekeeping gene GAPDH according to the formula $2^{-\Delta Ct}$ and expressed as number of molecules per 100,000 GAPDH molecules; * $p < 0.05$, ** $p < 0.01$.

RUNX2, a pivotal transcription factor that drives hypertrophy [41] was significantly reduced by NOTCH1 silencing, as well as transcription of aggrecan, that continues across the chondrogenesis-hypertrophy maturation. Concerning the key matrix degrading enzymes in OA [42], a profound yet not significant reduction of ADAMTS5 was found in 3-D cultures with NOTCH1 silencing while milder effects were observed with MMP13, possibly because of a high degree of patient variability together with the effects of pre-activated NF-κB and p38 MAPK in high density cultures [43].

Lastly, we observed reduced levels of IL8 and IL6 and significant reduced ($p = 0.018$, $n = 4$) levels of VEGF, the master angiogenetic factor, responsible for neovascularization of late OA cartilage, thus reproducing the status of terminally differentiated cartilage of growth plate [4].

2.4.2. Reduced Expression of RUNX2 Protein and Reduced Deposition of Glycosaminoglycan and Calcium

Given the importance of RUNX2 in the phenomena underlying OA progression [41], we further assessed the effect of NOTCH1 ablation on RUNX2 at the protein level (Figure 5).

The level of RUNX2 protein in 1 week old micromasses was significantly reduced, down to 60% of the level in control chondrocytes ($p < 0.05$, $n = 5$) as assessed by Western blot analysis with the normalization with reference to β-actin (Figure 5a). The reduced RUNX2 level paralleled that of HES1 in the 1w–3w maturation of N1 micromasses (Figure 5a right images). Consequently, the reduced RUNX2 determined a delayed maturation of the extracellular matrix, as shown by a markedly reduced glycosaminoglycan deposition at

1 week in N1 compared to NC micromasses. In parallel, alizarin red staining showed a markedly reduced deposition of calcium crystals, particularly evident at 1 week, but also maintained at 2 and 3 weeks. Supplementary Figure S8 shows the results of the image analysis of the pictures shown in Figure 5, performed with the Nikon Imaging Software (NIS).

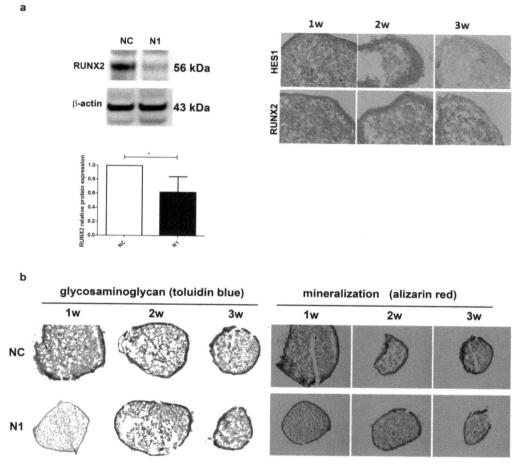

Figure 5. Effects of NOTCH1 silencing in the differentiation of chondrocytes in 3-D cultures. (**a**) NOTCH1 silencing impacts on RUNX2 expression: left, a representative Western blot indicates that RUNX2 protein is significantly reduced in NOTCH1 silenced 3-D cultures at 1 week as confirmed in the cumulative assessment shown in the lower graph ($n = 5$, * $p < 0.05$); right, immunohistochemistry imaging of the correlated reduced expression of RUNX2 and HES1 in micromass maturation across 1–3 weeks. (**b**) NOTCH1 silencing impacts on ECM maturation. Left, GAG deposition at 1, 2, and 3 weeks as evidenced by toluidin blue staining: GAG deposition resulted delayed in N1 KD 3-D constructs. Right: Alizarin Red staining on micromasses showed a markedly reduced calcium deposition at all time points in N1 KD micromasses. All images were obtained with a NIKON Eclipse 90i microscope equipped with 10× objective lens.

2.4.3. Reduced Release of Matrix Remodeling Enzymes

In keeping with the observed delayed maturation of 3-D chondrocyte cultures, we expected an effect on the repertoire of catabolic enzymes. The analysis was carried out in the supernatant of micromasses established with cells from four different patients. From each patient, triplicate micromasses were seeded and tested separately.

The regulation of ECM remodeling downstream N1 KD and across differentiation (1–3 week maturation) of the 3-D cultures was investigated evaluating the released MMP repertoire by means of the Bio-Plex Pro™ Human MMP Panel, 9-Plex (Biorad). High levels of MMP-2 were found in the supernatant of micromasses, but unaffected by NOTCH1 silencing. On the other hand, levels of MMP-9, -8, -7, and -12 were below the calibration curve. Therefore, we focused on comparison of the levels of MMP-1, 3, 10, and 13 (Figure 6). In most cases, reduction of MMP release was evident at the beginning of maturation. Quantification of major collagenases MMP-1 and 13 and of stromelysin 1 (MMP-3) and 2 (MMP-10) showed statistically significant reduction after NOTCH1 KD. In particular, the reduction of MMP-10 in the supernatant of N1 KD samples at 1 week of maturation, suggested a decreased activation of collagenases.

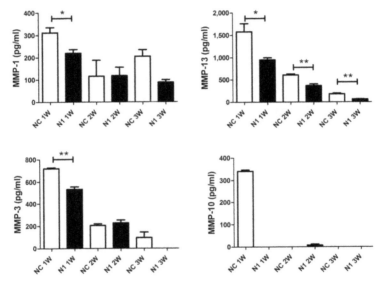

Figure 6. Effects of NOTCH1 silencing in the repertoire of MMPs released by chondrocytes cultured in 3-D. A representative patient out of four analyzed. Data are relative to triplicate micromasses at 1, 2, and 3 week maturation and are expressed as mean ± standard error of mean. Statistical analysis was performed by Student's t test; * $p < 0.05$, ** $p < 0.01$.

2.4.4. Reduced Terminal Differentiation and Increased Viability

We previously showed that in 3 weeks' time, chondrocytes cultured in 3-D recapitulate progression from hypertrophy to terminal differentiation with evidence of cell death that can be attenuated by means of selective targeting of critical effectors of progressed differentiation [29]. Therefore, to avoid biases connected to different viability we performed at 1 week maturation the assessment of the NOTCH1 dependent differential gene and protein expression of critical genes connected to hypertrophy. On the other hand, to maximize the effect of NOTCH1 silencing on terminal differentiation, we evaluated cell viability at 3 weeks as cell death is a hallmark of terminal differentiation (Figure 7). We found that NOTCH1 silencing significantly increases viability ($p = 0.0396$, $n = 3$) in chondrocytes cultured in 3-D compared to control chondrocytes, as evaluated by mean of the Cell Titer GLO 3D assay.

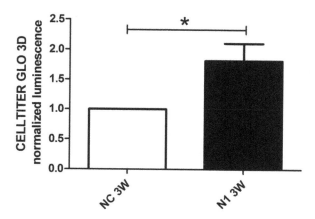

Figure 7. Effects of NOTCH1 silencing in the long term viability of chondrocytes cultured in 3-D. Assessment of cell viability in 3 week micromasses by means of the Cell Titer GLO 3D cell viability assay. N1 samples exhibited a statistically significant increased viability compared to NC. Data represent N1 luminescence normalized as fold change compared to NC values and are expressed as mean ± SD ($n = 3$). Statistical analysis was performed by Student's t test for paired samples; * $p < 0.05$.

3. Discussion

Previous evidence of the increased NOTCH1 expression in OA cartilage in human and animal models has supported the hypothesis that NOTCH1 inhibition could be therapeutic in OA management, but recent evidence has suggested that this issue should be carefully managed [17], since complete abrogation of this pathway via NOTCH1 antisense in all joint tissues in the DMM model instead exacerbated experimental OA. In keeping with the activity of NOTCH being both context and time specific other authors have shown that while sustained NOTCH1 activation promotes OA changes, transient NOTCH activation is chondroprotective and enhances ECM synthesis [24]. The crucial role of NOTCH in both development and OA disease has also been recently reported in arthritis of the temporomandibular joint in rats [44].

The aim of our work was to assess the effects of NOTCH1 silencing 2-D and 3-D cultures established with primary human osteoarthritic chondrocytes. The silencing strategy was chosen to selectively target NOTCH1 and therefore both its canonical (i.e., RBPJ-dependent) and non-canonical effects while sparing the NOTCH2 pathway which is quite highly expressed in articular chondrocytes [15]. The latter would have been affected by other possible strategies to dampen NOTCH1 pathway such as the use of RBPJ siRNA. Collectively, our results confirm that NOTCH1 inhibition is effective in reducing the major hallmarks of chondrocyte phenotypic dysregulation in OA cartilage: proliferation and differentiation progression to hypertrophy and terminal differentiation driven by extracellular matrix remodeling. The latter processes, that must be prevented in healthy cartilage but that are improperly triggered in OA, are also driven by re-expression of NOTCH1 [6]. NOTCH1 overexpression induces hypertrophy in condrocytes in vitro and in vivo [45]. In contrast, our data show that NOTCH1 silencing delays differentiation in 3-D, based on reduced gene expression of differentiation markers, reduced calcium deposition, and reduced cell death. Therefore, NOTCH1 signaling inhibition may represent one of the constraints that prevent progression of the differentiation of articular chondrocytes toward hypertrophy. Indeed, across chondrogenesis and endochondral ossification, the expression of NOTCH1 is time and space restricted. In endochondral ossification, NOTCH1 is switched on at the stage of pre-hypertrophic and early hypertrophic chondrocytes [6].

Our findings on chondrocyte proliferation show biphasic effects of NOTCH1 inhibition, further confirming the complexity of the pathway. At early time points (48 h) NOTCH1 KD elicit higher proliferation based on a higher chondrocyte yield and higher fraction of cycling (S-G$_2$M) cells. These findings are in keeping with those of Shang et al. [22], who showed that activation of the NOTCH1 signaling pathway via NICD1 transfection coordinately promoted cell cycle arrest (via Cyclin D1 inhibition and p57 induction) and chondrocyte hypertrophy (via SMAD1/5/8) [22]. However, findings at 48 h, based on cells collected after siRNA transfection are obtained before the completion of replication of primary chondrocyte cultures, since the estimated doubling time of chondrocyte cultures is 72 h [46,47]. On the other hand, at later times, NOTCH1 KD chondrocytes exhibited a lower proliferation, possibly because of a reduced expression of HES1, the main NOTCH1 target gene, known to be regulated by both NOTCH canonical and non-canonical pathways. Besides NOTCH, regulation of HES1 also involves other pathways [48], among which the Wnt-β-catenin and the Hedgehog pathways deserve to be mentioned for their role in chondrocyte differentiation. HES1 localizes in actively dividing cells confirming a role in controlling cell cycle progression, namely G$_1$/S transition (Reactome pathway analyzer, https://reactome.org/, accessed on 25 March 2021), in keeping with [49]. Moreover, the ability of HES1 of reducing p27 [37] and p57 [50], two cyclin-dependent kinase inhibitors, has previously been reported. Our findings are also in agreement with those of Karlsson et al. who found reduced proliferation of normal human chondrocytes after NOTCH1 signaling antagonism with a γ-secretase inhibitor [51].

The requirement of high NOTCH1 levels in "proliferating" 2-D compared to the "differentiating" 3-D cultures has been confirmed by our Western blot results that show a much higher expression of NICD1 in the former. Moreover, the evidence of differential impact and function of the pathway in 2-D or 3-D cultures is in keeping with findings of Karlsson et al. [51] who assessed the regulation of NOTCH using normal human chondrocytes during proliferation or across differentiation recapitulated in micromass and found reduction of NOTCH related proteins in differentiating pellet cultures [51], mimicking the levels found in cartilage biopsies.

The connection between NOTCH1 expression and chondrocyte proliferation has also been reported by Khan and coworkers who treated cartilage explants with the mitogen FGF-2 [52] and found increased expression of NOTCH1 and related genes (MMP-13, ADAMTS, and HES-1). The same authors proved that the role of NOTCH1 in the context of cell proliferation was a non-canonical activity being insensitive to γ-secretase inhibitors.

With regard to the effects on chondrocyte differentiation recapitulated in 3-D micromass cultures, globally our results confirm that NOTCH1 signaling inhibition delays the progression towards hypertrophy, via reduced expression of RUNX2 and ECM remodeling. OA onset and progression are sustained by changes in ECM remodeling [41]. Increased ECM remodeling may derive from increased MMP expression along with increased activation and/or decreased inhibition by the TIMPs. To our knowledge, few studies have investigated the relationship of NOTCH signaling with ECM degrading enzymes in articular chondrocytes, and mainly using murine chondrocytes. Indeed, in the latter settings, Sugita et al. described HES1 responsive elements in ADAMTS-5 and MMP-13 genes [23]. RBPJ, the primary nuclear mediator of NOTCH canonical activity upregulates RUNX2 promoter transcriptional activity [53]. NOTCH signaling in chondrocytes has been previously linked to increased MMP expression, particularly of MMP-13 that represents the pivotal collagenase in cartilage degradation [41]. A first study suggested a direct connection between MMP-13 and NOTCH: employing NOTCH signaling inhibition (DAPT) on murine chondrocytes a significant reduction of MMP-13 mRNA and protein was found [25], particularly in cells at later passages while MMP-2 resulted unaffected (as also found in supernatants from NC and N1 micromasses). A similar study was reproduced by Sassi et al. using human healthy articular chondrocytes from young donors. These cells do not express MMP-13 at early passages, while MMP-13 expression is induced by serial subculturing (at p3), together with that of Col1 and eNOS (dedifferentiation markers) preceded by that of

NOTCH1, found at p2. At the same time, expression of differentiation markers of "healthy chondrocytes" such as collagen 2 and aggrecan decreased, while the addition of DAPT was able to restore collagen 2 expression at p3 [27].

Blaise and Sassi therefore suggested that NOTCH signaling was pivotal in "chondrocyte dedifferentiation", but findings collected when the chondrocyte phenotype is lost, such as at the third passage, are less informative compared to those collected with primary chondrocytes cultured in 3-D [38,54], a culture model that allows for the recovery of the correct phenotype of the chondrocytes, in close relationship with their ECM [55,56]. Some differential cell reaction patterns of phenotypic modulation have been previously described in OA chondrocytes [57], but the current view is that rather than to "dedifferentiation", changes of chondrocyte features in OA are better related to a loss of maturational arrest, i.e., to a "progressed differentiation" into endochondral ossification and toward terminal differentiation [3,58], a process that can be reproduced dynamically in vitro in 3-D (micromass) cultures. Indeed, using this model and primary OA chondrocytes, we were previously able to show the effects of targeting critical effectors or signaling intermediates [29,59,60] of this process. The status of chondrocytes within 3-D cultures is similar to that of chondrocytes in cartilage explants but is more amenable for a large and multiplexed series of analyses [61].

The chondroprotective and anabolic effects of DAPT-dependent NOTCH1 inhibition was also confirmed in human cartilage: OA cartilage explants expressed MMP-13 but this expression was abrogated upon DAPT treatment, that was also able to rescue collagen II and aggrecan expression [27]. In the context of NOTCH1 pathway inhibition, it should be underlined that our data obtained with siRNA mediated NOTCH1 silencing are more selective compared to those obtained with DAPT, that at least also inhibits the other NOTCH receptors.

Other studies exploiting transfection of NICD in murine chondrocytes have shown that NOTCH1 induces MMP-13 via IL6-mediation [62]. Moreover, NOTCH signaling is involved in the expression of many other genes relevant in OA pathophysiology, such as IL-8 and MMP-9 [16].

The NOTCH-MMP-13 connection was confirmed with several other findings derived from both in vivo and in vitro studies. In a mouse model with selective inhibition of NOTCH signaling (via SOX-9-Cre; Rbpj fl/fl), a significant decrease was observed of markers related to endochondral ossification (MMP-13) and angiogenesis (VEGF-A), that paralleled the decrease of HES1, the master target gene of NOTCH1 [15]. A similar pattern of regulation was observed in an inducible and articular cartilage specific murine model (Col2a1-Cre; Rbpj fl/fl) where inactivation of Rbpj signaling was executed at skeletal maturity: this mouse was resistant to OA development as induced by means of surgical induction of joint instability, and this resistance was phenocopied with intraarticular delivery of DAPT [15]. More recently, it was shown that inducible and articular specific HES1 ablation in mice (in a Col2a1-CreERT; Rbpj fl/fl background) prevented OA progression, and inhibited expression of the key matrix degrading enzymes in OA, i.e., MMP-13 and ADAMTS-5 [23].

The NOTCH1 connection with chondrocyte hypertrophy and MMP-13 expression was shown in a recent study that used the murine chondrocytic cell line ATDC5. In these settings, transfection of NICD1 resulted in significant Sox9 reduction and Runx2 induction (and of alkaline phosphatase), suggesting that NOTCH1 signaling has profound effects on chondrocyte differentiation [22].

In agreement with our findings, a recent report of both in vitro and in vivo (rats) experiments has further addressed the relationship between NOTCH1, RUNX2, and MMP-13 [26] by either activating (with Jagged-1, the relevant ligand) or inhibiting (by DAPT treatment) the NOTCH1 pathway in conjunction with strategies of RUNX2 modulation via either silencing shRNA or overexpressing plasmids.

In our 3-D model, we observed reduced expression of RUNX2 and MMP-13 following NOTCH1 RNA interference. Moreover, our bioplex assay showed significantly reduced expression of MMP-1, the other collagenase relevant in OA [63], in NOTCH1 KD cells.

In addition, we observed markedly reduced expression of MMP-10, an enzyme that contributes to activation of collagenases in OA [64], besides decreased expression of MMP-3, a stromelysin included among the serum biomarkers of OA activity [65].

Some recent reports have also indicated the occurrence of relevant crosstalks in cartilage between the NOTCH1 and the NF-κB pathways [8,9], the latter exerting a fundamental role in OA onset and progression [66]. In addition, in 1 week micromasses established with NOTCH1 KD chondrocytes, we observed reduced gene expression of IKKα, a gene that we highlighted as having a role in OA pathophysiology [29,60,67,68] and that has also been included among the known NOTCH targets [39], although not much information is available with regard to human chondrocytes. IKKα might play multiple roles in OA pathophysiology. It contributes to NF-κB canonical activation [69], it is pivotal in NF-κB delayed non canonical activation, and also plays a peculiar role in chromatin remodeling required for NF-κB transcription [70,71]. In breast cancer cells, IKKα favors the chromatin recruitment of NOTCH1 transcriptional complex (NTC) and is recruited to the NTC itself in a NOTCH dependent manner [72]. Moreover, NOTCH1–IKKα interaction has been shown to exert an anti-apoptotic role [73]. In a rheumatoid arthritis mouse model, the IKKα-dependent non-canonical heterodimer relB-p52 enhances the transcriptional activity of NOTCH and Rbpj, required for the transcription of ADAMTS5 and MMP-13 [8]. In the latter disease context recent evidence has shown the feasibility of nanomedicine approaches for the intra-articular delivery of NOTCH1 siRNA-coupled micelles in a rheumatoid arthritis model developed in rats [74]. This approach is amenable to fine tuning in order to spare the chondroprotective and anabolic activities of the NOTCH1 pathway.

4. Materials and Methods

4.1. Establishment of Chondrocyte Cultures

Primary cultures of human osteoarthritic chondrocytes were established from knee cartilage derived from total knee replacement in OA patients. The study was conducted according to the guidelines of the Declaration of Helsinki and approved by the Ethics Committee of Istituto Ortopedico Rizzoli (ethic approval code: 0019715, approved on 28 September 2016), including documentation of written patient informed consent.

The patients (5 females and 1 male) had a mean $\pm$ SD age of 74 ± 2. The patients admitted to the study had to meet inclusion (patients undergoing total knee replacement, aged more than 18, and able to autonomously express the informed consent to participate to the study) and exclusion criteria (the latter criteria excluded patients with BMI higher than 35, or with complicating disease such as rheumatic diseases, diabetes, severe chronic infective diseases or malignancies, severe psychiatric diseases or use of steroid drugs or insulin). These patients had Kellgren-Lawrence (KL) grade 3 or 4.

After tissue retrieval, all patient identifiers were removed, and samples were coded by arbitrary designations to distinguish them solely for experimental purposes. Primary chondrocytes were isolated by mean of sequential enzymatic digestion (1 h with pronase (Sigma-Aldrich, Merck KGaA, Darmstadt, Germany)) and 1–2 h with 0.2% collagenase (Sigma-Aldrich) at 37 °C) from cartilage ($n = 6$, age = 73.8 ± 1.72, mean $\pm$ SD), as described in [75]. After recovery, isolated chondrocytes were filtered by 100 and 70 µm nylon meshes, washed, centrifuged, and counted. Chondrocytes were cultured in 10% FCS D-MEM (Sigma-Aldrich) with the addition of antibiotics in T150 flasks at an initial seeding density of 20.000 cells for cm^2 and left to grow until confluence. Only P_0 chondrocytes (i.e., cells that did not undergo subculturing and therefore retaining proper chondrocyte differentiation) were used for silencing experiments.

Some experiments were also performed with C28/I2 cells, an immortalized cell line widely used to mimic the behavior of primary chondrocytes [76].

4.2. Small Interfering RNA Mediated NOTCH1 Gene Silencing

NOTCH1 silencing of several chondrocyte cultures was obtained by mean of RNA interference (RNAi), using ON-TARGETplus SMARTpool with si-NOTCH1 or ON-TARGET plus Non-targeting Pool, Dharmacon (Horizon Discovery, Perkin Elmer, Cambridge, UK). The SMARTpool is a mixture of four siRNA providing advantages in both potency and specificity. Transient transfection was performed by Lipofectamine RNAiMAX Transfection Reagent (ThermoFisher Scientific, Waltham, MA, USA). Then, 48 h after siRNA delivery, chondrocytes were collected for count and evaluation of NOTCH1 knockdown (KD) at both gene and protein level, and for either monolayer or micromass seeding. Some cells were fixed in ethanol for subsequent cell cycle analysis. Given the high variability at the level of gene expression in the different primary cultures evaluated, the comparison was performed after variance normalization by using the Log_{10} of the values.

4.3. Cell Cycle Assessment

Flow cytometry was employed to evaluate cell cycle by means of DNA staining (Sytox green at 5 μM, Molecular Probes, ThermoFisher Scientific) of cells previously fixed with 70% ethanol and RNAse treated: 2.5 U RNAse One (Promega, Madison, WI, USA) plus 100 μg/mL RNAse A, Sigma-Aldrich). Analyses were performed using a FACS Canto II flow cytometer (Becton Dickinson Biosciences, Franklin Lakes, NJ, USA).

4.4. Chondrocyte Cultures

The 2-D culture was employed to evaluate the effect of NOTCH1 silencing on chondrocyte growth by means of the Picogreen assay as described below performed in combined NC and N1 cultures collected at 48 h after transfection.

The 3-D cultures established as described in [29] were allowed to mature across 3 weeks, with medium changes every second day to assess the effects of NOTCH1 silencing on differentiation progression. At selected time points (1w, 2w, and 3w) parallel samples were either embedded in OCT compound for immunohistochemistry and alizarin red or toluidine blue staining as described in [59] or dry frozen for subsequent Western blot or real time RT-PCR analysis or viability assay. Supernatants were also collected for MMP measurement. Noteworthy, for each experimental condition at least 4–6 replicate were established, and MMP assessment was carried out in triplicate for each of the four cultures assessed.

4.5. PicoGreen Assessment of Cell Growth

The analysis of cell growth was undertaken essentially as reported in [29], by means of a quantitative (Quant-IT PicoGreen dsDNA assay kit, Molecular Probes, ThermoFisher Scientific) DNA analysis of the proliferating cells. The fluorescence signal was collected from the bottom of the wells exploiting the well scan mode (3 × 3 areas) of the Spectra Max Gemini plate fluorometer (Molecular Devices, Sunnyvale, CA, USA).

NOTCH1 KD and control chondrocytes were seeded at low density (1000 cells per well in quintuplicate) in 96 well plates 48 h after transfection and cultured for 12 days. Parallel plates were established in order to measure the cell growth at times 0 (the day after seeding), 3, 7, 10, and 12, using one plate for each chondrocyte phenotype (NC or NOTCH1 KD) for each time point. At the selected time points, the plates were emptied and frozen at −20 °C until analysis, that was performed at the same time for cultures established from the same patient. To correct for differences in cell counts, values were calculated as the percentage increase over the starting (day 0) values [29]. Images of the wells were also obtained by using an inverted Nikon (Nikon Corporation, Tokio, Japan) Eclipse TS100 microscope equipped with a 465-495EX, 505DM, 515-555BA nm filter to collect the green signal of the stained nuclei.

4.6. Western Blot

Western blot was carried out to assess the differential NOTCH1 level in 2-D and 3-D cultures and to assess the level of KD efficiency, after siRNA delivery. The experimental details were essentially as described in [75]. Proteins from equal cell equivalents (150,000 cells) or micromasses (one half 1 w micromass per well, established with 250,000 cells) were extracted by means of Lysis buffer supplemented with benzonase to improve extraction of proteins bound to DNA, besides NaF, Na_3VO_4, PMSF, and Protease Inhibitor cocktail. In the case of 3-D cultures, improved extraction was achieved by using pestles connected to a pellet pestles cordless motor (Sigma-Aldrich). Extraction was carried out on ice (30 min), with 10 s vortexing every 10 min. At the end, the samples were centrifuged for 15 min at 10,000 rpm at 4 °C. The supernatants were collected and kept at −80 °C until analysis. Lysates corresponding to 150,000 cells (in 10 μL) or half micromasses (in 15 μL) were loaded in wells of NuPage pre-cast Bis-Tris 4–12% (ThermoFisher Scientific), after addition of LDS NuPage sample buffer and NuPage reducing agent and boiling to 100 °C for 10 min then transferred to ice. Electrophoretic run of proteins exploited MOPS or MES as a running buffer. In each gel, a molecular weight marker (Novex Sharp pre-stained protein standards, ThermoFisher Scientific) was loaded along the samples to allow accurate estimation of correct molecular weight. At the end of the run, the proteins were transferred to PVDF (Immobilon-P, Millipore, Merck) membranes exploiting the iBlot Dry Blotting system (ThermoFisher Scientific). To allow retention of proteins, the membranes were dried by immersing them in methanol, and stored at 4°C until use. At the time of analysis, the membranes were rehydrated by methanol and subjected to Western blot by means of the SNAP-ID 2.0 device (Millipore, Merck) or by conventional overnight incubation. Primary antibodies were as follows: NOTCH1 (polyclonal rabbit anti-human NOTCH1, sc-6014R used at 0.1 μg/mL, Santa Cruz Biotechnology, Dallas, TX, USA), cleaved Notch1 (Val1744) (rabbit monoclonal, #4147 used 1:1000, Cell Signaling Technology, Danvers, MA, USA), RUNX2 (polyclonal goat anti-human RUNX2, AF2006 used at 1:20,000, R&D Systems, Minneapolis, MN, USA). β-actin (mouse monoclonal, #A2228, clone AC-74, used at 0.8 μg/mL, Sigma-Aldrich) or GAPDH (mouse monoclonal, MAB374, used at 0.8 μg/mL, Sigma-Aldrich) were used as loading controls. Appropriate HRP conjugated anti secondary antibodies anti species (mouse, rabbit, goat) immunoglobulins were from Jackson ImmunoResearch Europe (Cambridge, UK) and the substrate was ECL-Select (Amersham, Cytiva, Marlborough, MA, USA). Signals were acquired by means of a ChemiDoc MP Imaging System (Bio-Rad Laboratories, Hercules, CA, USA). For accurate assessment of molecular weight, the signals were referred to the molecular weight marker stained with a chemiluminescent pen (Glow Writer, Sigma-Aldrich). With regard to NOTCH1, Western blot experiments showed occurrence of multiple bands, in keeping with the existence of intracellular enzymes in charge of cleavage and/or ubiquitination [77]. Therefore, for quantitative purposes we considered the intensity of the band corresponding to the NICD1 fragment, that in our hands resulted in 105-110 kDa. Semi-quantitative analysis of band intensity was performed considering "optical density" values and using Image Lab software (version 6.0, Bio-Rad). Samples were compared considering the expression level of the band of interest normalized to that of the housekeeping control.

4.7. Immunofluorescence and Immunohistochemistry

Immunofluorescence was carried out essentially as in [67] to disclose the pattern of NOTCH1 and HES1 in chondrocytes cultured on chamber slides, in relationship to mitosis or interphase.

For this purpose, NC and N1 chondrocytes at 72 h post-transfection were seeded onto chamber slides (8 well chamber slides, at a density of 10,000 cells per cm^2) and let to adhere for 72 h. Then, after a brief washing with PBS the cells were fixed with 100 μl of 4% paraformaldehyde (PFA) for 30 min at RT and washed again with PBS. The wells were filled with PBS and stored at 4 °C until the time of processing. The samples were pretreated for antigen unmasking with 0.02 U/mL Chondroitinase ABC (Sigma-Aldrich) in 50 mM pH 8.0 Tris/HCl solution for 20′ at 37 °C and permeabilized with 0.2% Triton in TBS (TRIS buffered saline) solution for 5 min at RT. After another wash with TBS, the nonspecific bindings were blocked with a 5% BSA (bovine serum albumin, Sigma-Aldrich), 5% Normal Donkey serum (Jackson ImmunoResearch Europe), and 0.1% Triton in TBS for 30′ at RT and washed again. Then, primary and control antibodies were delivered at a concentration of 5 μg/mL in TBS with 3% BSA 0.1% Tween and left overnight at 4 °C: anti NOTCH1 (rabbit anti NOTCH1 (NBP1-78292, Novus Biologicals, Centennial, CO, USA), anti-HES1 (rabbit anti-HES1, PA5-28802, ThermoFisher Scientific), or control antibody (normal rabbit immunoglobulins, AB105-C, R&D Systems). After rinsing in TBS, the signal was revealed by a 15 μg/mL donkey anti-rabbit Alexa Fluor 555 secondary antibody conjugate (ThermoFisher Scientific) in TBS with 3% BSA 0.1% Tween and incubated 30′ at RT together with 1μg/mL Hoechst 33342 (Sigma- Aldrich) for nuclear counterstaining. At the end, the samples were mounted with the addition of anti-fading (1% 1,4 Diazobicyclo (2.2.2) Octane (DABCO, Sigma-Aldrich) in 90% glycerol, in 0.1 M pH 8.0Tris-HCl), sealed with nail-polish and stored refrigerated and in the dark for subsequent analysis.

Images of these experiments were observed by mean of a NIKON (Nikon Corporation) Eclipse 90i microscope equipped with 540/25EX, 565DM, 605/55BA nm filters to evaluate NOTCH1 or HES1 stained with a red emitting fluorochrome while nuclear counterstaining with Hoechst 33342 was evaluated with 330-380EX, 400DM, 420BA nm filters.

Immunohistochemistry was instead carried out to assess the correlated expression levels of RUNX2 and HES1 along the maturation of N1 micromasses. To this end, 5 μm sections were obtained from micromasses established with NC or N1 chondrocytes and embedded in OCT compound. The slides were put on silanized glass slides and stored at −20 °C. At the time of processing, the slides were left to equilibrate to room temperature still wrapped with aluminum foil. The areas bearing the micromass slide for immunodetection were delimited with the pap pen and fixed with 4%PFA for 30 min at RT, followed by washing. Here again, a step of antigen unmasking was carried out with 0.02 U/mL Chondroitinase ABC (Sigma-Aldrich) followed by blocking of nonspecific bindings as detailed above. Then, primary antibodies and control antibodies were delivered at a concentration of 5μg/mL in TBS with 3% normal goat serum, 2% BSA, and 0.1% Triton and left 2 h at RT: anti RUNX2 (rat monoclonal MAB2006 used at 5 μg/mL, R&D Systems) and anti-HES1 (rabbit polyclonal PA5-28802 used at 5 μg/mL, ThermoFisher Scientific) or control rabbit antibody (normal rabbit immunoglobulins BD AB105-C, R&D Systems). In addition, a sample with only secondary antibody was set up, to control for nonspecific binding of immunodetection reagents. At the end of the incubation with primary antibodies two washings with TBS were performed, and immunodetection was carried out using the supersensitive IHC Detection System (BioGenex, Fremont, CA, USA) suitable to detect mouse, rat, or rabbit primary antibodies exploiting the avidin-biotin amplification system, to localize the alkaline phosphatase enzymes at antigen sites finally revealed with FAST RED substrate. At the end, the sections were washed and mounted with Aquamount. Pictures at 200× magnification (objective 20×) were obtained with Eclipse 90i Nikon.

To provide quantitative assessment of signal intensity, results of immunohistochemistry, toluidin blue, and alizarin red staining were analyzed with the Nikon Imaging Software (NIS, Nikon Corporation). For each signal, tissue areas underwent a thresholding using the intensity function of the software. NIS identified several areas (from tens to hundreds for each section with more areas in sections with higher staining) and produced an output with several calculated parameters, including mean intensity and area for each. These data were used in a statistical analysis (ANOVA) to compare the conditions. To emphasize the information that the cumulative area identified by NIS as "beyond the threshold" was variable according to the specific condition, we also included the graphical representation of the product of the mean intensity and the cumulative area.

4.8. MMPs Quantitative Assessment

Supernatants of micromasses derived from control siRNA (NC) or NOTCH1 siRNA (N1) chondrocytes were used to test the role of NOTCH1 on the expression of major matrix metalloproteinases, across micromass maturation.

To this end we used the Bio-Plex Pro™ Human MMP Panel, 9-Plex (Bio-Rad Laboratories, #171AM001M), a multiplex bead based sandwich immunoassay kit, with high sensitivity and dynamic range, to simultaneously evaluate the three collagenases (collagenase1/MMP-1, collagenase 2/MMP-8 and collagenase 3/MMP-13), the two stromelysins (stromelysin1/MMP-3 and stromelysin2/2MMP-10), the two gelatinase A (72 kDa, MMP-2) and B (92 kDa, MMP-9), the matrylisin/MMP-7, and the macrophage metalloelastase MMP-12.

4.9. Evaluation of Progressed Chondrocyte Terminal Differentiation/Cell Viability

Loss of maturational arrest leads to chondrocyte hypertrophy and terminal differentiation. This process can be recapitulated in vitro since 3w micromasses present a considerable number of dead cells that are reduced by selective targeting of effectors of chondrocyte hypertrophy [29]. Therefore, to test the effects of NOTCH1 silencing we used a recently developed assays: the CellTiter-Glo 3D Cell viability assay (Promega), that relies on the properties of a proprietary thermostable luciferase (Ultra-Glo™ Recombinant Luciferase), which generates a stable "glow-type" luminescent signal that is proportional to the amount of ATP present. The homogeneous "add-mix-measure" format results in cell lysis, "extraction" of intracellular ATP from healthy and viable cells, generation of a proportional luminescent signal, and good performance across a wide range of assay conditions.

Luminescence readings were collected from micromasses left to mature for 3 weeks and readings of NOTCH1 siRNA samples were normalized to their relative CTRLsiRNA samples. NOTCH1siRNA increased viability of 3 weeks samples of 1.82 ± 2.29 (mean $\pm$ standard deviation, $p = 0.04$, $n = 3$) fold.

4.10. Real-Time RT-PCR Analysis

Total RNA was extracted from cell pellets collected at 48 h from NOTCH1 silencing and micromasses (1w maturation), with TRIzol RNA isolating agent (ThermoFisher Scientific) according to manufacturer's instructions. Total RNA (1 µg) was reverse-transcribed using SuperScript VILO cDNA synthesis kit (ThermoFisher Scientific) following manufacturer's protocol. Real-time RT PCR analysis were performed employing QuantiTect SYBR Green PCR Kit (TaKaRa Bio inc., Shiga, Japan) and following standard protocol: Taqman DNA Polymerase activation 95° (45 cycles; denaturation 95°, amplification annealing temperature variable according to primers design, as indicated in Table 1). Results of mRNA quantification for both N1 and NC samples analysis were mRNA levels calculated for each target gene and normalized using the reference gene GAPDH according to the formula 2-ΔCt and expressed as a percentage of the reference gene. Primer specificity was established by evaluation of melting curves. Target gene primers sequences are shown below (Table 1).

Table 1. List of primers used for real time RT-PCR.

Gene	Forward Primer	Reverse Primer	Amplicon Size (Annealing T)
GAPDH	TGGTATCGTGGAAGGACTCA	GCAGGGATGAGTTCTGGA	123 bp (56 °C)
NOTCH1	CCTGAAGAACGGGGCTAACA	GATGTCCCGGTTGGCAAAGT	127 bp (60 °C)
HES1	AAGAAAGATAGCTCGCGGCA	TACTTCCCCAGCACACTTGG	134 bp (60 °C)
ADAMTS5	GCACTTCAGCCACCATCAC	AGGCGAGCACAGACATCC	187 bp (58 °C)
MMP-13	TCACGATGGCATTGCT	GCCGGTGTAGGTGTAGA	277 bp (58 °C)
ACAN	TCGAGGACAGCGAGGCC	TCGAGGGTGTAGCGTGTAGAGA	85 bp (60 °C)
RUNX2	GGAATGCCTCTGCTGTTATG	AGACGGTTATGGTCAAGGTG	105 bp (58 °C)
NFKB1	CAGGAGACGTGAAGATGCTG	AGTTGAGAATGAAGGTGGATGA	109 bp (60 °C)
CHUK (IKKα)	GCACAGAGATGGTGAAAATCATTG	CAACTTGCTCAAATGACCAAACAG	86 bp (60 °C)
IL6	TAGTGAGGAACAAGCCAGAG	GCGCAGAATGAGATGAGTTG	184 bp (60 °C)
IL8	CCAAACCTTTCCACCC	ACTTCTCCACAACCCT	153 bp (60 °C)
VEGFA	TGATGATTCTGCCCTCCTC	GCCTTGCCTTGCTGCTC	82 bp (58 °C)

4.11. Statistics

Data are represented as mean $\pm$ standard deviation (SD) and compared by means of two tailed Student's t test using the GraphPad Prism 5.0 software (GRAPHPAD SOFT-

WARE, La Jolla, CA, USA). Differences were considered significant when $p < 0.05$ with * $p < 0.05$; ** $p < 0.01$; *** $p < 0.001$.

Supplementary Materials: The following are available online at https://www.mdpi.com/article/10.3390/ijms222112012/s1, Figure S1: full blots used to derive the NICD1 and GAPDH results shown in Figure 1a of the main manuscript; Figure S2: full blots used to derive the NICD1 and β-actin results shown in Figure 1b of the main manuscript; Figure S3: full blots used to derive the NOTCH1/NICD1 and β-actin results useful to compare NOTCH1/NICD1 intensity in both C28/I2 immortalized chondrocytes and primary chondrocytes cultured at either low density (LD) or high density (HD); Figure S4: full blots used to compare the signal of Cleaved NOTCH1 (Val1744) in C28/I2 immortalized chondrocytes or primary chondrocytes in basal conditions or after 1 hour stimulation with either 5 mM EDTA or 2.5 ng/ml IL-1β; Figure S5: full blots used to derive the NICD1 and GAPDH results shown in Figure 2a of the main manuscript obtained with lysates of chondrocytes in either control (NC, control siRNA) or NOTCH1 KD conditions; Figure S6: full blots (used to derive the NICD1 and β-actin results) and real time PCR results useful to assess the persistence of NOTCH1 silencing across 1, 2 and 3 weeks' maturation of micromasses; Figure S7: full blots used to derive the RUNX-2 and β-actin results shown in Figure 5 of the main manuscript, obtained with lysates of chondrocytes cultured in 3-D, in either control (NC, control siRNA) or NOTCH1 KD (N1, NOTCH1 siRNA) conditions; Figure S8: image analysis of the immunohistochemistry (HES1 and RUNX2), toluidin blue and alizarin red results shown in Figure 5.

Author Contributions: Conceptualization, M.M. and R.M.B.; methodology, M.M., V.P. and R.M.B.; formal analysis, M.M., V.P., S.D. and R.M.B.; investigation, M.M., V.P., S.D., R.M.B.; resources, S.C., L.C., F.F., E.M. and R.M.B.; data curation, M.M., V.P., S.D., L.C. and R.M.B.; writing—original draft preparation, M.M., V.P. and R.M.B.; writing—review and editing, M.M., V.P., S.D., S.C., F.F. and R.M.B.; visualization, M.M., V.P. and R.M.B.; supervision, E.M. and R.M.B.; project administration, M.M., E.M. and R.M.B.; funding acquisition, E.M. and R.M.B. All authors have read and agreed to the published version of the manuscript.

Funding: This research was funded by by Ministero dell'Istruzione, dell'Università e della Ricerca, Italy (FIRB Grant: RBAP10KCNS); Ministero della Salute, Italy (Fondi Cinque per Mille). The APC was funded by Fondi Cinque per Mille.

Institutional Review Board Statement: The study was conducted according to the guidelines of the Declaration of Helsinki and approved by the Ethics Committee of Istituto Ortopedico Rizzoli (ethic approval code: 0019715, approved on 28 September 2016), including documentation of written patient informed consent.

Informed Consent Statement: Informed consent was obtained from all subjects involved in the study.

Data Availability Statement: Data reported in the study are available upon request to the corresponding author.

Conflicts of Interest: The authors declare no conflict of interest. The funders had no role in the design of the study; in the collection, analyses, or interpretation of data; in the writing of the manuscript, or in the decision to publish the results.

References

1. Jafarzadeh, S.R.; Felson, D.T. Updated Estimates Suggest a Much Higher Prevalence of Arthritis in United States Adults Than Previous Ones. *Arthritis Rheumatol.* **2018**, *70*, 185–192. [CrossRef]
2. Li, Z.; Huang, Z.; Bai, L. Cell Interplay in Osteoarthritis. *Front. Cell Dev. Biol.* **2021**, *9*, 720477. [CrossRef]
3. Van der Kraan, P.M.; van den Berg, W.B. Osteoarthritis in the context of ageing and evolution. Loss of chondrocyte differentiation block during ageing. *Ageing Res. Rev.* **2008**, *7*, 106–113. [CrossRef]
4. Aigner, T.; Gerwin, N. Growth plate cartilage as developmental model in osteoarthritis research–potentials and limitations. *Curr. Drug Targets* **2007**, *8*, 377–385. [CrossRef]
5. D'Adamo, S.; Cetrullo, S.; Panichi, V.; Mariani, E.; Flamigni, F.; Borzi, R.M. Nutraceutical Activity in Osteoarthritis Biology: A Focus on the Nutrigenomic Role. *Cells* **2020**, *9*, 1232. [CrossRef]
6. Green, J.D.; Tollemar, V.; Dougherty, M.; Yan, Z.; Yin, L.; Ye, J.; Collier, Z.; Mohammed, M.K.; Haydon, R.C.; Luu, H.H.; et al. Multifaceted signaling regulators of chondrogenesis: Implications in cartilage regeneration and tissue engineering. *Genes Dis.* **2015**, *2*, 307–327. [CrossRef] [PubMed]
7. Zanotti, S.; Canalis, E. Notch Signaling and the Skeleton. *Endocr. Rev.* **2016**, *37*, 223–253. [CrossRef] [PubMed]

8. Saito, T.; Tanaka, S. Molecular mechanisms underlying osteoarthritis development: Notch and NF-kappaB. *Arthritis Res. Ther.* **2017**, *19*, 94. [CrossRef]

9. Ottaviani, S.; Tahiri, K.; Frazier, A.; Hassaine, Z.N.; Dumontier, M.F.; Baschong, W.; Rannou, F.; Corvol, M.T.; Savouret, J.F.; Richette, P. Hes1, a new target for interleukin 1beta in chondrocytes. *Ann. Rheum. Dis.* **2010**, *69*, 1488–1494. [CrossRef]

10. Long, F.; Ornitz, D.M. Development of the endochondral skeleton. *Cold Spring Harb. Perspect. Biol.* **2013**, *5*, a008334. [CrossRef]

11. Mirando, A.J.; Liu, Z.; Moore, T.; Lang, A.; Kohn, A.; Osinski, A.M.; O'Keefe, R.J.; Mooney, R.A.; Zuscik, M.J.; Hilton, M.J. RBP-Jkappa-dependent Notch signaling is required for murine articular cartilage and joint maintenance. *Arthritis Rheum.* **2013**, *65*, 2623–2633. [PubMed]

12. Ustunel, I.; Ozenci, A.M.; Sahin, Z.; Ozbey, O.; Acar, N.; Tanriover, G.; Celik-Ozenci, C.; Demir, R. The immunohistochemical localization of notch receptors and ligands in human articular cartilage, chondroprogenitor culture and ultrastructural characteristics of these progenitor cells. *Acta Histochem.* **2008**, *110*, 397–407. [CrossRef] [PubMed]

13. Grogan, S.P.; Miyaki, S.; Asahara, H.; D'Lima, D.D.; Lotz, M.K. Mesenchymal progenitor cell markers in human articular cartilage: Normal distribution and changes in osteoarthritis. *Arthritis Res. Ther.* **2009**, *11*, R85. [CrossRef]

14. Guan, Y.J.; Li, J.; Yang, X.; Du, S.; Ding, J.; Gao, Y.; Zhang, Y.; Yang, K.; Chen, Q. Evidence that miR-146a attenuates aging- and trauma-induced osteoarthritis by inhibiting Notch1, IL-6, and IL-1 mediated catabolism. *Aging Cell* **2018**, *17*, e12752. [CrossRef]

15. Hosaka, Y.; Saito, T.; Sugita, S.; Hikata, T.; Kobayashi, H.; Fukai, A.; Taniguchi, Y.; Hirata, M.; Akiyama, H.; Chung, U.I.; et al. Notch signaling in chondrocytes modulates endochondral ossification and osteoarthritis development. *Proc. Natl. Acad. Sci. USA* **2013**, *110*, 1875–1880. [CrossRef]

16. Karlsson, C.; Brantsing, C.; Egell, S.; Lindahl, A. Notch1, Jagged1, and HES5 are abundantly expressed in osteoarthritis. *Cells Tissues Organs* **2008**, *188*, 287–298. [CrossRef]

17. Lin, N.Y.; Distler, A.; Beyer, C.; Philipi-Schobinger, A.; Breda, S.; Dees, C.; Stock, M.; Tomcik, M.; Niemeier, A.; Dell'Accio, F.; et al. Inhibition of Notch1 promotes hedgehog signalling in a HES1-dependent manner in chondrocytes and exacerbates experimental osteoarthritis. *Ann. Rheum. Dis.* **2016**, *75*, 2037–2044. [CrossRef]

18. Culley, K.L.; Dragomir, C.L.; Chang, J.; Wondimu, E.B.; Coico, J.; Plumb, D.A.; Otero, M.; Goldring, M.B. Mouse models of osteoarthritis: Surgical model of posttraumatic osteoarthritis induced by destabilization of the medial meniscus. *Methods Mol. Biol.* **2015**, *1226*, 143–173. [PubMed]

19. Glasson, S.S.; Blanchet, T.J.; Morris, E.A. The surgical destabilization of the medial meniscus (DMM) model of osteoarthritis in the 129/SvEv mouse. *Osteoarthr. Cartil.* **2007**, *15*, 1061–1069. [CrossRef]

20. Johnston, D.A.; Dong, B.; Hughes, C.C. TNF induction of jagged-1 in endothelial cells is NFkappaB-dependent. *Gene* **2009**, *435*, 36–44. [CrossRef]

21. Gardiner, M.D.; Vincent, T.L.; Driscoll, C.; Burleigh, A.; Bou-Gharios, G.; Saklatvala, J.; Nagase, H.; Chanalaris, A. Transcriptional analysis of micro-dissected articular cartilage in post-traumatic murine osteoarthritis. *Osteoarthr. Cartil.* **2015**, *23*, 616–628. [CrossRef] [PubMed]

22. Shang, X.; Wang, J.; Luo, Z.; Wang, Y.; Morandi, M.M.; Marymont, J.V.; Hilton, M.J.; Dong, Y. Notch signaling indirectly promotes chondrocyte hypertrophy via regulation of BMP signaling and cell cycle arrest. *Sci. Rep.* **2016**, *6*, 25594. [CrossRef]

23. Sugita, S.; Hosaka, Y.; Okada, K.; Mori, D.; Yano, F.; Kobayashi, H.; Taniguchi, Y.; Mori, Y.; Okuma, T.; Chang, S.H.; et al. Transcription factor Hes1 modulates osteoarthritis development in cooperation with calcium/calmodulin-dependent protein kinase 2. *Proc. Natl. Acad. Sci. USA* **2015**, *112*, 3080–3085. [CrossRef]

24. Liu, Z.; Chen, J.; Mirando, A.J.; Wang, C.; Zuscik, M.J.; O'Keefe, R.J.; Hilton, M.J. A dual role for NOTCH signaling in joint cartilage maintenance and osteoarthritis. *Sci. Signal.* **2015**, *8*, ra71. [CrossRef] [PubMed]

25. Blaise, R.; Mahjoub, M.; Salvat, C.; Barbe, U.; Brou, C.; Corvol, M.T.; Savouret, J.F.; Rannou, F.; Berenbaum, F.; Bausero, P. Involvement of the Notch pathway in the regulation of matrix metalloproteinase 13 and the dedifferentiation of articular chondrocytes in murine cartilage. *Arthritis Rheum.* **2009**, *60*, 428–439. [CrossRef]

26. Xiao, D.; Bi, R.; Liu, X.; Mei, J.; Jiang, N.; Zhu, S. Notch Signaling Regulates MMP-13 Expression via Runx2 in Chondrocytes. *Sci. Rep.* **2019**, *9*, 15596. [CrossRef]

27. Sassi, N.; Gadgadi, N.; Laadhar, L.; Allouche, M.; Mourali, S.; Zandieh-Doulabi, B.; Hamdoun, M.; Nulend, J.K.; Makni, S.; Sellami, S. Notch signaling is involved in human articular chondrocytes de-differentiation during osteoarthritis. *J. Recept. Signal Transduct. Res.* **2014**, *34*, 48–57. [CrossRef]

28. Minguzzi, M.; Panichi, V.; Cattini, L.; Filardo, G.; Mariani, E.; Borzì, R. Effects of notch-1 knockdown on the proliferation and the differentiation of human osteoarthritis chondrocytes. *Osteoarthr. Cartil.* **2018**, *26*, S110–S111. [CrossRef]

29. Olivotto, E.; Borzi, R.M.; Vitellozzi, R.; Pagani, S.; Facchini, A.; Battistelli, M.; Penzo, M.; Li, X.; Flamigni, F.; Li, J.; et al. Differential requirements for IKKalpha and IKKbeta in the differentiation of primary human osteoarthritic chondrocytes. *Arthritis Rheum.* **2008**, *58*, 227–239. [CrossRef]

30. Guidotti, S.; Minguzzi, M.; Platano, D.; Cattini, L.; Trisolino, G.; Mariani, E.; Borzi, R.M. Lithium Chloride Dependent Glycogen Synthase Kinase 3 Inactivation Links Oxidative DNA Damage, Hypertrophy and Senescence in Human Articular Chondrocytes and Reproduces Chondrocyte Phenotype of Obese Osteoarthritis Patients. *PLoS ONE* **2015**, *10*, e0143865. [CrossRef]

31. Lei, Y.; Guanghui, Z.; Xi, W.; Yingting, W.; Xialu, L.; Fangfang, Y.; Goldring, M.B.; Xiong, G.; Lammi, M.J. Cellular responses to T-2 toxin and/or deoxynivalenol that induce cartilage damage are not specific to chondrocytes. *Sci. Rep.* **2017**, *7*, 2231. [CrossRef]

32. Alabi, R.O.; Lora, J.; Celen, A.B.; Maretzky, T.; Blobel, C.P. Analysis of the Conditions That Affect the Selective Processing of Endogenous Notch1 by ADAM10 and ADAM17. *Int. J. Mol. Sci.* **2021**, *22*, 1846. [CrossRef]
33. Lee, C.R.; Park, Y.H.; Kim, Y.R.; Peterkofsky, A.; Seok, Y. Phosphorylation-Dependent Mobility Shift of Proteins on SDS-PAGE is Due to Decreased Binding of SDS. *Bull. Korean Chem. Soc.* **2013**, *34*, 2063–2066. [CrossRef]
34. Lee, H.J.; Kim, M.Y.; Park, H.S. Phosphorylation-dependent regulation of Notch1 signaling: The fulcrum of Notch1 signaling. *BMB Rep.* **2015**, *48*, 431–437. [CrossRef]
35. Bartlett, D.W.; Davis, M.E. Insights into the kinetics of siRNA-mediated gene silencing from live-cell and live-animal bioluminescent imaging. *Nucleic Acids Res.* **2006**, *34*, 322–333. [CrossRef] [PubMed]
36. Sarmento, L.M.; Huang, H.; Limon, A.; Gordon, W.; Fernandes, J.; Tavares, M.J.; Miele, L.; Cardoso, A.A.; Classon, M.; Carlesso, N. Notch1 modulates timing of G1-S progression by inducing SKP2 transcription and p27 Kip1 degradation. *J. Exp. Med.* **2005**, *202*, 157–168. [CrossRef] [PubMed]
37. Murata, K.; Hattori, M.; Hirai, N.; Shinozuka, Y.; Hirata, H.; Kageyama, R.; Sakai, T.; Minato, N. Hes1 directly controls cell proliferation through the transcriptional repression of p27Kip1. *Mol. Cell Biol.* **2005**, *25*, 4262–4271. [CrossRef] [PubMed]
38. Eglen, R.M.; Randle, D.H. Drug Discovery Goes Three-Dimensional: Goodbye to Flat High-Throughput Screening? *Assay Drug Dev. Technol.* **2015**, *13*, 262–265. [CrossRef]
39. Balistreri, C.R.; Madonna, R.; Melino, G.; Caruso, C. The emerging role of Notch pathway in ageing: Focus on the related mechanisms in age-related diseases. *Ageing Res. Rev.* **2016**, *29*, 50–65. [CrossRef] [PubMed]
40. Oeckinghaus, A.; Ghosh, S. The NF-kappaB family of transcription factors and its regulation. *Cold Spring Harb. Perspect Biol.* **2009**, *1*, a000034. [CrossRef]
41. Goldring, M.B.; Otero, M.; Plumb, D.A.; Dragomir, C.; Favero, M.; El Hachem, K.; Hashimoto, K.; Roach, H.I.; Olivotto, E.; Borzi, R.M.; et al. Roles of inflammatory and anabolic cytokines in cartilage metabolism: Signals and multiple effectors converge upon MMP-13 regulation in osteoarthritis. *Eur. Cell Mater.* **2011**, *21*, 202–220. [CrossRef] [PubMed]
42. Troeberg, L.; Nagase, H. Proteases involved in cartilage matrix degradation in osteoarthritis. *Biochim. Biophys. Acta* **2012**, *1824*, 133–145. [CrossRef]
43. Ulivi, V.; Giannoni, P.; Gentili, C.; Cancedda, R.; Descalzi, F. p38/NF-kB-dependent expression of COX-2 during differentiation and inflammatory response of chondrocytes. *J. Cell Biochem.* **2008**, *104*, 1393–1406. [CrossRef] [PubMed]
44. Ruscitto, A.; Scarpa, V.; Morel, M.; Pylawka, S.; Shawber, C.J.; Embree, M.C. Notch Regulates Fibrocartilage Stem Cell Fate and Is Upregulated in Inflammatory TMJ Arthritis. *J. Dent. Res.* **2020**, *99*, 1174–1181. [CrossRef]
45. Kohn, A.; Dong, Y.; Mirando, A.J.; Jesse, A.M.; Honjo, T.; Zuscik, M.J.; O'Keefe, R.J.; Hilton, M.J. Cartilage-specific RBPjkappa-dependent and -independent Notch signals regulate cartilage and bone development. *Development* **2012**, *139*, 1198–1212. [CrossRef]
46. Jakob, M.; Demarteau, O.; Schafer, D.; Stumm, M.; Heberer, M.; Martin, I. Enzymatic digestion of adult human articular cartilage yields a small fraction of the total available cells. *Connect. Tissue Res.* **2003**, *44*, 173–180. [CrossRef]
47. Kolettas, E.; Buluwela, L.; Bayliss, M.T.; Muir, H.I. Expression of cartilage-specific molecules is retained on long-term culture of human articular chondrocytes. *J. Cell Sci.* **1995**, *108*, 1991–1999. [CrossRef]
48. Rani, A.; Greenlaw, R.; Smith, R.A.; Galustian, C. HES1 in immunity and cancer. *Cytokine Growth Factor Rev.* **2016**, *30*, 113–117. [CrossRef]
49. Pfeuty, B. A computational model for the coordination of neural progenitor self-renewal and differentiation through Hes1 dynamics. *Development* **2015**, *142*, 477–485. [CrossRef]
50. Giovannini, C.; Gramantieri, L.; Minguzzi, M.; Fornari, F.; Chieco, P.; Grazi, G.L.; Bolondi, L. CDKN1C/P57 is regulated by the Notch target gene Hes1 and induces senescence in human hepatocellular carcinoma. *Am. J. Pathol.* **2012**, *181*, 413–422. [CrossRef]
51. Karlsson, C.; Jonsson, M.; Asp, J.; Brantsing, C.; Kageyama, R.; Lindahl, A. Notch and HES5 are regulated during human cartilage differentiation. *Cell Tissue Res.* **2007**, *327*, 539–551. [CrossRef]
52. Khan, I.M.; Palmer, E.A.; Archer, C.W. Fibroblast growth factor-2 induced chondrocyte cluster formation in experimentally wounded articular cartilage is blocked by soluble Jagged-1. *Osteoarthr. Cartil.* **2010**, *18*, 208–219. [CrossRef] [PubMed]
53. Wang, S.; Kawashima, N.; Sakamoto, K.; Katsube, K.; Umezawa, A.; Suda, H. Osteogenic differentiation of mouse mesenchymal progenitor cell, Kusa-A1 is promoted by mammalian transcriptional repressor Rbpj. *Biochem. Biophys. Res. Commun.* **2010**, *400*, 39–45. [CrossRef] [PubMed]
54. Caron, M.M.; Emans, P.J.; Coolsen, M.M.; Voss, L.; Surtel, D.A.; Cremers, A.; van Rhijn, L.W.; Welting, T.J. Redifferentiation of dedifferentiated human articular chondrocytes: Comparison of 2D and 3D cultures. *Osteoarthr. Cartil.* **2012**, *20*, 1170–1178. [CrossRef] [PubMed]
55. Otero, M.; Favero, M.; Dragomir, C.; Hachem, K.E.; Hashimoto, K.; Plumb, D.A.; Goldring, M.B. Human chondrocyte cultures as models of cartilage-specific gene regulation. *Methods Mol. Biol.* **2012**, *806*, 301–336.
56. Battistelli, M.; Borzi, R.M.; Olivotto, E.; Vitellozzi, R.; Burattini, S.; Facchini, A.; Falcieri, E. Cell and matrix morpho-functional analysis in chondrocyte micromasses. *Microsc. Res. Tech.* **2005**, *67*, 286–295. [CrossRef]
57. Sandell, L.J.; Aigner, T. Articular cartilage and changes in arthritis. An introduction: Cell biology of osteoarthritis. *Arthritis Res.* **2001**, *3*, 107–113. [CrossRef] [PubMed]
58. Drissi, H.; Zuscik, M.; Rosier, R.; O'Keefe, R. Transcriptional regulation of chondrocyte maturation: Potential involvement of transcription factors in OA pathogenesis. *Mol. Aspects Med.* **2005**, *26*, 169–179. [CrossRef] [PubMed]

59. Borzi, R.M.; Olivotto, E.; Pagani, S.; Vitellozzi, R.; Neri, S.; Battistelli, M.; Falcieri, E.; Facchini, A.; Flamigni, F.; Penzo, M.; et al. Matrix metalloproteinase 13 loss associated with impaired extracellular matrix remodeling disrupts chondrocyte differentiation by concerted effects on multiple regulatory factors. *Arthritis Rheum.* **2010**, *62*, 2370–2381. [CrossRef]

60. Olivotto, E.; Otero, M.; Astolfi, A.; Platano, D.; Facchini, A.; Pagani, S.; Flamigni, F.; Goldring, M.B.; Borzi, R.M.; Marcu, K.B. IKKalpha/CHUK regulates extracellular matrix remodeling independent of its kinase activity to facilitate articular chondrocyte differentiation. *PLoS ONE* **2013**, *8*, e73024. [CrossRef]

61. Guidotti, S.; Minguzzi, M.; Platano, D.; Santi, S.; Trisolino, G.; Filardo, G.; Mariani, E.; Borzi, R.M. Glycogen Synthase Kinase-3beta Inhibition Links Mitochondrial Dysfunction, Extracellular Matrix Remodelling and Terminal Differentiation in Chondrocytes. *Sci. Rep.* **2017**, *7*, 12059. [CrossRef]

62. Zanotti, S.; Canalis, E. Interleukin 6 mediates selected effects of Notch in chondrocytes. *Osteoarthr. Cartil.* **2013**, *21*, 1766–1773. [CrossRef]

63. Philipot, D.; Guerit, D.; Platano, D.; Chuchana, P.; Olivotto, E.; Espinoza, F.; Dorandeu, A.; Pers, Y.M.; Piette, J.; Borzi, R.M.; et al. p16INK4a and its regulator miR-24 link senescence and chondrocyte terminal differentiation-associated matrix remodeling in osteoarthritis. *Arthritis Res. Ther.* **2014**, *16*, R58. [CrossRef]

64. Barksby, H.E.; Milner, J.M.; Patterson, A.M.; Peake, N.J.; Hui, W.; Robson, T.; Lakey, R.; Middleton, J.; Cawston, T.E.; Richards, C.D.; et al. Matrix metalloproteinase 10 promotion of collagenolysis via procollagenase activation: Implications for cartilage degradation in arthritis. *Arthritis Rheum.* **2006**, *54*, 3244–3253. [CrossRef]

65. Martel-Pelletier, J.; Raynauld, J.P.; Mineau, F.; Abram, F.; Paiement, P.; Delorme, P.; Pelletier, J.P. Levels of serum biomarkers from a two-year multicentre trial are associated with treatment response on knee osteoarthritis cartilage loss as assessed by magnetic resonance imaging: An exploratory study. *Arthritis Res. Ther.* **2017**, *19*, 169. [CrossRef] [PubMed]

66. Marcu, K.B.; Otero, M.; Olivotto, E.; Borzi, R.M.; Goldring, M.B. NF-kappaB signaling: Multiple angles to target OA. *Curr. Drug Targets* **2010**, *11*, 599–613. [CrossRef]

67. Pagani, S.; Minguzzi, M.; Sicuro, L.; Veronesi, F.; Santi, S.; Scotto D'Abusco, A.; Fini, M.; Borzi, R.M. The N-Acetyl Phenylalanine Glucosamine Derivative Attenuates the Inflammatory/Catabolic Environment in a Chondrocyte-Synoviocyte Co-Culture System. *Sci. Rep.* **2019**, *9*, 13603. [CrossRef]

68. Veronesi, F.; Giavaresi, G.; Maglio, M.; Scotto d'Abusco, A.; Politi, L.; Scandurra, R.; Olivotto, E.; Grigolo, B.; Borzi, R.M.; Fini, M. Chondroprotective activity of N-acetyl phenylalanine glucosamine derivative on knee joint structure and inflammation in a murine model of osteoarthritis. *Osteoarthr. Cartil.* **2017**, *25*, 589–599. [CrossRef] [PubMed]

69. Zandi, E.; Rothwarf, D.M.; Delhase, M.; Hayakawa, M.; Karin, M. The IkappaB kinase complex (IKK) contains two kinase subunits, IKKalpha and IKKbeta, necessary for IkappaB phosphorylation and NF-kappaB activation. *Cell* **1997**, *91*, 243–252. [CrossRef]

70. Anest, V.; Hanson, J.L.; Cogswell, P.C.; Steinbrecher, K.A.; Strahl, B.D.; Baldwin, A.S. A nucleosomal function for IkappaB kinase-alpha in NF-kappaB-dependent gene expression. *Nature* **2003**, *423*, 659–663. [CrossRef] [PubMed]

71. Yamamoto, Y.; Verma, U.N.; Prajapati, S.; Kwak, Y.T.; Gaynor, R.B. Histone H3 phosphorylation by IKK-alpha is critical for cytokine-induced gene expression. *Nature* **2003**, *423*, 655–659. [CrossRef] [PubMed]

72. Hao, L.; Rizzo, P.; Osipo, C.; Pannuti, A.; Wyatt, D.; Cheung, L.W.; Sonenshein, G.; Osborne, B.A.; Miele, L. Notch-1 activates estrogen receptor-alpha-dependent transcription via IKKalpha in breast cancer cells. *Oncogene* **2010**, *29*, 201–213. [CrossRef] [PubMed]

73. Song, L.L.; Peng, Y.; Yun, J.; Rizzo, P.; Chaturvedi, V.; Weijzen, S.; Kast, W.M.; Stone, P.J.; Santos, L.; Loredo, A.; et al. Notch-1 associates with IKKalpha and regulates IKK activity in cervical cancer cells. *Oncogene* **2008**, *27*, 5833–5844. [CrossRef] [PubMed]

74. Zhao, G.; Zhang, H. Notch-1 siRNA and Methotrexate towards a Multifunctional Approach in Rhematoid Arthritis Management: A Nanomedicine Approach. *Pharm. Res.* **2018**, *35*, 123. [CrossRef]

75. Cavallo, C.; Merli, G.; Borzi, R.M.; Zini, N.; D'Adamo, S.; Guescini, M.; Grigolo, B.; di Martino, A.; Santi, S.; Filardo, G. Small Extracellular Vesicles from adipose derived stromal cells significantly attenuate in vitro the NF-kappaB dependent inflammatory/catabolic environment of osteoarthritis. *Sci. Rep.* **2021**, *11*, 1053. [CrossRef]

76. Finger, F.; Schorle, C.; Zien, A.; Gebhard, P.; Goldring, M.B.; Aigner, T. Molecular phenotyping of human chondrocyte cell lines T/C-28a2, T/C-28a4, and C-28/I2. *Arthritis Rheum.* **2003**, *48*, 3395–3403. [CrossRef]

77. Gupta-Rossi, N.; le Bail, O.; Gonen, H.; Brou, C.; Logeat, F.; Six, E.; Ciechanover, A.; Israel, A. Functional interaction between SEL-10, an F-box protein, and the nuclear form of activated Notch1 receptor. *J. Biol. Chem.* **2001**, *276*, 34371–34378. [CrossRef]

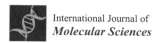

International Journal of
Molecular Sciences

MDPI

Article

Chondrocytes from Osteoarthritis Patients Adopt Distinct Phenotypes in Response to Central $T_H1/T_H2/T_H17$ Cytokines

Antti Pemmari [1], **Tiina Leppänen [1]**, **Mari Hämäläinen [1]**, **Teemu Moilanen [2]** and **Eeva Moilanen [1,*]**

[1] The Immunopharmacology Research Group, Faculty of Medicine and Health Technology, University of Tampere and Tampere University Hospital, 33100 Tampere, Finland; antti.pemmari@tuni.fi (A.P.); tiina.leppanen@tuni.fi (T.L.); mari.hamalainen@tuni.fi (M.H.)
[2] Coxa Hospital for Joint Replacement, 33520 Tampere, Finland; teemu.moilanen@coxa.fi
* Correspondence: eeva.moilanen@tuni.fi

Abstract: Chronic low-grade inflammation plays a central role in the pathogenesis of osteoarthritis (OA), and several pro- and anti-inflammatory cytokines have been implicated to mediate and regulate this process. Out of these cytokines, particularly IFNγ, IL-1β, IL-4 and IL-17 are associated with different phenotypes of T helper (T_H) cells and macrophages, both examples of cells known for great phenotypic and functional heterogeneity. Chondrocytes also display various phenotypic changes during the course of arthritis. We set out to study the hypothesis of whether chondrocytes might adopt polarized phenotypes analogous to T_H cells and macrophages. We studied the effects of IFNγ, IL-1β, IL-4 and IL-17 on gene expression in OA chondrocytes with RNA-Seq. Chondrocytes were harvested from the cartilage of OA patients undergoing knee replacement surgery and then cultured with or without the cytokines for 24 h. Total RNA was isolated and sequenced, and GO (Gene Ontology) functional analysis was performed. We also separately investigated genes linked to OA in recent genome wide expression analysis (GWEA) studies. The expression of more than 2800 genes was significantly altered in chondrocytes treated with IL-1β [in the C(IL-1β) phenotype] with a fold change (FC) > 2.5 in either direction. These included a large number of genes associated with inflammation, cartilage degradation and attenuation of metabolic signaling. The profile of genes differentially affected by IFNγ (the C(IFNγ) phenotype) was relatively distinct from that of the C(IL-1β) phenotype and included several genes associated with antigen processing and presentation. The IL-17-induced C(IL-17) phenotype was characterized by the induction of a more limited set of proinflammatory factors compared to C(IL-1β) cells. The C(IL-4) phenotype induced by IL-4 displayed a differential expression of a rather small set of genes compared with control, primarily those associated with TGFβ signaling and the regulation of inflammation. In conclusion, our results show that OA chondrocytes can adopt diverse phenotypes partly analogously to T_H cells and macrophages. This phenotypic plasticity may play a role in the pathogenesis of arthritis and open new therapeutic avenues for the development of disease-modifying treatments for (osteo)arthritis.

Keywords: chondrocyte; IL-1β; IFNγ; IL-17; IL-4; RNA-Seq

Citation: Pemmari, A.; Leppänen, T.; Hämäläinen, M.; Moilanen, T.; Moilanen, E. Chondrocytes from Osteoarthritis Patients Adopt Distinct Phenotypes in Response to Central $T_H1/T_H2/T_H17$ Cytokines. *Int. J. Mol. Sci.* **2021**, 22, 9463. https://doi.org/10.3390/ijms22179463

Academic Editor: Nicola Veronese

Received: 30 June 2021
Accepted: 6 August 2021
Published: 31 August 2021

Publisher's Note: MDPI stays neutral with regard to jurisdictional claims in published maps and institutional affiliations.

1. Introduction

Osteoarthritis (OA) is the most common form of arthritis. It has been estimated to affect up to a half of the elderly population, and therefore causes widespread disability and human suffering as well as an immense burden to healthcare systems [1]. Once thought as a mostly mechanical "wear and tear" disease, the chronic inflammatory component of osteoarthritis has been increasingly recognized during recent decades [2]. Constant low-grade inflammation in the joint contributes to pain, oxidative stress, increased catabolism, and the eventual breakdown of articular cartilage [3,4]. Despite intense research, no disease-modifying pharmacological treatments are currently available for OA [5], demonstrating that our understanding of the pathogenesis of the disease remains limited.

When comparing chondrocytes from OA patients with healthy cells, several changes in gene expression can be observed [6,7]. The potential causal roles of these changes in the pathogenesis of OA are currently largely unknown. However, some of them can be considered harmful (such as secretion of catabolic enzymes and proinflammatory cytokines) and others protective (e.g., the production of extracellular matrix [ECM] components) [8,9]. The changes in OA chondrocyte phenotype are thought to be caused by several physical and chemical factors, among them local proinflammatory cytokines [10].

The T helper (T_H) cell is probably the most well-known example of a cell capable of adopting distinct phenotypes in response to environmental factors. The different T_H phenotypes, in turn, are associated with different cytokines. The T_H1 phenotype drives inflammation and defense against intracellular pathogens. These cells are induced by interleukin 12 (IL-12) and produce mainly interferon gamma (IFNγ) as an effector cytokine [11]. In addition, they induce macrophages to produce IL-1β, which in turn promotes the proinflammatory effects of T_H1 cells [12]. T_H2 cells are induced by interleukins 2 and 4. They secrete various factors that promote humoral immunity and regulate inflammation, of which IL-4 is regarded as the central cytokine [11]. T_H17 cells are most closely associated with autoimmunity; they are induced by transforming growth factor beta (TGFβ) along with several proinflammatory cytokines, such as interleukins 6, 21 and 23, and they produce IL-17 as the central effector [13].

The macrophage is another cell type with well-defined differential phenotypes. The so-called "macrophage polarization" has two main phenotypes analogous to T_H1 and T_H2. The proinflammatory or "classically activated" M1 phenotype is associated with proinflammatory cytokines such as IL-1β and IFNγ, while the healing-promoting "alternatively activated" M2 phenotype is mainly linked to IL-4 [14]. The effects of IL-17 on macrophage phenotype have also attracted considerable interest. The M17 phenotype is not as well-defined as the M1 and M2 phenotypes; however, macrophages stimulated by IL-17 are characterized by the increased production of chemotactic and proinflammatory factors in the initial stages of the inflammatory response [15] and by the clearance of apoptotic cells and resolution of inflammation in the later phase [16].

Some authors have noted similarities between the variable functions and gene expression profiles of macrophages and chondrocytes in the setting of arthritis [17]. As another intriguing observation, major T_H1/2/17 cytokines have been shown to play roles in the development of different forms of arthritis. Of the cytokines that have been implicated in the development of OA, IL-1β is probably the most prominent. It has been shown to decrease the anabolic activity in chondrocytes and promote their apoptosis [18]. It also induces the expression of the proteolytic enzymes of the matrix metalloproteinase (MMP) and a disintegrin-like and metalloproteinase with trombospondin motifs (ADAMTS) families [19]. OA chondrocytes have been shown to upregulate the expression of IL-1 receptor (IL-1R) increasing their sensitivity to this cytokine [20]. Despite this, systemic treatment strategies specifically targeting IL-1β seem to have rather limited efficacy in OA [21], and none have reached clinical use.

Another major proinflammatory cytokine playing a role in the pathogenesis of arthritis is interleukin 17A (IL-17A) [22]. It promotes inflammation in concert with other proinflammatory cytokines [23], and its concentration in the synovial fluid correlates with radiographic severity of joint destruction [24]. In chondrocytes, it induces proinflammatory and catabolic factors and reduces proteoglycan synthesis [25–27]. Along with other proinflammatory cytokines, it also increases bone degradation by activating RANK ligand (RANKL) in osteoclasts [28]. In a murine model of collagen-induced arthritis, IL-17 deficiency has been shown to protect joints from the disease and IL-17 overexpression to exacerbate it [29,30]. Some functional gene expression analyses have actually implicated IL-17 signaling as a pathophysiological factor over IL-1β, the cytokine long known to drive OA [31].

In contrast to IL-1β and IL-17, the potential role of IFNγ as a causative factor in OA has attracted less interest. However, it has been found to be upregulated in chondrocytes by proinflammatory cytokines [32] as well as to be present in OA synovial fluid [33]. Some gene variants that affect the development of OA, particularly those of T-cell immunoglobulin and mucin-domain containing-3 (TIM-3), exert their effects via the modulation of IFNγ expression [34].

In the light of the above connections between the cytokines linked to major T helper cell/macrophage phenotypes and OA, it can be hypothesized that chondrocytes might also adopt phenotypes analogous to $T_H1/2/17$ or M1/2/17 cells, and that these phenotypes might play a role in the development of OA. In the present study, we investigated the effects of the central $T_H1/2/17$ cytokines on gene expression in OA chondrocytes. We sought to identify significantly differentially expressed genes and modulated pathways. The results were also compared to those of a recent genome-wide association study comparing degraded OA cartilage to preserved cartilage [35]. To our knowledge, this is the first study comparing the effects of the central $T_H1/2/17$ cytokines on OA chondrocytes and to characterize the resulting phenotypes.

2. Results

2.1. Effects of IL-1β on Chondrocyte Phenotype

After normalization and correction for multiple testing, a total of 2822 genes were found to be differentially expressed in IL-1β-treated chondrocytes [in the C(IL-1β) phenotype] versus controls in a statistically significant manner (FDR-corrected p-value < 0.05) and with a fold change (FC) 2.5 or more in either direction. Of these, 1092 were up- and 1730 downregulated. The list of the 20 most strongly upregulated genes contains several proinflammatory cyto- and chemokines, while the most strongly downregulated ones include several factors associated with regulation of gene expression, such as histone proteins (Table 1).

2.2. Effects of IL-17 on Chondrocyte Phenotype

Three hundred and eighty genes were differentially expressed in IL-17-treated chondrocytes [in the C(IL-17) phenotype] versus controls with FC > 2.5 in either direction, 314 of which were up- and 66 downregulated. Among the 20 most strongly upregulated genes were several associated with inflammation and chemotaxis, while the most strongly downregulated include genes involved in connective tissue development (Table 2).

2.3. Effects of IFNγ on Chondrocyte Phenotype

After normalization and correction for multiple testing, a total of 548 genes were found to be differentially expressed in IFNγ-treated chondrocytes [in the C(IFNγ) phenotype] versus controls in a statistically significant manner and FC 2.5 or more in either direction. Of these, 462 were up- and 86 downregulated. The 20 genes most strongly upregulated in C(IFNγ) cells included many associated with inflammation, antigen processing and presentation, and the regulation of proliferation. The most strongly downregulated genes included those involved in cell adhesion, proliferation and migration, and in Wnt signaling (Table 3).

2.4. Effects of IL-4 on Chondrocyte Phenotype

Twenty-six genes were upregulated by IL-4 with FC > 2.5 (Table S1). No genes were downregulated by IL-4 to a similar extent, but 10 genes were downregulated with FC < −1.5 (Table S2). In the C(IL-4) phenotype, the upregulated genes included those associated with the regulation of inflammation and TGFβ signaling as well as metabolism and cell adhesion, while several genes linked to cell proliferation were among the downregulated ones.

Table 1. Twenty most strongly up- and downregulated genes in interleukin 1-treated OA chondrocytes (IL1) relative to control (Co).

Gene	Name	Function	Mean (Co)	Mean (IL1)	Fold Change	adj. p
IL6	Interleukin 6	Inflammation	12.4	18,406.9	3685.72	$<1.0 \times 10^{-4}$
CXCL1	C-X-C motif chemokine ligand 1	Inflammation, chemotaxis	13.8	23,793.7	3457.68	$<1.0 \times 10^{-4}$
IL1B	Interleukin 1 beta	Inflammation	2.8	9575.7	3332.44	$<1.0 \times 10^{-4}$
CXCL8	C-X-C motif chemokine ligand 8	Inflammation, chemotaxis	329.5	855,146.3	2968.9	$<1.0 \times 10^{-4}$
CXCL6	C-X-C motif chemokine ligand 6	Inflammation, chemotaxis	2.8	4951.8	2352.02	$<1.0 \times 10^{-4}$
CXCL5	C-X-C motif chemokine ligand 5	Inflammation, chemotaxis	7.4	7352.4	1239.8	$<1.0 \times 10^{-4}$
CXCL2	C-X-C motif chemokine ligand 2	Inflammation, chemotaxis	3.9	4798.2	1198.05	$<1.0 \times 10^{-4}$
CXCL3	C-X-C motif chemokine ligand 3	Inflammation, chemotaxis	3.1	3154.6	1130.76	$<1.0 \times 10^{-4}$
CCL20	C-C motif chemokine ligand 20	Inflammation, chemotaxis	418	381,100.8	1128.35	$<1.0 \times 10^{-4}$
IL36RN	Interleukin 36 receptor antagonist	Regulation of inflammation	8.6	5863.8	914.19	$<1.0 \times 10^{-4}$
ADORA2A	Adenosine A2a receptor	Regulation of inflammation	5.5	1550.7	641.44	$<1.0 \times 10^{-4}$
IL36G	Interleukin 36 gamma	Inflammation	1.8	1065.5	562.03	$<1.0 \times 10^{-4}$
EREG	Epiregulin	Regulation of proliferation	31.9	13,697.7	506.87	$<1.0 \times 10^{-4}$
CSF3	Colony stimulating factor 3	Granulocyte-mediated inflammation	0.1	63.9	300.02	$<1.0 \times 10^{-4}$
VNN1	Vanin 1	T cell migration	9.2	2467.2	273.35	$<1.0 \times 10^{-4}$
CCL5	C-C motif chemokine ligand 5	Inflammation, chemotaxis	4.1	1134.2	271.85	$<1.0 \times 10^{-4}$
C15orf48	Chromosome 15 open reading frame 48	?	27.2	4669.1	253.13	$<1.0 \times 10^{-4}$
CCL3	C-C motif chemokine ligand 3	Inflammation, granulocyte activation	0.5	166.3	242.88	$<1.0 \times 10^{-4}$
FCAMR	Fc fragment of IgA and IgM receptor	Adaptive immunity, leukocyte migration	2.6	492	213.45	$<1.0 \times 10^{-4}$
SERPINB7	Serpin family B member 7	Endoproteinase inhibition	22.1	3747.9	205.63	$<1.0 \times 10^{-4}$
HRCT1	Histidine rich carboxyl terminus 1	?	105.8	4.1	−38.85	$<1.0 \times 10^{-4}$
LSP1	Lymphocyte specific protein 1	Regulation of neutrophil mobility	1749.6	58.1	−31.39	$<1.0 \times 10^{-4}$
HIST1H3G	Histone cluster 1 H3 family member g	Regulation of transcription	183.4	9.6	−28.26	$<1.0 \times 10^{-4}$
ACTC1	Actin, alpha, cardiac muscle 1	Heart muscle constituent	195.2	10.5	−24.79	$<1.0 \times 10^{-4}$
NXPH3	Neurexophilin 3	?	39.2	2.4	−23.89	$<1.0 \times 10^{-4}$
SCN2B	Sodium voltage-gated channel beta subunit 2	Cell adhesion and migration	167	8.7	−22.19	$<1.0 \times 10^{-4}$
HIST1H1A	Histone cluster 1 H1 family member a	?	908.5	47.2	−21.2	$<1.0 \times 10^{-4}$
GDF10	Growth differentiation factor 10	Skeletal system development	813.6	45.7	−20.57	$<1.0 \times 10^{-4}$
LINC02593	Long intergenic non-protein coding RNA 2593	?	68.3	3.4	−20.53	$<1.0 \times 10^{-4}$
HIST1H3B	Histone cluster 1 H3 family member b	Regulation of transcription	990.6	59.2	−20.46	$<1.0 \times 10^{-4}$
TMEM26	Transmembrane protein 26	?	403.7	21.4	−19.3	$<1.0 \times 10^{-4}$
PHYHIPL	Phytanoyl-CoA 2-hydroxylase interacting protein like	?	22	1.6	−19.19	$<1.0 \times 10^{-4}$
SARDH	Sarcosine dehydrogenase	Mitochondrial metabolism	25.8	2.4	−19.08	$<1.0 \times 10^{-4}$
HIST1H2BO	Histone cluster 1 H2B family member o	Regulation of transcription?	234.4	12.7	−18.99	$<1.0 \times 10^{-4}$

Table 1. *Cont.*

Gene	Name	Function	Mean (Co)	Mean (IL1)	Fold Change	adj. p
ID3	Inhibitor of DNA binding 3, HLH protein	Regulation of transcription	676.5	45.8	−18.32	<1.0 × 10^{-4}
HIST1H2AJ	Histone cluster 1 H2A family member j	Regulation of transcription?	857	47.1	−18.12	<1.0 × 10^{-4}
HIST1H1B	Histone cluster 1 H1 family member b	Regulation of transcription?	736	50.6	−17.69	<1.0 × 10^{-4}
MFAP2	Microfibril associated protein 2	ECM organization	33	3.2	−17.52	<1.0 × 10^{-4}
TNNT3	Troponin T3, fast skeletal type	Muscle constituent	95.6	6.4	−17.51	<1.0 × 10^{-4}
HIST1H2AL	Histone cluster 1 H2A family member l	Regulation of transcription?	321.4	21.2	−17.32	<1.0 × 10^{-4}

Red = upregulated genes; blue = downregulated genes.

Table 2. Twenty most strongly up- and downregulated genes in interleukin 17-treated OA chondrocytes (IL17) relative to control (Co).

Gene	Name	Function	Mean (Co)	Mean (IL17)	Fold Change	adj. p
SAA2	Serum amyloid A2	Chemotaxis	5.5	659.2	319.99	<1.0 × 10^{-4}
IL6	Interleukin 6	Inflammation	12.2	1431.4	250.15	<1.0 × 10^{-4}
SAA1	Serum amyloid A1	Inflammation, chemotaxis	63.7	3520.0	183.26	<1.0 × 10^{-4}
SAA2-SAA4	SAA2-SAA4 readthrough	Chemotaxis?	2.9	216.7	156.18	<1.0 × 10^{-4}
CXCL6	C-X-C motif chemokine ligand 6	Inflammation, chemotaxis	2.8	276.4	141.01	<1.0 × 10^{-4}
CXCL1	C-X-C motif chemokine ligand 1	Inflammation, chemotaxis	13.6	1170.5	136.48	<1.0 × 10^{-4}
VNN1	Vanin 1	T cell migration	9.1	820.5	84.13	<1.0 × 10^{-4}
CCL20	C-C motif chemokine ligand 20	Chemotaxis	412.8	26,508.9	73.49	<1.0 × 10^{-4}
TNFSF18	TNF superfamily member 18	T cell survival	4.2	470.3	73.05	<1.0 × 10^{-4}
IL36RN	Interleukin 36 receptor antagonist	Regulation of inflammation	8.5	468.0	69.09	<1.0 × 10^{-4}
VNN3	Vanin 3	?	1.8	130.3	66.35	<1.0 × 10^{-4}
ADORA2A	Adenosine A2a receptor	Inflammation, phagocytosis	5.4	105.9	64.74	<1.0 × 10^{-4}
CXCL2	C-X-C motif chemokine ligand 2	Inflammation, chemotaxis	3.9	220.3	55.90	<1.0 × 10^{-4}
CXCL8	C-X-C motif chemokine ligand 8	Inflammation, chemotaxis	324.8	14,116.5	48.18	<1.0 × 10^{-4}
C15orf48	Chromosome 15 open reading frame 48	Mitochondrial respiration?	26.9	820.3	46.34	<1.0 × 10^{-4}
PDZK1IP1	PDZK1 interacting protein 1	Regulation of apoptosis	5.2	206.9	41.18	<1.0 × 10^{-4}
NOS2	Nitric oxide synthase 2	Inflammation	137.9	3370.2	40.02	<1.0 × 10^{-4}
ODAPH	Odontogenesis associated phosphoprotein	Enamel production	1.4	41.9	37.29	<1.0 × 10^{-4}
SLC28A3	Solute carrier family 28 member 3	Nucleoside transport	4.3	150.4	35.34	<1.0 × 10^{-4}
CXCL5	C-X-C motif chemokine ligand 5	Inflammation, chemotaxis	7.3	207.5	34.25	<1.0 × 10^{-4}

Table 2. *Cont.*

Gene	Name	Function	Mean (Co)	Mean (IL17)	Fold Change	adj. p
ACTC1	Actin, alpha, cardiac muscle 1	Cardiac muscle component	191.7	26.7	−8.14	$<1.0 \times 10^{-4}$
TOX	Thymocyte selection associated high mobility group box	T cell development	14.6	3.9	−5.66	0.0010
TMEM26	Transmembrane protein 26	?	396.3	69.8	−5.47	$<1.0 \times 10^{-4}$
TNNT3	Troponin T3, fast skeletal type	Muscle component	93.9	17.9	−5.28	$<1.0 \times 10^{-4}$
TENT5B	Terminal nucleotidyltransferase 5B	Regulation of cell proliferation	152.5	39.7	−4.81	$<1.0 \times 10^{-4}$
TMEM26-AS1	TMEM26 antisense RNA 1	?	32.0	14.4	−4.77	3.8×10^{-4}
RCAN2	Regulator of calcineurin 2	Regulation of transcription	326.5	74.6	−4.74	$<1.0 \times 10^{-4}$
OPRL1	Opioid related nociceptin receptor 1	?	11.8	3.0	−4.51	0.0068
CSRNP3	Cysteine and serine rich nuclear protein 3	Regulation of apoptosis	59.7	19.7	−4.01	$<1.0 \times 10^{-4}$
ASPN	Asporin	Cartilage constituent	2011.2	505.2	−3.92	$<1.0 \times 10^{-4}$
HRCT1	Histidine rich carboxyl terminus 1	?	104.1	25.8	−3.85	$<1.0 \times 10{-4}$
AQP1	Aquaporin 1 (Colton blood group)	Regulation of osmotic pressure, angiogenesis, apoptosis	42.9	13.4	−3.69	$<1.0 \times 10^{-4}$
YWHAZP5	YWHAZ pseudogene 5		10.2	3.2	−3.68	0.013
MRAP2	Melanocortin 2 receptor accessory protein 2	cAMP signaling	1295.9	376.5	−3.62	$<1.0 \times 10^{-4}$
C1QTNF7	C1q and TNF related 7	?	63.4	20.1	−3.54	$<1.0 \times 10^{-4}$
MFAP2	Microfibril associated protein 2	Connective tissue organization	32.4	8.7	−3.47	$<1.0 \times 10^{-4}$
CLEC3A	C-type lectin domain family 3 member A	Skeletal system development	847.3	264.6	−3.46	$<1.0 \times 10^{-4}$
GREM1	Gremlin 1, DAN family BMP antagonist	Regulation of connective tissue development	5141.6	1566.4	−3.41	$<1.0 \times 10^{-4}$
CRISPLD1	Cysteine rich secretory protein LCCL domain containing 1	Morphogenesis	946.1	280.2	−3.39	$<1.0 \times 10^{-4}$
HRASLS5 (=PLAAT5)	HRAS like suppressor family member 5	Glycerophospholipid metabolism	12.8	3.6	−3.37	0.019

Red = upregulated genes; blue = downregulated genes.

Table 3. Twenty most strongly up- and downregulated genes in interferon gamma -treated OA chondrocytes (IFNγ) relative to control (Co).

Gene	Name	Function	Mean (Co)	Mean (IFNγ)	Fold change	adj. p
IDO1	Indoleamine 2,3-dioxygenase 1	Regulation of T cell -mediated immunity	17.5	42,320.0	4643.74	$<1.0 \times 10^{-4}$
LGALS17A	Galectin 14 pseudogene	?	0.4	1065.1	1750.58	$<1.0 \times 10^{-4}$
GBP1P1	Guanylate binding protein 1 pseudogene 1	?	2.6	2838.8	1245.34	$<1.0 \times 10^{-4}$
CXCL10	C-X-C motif chemokine ligand 10	Chemotaxis	2.2	2065.2	1117.91	$<1.0 \times 10^{-4}$
GBP5	Guanylate binding protein 5	Inflammasome activation	1.4	1518.3	1112.44	$<1.0 \times 10^{-4}$
CXCL9	C-X-C motif chemokine ligand 9	T cell chemotaxis	1.1	1069.9	1033.80	$<1.0 \times 10^{-4}$
GBP4	Guanylate binding protein 4	Inflammation?	30.9	27,565.6	955.57	$<1.0 \times 10^{-4}$

Table 3. *Cont.*

Gene	Name	Function	Mean (Co)	Mean (IFNγ)	Fold change	adj. p
IFI44L	Interferon induced protein 44 like	?	9.7	6185.8	694.66	$<1.0 \times 10^{-4}$
GBP1	Guanylate binding protein 1	Negative regulation of inflammation	124.3	54,562.1	454.62	$<1.0 \times 10^{-4}$
HLA-DRA	Major histocompatibility complex, class II, DR alpha	Antigen presentation	5.6	2338.3	408.93	$<1.0 \times 10^{-4}$
HLA-DRB1	Major histocompatibility complex, class II, DR beta 1	Antigen presentation	10.7	2430.7	383.18	$<1.0 \times 10^{-4}$
CD74	CD74 molecule	Antigen presentation	31.9	11,211.5	353.35	$<1.0 \times 10^{-4}$
RSAD2	Radical S-adenosyl methionine domain containing 2	Antiviral action	44.5	15,365.2	338.82	$<1.0 \times 10^{-4}$
RARRES3	Retinoic acid receptor responder 3	Phospholipid catabolism	33.1	8271.1	286.40	$<1.0 \times 10^{-4}$
BST2	Bone marrow stromal cell antigen 2	Antiviral action	10.1	2908.5	285.04	$<1.0 \times 10^{-4}$
GBP6	Guanylate binding protein family member 6	Inflammation	1.0	193.3	273.26	$<1.0 \times 10^{-4}$
HLA-DRB5	Major histocompatibility complex, class II, DR beta 5	Antigen presentation	4.4	825.4	253.47	$<1.0 \times 10^{-4}$
HLA-DRB6	Major histocompatibility complex, class II, DR beta 6 (pseudogene)	Antigen presentation?	0.3	125.7	226.68	$<1.0 \times 10^{-4}$
APOL4	Apolipoprotein L4	Lipid metabolism	2.6	500.8	225.95	$<1.0 \times 10^{-4}$
IFIT2	Interferon induced protein with tetratricopeptide repeats 2	Regulation of proliferation	96.2	20,648.8	225.79	$<1.0 \times 10^{-4}$
TNFRSF10D	TNF receptor superfamily member 10d	Inhibition of apoptosis	4135.1	501.9	−7.65	$<1.0 \times 10^{-4}$
ARHGAP9	Rho gtpase activating protein 9	?	10.7	2.4	−5.27	0.0028
NANOS1	Nanos C2HC-type zinc finger 1	Regulation of translation and cell migration	83.4	16.9	−4.94	$<1.0 \times 10^{-4}$
SNORD108	Small nucleolar RNA, C/D box 108	?	66.6	13.8	−4.81	$<1.0 \times 10^{-4}$
FAM189A2	Family with sequence similarity 189 member A2	?	13.6	4.3	−4.39	0.0033
PWAR6	Prader Willi/Angelman region RNA 6	?	34.0	7.9	−4.32	$<1.0 \times 10^{-4}$
GABRA4	Gamma-aminobutyric acid type A receptor alpha4 subunit	Synaptic transmission	2346.1	549.2	−4.28	$<1.0 \times 10^{-4}$
CORO2A	Coronin 2A	?	13.5	3.7	−4.11	0.020
WFDC1	WAP four-disulfide core domain 1	Regulation of proliferation	65.1	18.0	−4.06	$<1.0 \times 10^{-4}$
PRSS35	Serine protease 35	?	51.4	13.5	−4.01	$<1.0 \times 10^{-4}$
SLC16A14	Solute carrier family 16 member 14	Organic acid transport	40.2	13.3	−3.98	$<1.0 \times 10^{-4}$
PWAR5	Prader Willi/Angelman region RNA 5	?	359.7	91.4	−3.93	$<1.0 \times 10^{-4}$
MTURN	Maturin, neural progenitor differentiation regulator homolog	?	1857.1	519.7	−3.63	$<1.0 \times 10^{-4}$
C1QTNF5	C1q and TNF related 5	Cell adhesion	152.4	46.1	−3.47	$<1.0 \times 10^{-4}$
LONRF2	LON peptidase N-terminal domain and ring finger 2	?	206.8	59.5	−3.46	$<1.0 \times 10^{-4}$
FGFR4	Fibroblast growth factor receptor 4	Cell proliferation and migration	11.1	5.1	−3.31	0.045
TRABD2B	Trab domain containing 2B	Wnt signaling, proteolysis	14.2	5.5	−3.29	0.0014
TNNT3	Troponin T3, fast skeletal type	Muscle contraction	106.0	31.6	−3.26	$<1.0 \times 10^{-4}$
NCALD	Neurocalcin delta	Endocytosis	17.3	6.6	−3.24	0.029
CDH2	Cadherin 2	Cell adhesion	12.0	4.1	−3.23	0.0012

Red = upregulated genes; blue = downregulated genes.

2.5. Functional Gene Categories in Different Chondrocyte Phenotypes

Table 4 shows the Gene Ontology (GO) terms affected with a high significance (FDR-corrected p-value < 0.01) by at least one studied proinflammatory cytokine (IL-1β, IFNγ or IL-17). The C(IL-1β) phenotype was involved in the activation of a wide range of inflammatory terms and pathways, along with those related to cell adhesion as well as extracellular matrix production and degradation. The T_H17-associated cytokine IL-17 affected a partly overlapping, but smaller, set of inflammatory cytokines compared to IL-1β. The C(IFNγ) phenotype was quite distinct compared to the C(IL-1β) and C(IL-17) phenotypes; several terms related to antigen processing and presentation were affected by this cytokine alone. Nitric oxide synthase biosynthetic process and chemotaxis were among the functions involved solely in the C(IL-17) phenotype. In addition, many high-level GO terms related to inflammation were affected by all of the three proinflammatory cytokines.

In C(IL-4) cells, no significantly affected GO terms were detected when analyzing the genes with FC > 2.5 in either direction. When the FC threshold was lowered to 1.5, GO terms associated with cell division were among the significant ones (Table S3).

2.6. Comparing the Effects of Different Proinflammatory Cytokines

Next, we cross-compared the genes markedly upregulated (FC > 2.5) in the C(IL-1β), C(IFNγ) and C(IL-17) phenotypes to further characterize the differences and similarities between the resulting phenotypes. As shown in Figure 1A, a large portion (nearly 85%) of genes markedly upregulated in C(IL-17) cells were included in the large set of those similarly affected by IL-1β, but 45 genes were solely affected by IL-17, and the overlap of C(IL-17) and C(IFNγ) phenotypes was considerable smaller than that of C(IL-17) and C(IL-1β). The intersection of genes upregulated by both IL-17 and IFNγ was nearly completely contained in those upregulated by IL-1β (Figure 1A). Many central regulators of inflammation such as *IL6*, *PTGS2* (cyclo-oxygenase 2 or COX-2) and *NOS2* (inducible nitric oxide synthase or iNOS) were markedly upregulated by all the three T_H1/T_H17 cytokines, in line with the widespread activation of inflammatory pathways observed in the GO analysis (Table 5).

When comparing genes markedly downregulated (FC < −2.5) by the three proinflammatory cytokines, the large (>1000 genes) list of genes downregulated by IL-1β again contained a large proportion (85%) of those downregulated by IL-17 and a smaller amount (48%) of genes similarly affected by IFNγ (Figure 1B). Genes downregulated by all of the three cytokines are presented in Table 6 and include, for example, those associated with cell proliferation and skeletal system development.

2.7. Effects of the Cytokines on Genes Differentially Expressed in Degraded and Preserved OA Cartilage

Some previous studies have investigated the differences in gene expression between degraded and preserved OA cartilage. Of these, the study by Almeida et al. [35] is probably the most comprehensive. To see whether the studied cytokines shift chondrocyte phenotype towards either degraded or preserved cartilage, we compared the differentially expressed genes in the phenotypes observed in the present study to those differentially expressed in the study by Almeida et al. [35] As a very large number (over 2300) of significantly differentially expressed genes were identified in that study, we focused on those 84 genes which were most strongly upregulated (FC > 2.5 and FDR-corrected p-value < 0.01) in the degraded cartilage. Of those 84 genes, 38 were significantly affected by at least one of the proinflammatory cytokines (IL-1, IL-17 or IFNγ) in our data. A large majority (30) of these 38 genes were also upregulated by IL-1β, showing that the cytokine shifts chondrocyte phenotype towards the one observed in the degraded cartilage. Several mediators of inflammation, such as *LIF*, *CCL20* and *TREM1*, were especially strongly upregulated. Only four of the 84 genes (namely *CLIC3*, *ERFE*, *SLC27A2* and *ANK3*) were downregulated by IL-1β.

Table 4. GO terms affected by different proinflammatory cytokines. Genes with FC > 2.5 in either direction were analyzed with DAVID, and the resulting lists were reduced with REVIGO. GO terms significantly affected (with FDR-corrected *p*-value < 0.05) by a cytokine are marked with an X.

Term	IL1	IL17	IFNγ	Term	IL1	IL17	IFNγ
Inflammatory response	X	X	X	Nucleosome assembly	X		
Immune response	X	X	X	Chromosome segregation	X		
Response to lipopolysaccharide	X	X	X	Protein heterotetramerization	X		
Chemotaxis	X	X	X	Wound healing	X		
Negative regulation of viral entry into host cell	X	X	X	Regulation of cell proliferation	X		
				Cell migration	X		
Negative regulation of type I interferon production	X	X	X	Regulation of gene silencing	X		
				Positive regulation of interleukin-12 production	X		
Response to progesterone	X	X		Odontogenesis	X		
Cell-cell signaling	X	X		Cellular response to mechanical stimulus	X		
Angiogenesis	X	X		Peptidyl-tyrosine phosphorylation	X		
Negative regulation of growth	X	X		Collagen catabolic process	X		
Positive regulation of mitotic nuclear division	X	X		Positive regulation of cell division	X		
				Positive chemotaxis		X	
Negative regulation of cell proliferation	X	X		Positive regulation of nitric-oxide synthase biosynthetic process		X	
Signal transduction	X		X	Acute-phase response		X	
Response to virus	X		X	Positive regulation of cytosolic calcium ion concentration		X	
Positive regulation of interleukin-6 production	X		X	Positive regulation of gtpase activity			X
Response to hydrogen peroxide	X		X	Response to glucocorticoid			X
Positive regulation of I-kappab kinase/NF-kappab signaling	X		X	Response to wounding			X
				Positive regulation of NF-kappab transcription factor activity			X
Response to drug	X		X	Negative regulation of tumor necrosis factor production			X
Cellular response to zinc ion		X	X	Cellular response to organic cyclic compound			X
Response to toxic substance		X	X	Antigen processing and presentation			X
Tumor necrosis factor-mediated signaling pathway		X	X	Antigen processing and presentation of peptide or polysaccharide antigen via MHC class II			X
Cell division	X			Antigen processing and presentation of exogenous peptide antigen via MHC class I, TAP-independent			X
DNA replication	X						
Telomere organization	X			Response to interferon-beta			X
Positive regulation of gene expression	X			Response to interferon-alpha			X
				T cell costimulation			X
Cell adhesion	X			Positive regulation of T cell mediated cytotoxicity			X
Extracellular matrix organization	X			Defense response			X
Skeletal system development	X			Protein trimerization			X
Sister chromatid cohesion	X			Proteolysis			X
DNA replication initiation	X			Defense response to protozoan			X
Cellular protein metabolic process	X			Positive regulation of peptidyl-tyrosine phosphorylation			X
Cell proliferation	X			Protein polyubiquitination			X
Negative regulation of gene expression, epigenetic	X						

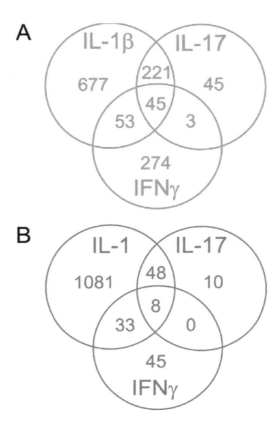

Figure 1. Venn diagrams of genes markedly upregulated (FC > 2.5) (**A**) or markedly downregulated (FC < 2.5) (**B**) by IL-1β, IL-17 and IFNγ. Red denotes up- and blue downregulated genes.

In the C(IFNγ) phenotype, 13 of the 84 genes associated with degraded cartilage (including *LIF* and *NGF*) were upregulated compared with control, but nearly as many (nine) were downregulated, including *TREM1*. This shows that the effects of IFNγ on chondrocyte phenotype in relation to the degraded/preserved cartilage are more ambiguous than those of IL-1β.

In C(IL-17) chondrocytes, 25 of the 84 genes associated with degraded cartilage were upregulated compared to naïve chondrocytes (including *CCL20* and *IL11*), and none were significantly downregulated. Nine genes, including *IGFBP1*, *LIF* and *GPR158*, were upregulated in all three inflammatory phenotypes C(IL-1β), C(IFNγ) and C(IL-17) and one (*ANK3*) was downregulated in all of them. (Figure 2 and Table S4).

Table 5. Genes upregulated by all studied proinflammatory cytokines with FC > 2.5. Shown are mean normalized expression levels in control (Co) and in C(IL1), C(IL17) and C(IFNγ) phenotypes, fold changes (FCs) for all comparisons vs. control and false discovery rate (FDR)-adjusted *p* values for them.

Gene	Name	Mean exp. (Co)	Mean exp. (IL1)	Mean exp. (IL17)	Mean exp. (IFNγ)	FC (IL1) vs. Co	adj. p (IL1) vs. Co	FC (IL17) vs. Co	adj. p (IL17) vs. Co	FC (IFNγ) vs. Co	adj. p (IFNγ) vs. Co
IL6	Interleukin 6	12.8	18,406.9	1431.4	94.2	3685.72	$<1.0 \times 10^{-4}$	250.15	$<1.0 \times 10^{-4}$	12.34	$<1.0 \times 10^{-4}$
IL36RN	Interleukin 36 receptor antagonist	8.9	5863.8	468.0	36.7	914.19	$<1.0 \times 10^{-4}$	69.09	$<1.0 \times 10^{-4}$	4.59	$<1.0 \times 10^{-4}$
ESM1	Endothelial cell specific molecule 1	276.7	37,984.1	1373.5	1449.2	157.25	$<1.0 \times 10^{-4}$	5.09	$<1.0 \times 10^{-4}$	4.70	$<1.0 \times 10^{-4}$
SAA2	Serum amyloid A2	5.8	371.4	659.2	27.1	149.11	$<1.0 \times 10^{-4}$	319.99	$<1.0 \times 10^{-4}$	8.73	$<1.0 \times 10^{-4}$
iNOS/NOS2	Inducible nitric oxide synthase/Nitric oxide synthase 2	144.2	12,704.9	3370.2	3046.1	131.22	$<1.0 \times 10^{-4}$	40.02	$<1.0 \times 10^{-4}$	30.16	$<1.0 \times 10^{-4}$
NOD2	Nucleotide binding oligomerization domain containing 2	7.6	919.4	96.7	43.9	116.73	$<1.0 \times 10^{-4}$	13.67	$<1.0 \times 10^{-4}$	5.61	$<1.0 \times 10^{-4}$
PTX3	Pentraxin 3	184.4	18,888.7	4615.3	479.6	113.19	$<1.0 \times 10^{-4}$	27.47	$<1.0 \times 10^{-4}$	2.60	$<1.0 \times 10^{-4}$
SAA1	Serum amyloid A1	66.6	2188.7	3520.0	227.6	94.66	$<1.0 \times 10^{-4}$	183.26	$<1.0 \times 10^{-4}$	6.46	$<1.0 \times 10^{-4}$
CD300E	CD300e molecule	3.6	316.9	32.7	71.6	72.79	$<1.0 \times 10^{-4}$	7.91	$<1.0 \times 10^{-4}$	17.15	$<1.0 \times 10^{-4}$
IL36B	Interleukin 36 beta	11.3	466.3	80.1	39.1	67.27	$<1.0 \times 10^{-4}$	9.65	$<1.0 \times 10^{-4}$	3.60	$<1.0 \times 10^{-4}$
TNFRSF1B	TNF receptor superfamily member 1B	40.0	2370.7	525.8	118.9	62.58	$<1.0 \times 10^{-4}$	14.66	$<1.0 \times 10^{-4}$	3.02	$<1.0 \times 10^{-4}$
TNFAIP6	TNF alpha induced protein 6	1176.4	42,950.3	5512.4	4561.2	36.87	$<1.0 \times 10^{-4}$	4.59	$<1.0 \times 10^{-4}$	3.59	$<1.0 \times 10^{-4}$
TMEM132A	Transmembrane protein 132A	10.3	328.1	165.0	32.6	33.90	$<1.0 \times 10^{-4}$	16.64	$<1.0 \times 10^{-4}$	3.18	$<1.0 \times 10^{-4}$
ICAM1	Intercellular adhesion molecule 1	1415.2	42,657.2	4388.3	8524.5	31.66	$<1.0 \times 10^{-4}$	3.15	$<1.0 \times 10^{-4}$	5.54	$<1.0 \times 10^{-4}$
C3AR1	Complement C3a receptor 1	2.2	66.2	11.4	11.2	28.15	$<1.0 \times 10^{-4}$	6.36	1.5×10^{-4}	5.32	4.9×10^{-4}
CLEC2B	C-type lectin domain family 2 member B	5.3	145.0	48.5	20.6	27.53	$<1.0 \times 10^{-4}$	9.35	$<1.0 \times 10^{-4}$	3.85	$<1.0 \times 10^{-4}$
COX-2/PTGS2	Cyclooxygenase-2/Prostaglandin-endoperoxide synthase 2	1310.7	37,281.5	4678.6	5349.2	26.96	$<1.0 \times 10^{-4}$	3.28	$<1.0 \times 10^{-4}$	3.57	$<1.0 \times 10^{-4}$
TLR2	Toll like receptor 2	134.9	3348.9	782.0	371.4	22.64	$<1.0 \times 10^{-4}$	5.02	$<1.0 \times 10^{-4}$	2.54	$<1.0 \times 10^{-4}$
CCL7	C-C motif chemokine ligand 7	2.1	36.7	20.6	24.4	20.66	$<1.0 \times 10^{-4}$	12.14	$<1.0 \times 10^{-4}$	10.56	$<1.0 \times 10^{-4}$
CCL2	C-C motif chemokine ligand 2	150.4	2475.0	815.0	430.6	19.42	$<1.0 \times 10^{-4}$	5.85	$<1.0 \times 10^{-4}$	2.61	$<1.0 \times 10^{-4}$
IRF4	Interferon regulatory factor 4	23.5	400.1	94.9	114.2	18.20	$<1.0 \times 10^{-4}$	4.62	$<1.0 \times 10^{-4}$	4.69	$<1.0 \times 10^{-4}$
CD274	CD274 molecule	61.8	1048.8	350.1	3845.7	17.56	$<1.0 \times 10^{-4}$	6.18	$<1.0 \times 10^{-4}$	60.08	$<1.0 \times 10^{-4}$
RBM47	RNA binding motif protein 47	8.8	122.3	30.6	22.8	14.96	$<1.0 \times 10^{-4}$	3.38	$<1.0 \times 10^{-4}$	2.67	0.040
CD38	CD38 molecule	9.8	133.8	74.3	211.4	14.81	$<1.0 \times 10^{-4}$	7.67	$<1.0 \times 10^{-4}$	20.76	$<1.0 \times 10^{-4}$
BDKRB1	Bradykinin receptor B1	29.0	401.5	129.6	105.0	13.95	$<1.0 \times 10^{-4}$	4.88	$<1.0 \times 10^{-4}$	3.19	$<1.0 \times 10^{-4}$
GCH1	GTP cyclohydrolase 1	591.7	7968.7	2212.7	3584.2	13.38	$<1.0 \times 10^{-4}$	3.90	$<1.0 \times 10^{-4}$	5.63	$<1.0 \times 10^{-4}$
LRRC38	Leucine rich repeat containing 38	11.2	132.1	44.4	35.8	11.59	$<1.0 \times 10^{-4}$	3.79	$<1.0 \times 10^{-4}$	2.98	$<1.0 \times 10^{-4}$
KIAA1217	KIAA1217	15.3	157.8	55.1	109.1	10.61	$<1.0 \times 10^{-4}$	3.80	$<1.0 \times 10^{-4}$	6.39	$<1.0 \times 10^{-4}$
SSTR2	Somatostatin receptor 2	90.0	971.2	1549.7	340.1	10.56	$<1.0 \times 10^{-4}$	16.11	$<1.0 \times 10^{-4}$	3.36	$<1.0 \times 10^{-4}$
DUSP5	Dual specificity phosphatase 5	77.3	746.8	302.4	236.1	10.54	$<1.0 \times 10^{-4}$	4.02	$<1.0 \times 10^{-4}$	2.90	$<1.0 \times 10^{-4}$
TYMP	Thymidine phosphorylase	311.3	3020.1	1275.1	9324.0	10.15	$<1.0 \times 10^{-4}$	4.24	$<1.0 \times 10^{-4}$	28.71	$<1.0 \times 10^{-4}$
GPR158	G protein-coupled receptor 158	6.9	38.0	22.0	21.5	9.98	$<1.0 \times 10^{-4}$	6.77	0.0018	5.55	7.6×10^{-4}
PRLR	Prolactin receptor	8.3	78.8	29.7	33.0	9.93	$<1.0 \times 10^{-4}$	3.05	0.0034	3.92	$<1.0 \times 10^{-4}$
GSAP	Gamma-secretase activating protein	122.2	1109.8	378.0	509.3	9.18	$<1.0 \times 10^{-4}$	3.26	$<1.0 \times 10^{-4}$	3.74	$<1.0 \times 10^{-4}$

Table 5. *Cont.*

Gene	Name	Mean exp. (Co)	Mean exp. (IL1)	Mean exp. (IL17)	Mean exp. (IFNγ)	FC (IL1 vs. Co)	adj. p (IL1 vs. Co)	FC (IL17 vs. Co)	adj. p (IL17 vs. Co)	FC (IFNγ vs. Co)	adj. p (IFNγ vs. Co)
GPR39	G protein-coupled receptor 39	15.4	110.6	39.1	41.4	9.17	$<1.0 \times 10^{-4}$	3.24	1.7×10^{-4}	2.71	$<1.0 \times 10^{-4}$
LYPD1	LY6/PLAUR domain containing 1	10.5	71.5	28.7	27.7	8.44	$<1.0 \times 10^{-4}$	3.31	5.6×10^{-4}	2.62	0.0023
ODF3B	Outer dense fiber of sperm tails 3B	34.6	261.0	106.0	773.8	7.98	$<1.0 \times 10^{-4}$	3.28	$<1.0 \times 10^{-4}$	21.57	$<1.0 \times 10^{-4}$
SLC15A3	Solute carrier family 15 member 3	16.3	119.4	54.7	607.4	7.63	$<1.0 \times 10^{-4}$	3.45	$<1.0 \times 10^{-4}$	35.59	$<1.0 \times 10^{-4}$
HAL	Histidine ammonia-lyase	6.2	44.1	28.7	47.4	7.57	$<1.0 \times 10^{-4}$	4.71	$<1.0 \times 10^{-4}$	6.97	$<1.0 \times 10^{-4}$
DOCK4	Dedicator of cytokinesis 4	44.0	306.8	144.9	139.2	6.94	$<1.0 \times 10^{-4}$	3.21	$<1.0 \times 10^{-4}$	2.91	$<1.0 \times 10^{-4}$
RAB27B	RAB27B, member RAS oncogene family	16.5	77.2	60.5	84.5	5.98	$<1.0 \times 10^{-4}$	3.85	$<1.0 \times 10^{-4}$	5.62	$<1.0 \times 10^{-4}$
CH25H	Cholesterol 25-hydroxylase	7.4	36.5	25.8	41.8	4.41	$<1.0 \times 10^{-4}$	3.27	0.022	6.32	$<1.0 \times 10^{-4}$
USP43	Ubiquitin specific peptidase 43	4.4	12.8	13.6	16.1	3.94	0.020	3.41	0.013	4.50	0.0091
AC104966.1	Ceruloplasmin (ferroxidase) (CP) pseudogene	16.5	47.6	57.3	53.7	3.39	$<1.0 \times 10^{-4}$	3.79	$<1.0 \times 10^{-4}$	3.36	$<1.0 \times 10^{-4}$
KLK10	Kallikrein related peptidase 10	14.0	37.1	33.0	43.1	3.11	0.022	3.29	0.0067	2.65	0.0028

Red = upregulated genes.

Table 6. Genes downregulated by all studied proinflammatory cytokines with FC < −2.5. Shown are mean normalized expression levels in control (Co), in C(IL1), C(IL17) and C(IFNγ) phenotypes, fold changes (FCs) for all comparisons vs. control and false discovery rate (FDR)-adjusted *p* values for them.

Gene	Name	Function	Mean exp. (Co)	Mean exp. (IL1)	Mean exp. (IL17)	Mean exp. (IFNγ)	FC (IL1 vs. Co)	adj. p (IL1 vs. Co)	FC (IL17 vs. Co)	adj. p (IL17 vs. Co)	FC (IFNγ vs. Co)	adj. p (IFNγ vs. Co)
SCN2B	Sodium voltage-gated channel beta subunit 2	Sodium ion transport	170.8	8.7	65.9	63.7	−22.19	$<1.0 \times 10^{-4}$	−2.59	$<1.0 \times 10^{-4}$	−2.90	$<1.0 \times 10^{-4}$
TNNT3	Troponin T3, fast skeletal type	Skeletal muscle constituent	97.8	6.4	17.9	31.6	−17.51	$<1.0 \times 10^{-4}$	−5.28	$<1.0 \times 10^{-4}$	−3.26	$<1.0 \times 10^{-4}$
MRAP2	Melanocortin 2 receptor accessory protein 2	Metabolism?	1348.7	91.1	376.5	572.0	−15.12	$<1.0 \times 10^{-4}$	−3.62	$<1.0 \times 10^{-4}$	−2.85	$<1.0 \times 10^{-4}$
WFDC1	WAP four-disulfide core domain 1	Negative regulation of cell growth	60.1	6.1	34.9	18.0	−12.06	$<1.0 \times 10^{-4}$	−2.68	0.0019	−4.06	$<1.0 \times 10^{-4}$
RANBP3L	RAN binding protein 3 like	Nuclear export	654.8	74.6	284.8	280.0	−9.40	$<1.0 \times 10^{-4}$	−2.54	$<1.0 \times 10^{-4}$	−2.60	$<1.0 \times 10^{-4}$
ASPN	Asporin	Skeletal system development, negative regulation of TGFβ signaling	2094.0	206.3	505.2	837.5	−8.28	$<1.0 \times 10^{-4}$	−3.92	$<1.0 \times 10^{-4}$	−2.77	$<1.0 \times 10^{-4}$
FGFR4	Fibroblast growth factor receptor 4	Cell proliferation and migration	10.3	2.3	3.1	5.1	−5.59	5.2×10^{-4}	−3.12	0.036	−3.31	0.045
PTGER3	Prostaglandin E receptor 3	Inflammation, cell death	494.1	173.6	162.3	188.8	−2.69	$<1.0 \times 10^{-4}$	−3.03	$<1.0 \times 10^{-4}$	−2.82	$<1.0 \times 10^{-4}$

blue = downregulated genes.

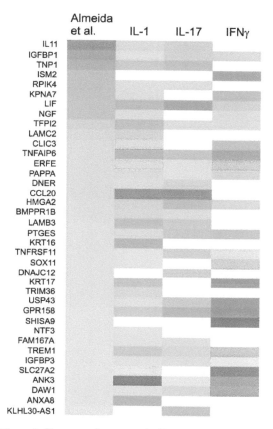

Figure 2. Heatmap of genes markedly upregulated (FC > 2.5) in degraded cartilage in the study by Almeida et al. [35] and significantly affected by at least one studied proinflammatory cytokine. Upregulated genes are marked with red, downregulated with blue, and genes with no significant fold change with white.

In the study by Almeida et al. [35], 52 genes were associated with preserved rather than degraded cartilage (i.e., significantly downregulated in degraded cartilage with FC < −2.5). Of these, 19 were significantly affected by at least one of the proinflammatory cytokines in our data. In C(IL-1β) cells, 13 of these 19 genes were significantly downregulated with *GDF10* displaying especially strong downregulation. In contrast, five of these genes were upregulated compared to control (including the especially strongly upregulated *C3* and *RSPO3*). This again shows that the net effect of IL-1β is to shift chondrocyte phenotype towards degraded cartilage. IFNγ showed a directionally similar, but less pronounced effect: seven of the genes associated with preserved cartilage were significantly downregulated and three upregulated in the C(IFNγ) phenotype. In C(IL-17) cells, eight genes associated with preserved cartilage were down- and four upregulated; *C3* once again displayed especially strong upregulation. Five genes, including *PTGER3* and *GDF10*, were downregulated in all of the three chondrocyte phenotypes. On the other hand, *RSPO3* and *PRLR*, both downregulated in degraded compared with preserved cartilage, were upregulated by all of the three cytokines. These data indicate that the C(IL-1β) and C(IL-17) phenotypes at least partly resemble the transcriptomic profile associated with degraded OA cartilage as identified by Almeida et al. [35]. In contrast, IFNγ seems to have a smaller effect on the genes directly linked to cartilage degradation in OA being instead characterized by the upregulation of genes associated with antigen processing and presentation. (Figure 3 and Table S5).

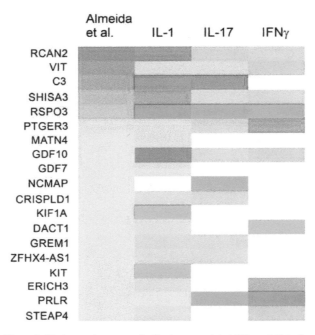

Figure 3. Heatmap of genes markedly downregulated (FC < −2.5) in degraded cartilage in the study by Almeida et al. [35] and significantly affected by at least one studied proinflammatory cytokine. Upregulated genes are marked with red, downregulated with blue, and genes with no significant fold change with white.

Relatively few genes were significantly affected by IL-4 in our data, and none of them were markedly (with FC > 2.5) associated with either degraded or preserved cartilage in the data of Almeida et al. [35]. However, looking at genes with a smaller proportional difference between degraded and preserved cartilage (FC > 1.5 in either direction) produced several genes that were significantly affected by IL-4. Ten genes (including *DUSP5* and *COL7A1*) were upregulated in degraded cartilage and also upregulated in C(IL-4) cells. In contrast, one gene associated with degraded cartilage (*HMMR*) was downregulated by IL-4, and seven genes (including *COL14A1*) associated with preserved cartilage were upregulated by IL-4. (Table S6)

To demonstrate that naïve chondrocytes can be affected by the cytokines studied, we separately studied the expression of their receptors. As shown in Table S7, receptors for all studied cytokines were expressed in unstimulated OA chondrocytes at meaningful levels.

3. Discussion

Chondrocytes from OA patients were found to adopt distinct phenotypes in response to the central $T_H1/T_H2/T_H17$ cytokines. The phenotype induced by the T_H1 cytokine interleukin 1 (IL-1β), the C(IL-1β) phenotype, can be characterized by widespread, strong upregulation of inflammation and catabolism as well as downregulation of metabolic signaling. The effects of the T_H17 cytokine IL-17 appear to be somewhat less widespread and partly overlapping those of IL-1β, with induction of inflammatory and chemotactic factors. The phenotype induced by the second T_H1 cytokine interferon gamma (IFNγ) seems to be distinct from both C(IL-1β) and C(IL-17) phenotypes, with a significant theme of antigen processing and presentation. The effects of the T_H2 cytokine IL-4 were much more modest; some factors involved in the regulation of inflammation and TGFβ signaling were upregulated, while the downregulated genes were mostly associated with cell proliferation and migration.

In T cells, the T_H1 phenotype drives inflammation and defense against intracellular pathogens (cell-mediated immunity) and is associated with the production of proinflammatory cytokines such as IFNγ and IL-1β [36]. Conversely, T_H2 cells promote humoral immunity, regulate inflammation and direct resolving and injury-healing responses [11]. Central T_H2 cytokines are IL-4 and IL-13. A third relatively well-established population of T_H cells is the T_H17 phenotype. These cells produce IL-17, drive autoimmune reactions and activate neutrophils. This contrasts with T_H1 cells that preferentially affect monocytes/macrophages, as well as T_H2 cells that are associated with eosinophils, basophils and mast cells [37].

The central $T_H1/T_H2/T_H17$ cytokines also induce loosely analogous macrophage phenotypes. Like T_H1 cells, M1 or "classically activated" macrophages are induced by proinflammatory cytokines such as IL-1β and IFNγ and promote inflammation by secreting further proinflammatory factors. M2 or "alternatively activated" macrophages are induced canonically by IL-4. In addition to functioning as antiparasite effectors, they attenuate inflammation, direct wound-healing processes and promote the resolution of inflammation. [38] IL-17 induces a less-studied macrophage phenotype characterized by increased chemotaxis and the production of proinflammatory factors such as cyclooxygenase 2 (COX-2), IL-6 and tumor necrosis factor alpha (TNFα) [15,39] as well as resolution-promoting effects in the later phases of inflammation [16].

The chondrocyte phenotypes induced by different cytokines in our study can be considered analogous to T_H cell and particularly macrophage phenotypes. IL-1β affects a very large number of genes and induces a phenotype characterized by the expression of inflammatory and matrix-degrading genes. The C(IL-17) phenotype appears likewise proinflammatory, but with a somewhat more limited repertoire of inflammatory genes. C(IFNγ) also appears to be a phenotype that is inflammatory, but is also characterized by genes linked to antigen presentation. The C(IL-4) phenotype is characterized by the expression of genes linked to TGFβ signaling and the regulation of inflammation.

The chondrocyte phenotypes induced by the $T_H1/T_H2/T_H17$ cytokines appeared to be quite distinct as only 45 genes were markedly (FC > 2.5) upregulated and eight markedly downregulated (FC < −2.5) by all three proinflammatory cytokines, considering that hundreds of genes were up- and dozens downregulated to a similar extent by each of the three cytokines. The factors upregulated by all of the three proinflammatory cytokines (IL-1β, IFNy and IL-17) include the well-known inflammatory mediators *IL6*, nitric oxide synthase 2/inducible nitric oxide synthase (*NOS2*/iNOS) and prostaglandin-endoperoxide synthase 2/cyclooxygenase 2 (*PTGS2*/COX-2). On this list were also included, for example, pentraxin 3 (*PTX3*), toll-like receptor 2 (*TLR2*), chemokine (C-C motif) ligand 2 (*CCL2*), interferon regulatory factor 4 (*IRF4*) and prolactin receptor (*PRLR*). Pentraxin 3 (*PTX*) promotes inflammation by activating the classical complement pathway and by facilitating antigen recognition by mononuclear phagocytes [40], and it has been shown to be elevated in the serum and synovial fluid of patients with rheumatoid arthritis [41]. *TLR2* is a pattern recognition receptor mediating innate immune activation by microbial particles. In osteoarthritis, it is activated by hyaluronan and aggrecan fragments leading to the activation of nuclear factor kappa-light-chain-enhancer of activated B cells (NF-κB) signaling, which may contribute to OA progression and pain [42,43]. *CCL2* is a monocyte-attracting chemokine that has been linked to OA development and pain [44,45]. *IRF4* has recently been associated with cartilage destruction and pain in OA via the induction of CCL17 [46]. Prolactin has been implicated to promote chondrocyte differentiation and attenuate apoptosis, and thus the upregulation of its receptor might promote cartilage survival [47,48].

Factors downregulated by all of the three proinflammatory cytokines include asporin (*ASPN*) and prostaglandin EP3 receptor (*PTGER3*). Asporin belongs to the family of leucine-rich repeat proteins and is associated with cartilage matrix, also bearing a similarity to decorin [49]. The potential role of asporin in OA appears to be unclear; several studies have linked the protein to the development of the disease, where it might impair chondrogenesis by inhibiting TGF-β signaling [50]. Polymorphisms of the asporin gene have also been linked to OA risk [51], even though the most recent meta-analysis failed to find evidence for this [52]. Prostaglandin E2 (PGE2)-induced *PTGER3* downregulation may contribute to cartilage inflammation and damage via NF-κB activation and IL-6 synthesis [53].

When the Gene Ontology (GO) terms significantly affected by the three different proinflammatory cytokines were studied, all three were found to affect those associated with inflammation. IL-1β was alone in significantly affecting several terms, such as cell adhesion, extracellular matrix metabolism and collagen catabolism, linking the chondrocyte phenotype induced by this cytokine to these functions. IL-17 solely affected nitric oxide synthase biosynthesis. This is intriguing, as the nitric oxide production is an important part of inflammatory response in chondrocytes [54]. The C(IFNγ) phenotype seems to be differentiated from others by activation of pathways related to antigen processing and presentation. Chondrocytes are not considered "professional" antigen-presenting cells, but they have, interestingly, been shown to present cartilage proteoglycans as antigens to CD8+ T cells, potentially contributing to local joint inflammation [55,56].

Previously published genome-wide expression analyses (GWEAs) have identified a number of differentially expressed genes between either damaged and intact OA cartilage or healthy and OA cartilage. These include genes involved in inflammation, skeletal system development, cell adhesion and monosaccharide metabolism [35,57–59]. When comparing our results to those of the comprehensive study by Almeida et al. [35], the C(IL-1β) phenotype most closely resembled degraded OA cartilage, while IL-17 upregulated a smaller number of proinflammatory factors associated with degraded cartilage in that study. Accordingly, some genes associated with preserved as opposed to degraded cartilage were also downregulated by these proinflammatory cytokines. Most of these genes are linked to cartilage anabolism. The effects of IFNγ and (especially) IL-4 on the genes identified by Almeida et al. [35] were more modest. It is important to note that the receptors for all cytokines studied were expressed at marked levels in our samples, which lends further validity to our results.

A potential limitation of the study is that whole thickness pieces of cartilage obtained from joint replacement surgery were used for chondrocyte isolation. Thus, the cells obtained are likely a mixture of chondrocytes from different layers of cartilage, and there might be some differences in the effects of cytokines between these groups. However, all chondrocytes can be expected to be exposed to cytokines diffused from the synovial fluid and/or produced by chondrocytes (in autocrine or paracrine manner). Thus, we think that the observed clear differences in the chondrocyte phenotypes in response to the major $T_H1/T_H2/T_H17$ cytokines are relevant for further understanding of chondrocyte biology and OA pathophysiology. In future studies, cartilage layer-specific cell isolation methods or single-cell RNA-Seq could be considered to unravel possible zone-specific responses.

Another limitation of the study is that the chondrocytes used were obtained from OA joints; therefore, some of the detected effects of the cytokines might differ from those observed in healthy chondrocytes. Studying the effects of the cytokines on healthy chondrocytes would be an interesting avenue of future study; however, obtaining healthy primary human chondrocytes presents a practical challenge (compared to OA chondrocytes which can be obtained from joint replacement surgery). In the present study, we observed similarities between the C(IL-1β) and C(Il-17) phenotypes and the gene expression profile of chondrocytes from degraded OA cartilage published by Almeida et al. [35]; C(IFNγ) and especially C(IL-4) bore less resemblance to that phenotype. This suggests that the cytokine-induced phenotypes observed in our data have relevance regarding OA pathogenesis.

In conclusion, OA chondrocytes, analogously to macrophages, can assume distinct phenotypes in response to the cytokines associated with the $T_H1/T_H2/T_H17$ phenotypes of T helper cells. These results provide novel information on chondrocyte biology and the pathogenesis of OA with further insights into the development of disease-modifying drugs for (osteo)arthritis.

4. Materials and Methods

4.1. Cartilage and Cell Culture

Leftover cartilage pieces were collected from nine patients undergoing total knee replacement surgery in Coxa Hospital for Joint Replacement, Tampere, Finland. All patients fulfilled the American College of Rheumatology classification criteria for knee OA [60]. Patients with diabetes mellitus were excluded from the study to avoid potential confounding effects on chondrocyte metabolism [61]. The study was approved by the Ethics Committee of Tampere University Hospital, Finland, and carried out in accordance with the Declaration of Helsinki. Written informed consent was obtained from the patients. Chondrocyte isolation and culture was carried out as previously described [62]. To ensure an adequate yield of chondrocytes, all available cartilage was removed aseptically using a scalpel from the bony parts received from joint replacement surgery and cut into small pieces. The pieces were first washed with phosphate buffered saline (PBS). After that, they were incubated for 24 h in the presence of Liberase enzyme (Roche, Mannheim, Germany) 0.25 mg/mL, diluted in serumless Dulbecco's modified Eagle's medium (DMEM, Sigma-Aldrich, St Louis, MO, USA) with glutamax-I containing penicillin (100 units/mL), streptomycin (100 µg/mL), and amphotericin B (250 ng/mL) (all three from Invitrogen, Carlsbad, CA, USA) at 37 °C. The resulting cell suspension was poured through a 70 µm nylon mesh and centrifuged for five minutes at 200 g. Cells were then washed twice and seeded on 24-well plates (0.2 million cells/mL) in DMEM supplemented with 10% heat-inactivated fetal bovine serum (Lonza) together with the aforementioned compounds. Confluent cultures were exposed to fresh culture medium alone, with 10 ng/mL IFNγ, with 100 pg/mL IL-1β, with 50 ng/mL IL-17 or with 10 ng/mL IL-4, for 24 h. The concentrations used were chosen based on our preliminary experiments with cultured chondrocytes.

4.2. RNA Isolation and Sample Preparation

Culture medium was removed at the indicated time points and total RNA of the chondrocytes was extracted with GenElute Mammalian Total RNA Miniprep kit (Sigma-Aldrich). The sample was treated with DNAse I (Fermentas UAB, Vilnius, Lithuania). RNA concentration and integrity were confirmed with the 2100 Bioanalyzer (Agilent Technologies, Santa Clara, CA, USA).

4.3. Next Generation Sequencing and Data Analysis

Sequencing of samples was performed in the Finnish Institute of Molecular Medicine (FIMM) sequencing core, Helsinki, Finland, using the Illumina HiSeq 2500 sequencing platform. Sequencing depth was 20 million paired-end reads 100 bp in length. Read quality was first assessed using FastQC [63], and the reads were trimmed using Trimmomatic [64]. Trimmed reads were aligned to reference human genome with STAR [65]. Count matrices were prepared with the featureCounts program [66]. Differential expression was assessed with DESeq2 [67]. Gene expression levels were given as DeSeq2-normalized counts, and genes with an average normalized count 10 or less across all samples were excluded from further analysis. For the purposes of further analysis, genes with a minimum of 2.5 fold change (FC) in abundance and FDR-corrected p-value < 0.05 were deemed biologically and statistically significant (unless otherwise indicated). Functional analysis was performed against the Gene Ontology (GO) database [68,69] using the DAVID tool [70], and REVIGO was used to reduce the resulting list [71].

4.4. Statistics

For NGS data analysis, normalization was performed and differential expression studied using a negative binomial model implemented in DESeq2.

Supplementary Materials: The following are available online at https://www.mdpi.com/article/10.3390/ijms22179463/s1.

Author Contributions: Conceptualization, A.P., T.L., M.H., T.M. and E.M.; funding acquisition, A.P. and E.M.; investigation, A.P., T.L., M.H. and T.M.; methodology, A.P., T.L., M.H., T.M. and E.M.; project administration, T.M. and E.M.; resources, T.M. and E.M.; supervision, E.M.; validation, A.P., T.L. and M.H.; visualization, A.P.; writing—original draft, A.P.; writing—review and editing, A.P., T.L., M.H., T.M. and E.M. All authors have read and agreed to the published version of the manuscript.

Funding: This study was supported by grants from the Finnish Society of Rheumatology, Tampere Rheumatism Foundation, the competitive research funding of Pirkanmaa Hospital District and the Scandinavian Rheumatology Research Foundation. The funders had no role in study design, data collection and analysis, decision to publish, or preparation of the manuscript.

Institutional Review Board Statement: This study was approved by the Ethics Committee of Tampere University Hospital, Finland (ref# ETL R09116).

Informed Consent Statement: This study was approved by the Ethics Committee of Tampere University Hospital, Finland. Written informed consent was obtained from all subjects involved in the study.

Data Availability Statement: Complete gene expression data for all samples are available from the corresponding author upon reasonable request.

Acknowledgments: We wish to thank research coordinator Heli Kupari for her skillful assistance with the cartilage samples. We are also thankful to Meiju Kukkonen and Salla Hietakangas for their excellent technical assistance in the laboratory, as well as Heli Määttä for great secretarial help.

Conflicts of Interest: The authors declare that they have no competing interests.

References

1. Hunter, D.J.; Bierma-Zeinstra, S. Osteoarthritis. *Lancet* **2019**, *393*, 1745–1759. [CrossRef]
2. Scanzello, C.R. Chemokines and inflammation in osteoarthritis: Insights from patients and animal models. *J. Orthop. Res.* **2017**, *35*, 735–739. [CrossRef] [PubMed]
3. Greene, M.A.; Loeser, R.F. Aging-related inflammation in osteoarthritis. *Osteoarth. Cartil.* **2015**, *23*, 1966–1971. [CrossRef] [PubMed]
4. Robinson, W.H.; Lepus, C.M.; Wang, Q.; Raghu, H.; Mao, R.; Lindstrom, T.M.; Sokolove, J. Low-grade inflammation as a key mediator of the pathogenesis of osteoarthritis. *Nat. Rev. Rheumatol.* **2016**, *12*, 580–592. [CrossRef]
5. Karsdal, M.A.; Michaelis, M.; Ladel, C.; Siebuhr, A.S.; Bihlet, A.R.; Andersen, J.R.; Guehring, H.; Christiansen, C.; Bay-Jensen, A.C.; Kraus, V.B. Disease-modifying treatments for osteoarthritis (DMOADs) of the knee and hip: Lessons learned from failures and opportunities for the future. *Osteoarthr. Cartil.* **2016**, *24*, 2013–2021. [CrossRef] [PubMed]
6. Aigner, T.; Fundel, K.; Saas, J.; Gebhard, P.M.; Haag, J.; Weiss, T.; Zien, A.; Obermayr, F.; Zimmer, R.; Bartnik, E. Large-scale gene expression profiling reveals major pathogenetic pathways of cartilage degeneration in osteoarthritis. *Arthritis Rheum.* **2006**, *54*, 3533–3544. [CrossRef] [PubMed]
7. Sandy, J.D.; Chan, D.D.; Trevino, R.L.; Wimmer, M.A.; Plaas, A. Human genome-wide expression analysis reorients the study of inflammatory mediators and biomechanics in osteoarthritis. *Osteoarthr. Cartil.* **2015**, *23*, 1939–1945. [CrossRef]
8. Hardingham, T. Extracellular matrix and pathogenic mechanisms in osteoarthritis. *Curr. Rheumatol. Rep.* **2008**, *10*, 30–36. [CrossRef] [PubMed]
9. Maldonado, M.; Nam, J. The Role of Changes in Extracellular Matrix of Cartilage in the Presence of Inflammation on the Pathology of Osteoarthritis. *BioMed Res. Int.* **2013**, *2013*, 284873. [CrossRef]
10. Loeser, R.F.; Collins, J.A.; Diekman, B.O. Ageing and the pathogenesis of osteoarthritis. *Nat. Rev. Rheumatol.* **2016**, *12*, 412–420. [CrossRef]
11. Zhu, J.; Paul, W.E. CD4 T cells: Fates, Functions, and Faults. *Blood, J. Am. Soc. Hematol.* **2008**, *112*, 1557–1569. [CrossRef] [PubMed]
12. Dinarello, C.A. Immunological and Inflammatory Functions of the Interleukin-1 Family [Internet]. *Annu. Rev. Immunol.* **2009**, *27*, 519–550. [CrossRef]

13. Harrington, L.E.; Hatton, R.D.; Mangan, P.R.; Turner, H.; Murphy, T.L.; Murphy, K.M.; Weaver, C.T. Interleukin 17-Producing CD4+ Effector T Cells Develop via a Lineage Distinct from the T Helper Type 1 and 2 Lineages. *Nat. Immunol.* **2005**, *6*, 1123–1132. [CrossRef] [PubMed]

14. Kang, S.; Kumanogoh, A. The Spectrum of Macrophage Activation by Immunometabolism [Internet]. *Int. Immunol.* **2020**, *32*, 467–473. [CrossRef]

15. Raucci, F.; Saviano, A.; Casillo, G.M.; Guerra-Rodriguez, M.; Mansour, A.A.; Piccolo, M.; Ferraro, M.G.; Panza, E.; Vellecco, V.; Irace, C.; et al. IL-17-Induced Inflammation Modulates the mPGES-1/PPAR-γ Pathway in Monocytes/Macrophages. *Br. J. Pharmacol.* **2021**. [CrossRef]

16. Zizzo, G.; Cohen, P.L. IL-17 Stimulates Differentiation of Human Anti-Inflammatory Macrophages and Phagocytosis of Apoptotic Neutrophils in Response to IL-10 and Glucocorticoids. *J. Immunol.* **2013**, *190*, 5237–5246. [CrossRef]

17. Minguzzi, M.; Cetrullo, S.; D'Adamo, S.; Silvestri, Y.; Flamigni, F.; Borzì, R.M. Emerging Players at the Intersection of Chondrocyte Loss of Maturational Arrest, Oxidative Stress, Senescence and Low-Grade Inflammation in Osteoarthritis. *Oxid. Med. Cell. Longev.* **2018**, *2018*, 3075293. [CrossRef]

18. López-Armada, M.J.; Caramés, B.; Lires-Deán, M.; Cillero-Pastor, B.; Ruiz-Romero, C.; Galdo, F.; Blanco, F.J. Cytokines, tumor necrosis factor-alpha and interleukin-1beta, differentially regulate apoptosis in osteoarthritis cultured human chondrocytes. *Osteoarthr. Cartil.* **2006**, *14*, 660–669. [CrossRef] [PubMed]

19. Daheshia, M.; Yao, J.Q. The interleukin 1beta pathway in the pathogenesis of osteoarthritis. *J. Rheumatol.* **2008**, *35*, 2306–2312. [CrossRef]

20. Martel-Pelletier, J.; McCollum, R.; DiBattista, J.; Faure, M.P.; Chin, J.A.; Fournier, S.; Sarfati, M.; Pelletier, J.P. The interleukin-1 receptor in normal and osteoarthritic human articular chondrocytes. Identification as the type I receptor and analysis of binding kinetics and biologic function. *Arthritis Rheum.* **1992**, *35*, 530–540. [CrossRef]

21. Jotanovic, Z.; Mihelic, R.; Sestan, B.; Dembic, Z. Role of Interleukin-1 Inhibitors in Osteoarthritis. *Drugs Aging* **2012**, *29*, 343–358. [CrossRef]

22. Yao, Z.; Painter, S.L.; Fanslow, W.C.; Ulrich, D.; Macduff, B.M.; Spriggs, M.K.; Armitage, R.J. Human IL-17: A novel cytokine derived from T cells. *J. Immunol.* **1995**, *155*, 5483–5486.

23. Miossec, P.; Korn, T.; Kuchroo, V.K. Interleukin-17 and Type 17 Helper T Cells. *N. Engl. J. Med.* **2009**, *361*, 888–898. [CrossRef]

24. Chen, B.; Deng, Y.; Tan, Y.; Qin, J.; Chen, L.-B. Association between severity of knee osteoarthritis and serum and synovial fluid interleukin 17 concentrations. *J. Int. Med. Res.* **2014**, *42*, 138–144. [CrossRef]

25. Martel-Pelletier, J.; Mineau, F.; Jovanovic, D.; Di Battista, J.A.; Pelletier, J.-P. Mitogen-activated protein kinase and nuclear factor κB together regulate interleukin-17-induced nitric oxide production in human osteoarthritic chondrocytes: Possible role of transactivating factor mitogen-activated protein kinase-activated protein kinase. *Arthritis Rheum.* **1999**, *42*, 2399–2409. [CrossRef]

26. Pacquelet, S.; Presle, N.; Boileau, C.; Dumond, H.; Netter, P.; Martel-Pelletier, J.; Pelletier, J.-P.; Terlain, B.; Jouzeau, J.-Y. Interleukin 17, a nitric oxide-producing cytokine with a peroxynitrite-independent inhibitory effect on proteoglycan synthesis. *J. Rheumatol.* **2002**, *29*, 2602–2610.

27. Benderdour, M.; Tardif, G.; Pelletier, J.-P.; Di Battista, J.A.; Reboul, P.; Ranger, P.; Martel-Pelletier, J. Interleukin 17 (IL-17) induces collagenase-3 production in human osteoarthritic chondrocytes via AP-1 dependent activation: Differential activation of AP-1 members by IL-17 and IL-1beta. *J. Rheumatol.* **2002**, *29*, 1262–1272. [PubMed]

28. Nakashima, T.; Kobayashi, Y.; Yamasaki, S.; Kawakami, A.; Eguchi, K.; Sasaki, H.; Sakai, H. Protein Expression and Functional Difference of Membrane-Bound and Soluble Receptor Activator of NF-κB Ligand: Modulation of the Expression by Osteotropic Factors and Cytokines. *Biochem. Biophys. Res. Commun.* **2000**, *275*, 768–775. [CrossRef] [PubMed]

29. Nakae, S.; Nambu, A.; Sudo, K.; Iwakura, Y. Suppression of immune induction of collagen-induced arthritis in IL-17-deficient mice. *J. Immunol.* **2003**, *171*, 6173–6177. [CrossRef] [PubMed]

30. Chabaud, M.; Lubberts, E.; Joosten, L.; van den Berg, W.; Miossec, P. IL-17 derived from juxta-articular bone and synovium contributes to joint degradation in rheumatoid arthritis. *Arthritis Res.* **2001**, *3*, 168. [CrossRef] [PubMed]

31. Xu, Y.; Barter, M.J.; Swan, D.C.; Rankin, K.S.; Rowan, A.D.; Santibanez-Koref, M.; Loughlin, J.; Young, D.A. Identification of the pathogenic pathways in osteoarthritic hip cartilage: Commonality and discord between hip and knee OA. *Osteoarthr. Cartil.* **2012**, *20*, 1029–1038. [CrossRef] [PubMed]

32. Santangelo, K.S.; Nuovo, G.J.; Bertone, A.L. In vivo reduction or blockade of interleukin-1β in primary osteoarthritis influences expression of mediators implicated in pathogenesis. *Osteoarthr. Cartil.* **2012**, *20*, 1610–1618. [CrossRef] [PubMed]

33. Hoff, P.; Buttgereit, F.; Burmester, G.-R.; Jakstadt, M.; Gaber, T.; Andreas, K.; Matziolis, G.; Perka, C.; Röhner, E. Osteoarthritis synovial fluid activates pro-inflammatory cytokines in primary human chondrocytes. *Int. Orthop.* **2013**, *37*, 145–151. [CrossRef]

34. Li, S.; Ren, Y.; Peng, D.; Yuan, Z.; Shan, S.; Sun, H.; Yan, X.; Xiao, H.; Li, G.; Song, H. TIM-3 Genetic Variations Affect Susceptibility to Osteoarthritis by Interfering with Interferon Gamma in CD4+ T Cells. *Inflammation* **2015**, *38*, 1857–1863. [CrossRef] [PubMed]

35. de Almeida, R.C.; Ramos, Y.F.; Mahfouz, A.; den Hollander, W.; Lakenberg, N.; Houtman, E.; van Hoolwerff, M.; Suchiman, H.E.D.; Rodríguez Ruiz, A.; Slagboom, P.E.; et al. RNA sequencing data integration reveals an miRNA interactome of osteoarthritis cartilage. *Ann. Rheum Dis.* **2019**, *78*, 270–277. [CrossRef]

36. Chizzolini, C.; Chicheportiche, R.; Burger, D.; Dayer, J.M. Human Th1 Cells Preferentially Induce Interleukin (IL)-1β While Th2 Cells Induce IL-1 Receptor Antagonist Production upon Cell/Cell Contact with Monocytes. *Eur. J. Immunol.* **1997**, *27*, 171–177. [CrossRef]

37. Weaver, C.T.; Elson, C.O.; Fouser, L.A.; Kolls, J.K. The Th17 Pathway and Inflammatory Diseases of the Intestines, Lungs and Skin. *Annu. Rev. Pathol.* **2013**, *8*, 477. [CrossRef] [PubMed]
38. Hume, D.A. The Many Alternative Faces of Macrophage Activation. *Front Immunol.* **2015**, *6*, 370. [CrossRef]
39. Alonso, M.N.; Wong, M.T.; Zhang, A.L.; Winer, D.; Suhoski, M.M.; Tolentino, L.L.; Gaitan, J.; Davidson, M.G.; Kung, T.H.; Galel, D.M.; et al. TH1, TH2, and TH17 Cells Instruct Monocytes to Differentiate into Specialized Dendritic Cell Subsets. *Blood J. Am. Soc. Hematol.* **2011**, *118*, 3311–3320. [CrossRef]
40. Diniz, S.N.; Nomizo, R.; Cisalpino, P.S.; Teixeira, M.M.; Brown, G.D.; Mantovani, A.; Gordon, S.; Reis, L.F.L.; Dias, A.A.M. PTX3 function as an opsonin for the dectin-1-dependent internalization of zymosan by macrophages. *J. Leukoc. Biol.* **2004**, *75*, 649–656. [CrossRef]
41. Sharma, A.; Khan, R.; Gupta, N.; Sharma, A.; Zaheer, M.S.; Abbas, M.; Khan, S.A. Acute phase reactant, Pentraxin 3, as a novel marker for the diagnosis of rheumatoid arthritis. *Clin. Chim. Acta* **2018**, *480*, 65–70. [CrossRef] [PubMed]
42. Liu, Y.-X.; Wang, G.-D.; Wang, X.; Zhang, Y.-L.; Zhang, T.-L. Effects of TLR-2/NF-κB signaling pathway on the occurrence of degenerative knee osteoarthritis: An in vivo and in vitro study. *Oncotarget* **2017**, *8*, 38602–38617. [CrossRef] [PubMed]
43. Miller, R.E.; Ishihara, S.; Tran, P.B.; Golub, S.B.; Last, K.; Miller, R.J.; Fosang, A.J.; Malfait, A.-M. An aggrecan fragment drives osteoarthritis pain through Toll-like receptor 2. *JCI Insight* **2018**, *3*, e95704. [CrossRef]
44. Raghu, H.; Lepus, C.M.; Wang, Q.; Wong, H.H.; Lingampalli, N.; Oliviero, F.; Punzi, L.; Giori, N.J.; Goodman, S.B.; Chu, C.R.; et al. CCL2/CCR2, but not CCL5/CCR5, mediates monocyte recruitment, inflammation and cartilage destruction in osteoarthritis. *Ann. Rheum. Dis.* **2017**, *76*, 914–922. [CrossRef]
45. Miller, R.J.; Malfait, A.M.; Miller, R.E. The Innate Immune Response as a Mediator of Osteoarthritis Pain [Internet]. *Osteoarthr. Cartil.* **2020**, *28*, 562–571. [CrossRef]
46. Lee, M.-C.; Saleh, R.; Achuthan, A.; Fleetwood, A.J.; Förster, I.; Hamilton, J.A.; Cook, A.D. CCL17 blockade as a therapy for osteoarthritis pain and disease. *Arthritis Res. Ther.* **2018**, *20*, 62. [CrossRef]
47. Adán, N.; Guzmán-Morales, J.; Ledesma-Colunga, M.G.; Perales-Canales, S.I.; Quintanar-Stéphano, A.; López-Barrera, F.; Méndez, I.; Moreno-Carranza, B.; Triebel, J.; Binart, N.; et al. Prolactin promotes cartilage survival and attenuates inflammation in inflammatory arthritis. *J. Clin. Investig.* **2013**, *123*, 3902–3913. [CrossRef]
48. Ogueta, S.; Muñoz, J.; Obregon, E.; Delgado-Baeza, E.; García-Ruiz, J.P. Prolactin Is a Component of the Human Synovial Liquid and Modulates the Growth and Chondrogenic Differentiation of Bone Marrow-Derived Mesenchymal Stem Cells. *Mol. Cell. Endocrinol.* **2002**, *190*, 51–63. [CrossRef]
49. Lorenzo, P.; Aspberg, A.; Onnerfjord, P.; Bayliss, M.T.; Neame, P.J.; Heinegard, D. Identification and characterization of asporin. a novel member of the leucine-rich repeat protein family closely related to decorin and biglycan. *J. Biol. Chem.* **2001**, *276*, 12201–12211. [CrossRef]
50. Xu, L.; Li, Z.; Liu, S.-Y.; Xu, S.-Y.; Ni, G.-X. Asporin and osteoarthritis. *Osteoarthr. Cartil.* **2015**, *23*, 933–939. [CrossRef] [PubMed]
51. Zhu, X.; Jiang, L.; Lu, Y.; Wang, C.; Zhou, S.; Wang, H.; Tian, T. Association of aspartic acid repeat polymorphism in the asporin gene with osteoarthritis of knee, hip, and hand. *Medicine (Baltimore)* **2018**, *97*, e0200. [CrossRef]
52. Wang, J.; Yang, A.; Zhang, J.; Sun, N.; Li, X.; Li, X.; Liu, Q.; Li, J.; Ren, X.; Ke, Z.; et al. Genetic polymorphism in the asporin gene is not a key risk factor for osteoarthritis: Evidence based on an updated cumulative meta-analysis. *Exp. Ther. Med.* **2018**, *15*, 3952–3966. [CrossRef]
53. Wang, P.; Zhu, F.; Lee, N.H.; Konstantopoulos, K. Shear-induced interleukin-6 synthesis in chondrocytes: Roles of E prostanoid (EP) 2 and EP3 in cAMP/protein kinase A- and PI3-K/Akt-dependent NF-kappaB activation. *J. Biol. Chem.* **2010**, *285*, 24793–24804. [CrossRef]
54. Eitner, A.; Müller, S.; König, C.; Wilharm, A.; Raab, R.; Hofmann, G.O.; Kamradt, T.; Schaible, H.G. Inhibition of Inducible Nitric Oxide Synthase Prevents il-1β-Induced Mitochondrial Dysfunction in Human Chondrocytes. *Int. J. Mol. Sci.* **2021**, *22*, 2477. [CrossRef]
55. Kuhne, M.; Erben, U.; Schulze-Tanzil, G.; Köhler, D.; Wu, P.; Richter, F.J.; John, T.; Radbruch, A.; Sieper, J.; Appel, H. HLA-B27-Restricted Antigen Presentation by Human Chondrocytes to CD8+ T Cells: Potential Contribution to Local Immunopathologic Processes in Ankylosing Spondylitis. *Arthritis Rheum.* **2009**, *60*, 1635–1646. [CrossRef] [PubMed]
56. Brennan, F.R.; Mikecz, K.; Buzás, E.I.; Glant, T.T. Interferon-Gamma but not Granulocyte/Macrophage Colony-Stimulating Factor Augments Proteoglycan Presentation by Synovial Cells and Chondrocytes to an Autopathogenic T Cell Hybridoma. *Immunol. Lett.* **1995**, *45*, 87–91. [CrossRef]
57. Lewallen, E.A.; Bonin, C.A.; Li, X.; Smith, J.; Karperien, M.; Larson, A.N.; Lewallen, D.G.; Cool, S.M.; Westendorf, J.J.; Krych, A.J.; et al. The synovial microenvironment of osteoarthritic joints alters RNA-seq expression profiles of human primary articular chondrocytes. *Gene* **2016**, *591*, 456–464. [CrossRef]
58. Dunn, S.L.; Soul, J.; Anand, S.; Schwartz, J.-M.; Boot-Handford, R.P.; Hardingham, T.E. Gene expression changes in damaged osteoarthritic cartilage identify a signature of non-chondrogenic and mechanical responses. *Osteoarthr. Cartil.* **2016**, *24*, 1431–1440. [CrossRef] [PubMed]
59. Ramos, Y.F.M.; den Hollander, W.; Bovée, J.V.M.G.; Bomer, N.; Breggen, R.; Lakenberg, N.; Keurentjes, J.C.; Goeman, J.J.; Slagboom, P.E.; Nelissen, R.G.H.H.; et al. Genes Involved in the Osteoarthritis Process Identified through Genome Wide Expression Analysis in Articular Cartilage; the RAAK Study. *PLoS ONE* **2014**, *9*, e103056. [CrossRef] [PubMed]

60. Altman, R.; Asch, E.; Bloch, D.; Bole, G.; Borenstein, D.; Brandt, K.; Christy, W.; Cooke, T.D.; Greenwald, R.; Hochberg, M.; et al. Development of criteria for the classification and reporting of osteoarthritis: Classification of osteoarthritis of the knee. *Arthritis Rheum.* **1986**, *29*, 1039–1049. [CrossRef]

61. Mobasheri, A.; Vannucci, S.J.; Bondy, C.A.; Carter, S.D.; Innes, J.F.; Arteaga, M.F.; Trujillo, E.; Ferraz, I.; Shakibaei, M.; Martín-Vasallo, P. Glucose transport and metabolism in chondrocytes: A key to understanding chondrogenesis, skeletal development and cartilage degradation in osteoarthritis. *Histol. Histopathol.* **2002**, *17*, 1239–1267. [PubMed]

62. Koskinen, A.; Juslin, S.; Nieminen, R.; Moilanen, T.; Vuolteenaho, K.; Moilanen, E. Adiponectin associates with markers of cartilage degradation in osteoarthritis and induces production of proinflammatory and catabolic factors through mitogen-activated protein kinase pathways. *Arthritis Res. Ther.* **2011**, *13*, R184. [CrossRef] [PubMed]

63. Andrews, S. FastQC: A Quality Control Tool for High Throughput Sequence Data. 2010. Available online: https://www.bioinformatics.babraham.ac.uk/projects/fastqc/ (accessed on 19 April 2021).

64. Bolger, A.M.; Lohse, M.; Usadel, B. Trimmomatic: A flexible trimmer for Illumina sequence data. *Bioinformatics* **2014**, *30*, 2114–2120. [CrossRef] [PubMed]

65. Dobin, A.; Davis, C.A.; Schlesinger, F.; Drenkow, J.; Zaleski, C.; Jha, S.; Batut, P.; Chaisson, M.; Gingeras, T.R. STAR: Ultrafast universal RNA-seq aligner. *Bioinformatics* **2013**, *29*, 15–21. [CrossRef]

66. Liao, Y.; Smyth, G.K.; Shi, W. featureCounts: An efficient general purpose program for assigning sequence reads to genomic features. *Bioinformatics* **2014**, *30*, 923–930. [CrossRef]

67. Love, M.I.; Huber, W.; Anders, S. Moderated estimation of fold change and dispersion for RNA-seq data with DESeq2. *Genome Biol.* **2014**, *15*, 550. [CrossRef]

68. Ashburner, M.; Ball, C.A.; Blake, J.A.; Botstein, D.; Butler, H.; Cherry, J.M.; Davis, A.P.; Dolinski, K.; Dwight, S.S.; Eppig, J.T.; et al. Gene Ontology: Tool for the unification of biology. *Nat. Genet.* **2000**, *25*, 25–29. [CrossRef]

69. The Gene Ontology Consortium. Expansion of the Gene Ontology knowledgebase and resources. *Nucleic Acids Res.* **2017**, *45*, D331–D338. [CrossRef]

70. Huang, D.W.; Sherman, B.T.; Lempicki, R.A. Systematic and Integrative Analysis of Large Gene Lists Using DAVID Bioinformatics Resources. *Nat. Protoc.* **2009**, *4*, 44–57. [CrossRef]

71. Supek, F.; Bošnjak, M.; Škunca, N.; Šmuc, T. REVIGO Summarizes and Visualizes Long Lists of Gene Ontology Terms. *PLoS ONE* **2011**, *6*, e21800. [CrossRef]

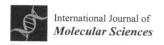

International Journal of
Molecular Sciences

MDPI

Review

Cytokines and Chemokines Involved in Osteoarthritis Pathogenesis

Vilim Molnar [1,2,3], Vid Matišić [1,2], Ivan Kodvanj [4], Roko Bjelica [1,2], Željko Jelec [1,2,5], Damir Hudetz [1,2,3,6], Eduard Rod [1,2], Fabijan Čukelj [1,2,7,8,9], Trpimir Vrdoljak [1,2,6], Dinko Vidović [1,2,7], Mario Starešinić [10], Srećko Sabalić [7], Borut Dobričić [1,2,11], Tadija Petrović [1,2,8], Darko Antičević [1,2,12], Igor Borić [1,2,9,10,13,14], Rok Košir [15], Uršula Prosenc Zmrzljak [15] and Dragan Primorac [1,2,3,10,12,13,14,16,17,18,*]

1 St. Catherine Specialty Hospital, 49210 Zabok, Croatia; vilim.molnar@svkatarina.hr (V.M.);
   vid.matisic@svkatarina.hr (V.M.); roko.bjelica@gmail.com (R.B.); zeljko.jelec@svkatarina.hr (Ž.J.);
   ortohud@gmail.com (D.H.); eduard.rod@svkatarina.hr (E.R.); fabijan.cukelj@svkatarina.hr (F.Č.);
   trpimir.vrdoljak@svkatarina.hr (T.V.); dinko.vidovic@gmail.com (D.V.); dobricic_borut@yahoo.de (B.D.);
   tadijap@gmail.com (T.P.); darko.anticevic@gmail.com (D.A.); igor.boric@svkatarina.hr (I.B.)
2 St. Catherine Specialty Hospital, 10000 Zagreb, Croatia
3 Faculty of Medicine, Josip Juraj Strossmayer University of Osijek, 31000 Osijek, Croatia
4 Department of Pharmacology, School of Medicine, University of Zagreb, 10000 Zagreb, Croatia;
   ikodvanj@gmail.com
5 Department of Nursing, University North, 48000 Varaždin, Croatia
6 Department of Orthopaedic Surgery, Clinical Hospital "Sveti Duh", 10000 Zagreb, Croatia
7 University Hospital "Sisters of Mercy", Clinic for Traumatology, Draškovićeva 19, 10000 Zagreb, Croatia;
   ssabalic@gmail.com
8 Department of Health Studies, University of Split, 21000 Split, Croatia
9 Department of Traumatology, Medical University Merkur Hospital, 10000 Zagreb, Croatia
10 Medical School, University of Split, 21000 Split, Croatia; mstaresinic@yahoo.com
11 Department of Orthopaedics and Traumatology, University Hospital Dubrava, 10000 Zagreb, Croatia
12 Faculty of Dental Medicine and Health, Josip Juraj Strossmayer University of Osijek, 31000 Osijek, Croatia
13 Medical School, University of Mostar, 88000 Mostar, Bosnia and Herzegovina
14 Medical School, University of Rijeka, 51000 Rijeka, Croatia
15 Molecular Biology Laboratory, BIA Separations CRO, Labena Ltd., 1000 Ljubljana, Slovenia;
   rok.kosir@labena.si (R.K.); ursula.prosenc@biaseparationscro.com (U.P.Z.)
16 Medical School REGIOMED, 96450 Coburg, Germany
17 Eberly College of Science, State College, The Pennsylvania State University, University Park, PA 16802, USA
18 The Henry C. Lee College of Criminal Justice and Forensic Sciences, University of New Haven,
   West Haven, CT 06516, USA
* Correspondence: draganprimorac2@gmail.com; Tel.: +385-98-470-710

Citation: Molnar, V.; Matišić, V.;
Kodvanj, I.; Bjelica, R.; Jelec, Ž.;
Hudetz, D.; Rod, E.; Čukelj, F.;
Vrdoljak, T.; Vidović, D.; et al.
Cytokines and Chemokines Involved
in Osteoarthritis Pathogenesis. *Int. J.
Mol. Sci.* 2021, 22, 9208. https://
doi.org/10.3390/ijms22179208

Academic Editor: Alfonso Baldi

Received: 30 June 2021
Accepted: 24 August 2021
Published: 26 August 2021

Publisher's Note: MDPI stays neutral
with regard to jurisdictional claims in
published maps and institutional affiliations.

Abstract: Osteoarthritis is a common cause of disability worldwide. Although commonly referred to as a disease of the joint cartilage, osteoarthritis affects all joint tissues equally. The pathogenesis of this degenerative process is not completely understood; however, a low-grade inflammation leading to an imbalance between anabolic and katabolic processes is a well-established factor. The complex network of cytokines regulating these processes and cell communication has a central role in the development and progression of osteoarthritis. Concentrations of both proinflammatory and anti-inflammatory cytokines were found to be altered depending on the osteoarthritis stage and activity. In this review, we analyzed individual cytokines involved in the immune processes with an emphasis on their function in osteoarthritis.

Keywords: osteoarthritis; cytokines; chemokines; pathogenesis; inflammation; biomarker

1. Introduction

Osteoarthritis (OA) is the most common musculoskeletal condition and the largest cause of disability in the world [1]. The knee is predominantly affected in OA. A recent study concluded that knee OA globally affects 16% of the population, more often women, and that its prevalence, due to today's lifestyle, higher obesity rates and higher average life expectancy, is constantly increasing [2]. Although OA is often referred to as a joint disease with damage and loss of cartilage, OA is a much more diverse disease with complex pathogenesis that affects all tissues within the joint [3].

One of the most important factors in the pathogenesis of OA is a disturbed cytokine balance in favor of proinflammatory cytokines that by their action initiate a vicious cycle that leads to final effects such as damage to cartilage and other intra-articular structures by activating catabolic enzymes (matrix metalloproteinases (MMPs) and ADAMTS (a disintegrin-like and metalloproteinase with thrombospondin motif)) (Figure 1) [4]. The most important inflammatory mediators in the pathogenesis of OA are IL-1β, TNF-α and IL-6. They are activators of a plethora of different signaling pathways that activate other cytokines and pathologic processes. Part of this unstoppable process are chemokines that, stimulated by cytokines, attract inflammatory cells to the joint that further promote the secretion of inflammatory factors and disease progression [5]. The aim of this review was to describe the mechanisms of action of the most important cytokines and chemokines involved in OA pathogenesis, with emphasis on knee OA.

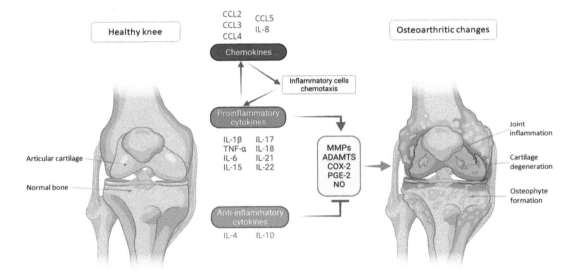

Figure 1. Schematic representation of key inflammatory processes and factors in osteoarthritis pathogenesis. The disturbed balance of proinflammatory and anti-inflammatory cytokines (in favor of proinflammatory cytokines) is responsible for the secretion of enzymes and other inflammatory factors involved in the pathogenesis of osteoarthritis leading to morphological changes within the joint such as cartilage degeneration, osteophyte formation and other inflammatory changes such as synovitis. Chemokines also contribute to inflammatory processes, stimulating the chemotaxis of inflammatory cells that then further secrete proinflammatory cytokines, thus creating a vicious circle that poses a major challenge in treating and slowing the progression of osteoarthritis. IL—interleukin; CCL-CC—chemokine ligand; TNF-α—tumor necrosis factor α; MMPs—matrix metalloproteinases (MMPs); ADAMTS—a disintegrin-like and metalloproteinase with thrombospondin motif; COX-2—cyclooxygenase-2; PGE-2—prostaglandin E2; NO—nitric oxide.

2. Cytokines and Chemokines Involved in Knee Osteoarthritis Pathogenesis

2.1. Proinflammatory Cytokines

2.1.1. IL-1β

IL-1β is one of the main proinflammatory cytokines involved in the pathogenesis of numerous diseases and a member of the IL-1 superfamily, which consists of IL-1α,

IL-1β, IL36α, IL-36β, IL-36γ, IL-36RA, IL-37, IL-38 and IL-1Ra (IL-1 receptor antagonist). It achieves its effects by binding to the receptor named type I IL-1 receptor I (IL-1RI), a type I transmembrane protein that is the binding site of IL-1α and IL-1Ra as well [6]. IL-1Ra competes for an IL-1RI binding site with IL-1β with antagonistic activity. These receptors are expressed on a number of cell types in the knee joint, including chondrocytes, synoviocytes, osteoblasts, osteoclasts and inflammatory cells such as macrophages [7]. Furthermore, it has been observed that the number of IL-1RI is increased in isolated human OA chondrocytes in vitro [8]. By binding to the receptor, IL-1β activates several signaling pathways, which, combined, lead to the progression of OA. IL-1Ra binds to the same receptors as IL-1β and acts as its competitive antagonist, thus blocking IL-1β proinflammatory effects. Although IL-1Ra is an anti-inflammatory mediator, its plasma levels have been found to correlate with the radiological stage of symptomatic OA and its progression, regardless of risk factors such as age, sex and body mass index, confirming the idea of a constant competition of proinflammatory and anti-inflammatory factors in OA [9].

Through mitogen-activated protein kinase (MAPK) signaling, IL-1β induces catabolic events such as cartilage degradation, as the most dominant process in OA. MAPK consists of three families: extracellular signal-regulated kinases (ERKs), c-Jun N-terminal kinases (JNKs) and p38 MAPKs. By downregulating type II collagen and aggrecan gene expression, ERK activation by IL-1β reduces cartilage extracellular matrix (ECM) production [10]. JNK signaling also inhibits collagen synthesis through SOX-9 suppression [11]. Furthermore, IL-1β leads to ECM degradation by inducing collagenases and aggrecanases such as MMP-1 (via ERK, p38, JNK), MMP-3 (via ERK), MMP-13 (via ERK, p38, JNK), ADAMTS-4 (via ERK, p38, JNK) and ADAMTS-5 (via JNK) [12]. These catabolic events result in chondrocyte hypertrophy, dedifferentiation and, finally, apoptosis [13]. Through all three MAPK signaling pathways, IL-1β stimulates the secretion of IL-6, LIF and other proinflammatory cytokines, which potentiate the catabolic effects of IL-1β and at the same time serve as catabolic mediators on their own [12]. In that way, IL-1β can upregulate itself through a positive feedback mechanism. ERK-mediated effects can also be activated by PGE-2 (prostaglandin E2), NO (nitric oxide) and COX-2 (cyclooxygenase-2), inflammatory mediators that are, again, induced by IL-1β [14]. These mediators also contribute to synovial inflammation, which additionally enhances the secretion of IL-1β and other cytokines and aggravates the vicious circle of OA progression [15].

Another important signaling pathway in IL-1β mediated OA progression is NF-κB, which, when activated, leads to inhibition of type II collagen expression, increased production of matrix metalloproteinases (MMP-1, MMP-2, MMP-3, MMP-7, MMP-8, MMP-9 and MMP-13) and aggrecanases (ADAMTS4 and ADAMTS5), but also COX-2, iNOS, PGE-2 and NO [16,17]. Additionally, the IL-1β-activated NF-κB pathway supports proinflammatory cytokines synthesis and secretion, such as IL-6 and TNF-α [16].

Furthermore, IL-1β-mediated NF-κB activation stimulates the production of various chemokines including IL-8, monocyte chemoattractant protein-1 (MCP-1 or CCL2), CCL5, also known as RANTES (regulated on activation, normal T cell expressed and secreted) and macrophage inflammatory protein-1a (MIP-1a), which, by attracting additional inflammatory cells, potentiate the inflammatory state in the joint [4]. In addition, activated macrophages, attracted to the synovial tissue due to the effects of chemokines, are the primary source of IL-1β secretion in the synovium, which once again confirms the complexity of the vicious inflammatory cycle in OA [12]. A schematic representation of the mechanism of action and effects of IL-1β is shown in Figure 2.

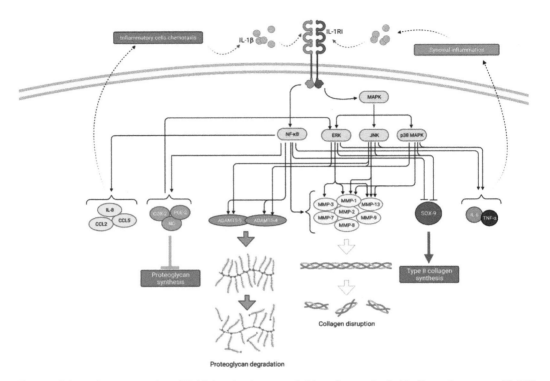

Figure 2. Schematic representation of IL-1β function in osteoarthritis pathogenesis. By binding to its receptor (IL-1RI), IL-1β activates signaling pathways (NF-κB and MAPK) that, by raising the expression of enzymes (ADAMTS and MMPs), lead to catabolic reactions, i.e., proteoglycan degradation and collagen disruption. Furthermore, via the same signaling pathways, IL-1β inhibits type II collagen synthesis through SOX-9 suppression but also proteoglycan synthesis by increasing the synthesis of COX-2, PGE-2 and NO. In addition, IL-1β increases the expression of chemokines such as IL-8, CCL2 and CCL5, as well as the cytokines IL-6 and TNF-α, which attract inflammatory cells and cause synovial inflammation, respectively, resulting in the even greater production and secretion of IL-1β. IL-1β—interleukin 1β; IL-1RI—interleukin 1 receptor 1; MAPK—mitogen-activated protein kinase; ERK—extracellular signal-regulated kinases; JNK—c-Jun N-terminal kinases; NF-κB—nuclear factor kappa-light-chain-enhancer of activated B cells; MMPs—matrix metalloproteinases (MMPs); ADAMTS—a disintegrin-like and metalloproteinase with thrombospondin motif; COX-2—cyclooxygenase-2; PGE—prostaglandin E2; NO—nitric oxide; IL-8—interleukin 8; CCL2—chemokine ligand 2; CCL—chemokine ligand 5; SOX-9—SRY-Box Transcription Factor 9; IL-6—interleukin 6; TNF-α—tumor necrosis factor α.

Due to its significant proinflammatory effects and ability to activate a number of signaling pathways in the pathogenesis of OA, the suppression of IL-1β action has been studied as a potential therapeutic method in treating OA and stopping its progression. However, IL-1β inhibition did not produce the desired effects of preventing OA progression; therefore, the negative results led to the idea that IL-1β does not likely drive OA progression [18–21]. With that in mind, researchers should consider that the pathogenesis of OA does not depend on a single cytokine; rather, the same signaling pathways can be activated by different cytokines, and the interplay of multiple factors is crucial in the onset and progression of the disease.

2.1.2. TNF-α

TNF-α is a potent proinflammatory cytokine that plays an important role in the inflammatory response. As such, it is involved in cell differentiation, proliferation and apoptosis [22]. TNF-α was discovered in 1975 by Carswell et al. as a protein that showed cytotoxic activity and caused the necrotic regression of certain tumor types. Alongside IL-1β, this cytokine is considered the key proinflammatory cytokine in the pathogenesis of OA [23].

It is a part of the tumor necrosis factors superfamily, together with 18 other ligands [24]. The TNF superfamily members are type II transmembrane proteins that can be expressed in soluble and membrane-bound forms [25]. TNF-α is a homotrimeric, cone-shaped protein secreted in two forms, as mentioned above. The membrane-bound form (tmTNF-α) differs from the soluble form (sTNF-α) in its biological activity and is considered more active [26]. TNF-α binds to two isotypes of membrane receptors present on almost all known cell types except erythrocytes and unstimulated T lymphocytes. Tumor necrosis factor receptor 1 (TNRF-1) can be activated by both TNF-α forms, while TNRF-2 is mainly activated by the membrane form. Westacott et al. claim that TNRF-1 activity has a greater impact on local cartilaginous tissue loss, but both receptors are involved in signal transduction related to the pathogenesis of OA [27]. Due to their differences and unique structural features, both receptors are able to participate in different signal pathways [28]. Ligands can induce two different signaling complexes by binding to TNRF-1 receptors. Complex 1 leads to the stimulation of cell survival and the expression of pro-inflammatory genes and complex 2 leads to apoptosis and cell death. Complex 1 is associated with TNFR-1 associated death domain protein (TRADD), which allows for the binding of another two adapter proteins—receptor interacting protein-1 (RIP-1) and TNF receptor-associated factor-2 (TRAF-2). The most important transcription pathways are NF-κB and AP-1. Furthermore, another important signaling pathway is activated by mitogen-activated protein kinases (MAPK), more precisely by its three independent pathways (ERK, JNK and p38 MAPK). On the contrary, signaling complex 2 is directed towards cell death or apoptosis [28,29]. The formation of FADD (Fas-associated death domain protein), procaspase 8/10 and caspase 3 are responsible for programmed cell death. Not so long ago, TNRF-2 initiated signaling was considered less investigated than those initiated by the activation of TNRF-1 receptors. It is claimed that TNRF-2 stimulation notably supports cell activation, migration and proliferation [29]. It activates the JNK kinase and the transcription factor NF-κB. It is worth mentioning that polymorphism in the gene (*M196R*) encoding TNFR-2 may predetermine the development of OA by increasing the number of receptor proteins on the surface of chondrocytes [28]. The mechanism of action of TNF-α is shown in Figure 3.

The activation of the same signaling pathways as IL-1ß results in synergism between these two cytokines [30]. Chondrocytes' synthesis of proteoglycan components and type II collagen is blocked by TNF-α [31]. TNF-α also leads to extracellular matrix (ECM) degradation by inducing collagenases and aggrecanases including MMP-1, MMP-3, MMP-13 and ADAMTS-4, which coincides with IL-1β [32]. The possibility of cartilage repair is vastly reduced because of the earlier mentioned complex 2 signaling pathway and consequent cell apoptosis. Furthermore, TNF-α increases the synthesis of IL-6, IL-8, RANTES and VEGF. Together with the already mentioned IL-1β, TNF-α induces the production of iNOS, COX-2 and PGE-2 synthase, which further upregulates IL-1β and TNF-α production [28]. Considering its proinflammatory nature, it is important to mention that the inhibition of TNF-α could be a sufficient therapeutic option in treating OA. Present data suggest that monoclonal antibodies may exhibit a favorable risk-benefit ratio considering future targeted therapeutic methods. However, current monoclonal antibodies targeting TNF-α such as adalimumab, infliximab and etanercept have shown poor results in clinical studies of general OA patients. They demonstrated only limited benefits in pain reduction and no significant disease modification [33].

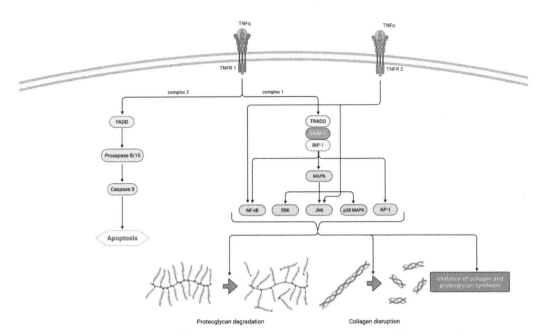

Figure 3. Schematic representation of TNF-α function in osteoarthritis pathogenesis. TNF-α can bind to two receptors, TNRF-1 and TNRF-2. By binding to TNRF-1, TNF-α can induce two different signaling complexes. Complex 1 leads to the stimulation of cell survival and the expression of NF-κB, MAPK and AP-1, which results in proteoglycan degradation, collagen disruption and the inhibition of proteoglycan and collagen synthesis. On the other hand, the activation of complex 2 leads to a cascade of reactions, which include the formation of FADD and the activation of procaspase 8/10 and caspase 3, which consequently leads to cell apoptosis. Additionally, the binding of TNF-α to TNRF-2 activates NF-κB and JNK. In summation, TNF-α leads to degeneration of cartilage and other joint structures, thus contributing to the onset and progression of osteoarthritis. TNF-α—tumor necrosis factor α; TNRF-1—Tumor necrosis factor receptor 1; TNRF-2—Tumor necrosis factor receptor 2; TRADD—TNFR-1 associated death domain protein; RIP-1—receptor interacting protein-1; TRAF-2—TNF receptor-associated factor-2; MAPK—mitogen-activated protein kinase; ERK—extracellular signal-regulated kinases; JNK—c-Jun N-terminal kinases; NF-κB—nuclear factor kappa-light-chain-enhancer of activated B cells; AP-1—activator protein 1; FADD—Fas-associated death domain protein.

2.1.3. IL-6

Classic immunology textbooks commonly depict interleukin-6 (IL-6) as a proinflammatory cytokine important in many inflammatory diseases [34,35]. Contrary to this, the biological role of IL-6 is far more complex.

In 1986, the molecular cloning and structural analysis of B-cell differentiation factor (BCDF) was first reported [36]. Today, BCDF is known as interleukin-6, and as its name suggests, IL-6 is a protein that is essential for the communication between leukocyte cells [37]. IL-6 is a member of the IL-6 family (IL-11, ciliary neurotrophic factor, leukemia inhibitory factor, oncostatin M, cardiotrophin 1, cardiotrophin-like cytokine and IL-27), a group of cytokines that share a common signal-transducing protein gp130 that signals through various signaling pathways, including JAK/STAT (Janus kinase/signal transducers and activators of transcription) and MAPK, PI3K (phosphoinositide 3-kinases), and to which IL-6 has no binding affinity [38,39]. Although it is most commonly mentioned in the context of immune system functioning, IL-6 is essential for various organ systems, including the hematopoietic, endocrine and nervous system, and it is classified as an adipokine and myokine [40,41]. It is produced by a number of cells, including T cells, B cells, granulocytes, smooth muscle cells, eosinophils, mast cells, glial cells and keratinocytes, but in the context of OA, chondrocytes, osteoblasts and synoviocytes are the most important to mention [42,43].

IL-6 acts by binding to the IL-6 receptors, either membrane-bound (mbIL-6R) or soluble (sIL-6R). The binding of IL-6 to sIL-6R forms a complex that associates with ubiquitously expressed gp130 protein and activates *trans*-signaling responsible for the proinflammatory action of IL-6 [44]. On the other hand, the binding of IL-6 and selectively expressed mbIL-6R is considered to form a complex that activates *classic*-signaling responsible for the anti-inflammatory and regenerative properties of IL-6 [44]. Trans-signaling affects virtually all cell types since gp130 is ubiquitously expressed, while classic signaling only affects cells that express mbIL-6R, namely, the hepatocytes, neutrophils, monocytes, macrophages, osteocytes, chondrocytes and some lymphocytes [45–47]. The concentration of sIL-6R is considered a determining factor of *trans*- or classic signaling dominance [48,49]. sIL-6R is considered to be produced as a result of the alternative splicing of mRNA and, to a greater extent, by the proteolytic cleavage of mbIL-6R mediated by metzincin type proteases that are known to have increased expression in OA, specifically a disintegrin and metalloproteinases 10 and 17 (ADAM10 and ADAM17) [50,51]. Furthermore, the endogenous soluble form of gp130 (sgp130) has the ability to bind and stabilize IL-6 and sIL-6R. Although it was initially claimed that this could suppress *trans*-signaling without affecting the classic signaling, newer studies have shown that inhibition of classic signaling can occur as well when there is a molar excess of sIL-6R over IL-6 [52–54]. Interestingly, ADAM10 and 17 can also shed membrane-bound gp130, but their affinity for gp130 is small and thus their proteolytic activity against gp130 is likely not biologically significant [55].

IL-6's exact role in OA is difficult to define, as there are beneficial and detrimental effects of IL-6. In vitro studies on chondrocytes have shown that IL-6 alone can induce TIMP-1, with the effect even more pronounced when chondrocytes are co-treated with sIL-6R [56,57]. Some studies have shown that IL-6, with and without sIL-6R, increases the expression of collagen type 2, while others have shown that IL-6 or IL-6 + sIL-6R treatment inhibits collagen type 2 production via transcriptional control [58]. The combination of IL-6 and sIL-6R induces the expression of MMP-1, 3 and 13 and ADAMTS-4, 5/11 [57]. On the other hand, animal studies have shown that IL-6 knockout mice develop OA in higher prevalence and severity than wild-type mice and that IL-6 intraarticular injection induces OA-like cartilage lesions [45,59]. Conversely, the systemic treatment using anti-IL-6 or STAT-3 alleviated experimental OA in mice [57].

When compared with healthy controls, patients with end-stage OA have a significantly higher concentration of IL-6 in synovial fluid (median 4.8 vs. 196.9 pg/mL), and the concentration of IL-6 in synovial fluid is known to correlate with the pain experienced by patients with OA [60,61]. Additionally, IL-6 seems to have a predictive value as well. In a prospective cohort study conducted on 163 subjects aged 50–79, disease severity assessment and IL-6 and TNF-α serum measurements were performed at baseline and a 3-year follow-up. The findings of both univariate and multivariate analyses suggest that increased IL-6 and TNF-α concentration at baseline are associated with an increased loss of cartilage volume [62]. Furthermore, the decreased innate production of IL-6 has also been associated with a decreased risk for developing hand OA, and a trend of decreased risk can be observed for knee and hip OA as well [63]. IL-6 might also be an important link between obesity and OA. It has been shown that infrapatellar fat, and to a lesser extent subcutaneous adipose tissue, can induce the expression of IL-6 in fibroblast-like synoviocytes [64]. Moreover, obese OA patients are known to have higher IL-6 and sIL-6R than non-obese patients with OA [65].

Thus, it is clear that the interpretation of IL-6 role in OA should not be based solely on the concentration of IL-6 but also on the concentration of sIL-6R and sgp130 and on the assessment of *trans*- and *classic*-IL-6 signaling. This is often overlooked in studies, making it hard to demystify the pathophysiological role of IL-6 in OA. A schematic representation of the mechanism of action and effects of IL-6 is shown in Figure 4.

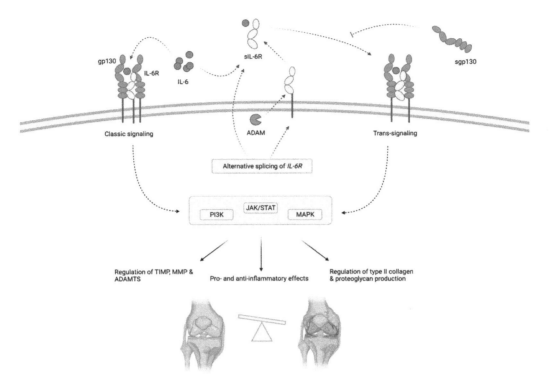

Figure 4. Schematic representation of IL-6 function in osteoarthritis pathogenesis. IL-6 acts by binding membrane-bound IL-6R or sIL-6R that associates with gp130. Gp130 initiates intracellular signaling that regulates the inflammation and expression of enzymes, collagen and proteoglycans. sIL-6R is produced by means of alternative splicing or the shedding of membrane-bound IL-6R. sgp130 can inhibit IL-6 signaling. Through classic and trans-signaling, IL-6 activates the PI3K, JAK/STAT and MAPK signaling pathways that regulate enzymes production (TIMP, MMPs and ADAMTS) and type II collagen and proteoglycan synthesis. Thus, IL-6 balances between anti-inflammatory and proinflammatory effects, but the latter predominates, ultimately leading to the progression of osteoarthritis. ADAM—a disintegrin and metalloproteinase; ADAMTS—a disintegrin-like and metalloproteinase with thrombospondin motifs; gp130—glycoprotein 130; IL-6—interleukin-6; MMP—matrix metalloproteinases; sgp130—soluble glycoprotein 130; sIL-6R—soluble IL-6 receptor; TIMP—tissue inhibitor of metalloproteinase; JAK/STAT—Janus kinase/signal transducers and activators of transcription; PI3K—phosphoinositide 3-kinases; MAPK—mitogen-activated protein kinase.

2.1.4. IL-15

IL-15 is a proinflammatory cytokine produced by various cell types such as fibroblasts, synoviocytes, phagocytes, skeletal muscle, inflammatory cells and many others [66,67]. Although the role of inflammation in the development of the disease has largely been studied in rheumatoid arthritis (RA), recent findings suggest inflammation as an important factor in the pathogenesis of OA. The division of OA into phenotypes speaks in favor of this, defining the inflammatory phenotype of OA among other forms [68]. Likewise, IL-15 has been studied more in the pathogenesis of RA because of its effect on the activation, differentiation and proliferation of T lymphocytes and NK cells [67,69]. However, a study comparing cytokine expressions in synovial fluid of the knee joints of patients with OA and RA showed no significant difference in IL-15 concentrations between OA and RA [70]. Furthermore, according to a study by Scanzello et al., higher concentrations of IL-15 were found in the synovial fluid of patients with early-stage OA compared to patients with late-stage disease, independently of age, gender and BMI [71]. Also, the study found that IL-15 was detectable in all patients with early-stage OA included in the study, indicating its importance in disease progression [71]. Another study found increased IL-15 levels in the serum of patients with OA compared with healthy controls [72,73]. In addition, serum IL-15 correlated with patient-reported pain severity measured by the WOMAC pain score, independently of age, gender and BMI [72].

The exact mechanism by which IL-15 affects the onset and progression of OA is not yet known, but it is known that IL-15 enhances the production of MMPs, as is the case with MMP-9 [74]. It was also shown that the concentration of IL-15 in the synovial fluid of the knee correlates with the concentrations of MMP-1 and MMP-3 and that the concentration of IL-15 in the serum correlates with the concentration of MMP-7 in the serum [71,73]. Despite the association of IL-15 with the enhanced production of matrix-degrading enzymes, an association with the radiological severity of OA has not been established [75]. Precisely because of the unclear mechanism of action, further research is needed to elucidate the role of IL-15 in the development of OA. Elevated concentrations in the early stages of the disease suggest a potential role for IL-15 as a biomarker for the early diagnosis of OA. The confirmation of these findings would be an excellent tool in stopping disease progression in a timely fashion.

2.1.5. IL-17

IL-17, also named IL-17A, is considered a proinflammatory cytokine and a member of the IL-17 cytokine family that includes IL-17B, IL-17C, IL-17D and IL-17E [76]. IL-17A is the most extensively researched cytokine of the IL-17 family, and it has been shown to induce the most potent changes of all IL-17 family cytokines in the transcriptome of synovium and chondrocytes of patients with OA [76,77].

Multiple types of cells secrete IL-17, but little is known about the particular role of these cells in OA and their contribution to IL-17 production in OA. In general, IL-17 is prominently produced by the Th17 subtype of T helper (Th) cells [78]. These cells can act as either pathogenic (responsible for the development of autoinflammatory (AI) diseases, including AI diseases of the joint) or non-pathogenic (protective), depending on the cytokine milieu that stimulates them [78]. The most prominent influence on them is exhibited by IL-23, which is induced in fibroblast-like synoviocytes by IL-17 in RA patients [79]. However, only several studies measured these cells in OA patients, and their explicit role in OA is unclear. Another important source of IL-17 are $\gamma\delta$ T cells. These cells are abundant in mucosal tissue and essential in microorganism sensing but also seem to be implicated in bone healing [80,81]. Nevertheless, $\gamma\delta$ T cells do not seem altered in the synovial tissue in patients with OA, and we could not find relevant articles investigating $\gamma\delta$ T cells' contribution to IL-17 production in OA [82]. Other known sources of IL-17 include natural killer (NK) cells and macrophages. The abundance of NK cells is present in the synovium and synovial fluid of OA patients [83,84]. Additionally, the enrichment of CD56 [bright] CD16 (-) subtypes of NK cells in the synovial fluid, and their numbers, correlate with the concentration of IL-6 [84]. The same cells also accumulate in inflamed tissue and in the interplay with monocytes. They are prone to stimulation by IL-12, IL-15 and IL-18 secreted by monocytes and recurrently stimulate TNF-α secretion in monocytes [85]. These findings accentuate the importance of the inflammatory component to OA, but whether NK cells are a significant source of IL-17 in OA is unknown (unmeasured).

IL-17 signals by binding to the heterodimeric receptors IL17RA and IL17RC to activate downstream NF-κB, MAPK and C/EBP pathways. Although it is a weak activator of NF-κB, IL-17 TRAF-mediated signaling can stabilize the mRNAs of proinflammatory cytokines [86]. IL-17RA and IL-17RC, the main targets for IL-17, are both found on chondrocytes and synovial fibroblasts, with IL-17RA more expressed on the synovial fibroblasts of OA patients with highly inflamed synovium [87]. Furthermore, IL-17 has been found to upregulate catabolic factors (MMP 1, 3 and 13) and downregulate anabolic factors (TIMP3, COL2A1 and SOX9) in chondrocytes isolated from the cartilage of patients with OA and induce cartilage degradation in bovine full depth explant [88,89]. It has also been shown that IL-17 can increase IL-6 and TNF-α production in OA [87]. OA-prone guinea pigs had a higher concentration of IL-17 in comparison to OA-resistant guinea pigs [90]. Moreover, a weak correlation was observed in a longitudinal study of serum cytokines in Hartley guinea pig OA between serum IL-17 and histological score ($R2 = 0.16$, $p = 0.047$) [91]. Furthermore, a single intra-articular IL-17 injection induces the depletion of proteoglycans with no signs of inflammation, whereas repeated injection induces both inflammation and proteoglycan degradation [92].

There are multiple studies with conflicting results investigating IL-17 in the serum and synovial fluid of OA patients. We identified two studies that failed to demonstrate the difference in concentration of IL-17 and the presence of Th17 cells in the serum of patients with OA and the healthy control [93,94]. On the other hand, Qi et al. identified a statistically significant increase in IL-17 concentration in the serum of OA patients. However, the difference between OA and healthy controls is minor (approximately 2 pg/mL, based on Figure 4) [95]. Similarly, Liu et al. have found slightly increased serum IL-17 in OA patients (2.17 pg/mL in control vs. 6.04, 6.35, 6.00 and 5.85 in KL grades 1–4 of OA, respectively). Although not statistically significant, a slight decrease in IL-17 serum concentration is present in KL grade 4 vs. KL grade 1, 2 and 3 [96]. Conversely, another study identified an increase in serum IL-17 only in patients with KL grade 4 OA compared to control (6.161 vs. 4.173 pg/mL), suggesting that IL-17 is increased in patients with more severe OA [97]. We identified two more studies that demonstrated an increase in IL-17 in patients with OA; however, the IL-17 concentration measured in the serum was remarkably higher than in the previous studies (mean values of 106.24 and 134.89 vs. 63.46 and 67.37 pg/mL) [98,99]. Furthermore, IL-17 seems to be negatively associated with infrapatellar fat pat volume and positively associated with the severity of infrapatellar fat pad signal intensity alteration [100]. Both variables are associated with OA, but the observed association with IL-17 is rather tiny. In summation, these results demonstrate high variance, and it is not clear whether IL-17 is altered in OA patients or not. More importantly, the significance of a slight change in the serum IL-17 observed in most of the studies is questionable, especially when changes in the IL-17 target receptors and the other molecules affecting IL-17 signaling are unknown (unmeasured).

Regarding IL-17 in the synovial fluid, Chen et al. reported that IL-17 concentration from synovial fluid increases from KL grade 2 to KL grade 4, ranging from 5.565 to 8.701 pg/mL, and correlates with the severity of the knee OA graded using the Lequesne index. Although the authors did not specifically comment on this, we observe that the concentration of the IL-17 in the synovial fluid is insignificantly higher than the concentration in the serum [97]. Similarly, two studies reported no difference in the IL-17 measured in the synovial fluid and the peripheral blood [84,101]. A recent study performed measurements of several cytokines in the synovial fluid of patients that underwent total hip or knee arthroplasty, including IL-17, and successfully detected IL-17 in only 14 out of 152 (9.6%). However, the authors suggest that IL-17 identifies an inflammatory OA type based on observed increased IL-6, leptin, resistin, CCL7 and NGF in patients with detectable IL-17 [102]. Similarly, it was reported that the serum IL-17 levels were not significantly associated with cartilage defects and bone marrow lesions, except in a subgroup of patients with hs-CRP of > 2.45 pg/mL, where a moderate association was demonstrated [103].

To date, numerous studies have investigated the association between *IL-17* polymorphism and OA. Lee and Song conducted a meta-analysis and concluded that rs2275913 and rs763780 polymorphism is a risk factor for developing OA [104,105].

2.1.6. IL-18

IL-18, a cytokine primarily identified as an IFN-γ-inducing factor, is a member of the IL-1 family. It is produced, as a biologically inactive precursor (pro-IL-18), by a variety of cells, including chondrocytes, osteoblasts, synoviocytes, macrophages, keratinocytes, dendritic cells, astrocytes, microglia, respiratory epithelial cells and osteoblasts [106,107].

The enzyme responsible for obtaining the active form of IL-18 is caspase-I, known as IL-1 converting enzyme [108].

IL-18 was found in elevated concentrations in the plasma, synovial fluid, and articular cartilage of patients with OA compared with healthy controls, indicating the increased local and systemic production of IL-18 in OA [106]. Furthermore, IL-18 levels, either from plasma, synovial fluid or articular cartilage, were higher in advanced OA than in early-stage OA; that is, they correlated with the radiographic severity of the disease [106]. Furthermore, a more recent study found that synovial fluid IL-18 levels correlated with the severity of post-traumatic OA [109].

IL-18 achieves its effects by various mechanisms of action, which begin when IL-18 binds to its receptors, IL-18Rα and IL-18Rβ, both of which are expressed on chondrocytes [110]. Moreover, IL-18 induces an increase in the number of receptors on the chondrocyte surface and the synthesis of metalloproteinases, MMP-1, MMP-3 and MMP-13, the key enzymes responsible for cartilage degradation [111]. Similar to IL-1β, IL-18 triggers signal transduction via the NF-κB and MAPK-p38-AP1 signaling pathways and thus upregulates COX-2 expression, thereby increasing PGE-2 synthesis in chondrocytes, which inhibits proteoglycan production and aggrecan synthesis but also upregulates MMPs, leading to cartilage degradation [107,112–114]. In addition, IL-18 increases the production of NO, a cytotoxic free radical that is an independent factor in cartilage degradation and, unlike the PGE-2 mechanism, is not inhibited by the use of anti-inflammatory drugs [113].

As OA is not a disease of the cartilage but rather of the whole joint, the effects of inflammatory mediators in other tissues within the joint are also important [3]. Thus, COX-2, NO and PGE-2 stimulate both catabolic and anabolic processes in the bone, leading to bone resorption and the formation of osteophytes, respectively [115,116].

Furthermore, IL-18 induces the enhanced expression of genes for the synthesis of IL-6 and TNF-α in chondrocytes and synoviocytes, which further contributes to the fact that one of the most important factors in the pathogenesis of OA is a complex vicious circle of proinflammatory cytokines and other inflammatory mediators [110].

2.1.7. IL-21

Produced by NK cells, Th17 and follicular T-cells, IL-21 is another pleiotropic cytokine involved in immune processes, including OA. The IL-21 signal is transduced when it binds to its receptor (IL-21R) and the common cytokine receptor γ-chain, γc (shared by the receptors for IL-2, IL-4, IL-7, IL-9 and IL-15), which are found in a variety of cell types [117]. The effect of IL-21 has been thoroughly explored in studies on RA, where its immunologic function is used as a potential drug target [118,119]. In RA, IL-21 levels correlate with IL-17 levels in the sera and synovial fluid of these patients, promoting the production of T$_h$17 cells that perpetuate the immune reaction. IL-21 levels also correlate with IL-6 levels, and the inhibition of IL-6 lowers the concentration of IL-21 as well [117]. However, in OA, its place in the underlying immunologic mechanism is still to be defined. In a study by Scanzello et al. IL-21 was found in the majority of synovial fluid samples of patients with cartilage degeneration [71]. A more recent study by Shan et al. increased the levels of IL-21 and IL-21–follicular helper T-cells were found, which correlated with OA severity measured by WOMAC scores and CRP levels, indicating the potential role of IL-21 as a biomarker of OA [120].

2.1.8. IL-22

IL-22 is a member of the IL-10 family produced primarily by Th17 and NK cells. Other cells producing IL-22 include macrophages, neutrophils and fibroblasts [121]. Higher IL-22 concentrations were found In RA and OA joints when there was active synovial inflammation, a common feature of RA but found in OA as well [122]. In OA patients, IL-22 was increased in the synovial fluid and fibroblast-like synoviocytes, and IL-22 receptors were elevated almost tenfold in chondrocytes. Conversely, no difference in IL-22 concentration was observed in the serum of OA patients [123]. Constitutively expressed by fibroblast-like synoviocytes, IL-22 plays an important role in the pathophysiologic mechanism of OA by promoting MMP-1 activity. The potential therapeutic strategy includes blocking this signaling pathway, since it was shown that blocking JAK 2 and JAK 3 decreased the effect of IL-22 on S100A8/A9 [124]. Indeed, in the experimental model of OA, IL-22R neutralizing antibodies proved beneficial [123].

2.2. Anti-Inflammatory Cytokines

2.2.1. IL-4

IL-4 is a potent regulator of the immune system and is often called the prototypic immunoregulatory cytokine. It is secreted by Th2 cells, eosinophils, basophils and mast cells [125]. IL-4 is a protein consisting of 129 amino acids, and it takes the form of a four-helix bundle [28].

Its biological effect is achieved by binding to a multimeric receptor system shared with some other cytokines, such as IL-2 and IL-13. There are two different receptor type complexes. Type 1 complex is formed by the dimerization of IL-4Rα and IL-2Rγc and enables the attachment of IL-4, while the interaction between IL-4Rα and IL-13Rα1 forms type 2 complex, which enables the attachment of both IL-4 and IL-13 [28]. The exact signaling pathway of IL-4 is still not clearly described, although there is some relevant information regarding the initial intracellular events. It is known that the gradual phosphorylation of the IL-4Rα/JAK1/STAT3/STAT6 cascade leads to the expression of several proinflammatory genes [126].

There is evidence that polymorphism within the functional candidate gene *IL4R* is associated with OA of the hand, knee and hip [127]. Silvestri et al. found that serum soluble interleukin-4 receptor (sIL-4R) concentration was significantly higher in all OA patients compared to the healthy control group. IL-4 concentration within the synovial fluid and synovial cells was also increased [128,129]. CD4$^+$ T-cells were detected in the sublining layer of the synovium of patients with OA, and their number was significantly higher than that of those in the same layer of healthy control. This suggests that the production of IL-4 is primarily determined by T cells (Th2) infiltrating the synovium of the joint [130]. It is worth mentioning that IL-4 has a noticeable chondroprotective effect. It inhibits the secretion of MMPs metalloproteinases, reduces the variation in the production of proteoglycans that are visible in the course of OA and, consequently, has an inhibiting effect on the degradation of proteoglycans in the articular cartilage [131,132]. Furthermore, IL-4 alone or in combination with IL-10 protects against blood-induced cartilage damage and inhibits the apoptosis of both the chondrocytes and FLS [28,133]. Considering its chondroprotective effect and the effect on other cell lineages, it is not surprising that IL-4 decreases the synthesis of inflammatory cytokines such as IL-1β, TNF-α and IL-6 [134]. In addition, IL-4 also decreases the secretion of other inflammatory mediators such as PGE-2, COX-2, PLA2 and iNOS [28].

2.2.2. IL-10

Another cytokine with pleiotropic anti-inflammatory properties is IL-10. IL-10, structurally related to interferons, initiates its effect by binding to its receptor IL-10R—a heterodimer composed of IL-10R1 and IL-10R2 subunits. Mainly produced by immune cells, IL-10 is also synthesized by chondrocytes, where it has a role in the complex mechanism of cartilage extracellular matrix turnover [135]. Upon binding, IL-10R activates the JAK-STAT kinase intracellular pathway and stimulates the expression of genes dependent on IL-10 [28]. The end product of this stimulation is a net chondroprotective, antiapoptotic and anti-inflammatory effect caused by the stimulation of type II collagen and aggrecan synthesis, as well as the inhibition of MMP synthesis [135,136]. Alternatively, IL-10 expresses its profound anti-inflammatory properties by the stimulation of IL-1β antagonist synthesis by macrophages and the inhibition of TNFα, IL-6 and IL-12, thus opposing their proinflammatory effect [28,137]. In vitro IL-10 treatment of cartilage injury model demonstrated a chondroprotective effect and increased glycosaminoglycan content (GAG).

Autologous chondrocyte implant grafts treated with IL-10 also demonstrated an improvement in chondrocyte differentiation and cartilage matrix formation [138]. A recent study observed decreased serum levels of IL-10 and the decreased IL-10/TNFα ratio in patients with high-stage knee OA (Kellgren-Lawrence 4) compared with patients with moderate knee OA (Kellgren-Lawrence 3), potentially indicating its prognostic value [139]. The therapeutic effect of physical activity is often taken as an axiom in modern medicine. A clinical study exploring the effect of physical activity on IL levels in 31 female OA patients found increased levels of IL-10 intra- and periarticularly in a 3-h post-exercise period, while IL-6 and IL-8 levels remained stable throughout, thus strengthening the recommendation of physical activity for OA patients [140]. Studies also demonstrated that physical activity promotes M" anti-inflammatory macrophage phenotype differentiation, which in turn produces IL-10 and other anti-inflammatory chemokines and helps in achieving a chondroprotective anabolic joint environment [141]. The effect of mesenchymal stem cell (MSC) therapy on M2 macrophage differentiation has been established as one of the mechanisms by which they stabilize micro-inflammation in knee OA [3,141,142]. Targeted intraarticular plasmid DNA therapy was found to be safe and effective in a canine OA study, highlighting a potential for further treatment options based on IL-10 activity in knee OA [143].

2.3. Chemokines

Chemokines, also known as chemotactic cytokines, are small molecules with the ability to induce chemotaxis in a wide variety of cells. They are best known for their effect on the trafficking and guiding of immune effector cells to sites of infection or inflammation. Their wide range of action affects the proliferation, differentiation and activation of cellular responses. Thus, chemokines play an important role in persistent and ongoing inflammation in OA joints [5].

These small (8–12 kDa) protein ligands are divided into four families based on the positioning of the N-terminal cysteine residues: C, CC, CXC and CX3C. In the CC family, the cysteine residues are adjacent to each other. On the contrary, the CXC family is characterized by the separation of the two cysteine residues by an amino acid. The vast majority of known chemokines belong to these two families. The third identified chemokine family is the C family, containing a single cysteine residue in the conserved position. Finally, in the CX3C family, cysteine residues are separated similarly to the CXC family but by three variable amino acids instead of one [144]. Chemokines achieve their effects by binding to G-protein coupled cell-surface receptors. These receptors show different levels of binding specificity and promiscuity, but they do not bind different groups of chemokines. For example, CCR receptors bind only CCL chemokine ligands and CXCR receptors bind CXCL ligands. In order to understand the importance of chemokines in the course of OA, it is inevitable to mention their role in driving cellular motility during the inflammatory response. Leukocytes express a specific set of chemokine receptors and migrate to sites of infection or tissue damage along the gradients of their cognate chemokine ligands. Furthermore, chemokines arrange the recruitment of pluripotent cell types to sites of tissue repair. They perform a variety of functions aside from chemotaxis, including T helper cell differentiation and function as well as angiogenesis, and have a pleiotropic effect on multiple cell types related to the pathogenesis of OA [5,145].

The most important CC family chemokines that are related to OA are CCL2, CCL3, CCL4 and CCL5 [5]. The monocyte chemoattractant protein-1 (MCP-1/CCL2) is a potent chemotactic factor for monocytes that also recruits memory T-lymphocytes and natural killer (NK) cells. Its effects are primarily associated with its binding to the CCR2 receptor [146]. Elevated levels of CCL2 were found in the synovial fluid of patients with both knee injuries and knee OA [147,148]. Miller et al. found that both CCL2 and CCR2 were upregulated in the innervating dorsal root ganglia (DRG) of the knee 8 weeks after surgical injury in a murine model [149]. The same authors did a follow-up study and reported that CCL2 production by murine DRG neurons was induced by alarmin S100A8 and the plasma protein α2 macroglobulin, which are molecular "danger signals" strongly involved in OA pathogenesis [150]. CCL2 (MCP-1) production is dependent on Toll-like receptor-4 (TLR-4) signaling. These findings imply that products of tissue damage and inflammation during OA could stimulate nociceptive pathways. Genetic variation in the CCL2 gene may be associated with knee OA [151]. CCL2 increases MMP-3 expression, which results in proteoglycan loss and the degradation of cartilaginous tissue [152].

CCL3 (MIP-1α), CCL4 (MIP-1β), and CCL5 (RANTES) are other members of the CC family that are also upregulated in OA. Zhao et al. investigated chemokine levels in the plasma of 181 patients (75 control patients, 47 pre-radiographic knee OA patients and 50 radiographic knee OA patients) [153]. CCL3 in plasma showed the highest ability to discriminate pre-radiographic knee OA patients from the control group. Levels in plasma increased with the radiographic severity of the disease. Beekhuizen et al. found that CCL5 levels were among the most significantly elevated mediators in OA synovial fluid compared with controls [60]. Another study that confirms this statement documented CCL5 levels elevation in 18 additional patients [147]. It is worth mentioning that all of these three chemokines are ligands for CCR5. Consequently, Takabe et al. found that CCR5 deficient mice were partially protected against post-traumatic cartilage erosion [154]. There were no signs of bone remodeling or synovial response to surgery, suggesting that CCR5 functions primarily in cartilage during the development of post-traumatic OA. IL-1β-treated human chondrocytes showed the significant upregulation of CCL3, CCL4 and CCL5 [155].

Chemokines from the CXC family that play a significant role in the pathogenesis of OA are CXCL8 (IL-8) and CXCL12. IL-8 is a chemokine molecule, first described as a chemoattractant of neutrophils. Today it is known that IL-8 exhibits effects on many different cells, and it is researched in numerous diseases [156]. It is expressed by cells of the immune system, most prominently CD8$^+$ T cells, macrophages and monocytes, but also by keratinocytes, fibroblasts, epithelial cells, hepatocytes and synovial cells [156]. It acts on CXCR1 and CXCR2 receptors expressed not only on leukocytes but also on chondrocytes, osteoclasts, fibroblasts, epithelial and endothelial cells and on the cells of the nervous system [156–158].

It has been shown on the human chondrocyte cell line (CHON-002) that IL-8 can be upregulated by TNF-α [159]. Furthermore, IL-8 production is stimulated by advanced glycation end products (AGEs) through NF-κB signaling, which are known to accumulate in cartilage with age and stimulate catabolic metabolism in chondrocytes [160]. Additionally, it has been shown that in human OA chondrocytes, IL-8 is regulated by DNA demethylation that is affected by IL-1b signaling [161]. Free fatty acids also increase the production of IL-8 in the osteoblasts of patients with OA but have little effect on IL-8 secretion in osteoclasts [162]. Osteopontin is yet another molecule involved in the regulation of IL-8 expression, and it is known to stimulate IL-8 in chondrocytes [163]. The mechanical load also increases IL-8 secretion in the chondrocytes of OA patients [164].

Without a doubt, IL-8 is significantly more expressed in the synovial tissue and synovial fluid of patients with RA than in OA [165–170]. OA patients undergoing surgery had 37-fold higher IL-8 expression in chondrocytes than patients undergoing surgery due to a fracture of the neck of the femur (likely due to osteoporosis) [161]. Koh et al. have shown that IL-8 is higher in the synovial fluid of OA patients than in young patients with ligament injury [171]. This is also supported by animal studies demonstrating increased IL-8 in dogs with OA [172,173]. Furthermore, it has been shown that IL-8 is also slightly higher in the serum of OA patients than in healthy control [167,171]. IL-8 in synovial fluid has been shown to correlate with the clinical severity of OA, but IL-8 in serum has not [174]. On the other hand, Ruan et al. have demonstrated a certain correlation between serum IL-8 and the clinically and radiologically assessed severity of OA [174,175].

IL-8 is also known to increase collagen I, MMP1- and MMP-13 protein concentration and to enhance the phosphorylation of STAT3 and NF-Kb subunit p65 [159]. It can also affect chondrocyte morphology by decreasing endogenous GTP-Cdc42 and increasing stress fibers. HA concentration in the knee negatively correlates with IL-8 in synovial fluid [170]. In patients with a good response to sodium hyaluronate treatment in terms of improvement of hydrarthrosis, there was a prominent reduction of IL-8 and IL-6 concentration following the treatment [170]. IL-8 also stimulates the hypertrophy of chondrocytes and the calcifications of the matrix [157]. Further studies by the same group have shown that IL-8 increases the expression of PiT-1 expression and stimulates the uptake of inorganic phosphate in chondrocytes [176].

CXCL12, also known as stromal cell-derived factor-1 (SDF-1), is a chemokine that plays a key role in tissue regeneration. It mobilizes mesenchymal stem cells (MSCs) to sites of injury by binding to CXCR4 [177]. Shen et al. confirmed this statement by studying the effects of human meniscus-derived stem/progenitor cells (hMeSPCs) in a rat meniscectomy model [178]. hMeSPCs were injected intra-articularly after meniscectomy and homed to the injured meniscus. The meniscal repair was superior in the hMeSPCs-treated mice, with significantly reduced cartilage degeneration. In a study consisting of 252 patients with knee OA and 144 healthy controls, CXCL12 levels in the synovial fluid were closely related to the radiographic severity of OA [179]. Besides their effect on MSCs, there is evidence that articular chondrocytes express CXCR4, and CXCL12 also induces MMP13 and some other catabolic mediators. The disruption of these catabolic events could be achieved by the pharmacological blockade of CXCL2/CXCR4 signaling. Thus, the disruption of the CXCL12/CXCR4 signaling can be used as a therapeutic approach to attenuate cartilage degeneration in OA [180]. Taking into consideration all of the above, it is obvious that CXCL12 has diverse effects that depend on cellular targets.

3. Conclusions

The pathogenesis of OA is largely determined by the imbalance of proinflammatory and anti-inflammatory mediators, leading to low-grade inflammation, which is responsible for cartilage degradation, bone remodeling and synovial proliferation [181]. Many cytokines, by activating multiple signaling pathways, increase COX-2 expression and consequently PGE-2, which subsequently affects cartilage degradation and osteophyte formation. COX-2 inhibitors such as nonsteroidal anti-inflammatory drugs, which are generally listed as first-line drugs in the relevant guidelines, do not slow down disease progression [182]. The potential answer to this problem lies in the finding that the activation of signaling pathways such as NF-κB and MAPK also activates other mechanisms that lead to OA progression that are not affected by NSAIDs. However, changes in lifestyle habits, such as diet, supplementation and physical activity, can lead to improvements in OA symptoms, even before drug therapies, and it would be of great value to continue research on the mechanism of lifestyle changes on cytokines modulation and slowing OA progression, as it could provide valuable new findings [183–186]. Furthermore, targeting major cytokines in the development of OA, such as IL-1β and TNF-α, and suppressing their effects did not offer the expected results in clinical studies [18–20,187,188]. Since in OA the effects of one cytokine are not necessarily dependent on the activation of another, the suppression of one cytokine may not sufficiently contribute to stopping the inflammation and the production of matrix-degrading enzymes. Therefore, biological treatment methods such as the application of mesenchymal stem cells, which have various anti-inflammatory effects and have obtained significant clinical effects in numerous studies, deserve attention in future research in terms of proving the role of certain anti-inflammatory factors in suppressing OA progression [189–195]. This potential future research should take into consideration the effect of these therapeutic options on the interplay between different cytokines. Therefore, it would be imprudent to choose a single cytokine to measure the therapeutic effect, as the change of a single variable does not necessarily reflect the change at the level of cellular interactions.

In conclusion, much further research is needed to fully understand the role of cytokines and chemokines in the onset and progression of OA. The epigenetic regulation of cytokine synthesis is also an interesting area to be explored and could offer new solutions in OA management. A sound biological understanding is necessary for any therapeutic intervention to be successful in treating OA patients.

Author Contributions: Conceptualization, V.M. (Vilim Molnar) and V.M. (Vid Matišić); writing—original draft preparation, V.M. (Vilim Molnar), V.M. (Vid Matišić), I.K., R.B., Ž.J., D.H., E.R., F.Č., T.V., D.V., M.S., S.S., B.D., T.P., D.A. and I.B.; writing—review and editing, V.M.(Vilim Molnar), V.M.(Vid Matišić), I.K., R.B., R.K., U.P.Z. and D.P.; visualization, V.M.(Vilim Molnar) and I.K.; supervision, V.M.(Vilim Molnar) and D.P. All authors have read and agreed to the published version of the manuscript.

Funding: This research received no external funding.

Institutional Review Board Statement: Not applicable.

Informed Consent Statement: Not applicable.

Acknowledgments: All figures were made in Biorender (https://biorender.com/; last accessed on 29 June 2021).

Conflicts of Interest: The authors declare no conflict of interest.

References

1. Neogi, T. The epidemiology and impact of pain in osteoarthritis. *Osteoarthr. Cartil.* **2013**, *21*, 1145–1153. [CrossRef]
2. Cui, A.; Li, H.; Wang, D.; Zhong, J.; Chen, Y.; Lu, H. Global, regional prevalence, incidence and risk factors of knee osteoarthritis in population-based studies. *EClinicalMedicine* **2020**, *29–30*, 100587. [CrossRef]
3. Primorac, D.; Molnar, V.; Rod, E.; Jeleč, Ž.; Čukelj, F.; Matišić, V.; Vrdoljak, T.; Hudetz, D.; Hajsok, H.; Borić, I. Knee Osteoarthritis: A Review of Pathogenesis and State-Of-The-Art Non-Operative Therapeutic Considerations. *Genes* **2020**, *11*, 854. [CrossRef]
4. Kapoor, M.; Martel-Pelletier, J.; Lajeunesse, D.; Pelletier, J.-P.P.; Fahmi, H. Role of proinflammatory cytokines in the pathophysiology of osteoarthritis. *Nat. Rev. Rheumatol.* **2011**, *7*, 33–42. [CrossRef] [PubMed]
5. Scanzello, C.R. Chemokines and inflammation in osteoarthritis: Insights from patients and animal models. *J. Orthop. Res.* **2017**, *35*, 735–739. [CrossRef] [PubMed]
6. Fields, J.K.; Günther, S.; Sundberg, E.J. Structural Basis of IL-1 Family Cytokine Signaling. *Front. Immunol.* **2019**, *10*, 1412. [CrossRef]
7. Boraschi, D.; Italiani, P.; Weil, S.; Martin, M.U. The family of the interleukin-1 receptors. *Immunol. Rev.* **2018**, *281*, 197–232. [CrossRef]
8. Martel-Pelletier, J.; Mccollum, R.; Dibattista, J.; Faure, M.-P.; Chin, J.A.; Fournier, S.; Sarfati, M.; Pelletier, J.-P. The interleukin-1 receptor in normal and osteoarthritic human articular chondrocytes. Identification as the type I receptor and analysis of binding kinetics and biologic function. *Arthritis Rheum.* **1992**, *35*, 530–540. [CrossRef]
9. Attur, M.; Statnikov, A.; Samuels, J.; Li, Z.; Alekseyenko, A.V.; Greenberg, J.D.; Krasnokutsky, S.; Rybak, L.; Lu, Q.A.; Todd, J.; et al. Plasma levels of interleukin-1 receptor antagonist (IL1Ra) predict radiographic progression of symptomatic knee osteoarthritis. *Osteoarthr. Cartil.* **2015**, *23*, 1915–1924. [CrossRef]
10. Wang, X.; Li, F.; Fan, C.; Wang, C.; Ruan, H. Effects and relationship of ERK1 and ERK2 in interleukin-1β-induced alterations in MMP3, MMP13, type II collagen and aggrecan expression in human chondrocytes. *Int. J. Mol. Med.* **2011**, *27*, 583–589. [CrossRef] [PubMed]
11. Hwang, S.-G.; Yu, S.-S.; Poo, H.; Chun, J.-S. c-Jun/Activator Protein-1 Mediates Interleukin-1β-induced Dedifferentiation but Not Cyclooxygenase-2 Expression in Articular Chondrocytes. *J. Biol. Chem.* **2005**, *280*, 29780–29787. [CrossRef]
12. Jenei-Lanzl, Z.; Meurer, A.; Zaucke, F. Interleukin-1β signaling in osteoarthritis—chondrocytes in focus. *Cell. Signal.* **2019**, *53*, 212–223. [CrossRef]
13. Hwang, H.; Kim, H. Chondrocyte Apoptosis in the Pathogenesis of Osteoarthritis. *Int. J. Mol. Sci.* **2015**, *16*, 26035–26054. [CrossRef]
14. Wang, X.; Li, F.; Fan, C.; Wang, C.; Ruan, H. Analysis of isoform specific ERK signaling on the effects of interleukin-1β on COX-2 expression and PGE2 production in human chondrocytes. *Biochem. Biophys. Res. Commun.* **2010**, *402*, 23–29. [CrossRef] [PubMed]
15. Chow, Y.Y.; Chin, K.-Y. The Role of Inflammation in the Pathogenesis of Osteoarthritis. *Mediat. Inflamm.* **2020**, *2020*, 1–19. [CrossRef] [PubMed]
16. Choi, M.C.; Jo, J.; Park, J.; Kang, H.K.; Park, Y. NF-B Signaling Pathways in Osteoarthritic Cartilage Destruction. *Cells* **2019**, *8*, 734. [CrossRef]
17. Lepetsos, P.; Papavassiliou, K.A.; Papavassiliou, A.G. Redox and NF-κB signaling in osteoarthritis. *Free Radic. Biol. Med.* **2019**, *132*, 90–100. [CrossRef]
18. Chevalier, X.; Eymard, F.; Richette, P. Biologic agents in osteoarthritis: Hopes and disappointments. *Nat. Rev. Rheumatol.* **2013**, *9*, 400–410. [CrossRef]

19. Chevalier, X.; Goupille, P.; Beaulieu, A.D.; Burch, F.X.; Bensen, W.G.; Conrozier, T.; Loeuille, D.; Kivitz, A.J.; Silver, D.; Appleton, B.E. Intraarticular injection of anakinra in osteoarthritis of the knee: A multicenter, randomized, double-blind, placebo-controlled study. *Arthritis Care Res.* **2009**, *61*, 344–352. [CrossRef]

20. Chevalier, X.; Eymard, F. Anti-IL-1 for the treatment of OA: Dead or alive? *Nat. Rev. Rheumatol.* **2019**, *15*, 191–192. [CrossRef] [PubMed]

21. Theeuwes, W.F.; van den Bosch, M.H.J.; Thurlings, R.M.; Blom, A.B.; van Lent, P.L.E.M. The role of inflammation in mesenchymal stromal cell therapy in osteoarthritis, perspectives for post-traumatic osteoarthritis: A review. *Rheumatology* **2021**, *60*, 1042–1053. [CrossRef]

22. Baud, V.; Karin, M. Signal transduction by tumor necrosis factor and its relatives. *Trends Cell Biol.* **2001**, *11*, 372–377. [CrossRef]

23. Bodmer, J.L.; Schneider, P.; Tschopp, J. The molecular architecture of the TNF superfamily. *Trends Biochem. Sci.* **2002**, *27*, 19–26. [CrossRef]

24. Kriegler, M.; Perez, C.; DeFay, K.; Albert, I.; Lu, S.D. A novel form of TNF/cachectin is a cell surface cytotoxic transmembrane protein: Ramifications for the complex physiology of TNF. *Cell* **1988**, *53*, 45–53. [CrossRef]

25. Zhou, T.; Mountz, J.D.; Kimberly, R.P. Immunobiology of tumor necrosis factor receptor superfamily. *Immunol. Res.* **2002**, *26*, 323–336. [CrossRef]

26. Appay, V.; Sauce, D. Immune activation and inflammation in HIV-1 infection: Causes and consequences. *J. Pathol.* **2008**, *214*, 231–241. [CrossRef] [PubMed]

27. Westacott, C.I.; Barakat, A.F.; Wood, L.; Perry, M.J.; Neison, P.; Bisbinas, I.; Armstrong, L.; Millar, A.B.; Elson, C.J. Tumor necrosis factor alpha can contribute to focal loss of cartilage in osteoarthritis. *Osteoarthr. Cartil.* **2000**, *8*, 213–221. [CrossRef]

28. Wojdasiewicz, P.; Poniatowski, Ł.A.; Szukiewicz, D. The Role of Inflammatory and Anti-Inflammatory Cytokines in the Pathogenesis of Osteoarthritis. *Mediat. Inflamm.* **2014**, *2014*, 1–19. [CrossRef] [PubMed]

29. Zelová, H.; Hošek, J. TNF-α signalling and inflammation: Interactions between old acquaintances. *Inflamm. Res.* **2013**, *62*, 641–651. [CrossRef]

30. Henderson, B.; Pettipher, E.R. Arthritogenic actions of recombinant IL-1 and tumour necrosis factor α in the rabbit: Evidence for synergistic interactions between cytokines in vivo. *Clin. Exp. Immunol.* **1989**, *75*, 306–310. [PubMed]

31. Séguin, C.A.; Bernier, S.M. TNFα Suppresses Link Protein and Type II Collagen Expression in Chondrocytes: Role of MEK1/2 and NF-κB Signaling Pathways. *J. Cell. Physiol.* **2003**, *197*, 356–369. [CrossRef]

32. Xue, J.; Wang, J.; Liu, Q.; Luo, A. Tumor necrosis factor-α induces ADAMTS-4 expression in human osteoarthritis chondrocytes. *Mol. Med. Rep.* **2013**, *8*, 1755–1760. [CrossRef]

33. Oo, W.M.; Yu, S.P.-C.; Daniel, M.S.; Hunter, D.J. Disease-modifying drugs in osteoarthritis: Current understanding and future therapeutics. *Expert Opin. Emerg. Drugs* **2018**, *23*, 331–347. [CrossRef] [PubMed]

34. Abul, K.; Abbas, M.; Lichtman, A.H.; Shiv Pillai, M. *Cellular and Molecular Immunology*; Elsevier: Philadeplphia, PA, USA, 2021.

35. Murphy, K.M.; Weaver, C. *Janeway's Immunobiology: Ninth International Student Edition*; Garland Science, Taylor & Francis Group, LLC: New York, NY, USA, 2017.

36. Hirano, T.; Yasukawa, K.; Harada, H.; Taga, T.; Watanabe, Y.; Matsuda, T.; Kashiwamura, S.; Nakajima, K.; Koyama, K.; Iwamatsu, A.; et al. Complementary DNA for a novel human interleukin (BSF-2) that induces B lymphocytes to produce immunoglobulin. *Nature* **1986**, *324*, 73–76. [CrossRef]

37. Hirano, T. Revisiting the 1986 Molecular Cloning of Interleukin 6. *Front. Immunol.* **2014**, *5*, 456. [CrossRef] [PubMed]

38. Rose-John, S. Interleukin-6 Family Cytokines. *Cold Spring Harb. Perspect. Biol.* **2018**, *10*, a028415. [CrossRef]

39. Baran, P.; Hansen, S.; Waetzig, G.H.; Akbarzadeh, M.; Lamertz, L.; Huber, H.J.; Ahmadian, M.R.; Moll, J.M.; Scheller, J. The balance of interleukin (IL)-6, IL-6·soluble IL-6 receptor (sIL-6R), and IL-6·sIL-6R·sgp130 complexes allows simultaneous classic and trans-signaling. *J. Biol. Chem.* **2018**, *293*, 6762–6775. [CrossRef]

40. Lutosławska, G. Interleukin-6 As An Adipokine And Myokine: The Regulatory Role Of Cytokine In Adipose Tissue And Skeletal Muscle Metabolism. *Hum. Mov.* **2012**, *13*, 372–379. [CrossRef]

41. Pal, M.; Febbraio, M.A.; Whitham, M. From cytokine to myokine: The emerging role of interleukin-6 in metabolic regulation. *Immunol. Cell Biol.* **2014**, *92*, 331–339. [CrossRef]

42. Akdis, M.; Burgler, S.; Crameri, R.; Eiwegger, T.; Fujita, H.; Gomez, E.; Klunker, S.; Meyer, N.; O'Mahony, L.; Palomares, O.; et al. Interleukins, from 1 to 37, and interferon-γ: Receptors, functions, and roles in diseases. *J. Allergy Clin. Immunol.* **2011**, *127*, 701–721.e70. [CrossRef]

43. Sanchez, C.; Gabay, O.; Salvat, C.; Henrotin, Y.E.; Berenbaum, F. Mechanical loading highly increases IL-6 production and decreases OPG expression by osteoblasts. *Osteoarthr. Cartil.* **2009**, *17*, 473–481. [CrossRef] [PubMed]

44. Scheller, J.; Chalaris, A.; Schmidt-Arras, D.; Rose-John, S. The pro- and anti-inflammatory properties of the cytokine interleukin-6. *Biochim. Biophys. Acta- Mol. Cell Res.* **2011**, *1813*, 878–888. [CrossRef] [PubMed]

45. Ryu, J.-H.; Yang, S.; Shin, Y.; Rhee, J.; Chun, C.-H.; Chun, J.-S. Interleukin-6 plays an essential role in hypoxia-inducible factor 2α-induced experimental osteoarthritic cartilage destruction in mice. *Arthritis Rheum.* **2011**, *63*, 2732–2743. [CrossRef] [PubMed]

46. Rose-John, S.; Scheller, J.; Elson, G.; Jones, S.A. Interleukin-6 biology is coordinated by membrane-bound and soluble receptors: Role in inflammation and cancer. *J. Leukoc. Biol.* **2006**, *80*, 227–236. [CrossRef]

47. McGregor, N.E.; Murat, M.; Elango, J.; Poulton, I.J.; Walker, E.C.; Crimeen-Irwin, B.; Ho, P.W.M.; Gooi, J.H.; Martin, T.J.; Sims, N.A. IL-6 exhibits both cis- and trans-signaling in osteocytes and osteoblasts, but only trans-signaling promotes bone formation and osteoclastogenesis. *J. Biol. Chem.* **2019**, *294*, 7850–7863. [CrossRef]

48. Reeh, H.; Rudolph, N.; Billing, U.; Christen, H.; Streif, S.; Bullinger, E.; Schliemann-Bullinger, M.; Findeisen, R.; Schaper, F.; Huber, H.J.; et al. Response to IL-6 trans- and IL-6 classic signalling is determined by the ratio of the IL-6 receptor α to gp130 expression: Fusing experimental insights and dynamic modelling. *Cell Commun. Signal.* **2019**, *17*, 46. [CrossRef]

49. Rose-John, S. The soluble interleukin-6 receptor and related proteins. *Best Pract. Res. Clin. Endocrinol. Metab.* **2015**, *29*, 787–797. [CrossRef]

50. Yang, C.-Y.; Chanalaris, A.; Troeberg, L. ADAMTS and ADAM metalloproteinases in osteoarthritis—Looking beyond the 'usual suspects'. *Osteoarthr. Cartil.* **2017**, *25*, 1000–1009. [CrossRef] [PubMed]

51. Chalaris, A.; Garbers, C.; Rabe, B.; Rose-John, S.; Scheller, J. The soluble Interleukin 6 receptor: Generation and role in inflammation and cancer. *Eur. J. Cell Biol.* **2011**, *90*, 484–494. [CrossRef]

52. Garbers, C.; Thaiss, W.; Jones, G.W.; Waetzig, G.H.; Lorenzen, I.; Guilhot, F.; Lissilaa, R.; Ferlin, W.G.; Grötzinger, J.; Jones, S.A.; et al. Inhibition of Classic Signaling Is a Novel Function of Soluble Glycoprotein 130 (sgp130), Which Is Controlled by the Ratio of Interleukin 6 and Soluble Interleukin 6 Receptor. *J. Biol. Chem.* **2011**, *286*, 42959–42970. [CrossRef]

53. Narazaki, M.; Yasukawa, K.; Saito, T.; Ohsugi, Y.; Fukui, H.; Koishihara, Y.; Yancopoulos, G.D.; Taga, T.; Kishimoto, T. Soluble forms of the interleukin-6 signal-transducing receptor component gp130 in human serum possessing a potential to inhibit signals through membrane-anchored gp130. *Blood* **1993**, *82*, 1120–1126. [CrossRef] [PubMed]

54. Jostock, T.; Müllberg, J.; Özbek, S.; Atreya, R.; Blinn, G.; Voltz, N.; Fischer, M.; Neurath, M.F.; Rose-John, S. Soluble gp130 is the natural inhibitor of soluble interleukin-6 receptor transsignaling responses. *Eur. J. Biochem.* **2001**, *268*, 160–167. [CrossRef] [PubMed]

55. Wolf, J.; Waetzig, G.H.; Chalaris, A.; Reinheimer, T.M.; Wege, H.; Rose-John, S.; Garbers, C. Different Soluble Forms of the Interleukin-6 Family Signal Transducer gp130 Fine-tune the Blockade of Interleukin-6 Trans-signaling. *J. Biol. Chem.* **2016**, *291*, 16186–16196. [CrossRef] [PubMed]

56. Silacci, P.; Dayer, J.-M.; Desgeorges, A.; Peter, R.; Manueddu, C.; Guerne, P.-A. Interleukin (IL)-6 and Its Soluble Receptor Induce TIMP-1 Expression in Synoviocytes and Chondrocytes, and Block IL-1-induced Collagenolytic Activity. *J. Biol. Chem.* **1998**, *273*, 13625–13629. [CrossRef]

57. Latourte, A.; Cherifi, C.; Maillet, J.; Ea, H.-K.; Bouaziz, W.; Funck-Brentano, T.; Cohen-Solal, M.; Hay, E.; Richette, P. Systemic inhibition of IL-6/Stat3 signalling protects against experimental osteoarthritis. *Ann. Rheum. Dis.* **2017**, *76*, 748–755. [CrossRef]

58. Porée, B.; Kypriotou, M.; Chadjichristos, C.; Beauchef, G.; Renard, E.; Legendre, F.; Melin, M.; Gueret, S.; Hartmann, D.-J.J.; Malléin-Gerin, F.; et al. Interleukin-6 (IL-6) and/or soluble IL-6 receptor down-regulation of human type II collagen gene expression in articular chondrocytes requires a decrease of Sp1·Sp3 ratio and of the binding activity of both factors to the COL2A1 promoter. *J. Biol. Chem.* **2008**, *283*, 4850–4865. [CrossRef]

59. De Hooge, A.S.K.; van de Loo, F.A.J.; Bennink, M.B.; Arntz, O.J.; de Hooge, P.; van den Berg, W.B. Male IL-6 gene knock out mice developed more advanced osteoarthritis upon aging. *Osteoarthr. Cartil.* **2005**, *13*, 66–73. [CrossRef] [PubMed]

60. Beekhuizen, M.; Gierman, L.M.M.; van Spil, W.E.E.; Van Osch, G.J.V.M.J.V.M.; Huizinga, T.W.J.W.J.; Saris, D.B.F.B.F.; Creemers, L.B.B.; Zuurmond, A.-M.M. An explorative study comparing levels of soluble mediators in control and osteoarthritic synovial fluid. *Osteoarthr. Cartil.* **2013**, *21*, 918–922. [CrossRef]

61. Li, L.; Li, Z.; Li, Y.; Hu, X.; Zhang, Y.; Fan, P. Profiling of inflammatory mediators in the synovial fluid related to pain in knee osteoarthritis. *BMC Musculoskelet. Disord.* **2020**, *21*, 99. [CrossRef]

62. Stannus, O.; Jones, G.; Cicuttini, F.; Parameswaran, V.; Quinn, S.; Burgess, J.; Ding, C. Circulating levels of IL-6 and TNF-α are associated with knee radiographic osteoarthritis and knee cartilage loss in older adults. *Osteoarthr. Cartil.* **2010**, *18*, 1441–1447. [CrossRef] [PubMed]

63. Goekoop, R.J.; Kloppenburg, M.; Kroon, H.M.; Frölich, M.; Huizinga, T.W.J.; Westendorp, R.G.J.; Gussekloo, J. Low innate production of interleukin-1β and interleukin-6 is associated with the absence of osteoarthritis in old age. *Osteoarthr. Cartil.* **2010**, *18*, 942–947. [CrossRef]

64. Eymard, F.; Pigenet, A.; Citadelle, D.; Flouzat-Lachaniette, C.-H.; Poignard, A.; Benelli, C.; Berenbaum, F.; Chevalier, X.; Houard, X. Induction of an Inflammatory and Prodegradative Phenotype in Autologous Fibroblast-like Synoviocytes by the Infrapatellar Fat Pad From Patients With Knee Osteoarthritis. *Arthritis Rheumatol.* **2014**, *66*, 2165–2174. [CrossRef]

65. Pearson, M.J.; Herndler-Brandstetter, D.; Tariq, M.A.; Nicholson, T.A.; Philp, A.M.; Smith, H.L.; Davis, E.T.; Jones, S.W.; Lord, J.M. IL-6 secretion in osteoarthritis patients is mediated by chondrocyte-synovial fibroblast cross-talk and is enhanced by obesity. *Sci. Rep.* **2017**, *7*, 3451. [CrossRef] [PubMed]

66. Waldmann, T.A. IL-15 in the life and death of lymphocytes: Immunotherapeutic implications. *Trends Mol. Med.* **2003**, *9*, 517–521. [CrossRef] [PubMed]

67. Allard-Chamard, H.; Mishra, H.K.; Nandi, M.; Mayhue, M.; Menendez, A.; Ilangumaran, S.; Ramanathan, S. Interleukin-15 in autoimmunity. *Cytokine* **2020**, *136*, 155258. [CrossRef] [PubMed]

68. Dell'Isola, A.; Steultjens, M. Classification of patients with knee osteoarthritis in clinical phenotypes: Data from the osteoarthritis initiative. *PLoS ONE* **2018**, *13*, e0191045. [CrossRef] [PubMed]

69. McInnes, I.B.; Al-Mughales, J.; Field, M.; Leung, B.P.; Huang, F.; Dixon, R.; Sturrock, R.D.; Wilkinson, P.C.; Liew, F.Y. The role of interleukin–15 in T–cell migration and activation in rheumatoid arthritis. *Nat. Med.* **1996**, *2*, 175–182. [CrossRef]

70. Savio, A.S.; Diaz, A.C.M.; Capote, A.C.; Navarro, J.M.; Alvarez, Y.R.; Pérez, R.B.; del Toro, M.E.; Nieto, G.E.G. Differential expression of pro-inflammatory cytokines IL-15Ralpha, IL-15, IL-6 and TNFalpha in synovial fluid from Rheumatoid arthritis patients. *BMC Musculoskelet. Disord.* **2015**, *16*, 51. [CrossRef]

71. Scanzello, C.R.R.; Umoh, E.; Pessler, F.; Diaz-Torne, C.; Miles, T.; DiCarlo, E.; Potter, H.G.G.; Mandl, L.; Marx, R.; Rodeo, S.; et al. Local cytokine profiles in knee osteoarthritis: Elevated synovial fluid interleukin-15 differentiates early from end-stage disease. *Osteoarthr. Cartil.* **2009**, *17*, 1040–1048. [CrossRef]

72. Sun, J.-M.; Sun, L.-Z.; Liu, J.; Su, B.; Shi, L. Serum Interleukin-15 Levels Are Associated with Severity of Pain in Patients with Knee Osteoarthritis. *Dis. Markers* **2013**, *35*, 203–206. [CrossRef]

73. Tao, Y.; Qiu, X.; Xu, C.; Sun, B.; Shi, C. Expression and correlation of matrix metalloproteinase-7 and interleukin-15 in human osteoarthritis. *Int. J. Clin. Exp. Pathol.* **2015**, *8*, 9112–9118. [PubMed]

74. Constantinescu, C.S.; Grygar, C.; Kappos, L.; Leppert, D. Interleukin 15 stimulates production of matrix metalloproteinase-9 and tissue inhibitor of metalloproteinase-1 by human peripheral blood mononuclear cells. *Cytokine* **2001**, *13*, 244–247. [CrossRef] [PubMed]

75. Warner, S.C.; Nair, A.; Marpadga, R.; Chubinskaya, S.; Doherty, M.; Valdes, A.M.; Scanzello, C.R. IL-15 and IL15RA in Osteoarthritis: Association With Symptoms and Protease Production, but Not Structural Severity. *Front. Immunol.* **2020**, *11*, 1385. [CrossRef] [PubMed]

76. Jin, W.; Dong, C. IL-17 cytokines in immunity and inflammation. *Emerg. Microbes Infect.* **2013**, *2*, 1–5. [CrossRef] [PubMed]

77. Mimpen, J.Y.; Baldwin, M.J.; Cribbs, A.P.; Philpott, M.; Carr, A.J.; Dakin, S.G.; Snelling, S.J.B. Interleukin-17A causes osteoarthritis-like transcriptional changes in human osteoarthritis-derived chondrocytes and synovial fibroblasts in vitro. *bioRxiv* **2021**. [CrossRef]

78. Wu, X.; Tian, J.; Wang, S. Insight Into Non-Pathogenic Th17 Cells in Autoimmune Diseases. *Front. Immunol.* **2018**, *9*, 1112. [CrossRef]

79. Goldberg, M.; Nadiv, O.; Luknar-Gabor, N.; Agar, G.; Beer, Y.; Katz, Y. Synergism between tumor necrosis factor alpha and interleukin-17 to induce IL-23 p19 expression in fibroblast-like synoviocytes. *Mol. Immunol.* **2009**, *46*, 1854–1859. [CrossRef]

80. Ribot, J.C.; Lopes, N.; Silva-Santos, B. γδ T cells in tissue physiology and surveillance. *Nat. Rev. Immunol.* **2021**, *21*, 221–232. [CrossRef]

81. Ono, T.; Okamoto, K.; Nakashima, T.; Nitta, T.; Hori, S.; Iwakura, Y.; Takayanagi, H. IL-17-producing γδ T cells enhance bone regeneration. *Nat. Commun.* **2016**, *7*, 10928. [CrossRef]

82. Li, J.; Luo, W.; Zhu, S.; Lei, G. T Cells in Osteoarthritis: Alterations and Beyond. *Front. Immunol.* **2017**, *8*, 356. [CrossRef] [PubMed]

83. Huss, R.S.; Huddleston, J.I.; Goodman, S.B.; Butcher, E.C.; Zabel, B.A. Synovial tissue-infiltrating natural killer cells in osteoarthritis and periprosthetic inflammation. *Arthritis Rheum.* **2010**, *62*, 3799–3805. [CrossRef] [PubMed]

84. Jaime, P.; García-Guerrero, N.; Estella, R.; Pardo, J.; García-Álvarez, F.; Martinez-Lostao, L. CD56+/CD16− Natural Killer cells expressing the inflammatory protease granzyme A are enriched in synovial fluid from patients with osteoarthritis. *Osteoarthr. Cartil.* **2017**, *25*, 1708–1718. [CrossRef] [PubMed]

85. Dalbeth, N.; Gundle, R.; Davies, R.J.O.; Lee, Y.C.G.; McMichael, A.J.; Callan, M.F.C. CD56 bright NK Cells Are Enriched at Inflammatory Sites and Can Engage with Monocytes in a Reciprocal Program of Activation. *J. Immunol.* **2004**, *173*, 6418–6426. [CrossRef]

86. Gu, C.; Wu, L.; Li, X. IL-17 family: Cytokines, receptors and signaling. *Cytokine* **2013**, *64*, 477–485. [CrossRef] [PubMed]

87. Mimpen, J.Y.; Carr, A.J.; Dakin, S.G.; Snelling, S.J. Inhibition of interleukin-17-induced effects in osteoarthritis—An in vitro study. *Osteoarthr. Cartil.* **2018**, *26*, S118. [CrossRef]

88. Na, H.S.; Park, J.-S.; Cho, K.-H.; Kwon, J.Y.; Choi, J.; Jhun, J.; Kim, S.J.; Park, S.-H.; Cho, M.-L. Interleukin-1-Interleukin-17 Signaling Axis Induces Cartilage Destruction and Promotes Experimental Osteoarthritis. *Front. Immunol.* **2020**, *11*, 730. [CrossRef]

89. Sinkeviciute, D.; Aspberg, A.; He, Y.; Bay-Jensen, A.-C.; Önnerfjord, P. Characterization of the interleukin-17 effect on articular cartilage in a translational model: An explorative study. *BMC Rheumatol.* **2020**, *4*, 30. [CrossRef] [PubMed]

90. Huebner, J.L.; Kraus, V.B. Assessment of the utility of biomarkers of osteoarthritis in the guinea pig. *Osteoarthr. Cartil.* **2006**, *14*, 923–930. [CrossRef]

91. Huebner, J.L.; Seifer, D.R.; Kraus, V.B. A longitudinal analysis of serum cytokines in the Hartley guinea pig model of osteoarthritis. *Osteoarthr. Cartil.* **2007**, *15*, 354–356. [CrossRef]

92. Chabaud, M.; Lubberts, E.; Joosten, L.; van Den Berg, W.; Miossec, P. IL-17 derived from juxta-articular bone and synovium contributes to joint degradation in rheumatoid arthritis. *Arthritis Res.* **2001**, *3*, 168–177. [CrossRef]

93. Zhang, L.; Li, Y.; Li, Y.; Qi, L.; Liu, X.; Yuan, C.; Hu, N.; Ma, D.; Li, Z.; Yang, Q.; et al. Increased Frequencies of Th22 Cells as well as Th17 Cells in the Peripheral Blood of Patients with Ankylosing Spondylitis and Rheumatoid Arthritis. *PLoS ONE* **2012**, *7*, e31000. [CrossRef]

94. Zhang, L.; Li, J.; Liu, X.; Ma, D.; Hu, N.; Li, Y.; Li, W.; Hu, Y.; Yu, S.; Qu, X.; et al. Elevated Th22 Cells Correlated with Th17 Cells in Patients with Rheumatoid Arthritis. *J. Clin. Immunol.* **2011**, *31*, 606–614. [CrossRef]

95. Qi, C.; Shan, Y.; Wang, J.; Ding, F.; Zhao, D.; Yang, T.; Jiang, Y. Circulating T helper 9 cells and increased serum interleukin-9 levels in patients with knee osteoarthritis. *Clin. Exp. Pharmacol. Physiol.* **2016**, *43*, 528–534. [CrossRef]

96. Wei, M. Correlation of IL-17 Level in Synovia and Severity of Knee Osteoarthritis. *Med. Sci. Monit.* **2015**, *21*, 1732–1736. [CrossRef] [PubMed]

97. Chen, B.; Deng, Y.; Tan, Y.; Qin, J.; Chen, L.-B. Bin Association between severity of knee osteoarthritis and serum and synovial fluid interleukin 17 concentrations. *J. Int. Med. Res.* **2014**, *42*, 138–144. [CrossRef] [PubMed]
98. Askari, A.; Naghizadeh, M.M.; Homayounfar, R.; Shahi, A.; Afsarian, M.H.; Paknahad, A.; Kennedy, D.; Ataollahi, M.R. Increased Serum Levels of IL-17A and IL-23 Are Associated with Decreased Vitamin D3 and Increased Pain in Osteoarthritis. *PLoS ONE* **2016**, *11*, e0164757. [CrossRef]
99. Jiang, L.; Zhou, X.; Xiong, Y.; Bao, J.; Xu, K.; Wu, L. Association between interleukin-17A/F single nucleotide polymorphisms and susceptibility to osteoarthritis in a Chinese population. *Medicine* **2019**, *98*, e14944. [CrossRef] [PubMed]
100. Wang, K.; Xu, J.; Cai, J.; Zheng, S.; Han, W.; Antony, B.; Ding, C. Serum levels of interleukin-17 and adiponectin are associated with infrapatellar fat pad volume and signal intensity alteration in patients with knee osteoarthritis. *Arthritis Res. Ther.* **2016**, *18*, 1–7. [CrossRef] [PubMed]
101. Babaei, M.; Javadian, Y.; Narimani, H.; Ranaei, M.; Heidari, B.; Basereh, H.; Gholinia, H.; Firouzjahi, A. Correlation between systemic markers of inflammation and local synovitis in knee osteoarthritis. *Casp. J. Intern. Med.* **2019**, *10*, 383–387. [CrossRef]
102. Snelling, S.J.B.B.; Bas, S.; Puskas, G.J.; Dakin, S.G.; Suva, D.; Finckh, A.; Gabay, C.; Hoffmeyer, P.; Carr, A.J.; Lübbeke, A. Presence of IL-17 in synovial fluid identifies a potential inflammatory osteoarthritic phenotype. *PLoS ONE* **2017**, *12*, e0175109. [CrossRef]
103. Wang, K.; Xu, J.; Cai, J.; Zheng, S.; Yang, X.; Ding, C. Serum levels of resistin and interleukin-17 are associated with increased cartilage defects and bone marrow lesions in patients with knee osteoarthritis. *Mod. Rheumatol.* **2017**, *27*, 339–344. [CrossRef]
104. Lee, Y.H.; Song, G.G. Association between IL-17 gene polymorphisms and circulating IL-17 levels in osteoarthritis: A meta-analysis. *Z. Rheumatol.* **2020**, *79*, 482–490. [CrossRef] [PubMed]
105. Yang, H.-Y.; Liu, Y.-Z.; Zhou, X.-D.; Huang, Y.; Xu, N.-W. Role of IL-17 gene polymorphisms in osteoarthritis: A meta-analysis based on observational studies. *World J. Clin. Cases* **2020**, *8*, 2280–2293. [CrossRef] [PubMed]
106. Wang, Y.; Xu, D.; Long, L.; Deng, X.; Tao, R.; Huang, G. Correlation between plasma, synovial fluid and articular cartilage Interleukin-18 with radiographic severity in 33 patients with osteoarthritis of the knee. *Clin. Exp. Med.* **2014**, *14*, 297–304. [CrossRef] [PubMed]
107. Inoue, H.; Hiraoka, K.; Hoshino, T.; Okamoto, M.; Iwanaga, T.; Zenmyo, M.; Shoda, T.; Aizawa, H.; Nagata, K. High levels of serum IL-18 promote cartilage loss through suppression of aggrecan synthesis. *Bone* **2008**, *42*, 1102–1110. [CrossRef]
108. Kaplanski, G. Interleukin-18: Biological properties and role in disease pathogenesis. *Immunol. Rev.* **2018**, *281*, 138–153. [CrossRef] [PubMed]
109. Panina, S.B.; Krolevets, I.V.; Milyutina, N.P.; Sagakyants, A.B.; Kornienko, I.V.; Ananyan, A.A.; Zabrodin, M.A.; Plotnikov, A.A.; Vnukov, V.V. Circulating levels of proinflammatory mediators as potential biomarkers of post-traumatic knee osteoarthritis development. *J. Orthop. Traumatol.* **2017**, *18*, 349–357. [CrossRef]
110. Fu, Z.; Liu, P.; Yang, D.; Wang, F.; Yuan, L.; Lin, Z.; Jiang, J. Interleukin-18-induced inflammatory responses in synoviocytes and chondrocytes from osteoarthritic patients. *Int. J. Mol. Med.* **2012**, *30*, 805–810. [CrossRef]
111. Dai, S.-M. Implication of interleukin 18 in production of matrix metalloproteinases in articular chondrocytes in arthritis: Direct effect on chondrocytes may not be pivotal. *Ann. Rheum. Dis.* **2005**, *64*, 735–742. [CrossRef]
112. Olee, T.; Hashimoto, S.; Quach, J.; Lotz, M. IL-18 is produced by articular chondrocytes and induces proinflammatory and catabolic responses. *J. Immunol.* **1999**, *162*, 1096–1100.
113. Futani, H.; Okayama, A.; Matsui, K.; Kashiwamura, S.; Sasaki, T.; Hada, T.; Nakanishi, K.; Tateishi, H.; Maruo, S.; Okamura, H. Relation Between Interleukin-18 and PGE2 in Synovial Fluid of Osteoarthritis: A Potential Therapeutic Target of Cartilage Degradation. *J. Immunother.* **2002**, *25*, S61–S64. [CrossRef]
114. Lee, J.-K.; Kim, S.-H.; Lewis, E.C.; Azam, T.; Reznikov, L.L.; Dinarello, C.A. Differences in signaling pathways by IL-1 and IL-18. *Proc. Natl. Acad. Sci. USA* **2004**, *101*, 8815–8820. [CrossRef]
115. Miyaura, C.; Inada, M.; Suzawa, T.; Sugimoto, Y.; Ushikubi, F.; Ichikawa, A.; Narumiya, S.; Suda, T. Impaired bone resorption to prostaglandin E2 in prostaglandin E receptor EP4-knockout mice. *J. Biol. Chem.* **2000**, *275*, 19819–19823. [CrossRef] [PubMed]
116. Scharstuhl, A.; Glansbeek, H.L.; van Beuningen, H.M.; Vitters, E.L.; van der Kraan, P.M.; van den Berg, W.B. Inhibition of Endogenous TGF-β During Experimental Osteoarthritis Prevents Osteophyte Formation and Impairs Cartilage Repair. *J. Immunol.* **2002**, *169*, 507–514. [CrossRef]
117. Spolski, R.; Leonard, W.J. Interleukin-21: A double-edged sword with therapeutic potential. *Nat. Rev. Drug Discov.* **2014**, *13*, 379–395. [CrossRef]
118. Xing, R.; Yang, L.; Jin, Y.; Sun, L.; Li, C.; Li, Z.; Zhao, J.; Liu, X. Interleukin-21 Induces Proliferation and Proinflammatory Cytokine Profile of Fibroblast-like Synoviocytes of Patients with Rheumatoid Arthritis. *Scand. J. Immunol.* **2016**, *83*, 64–71. [CrossRef]
119. Li, J.; Shen, W.; Kong, K.; Liu, Z. Interleukin-21 Induces T-cell Activation and Proinflammatory Cytokine Secretion in Rheumatoid Arthritis. *Scand. J. Immunol.* **2006**, *64*, 515–522. [CrossRef]
120. Shan, Y.; Qi, C.; Liu, Y.; Gao, H.; Zhao, D.; Jiang, Y. Increased frequency of peripheral blood follicular helper T cells and elevated serum IL-21 levels in patients with knee osteoarthritis. *Mol. Med. Rep.* **2017**, *15*, 1095–1102. [CrossRef] [PubMed]
121. Dudakov, J.A.; Hanash, A.M.; van den Brink, M.R.M. Interleukin-22: Immunobiology and Pathology. *Annu. Rev. Immunol.* **2015**, *33*, 747–785. [CrossRef]
122. Deligne, C.; Casulli, S.; Pigenet, A.; Bougault, C.; Campillo-Gimenez, L.; Nourissat, G.; Berenbaum, F.; Elbim, C.; Houard, X. Differential expression of interleukin-17 and interleukin-22 in inflamed and non-inflamed synovium from osteoarthritis patients. *Osteoarthr. Cartil.* **2015**, *23*, 1843–1852. [CrossRef] [PubMed]

123. Yi, C.; Yi, Y.; Wei, J.; Jin, Q.; Li, J.; Sacitharan, P.K. Targeting IL-22 and IL-22R protects against experimental osteoarthritis. *Cell. Mol. Immunol.* **2021**, *18*, 1329–1331. [CrossRef] [PubMed]

124. Carrión, M.; Juarranz, Y.; Martínez, C.; González-Álvaro, I.; Pablos, J.L.; Gutiérrez-Cañas, I.; Gomariz, R.P. IL-22/IL-22R1 axis and S100A8/A9 alarmins in human osteoarthritic and rheumatoid arthritis synovial fibroblasts. *Rheumatology* **2013**, *52*, 2177–2186. [CrossRef]

125. Brown, M.A.; Hural, J. Functions of IL-4 and control of its expression. *Crit. Rev. Immunol.* **2017**, *37*, 181–212. [CrossRef] [PubMed]

126. Bhattacharjee, A.; Shukla, M.; Yakubenko, V.P.; Mulya, A.; Kundu, S.; Cathcart, M.K. IL-4 and IL-13 employ discrete signaling pathways for target gene expression in alternatively activated monocytes/macrophages. *Free Radic. Biol. Med.* **2013**, *54*, 1–16. [CrossRef]

127. Forster, T.; Chapman, K.; Loughlin, J. Common variants within the interleukin 4 receptor α gene (IL4R) are associated with susceptibility to osteoarthritis. *Hum. Genet.* **2004**, *114*, 391–395. [CrossRef]

128. Schlaak, J.F.; Pfers, I.; Meyer Zum Büschenfelde, K.H.; Märker-Hermann, E. Different cytokine profiles in the synovial fluid of patients with osteoarthritis, rheumatoid arthritis and seronegative spondylarthropathies. *Clin. Exp. Rheumatol.* **1996**, *14*, 155–162.

129. Wagner, S.; Fritz, P.; Einsele, H.; Sell, S.; Saal, J.G. Evaluation of synovial cytokine patterns in rheumatoid arthritis and osteoarthritis by quantitative reverse transcription polymerase chain reaction. *Rheumatol. Int.* **1997**, *16*, 191–196. [CrossRef]

130. Ishii, H.; Tanaka, H.; Katoh, K.; Nakamura, H.; Nagashima, M.; Yoshino, S. Characterization of infiltrating T cells and Th1/Th2-type cytokines in the synovium of patients with osteoarthritis. *Osteoarthr. Cartil.* **2002**, *10*, 277–281. [CrossRef]

131. Yeh, L.A.; Augustine, A.J.; Lee, P.; Riviere, L.R.; Sheldon, A. Interleukin-4, an inhibitor of cartilage breakdown in bovine articular cartilage explants. *J. Rheumatol.* **1995**, *22*, 1740–1746.

132. Doi, H.; Nishida, K.; Yorimitsu, M.; Komiyama, T.; Kadota, Y.; Tetsunaga, T.; Yoshida, A.; Kubota, S.; Takigawa, M.; Ozaki, T. Interleukin-4 downregulates the cyclic tensile stress-induced matrix metalloproteinases-13 and cathepsin B expression by rat normal chondrocytes. *Acta Med. Okayama* **2008**, *62*, 119–126. [CrossRef] [PubMed]

133. Van Meegeren, M.E.R.; Roosendaal, G.; Jansen, N.W.D.; Wenting, M.J.G.; Van Wesel, A.C.W.; Van Roon, J.A.G.; Lafeber, F.P.J.G. IL-4 alone and in combination with IL-10 protects against blood-induced cartilage damage. *Osteoarthr. Cartil.* **2012**, *20*, 764–772. [CrossRef]

134. Schuerwegh, A.J.; Dombrecht, E.J.; Stevens, W.J.; Van Offel, J.F.; Bridts, C.H.; De Clerck, L.S. Influence of pro-inflammatory (IL-1α, IL-6, TNF-α, IFN-γ) and anti-inflammatory (IL-4) cytokines on chondrocyte function. *Osteoarthr. Cartil.* **2003**, *11*, 681–687. [CrossRef]

135. Schulze-Tanzil, G.; Zreiqat, H.; Sabat, R.; Kohl, B.; Halder, A.; Muller, R.; John, T. Interleukin-10 and Articular Cartilage: Experimental Therapeutical Approaches in Cartilage Disorders. *Curr. Gene Ther.* **2009**, *9*, 306–315. [CrossRef]

136. Mostafa, E.; Chollet-martin, S.; Oudghiri, M.; Laquay, N.; Jacob, M.; Michel, J.; Feldman, L.J. Effects of interleukin-10 on monocyte / endothelial cell adhesion and MMP-9/TIMP-1 secretion. *Cardiovasc. Res.* **2001**, *49*, 882–890. [CrossRef]

137. Wang, Y.S.; Wang, Y.H.; Zhao, G.Q.; Li, Y.B. Osteogenic potential of human calcitonin gene-related peptide alpha gene-modified bone marrow mesenchymal stem cells. *Chin. Med. J.* **2011**, *124*, 3976–3981. [CrossRef]

138. Behrendt, P.; Feldheim, M.; Preusse-Prange, A.; Weitkamp, J.T.; Haake, M.; Eglin, D.; Rolauffs, B.; Fay, J.; Seekamp, A.; Grodzinsky, A.J.; et al. Chondrogenic potential of IL-10 in mechanically injured cartilage and cellularized collagen ACI grafts. *Osteoarthr. Cartil.* **2018**, *26*, 264–275. [CrossRef]

139. Barker, T.; Rogers, V.E.; Henriksen, V.T.; Trawick, R.H.; Momberger, N.G.; Lynn Rasmussen, G. Circulating IL-10 is compromised in patients predisposed to developing and in patients with severe knee osteoarthritis. *Sci. Rep.* **2021**, *11*, 1–10. [CrossRef] [PubMed]

140. Helmark, I.C.; Mikkelsen, U.R.; Børglum, J.; Rothe, A.; Petersen, M.C.; Andersen, O.; Langberg, H.; Kjaer, M. Exercise increases interleukin-10 levels both intraarticularly and peri-synovially in patients with knee osteoarthritis: A randomized controlled trial. *Arthritis Res. Ther.* **2010**, *12*, R126. [CrossRef]

141. Fernandes, T.L.; Gomoll, A.H.; Lattermann, C.; Hernandez, A.J.; Bueno, D.F.; Amano, M.T. Macrophage: A Potential Target on Cartilage Regeneration. *Front. Immunol.* **2020**, *11*, 111. [CrossRef] [PubMed]

142. Zhang, J.; Rong, Y.; Luo, C.; Cui, W. Bone marrow mesenchymal stem cell-derived exosomes prevent osteoarthritis by regulating synovial macrophage polarization. *Aging* **2020**, *12*, 25138–25152. [CrossRef]

143. Watkins, L.R.; Chavez, R.A.; Landry, R.; Fry, M.; Green-Fulgham, S.M.; Coulson, J.D.; Collins, S.D.; Glover, D.K.; Rieger, J.; Forsayeth, J.R. Targeted interleukin-10 plasmid DNA therapy in the treatment of osteoarthritis: Toxicology and pain efficacy assessments. *Brain. Behav. Immun.* **2020**, *90*, 155–166. [CrossRef]

144. Borish, L.C.; Steinke, J.W. 2. Cytokines and chemokines. *J. Allergy Clin. Immunol.* **2003**, *111*, S460–S475. [CrossRef] [PubMed]

145. Turner, M.D.; Nedjai, B.; Hurst, T.; Pennington, D.J. Cytokines and chemokines: At the crossroads of cell signalling and inflammatory disease. *Biochim. Biophys. Acta- Mol. Cell Res.* **2014**, *1843*, 2563–2582. [CrossRef] [PubMed]

146. Deshmane, S.L.; Kremlev, S.; Amini, S.; Sawaya, B.E. Monocyte chemoattractant protein-1 (MCP-1): An overview. *J. Interf. Cytokine Res.* **2009**, *29*, 313–325. [CrossRef]

147. Monibi, F.; Roller, B.L.; Stoker, A.; Garner, B.; Bal, S.; Cook, J.L. Identification of Synovial Fluid Biomarkers for Knee Osteoarthritis and Correlation with Radiographic Assessment. *J. Knee Surg.* **2016**, *29*, 242–247. [CrossRef] [PubMed]

148. Watt, F.E.; Paterson, E.; Freidin, A.; Kenny, M.; Judge, A.; Saklatvala, J.; Williams, A.; Vincent, T.L. Acute Molecular Changes in Synovial Fluid Following Human Knee Injury: Association With Early Clinical Outcomes. *Arthritis Rheumatol.* **2016**, *68*, 2129–2140. [CrossRef]

149. Miller, R.E.; Tran, P.B.; Das, R.; Ghoreishi-Haack, N.; Ren, D.; Miller, R.J.; Malfait, A.M. CCR2 chemokine receptor signaling mediates pain in experimental osteoarthritis. *Proc. Natl. Acad. Sci. USA* **2012**, *109*, 20602–20607. [CrossRef]
150. Miller, R.E.; Belmadani, A.; Ishihara, S.; Tran, P.B.; Ren, D.; Miller, R.J.; Malfait, A.M. Damage-associated molecular patterns generated in osteoarthritis directly excite murine nociceptive neurons through toll-like receptor 4. *Arthritis Rheumatol.* **2015**, *67*, 2933–2943. [CrossRef] [PubMed]
151. Hulin-Curtis, S.L.; Bidwell, J.L.; Perry, M.J. Association between CCL2 haplotypes and knee osteoarthritis. *Int. J. Immunogenet.* **2013**, *40*, 280–283. [CrossRef] [PubMed]
152. Borzí, R.M.; Mazzetti, I.; Cattini, L.; Uguccioni, M.; Baggiolini, M.; Facchini, A. Human chondrocytes express functional chemokine receptors and release matrix-degrading enzymes in response to C-X-C and C-C chemokines. *Arthritis Rheum.* **2000**, *43*, 1734–1741. [CrossRef]
153. Zhao, X.Y.; Yang, Z.B.; Zhang, Z.J.; Zhang, Z.Q.; Kang, Y.; Huang, G.X.; Wang, S.W.; Huang, H.; Liao, W.M. CCL3 serves as a potential plasma biomarker in knee degeneration (osteoarthritis). *Osteoarthr. Cartil.* **2015**, *23*, 1405–1411. [CrossRef]
154. Takebe, K.; Rai, M.F.; Schmidt, E.J.; Sandell, L.J. The chemokine receptor CCR5 plays a role in post-traumatic cartilage loss in mice, but does not affect synovium and bone. *Osteoarthr. Cartil.* **2015**, *23*, 454–461. [CrossRef] [PubMed]
155. Sandell, L.J.; Xing, X.; Franz, C.; Davies, S.; Chang, L.W.; Patra, D. Exuberant expression of chemokine genes by adult human articular chondrocytes in response to IL-1β. *Osteoarthr. Cartil.* **2008**, *16*, 1560–1571. [CrossRef] [PubMed]
156. Russo, R.C.; Garcia, C.C.; Teixeira, M.M.; Amaral, F.A. The CXCL8/IL-8 chemokine family and its receptors in inflammatory diseases. *Expert Rev. Clin. Immunol.* **2014**, *10*, 593–619. [CrossRef]
157. Merz, D.; Liu, R.; Johnson, K.; Terkeltaub, R. IL-8/CXCL8 and Growth-Related Oncogene α/CXCL1 Induce Chondrocyte Hypertrophic Differentiation. *J. Immunol.* **2003**, *171*, 4406–4415. [CrossRef] [PubMed]
158. Galliera, E.; Locati, M.; Mantovani, A.; Corsi, M.M. Chemokines and bone remodeling. *Int. J. Immunopathol. Pharmacol.* **2008**, *21*, 485–491. [CrossRef] [PubMed]
159. Sun, F.; Zhang, Y.; Li, Q. Therapeutic mechanisms of ibuprofen, prednisone and betamethasone in osteoarthritis. *Mol. Med. Rep.* **2017**, *15*, 981–987. [CrossRef]
160. Rasheed, Z.; Akhtar, N.; Haqqi, T.M. Advanced glycation end products induce the expression of interleukin-6 and interleukin-8 by receptor for advanced glycation end product-mediated activation of mitogen-activated protein kinases and nuclear factor-κB in human osteoarthritis chondrocytes. *Rheumatology* **2011**, *50*, 838–851. [CrossRef]
161. Takahashi, A.; de Andrés, M.C.; Hashimoto, K.; Itoi, E.; Oreffo, R.O.C. Epigenetic regulation of interleukin-8, an inflammatory chemokine, in osteoarthritis. *Osteoarthr. Cartil.* **2015**, *23*, 1946–1954. [CrossRef]
162. Frommer, K.W.; Hasseli, R.; Schäffler, A.; Lange, U.; Rehart, S.; Steinmeyer, J.; Rickert, M.; Sarter, K.; Zaiss, M.M.; Culmsee, C.; et al. Free Fatty Acids in Bone Pathophysiology of Rheumatic Diseases. *Front. Immunol.* **2019**, *10*, 2757. [CrossRef]
163. Yang, Y.; Gao, S.G.; Zhang, F.J.; Luo, W.; Xue, J.X.; Lei, G.H. Effects of osteopontin on the expression of IL-6 and IL-8 inflammatory factors in human knee osteoarthritis chondrocytes. *Eur. Rev. Med. Pharmacol. Sci.* **2014**, *18*, 3580–3586.
164. Sakao, K.; Takahashi, K.A.; Arai, Y.; Saito, M.; Honjo, K.; Hiraoka, N.; Asada, H.; Shin-Ya, M.; Imanishi, J.; Mazda, O.; et al. Osteoblasts derived from osteophytes produce interleukin-6, interleukin-8, and matrix metalloproteinase-13 in osteoarthritis. *J. Bone Miner. Metab.* **2009**, *27*, 412–423. [CrossRef]
165. Remick, D.G.; DeForge, L.E.; Sullivan, J.F.; Showell, H.J. Profile of cytokines in synovial fluid specimens from patients with arthritis. *Immunol. Invest.* **1992**, *21*, 321–327. [CrossRef] [PubMed]
166. Lee, Y.A.; Choi, H.M.; Lee, S.H.; Yang, H.I.; Yoo, M.C.; Hong, S.J.; Kim, K.S. Synergy between adiponectin and interleukin-1β on the expression of interleukin-6, interleukin-8, and cyclooxygenase-2 in fibroblast-like synoviocytes. *Exp. Mol. Med.* **2012**, *44*, 440–447. [CrossRef] [PubMed]
167. Furuzawa-Carballeda, J.; Alcocer-Varela, J. Interleukin-8, interleukin-10, intercellular adhesion molecule-1 and vascular cell adhesion molecule-1 expression levels are higher in synovial tissue from patients with rheumatoid arthritis than in osteoarthritis. *Scand. J. Immunol.* **1999**, *50*, 215–222. [CrossRef] [PubMed]
168. Bertazzolo, N.; Punzi, L.; Stefani, M.P.; Cesaro, G.; Pianon, M.; Finco, B.; Todesco, S. Interrelationships between interleukin (IL)-1, IL-6 and IL-8 in synovial fluid of various arthropathies. *Agents Actions* **1994**, *41*, 90–92. [CrossRef]
169. Valcamonica, E.; Chighizola, C.B.; Comi, D.; De Lucia, O.; Pisoni, L.; Murgo, A.; Salvi, V.; Sozzani, S.; Meroni, P.L. Levels of chemerin and interleukin 8 in the synovial fluid of patients with inflammatory arthritides and osteoarthritis. *Clin. Exp. Rheumatol.* **2014**, *32*, 243–250.
170. Kaneko, S.; Satoh, T.; Chiba, J.; Ju, C.; Inoue, K.; Kagawa, J. Interleukin-6 and interleukin-8 levels in serum and synovial fluid of patients with osteoarthritis. *Cytokines Cell. Mol. Ther.* **2000**, *6*, 71–79. [CrossRef]
171. Koh, S.M.M.; Chan, C.K.K.; Teo, S.H.H.; Singh, S.; Merican, A.; Ng, W.M.M.; Abbas, A.; Kamarul, T. Elevated plasma and synovial fluid interleukin-8 and interleukin-18 may be associated with the pathogenesis of knee osteoarthritis. *Knee* **2020**, *27*, 26–35. [CrossRef] [PubMed]
172. Allen, P.I.; Conzemius, M.G.; Evans, R.B.; Kiefer, K. Correlation between synovial fluid cytokine concentrations and limb function in normal dogs and in dogs with lameness from spontaneous osteoarthritis. *Vet. Surg.* **2019**, *48*, 770–779. [CrossRef] [PubMed]
173. Kleine, S.A.; Gogal, R.M.; George, C.; Thaliath, M.; Budsberg, S.C. Elevated Synovial Fluid Concentration of Monocyte Chemoattractant Protein-1 and Interleukin-8 in Dogs with Osteoarthritis of the Stifle. *Vet. Comp. Orthop. Traumatol.* **2020**, *33*, 147–150. [CrossRef]

174. García-Manrique, M.; Calvet, J.; Orellana, C.; Berenguer-Llergo, A.; Garcia-Cirera, S.; Llop, M.; Albiñana-Giménez, N.; Galisteo-Lencastre, C.; Gratacós, J. Synovial fluid but not plasma interleukin-8 is associated with clinical severity and inflammatory markers in knee osteoarthritis women with joint effusion. *Sci. Rep.* **2021**, *11*, 1–7. [CrossRef] [PubMed]

175. Ruan, G.; Xu, J.; Wang, K.; Zheng, S.; Wu, J.; Bian, F.; Chang, B.; Zhang, Y.; Meng, T.; Zhu, Z.; et al. Associations between serum IL-8 and knee symptoms, joint structures, and cartilage or bone biomarkers in patients with knee osteoarthritis. *Clin. Rheumatol.* **2019**, *38*, 3609–3617. [CrossRef]

176. Cecil, D.L.; Rose, D.M.; Terkeltaub, R.; Liu-Bryan, R. Role of interleukin-8 in PiT-1 expression and CXCR1-mediated inorganic phosphate uptake in chondrocytes. *Arthritis Rheum.* **2005**, *52*, 144–154. [CrossRef]

177. Marquez-Curtis, L.A.; Janowska-Wieczorek, A. Enhancing the migration ability of mesenchymal stromal cells by targeting the SDF-1/CXCR4 axis. *Biomed. Res. Int.* **2013**, *2013*, 1–15. [CrossRef]

178. Shen, W.; Chen, J.; Zhu, T.; Chen, L.; Zhang, W.; Fang, Z.; Heng, B.C.; Yin, Z.; Chen, X.; Ji, J.; et al. Intra-Articular Injection of Human Meniscus Stem/Progenitor Cells Promotes Meniscus Regeneration and Ameliorates Osteoarthritis Through Stromal Cell-Derived Factor-1/CXCR4-Mediated Homing. *Stem Cells Transl. Med.* **2014**, *3*, 387–394. [CrossRef] [PubMed]

179. Gao, F.; Tian, J.; Pan, H.; Gao, J.; Yao, M. Association of CCL13 levels in serum and synovial fluid with the radiographic severity of knee osteoarthritis. *J. Investig. Med.* **2015**, *63*, 545–547. [CrossRef]

180. Wei, F.; Moore, D.C.; Wei, L.; Li, Y.; Zhang, G.; Wei, X.; Lee, J.K.; Chen, Q. Correction: Attenuation of osteoarthritis via blockade of the SDF-1/CXCR4 signaling pathway. *Arthritis Res. Ther.* **2013**, *15*, 410. [CrossRef]

181. Robinson, W.H.; Lepus, C.M.; Wang, Q.; Raghu, H.; Mao, R.; Lindstrom, T.M.; Sokolove, J. Low-grade inflammation as a key mediator of the pathogenesis of osteoarthritis. *Nat. Rev. Rheumatol.* **2016**, *12*, 580–592. [CrossRef] [PubMed]

182. Primorac, D.; Molnar, V.; Matišić, V.; Hudetz, D.; Jeleč, Ž.; Rod, E.; Čukelj, F.; Vidović, D.; Vrdoljak, T.; Dobričić, B.; et al. Comprehensive Review of Knee Osteoarthritis Pharmacological Treatment and the Latest Professional Societies' Guidelines. *Pharmaceuticals* **2021**, *14*, 205. [CrossRef]

183. Messina, O.D.; Vidal Wilman, M.; Vidal Neira, L.F. Nutrition, osteoarthritis and cartilage metabolism. *Aging Clin. Exp. Res.* **2019**, *31*, 807–813. [CrossRef] [PubMed]

184. Malorgio, A.; Malorgio, M.; Benedetti, M.; Casarosa, S.; Cannataro, R. High intensity resistance training as intervention method to knee osteoarthritis. *Sport. Med. Health Sci.* **2021**, *3*, 46–48. [CrossRef]

185. Hill, C.L.; March, L.M.; Aitken, D.; Lester, S.E.; Battersby, R.; Hynes, K.; Fedorova, T.; Proudman, S.M.; James, M.; Cleland, L.G.; et al. Fish oil in knee osteoarthritis: A randomised clinical trial of low dose versus high dose. *Ann. Rheum. Dis.* **2016**, *75*, 23–29. [CrossRef]

186. Schell, J.; Scofield, R.; Barrett, J.; Kurien, B.; Betts, N.; Lyons, T.; Zhao, Y.; Basu, A. Strawberries Improve Pain and Inflammation in Obese Adults with Radiographic Evidence of Knee Osteoarthritis. *Nutrients* **2017**, *9*, 949. [CrossRef]

187. Cohen, S.B.; Proudman, S.; Kivitz, A.J.; Burch, F.X.; Donohue, J.P.; Burstein, D.; Sun, Y.N.; Banfield, C.; Vincent, M.S.; Ni, L.; et al. A randomized, double-blind study of AMG 108 (a fully human monoclonal antibody to IL-1R1) in patients with osteoarthritis of the knee. *Arthritis Res. Ther.* **2011**, *13*, R125. [CrossRef] [PubMed]

188. Verbruggen, G.; Wittoek, R.; Vander Cruyssen, B.; Elewaut, D. Tumour necrosis factor blockade for the treatment of erosive osteoarthritis of the interphalangeal finger joints: A double blind, randomised trial on structure modification. *Ann. Rheum. Dis.* **2012**, *71*, 891–898. [CrossRef]

189. Cosenza, S.; Ruiz, M.; Toupet, K.; Jorgensen, C.; Noël, D. Mesenchymal stem cells derived exosomes and microparticles protect cartilage and bone from degradation in osteoarthritis. *Sci. Rep.* **2017**, *7*, 1–12. [CrossRef]

190. Petryk, N.; Shevchenko, O. Mesenchymal stem cells anti-inflammatory activity in rats: Proinflammatory cytokines. *J. Inflamm. Res.* **2020**, *13*, 293–301. [CrossRef]

191. Kyurkchiev, D. Secretion of immunoregulatory cytokines by mesenchymal stem cells. *World J. Stem Cells* **2014**, *6*, 552. [CrossRef]

192. Hudetz, D.; Borić, I.; Rod, E.; Jeleč, Ž.; Radić, A.; Vrdoljak, T.; Skelin, A.; Lauc, G.; Trbojević-Akmačić, I.; Plečko, M.; et al. The effect of intra-articular injection of autologous microfragmented fat tissue on proteoglycan synthesis in patients with knee osteoarthritis. *Genes* **2017**, *8*, 270. [CrossRef]

193. Hudetz, D.; Borić, I.; Rod, E.; Jeleč, Ž.; Kunovac, B.; Polašek, O.; Vrdoljak, T.; Plečko, M.; Skelin, A.; Polančec, D.; et al. Early results of intra-articular micro-fragmented lipoaspirate treatment in patients with late stages knee osteoarthritis: A prospective study. *Croat. Med. J.* **2019**, *60*, 227–236. [CrossRef] [PubMed]

194. Polancec, D.; Zenic, L.; Hudetz, D.; Boric, I.; Jelec, Z.; Rod, E.; Primorac, D. Immunophenotyping of a Stromal Vascular Fraction from Microfragmented Lipoaspirate Used in Osteoarthritis Cartilage Treatment and Its Lipoaspirate Counterpart. *Genes* **2019**, *10*, 474. [CrossRef] [PubMed]

195. Borić, I.; Hudetz, D.; Rod, E.; Jeleč, Ž.; Vrdoljak, T.; Skelin, A.; Polašek, O.; Plečko, M.; Trbojević-Akmačić, I.; Lauc, G.; et al. A 24-month follow-up study of the effect of intra-articular injection of autologous microfragmented fat tissue on proteoglycan synthesis in patients with knee osteoarthritis. *Genes* **2019**, *10*, 1051. [CrossRef] [PubMed]

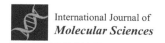

International Journal of
Molecular Sciences

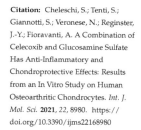

Article

A Combination of Celecoxib and Glucosamine Sulfate Has Anti-Inflammatory and Chondroprotective Effects: Results from an In Vitro Study on Human Osteoarthritic Chondrocytes

Sara Cheleschi [1], Sara Tenti [1], Stefano Giannotti [2], Nicola Veronese [3,*], Jean-Yves Reginster [4] and Antonella Fioravanti [1]

[1] Rheumatology Unit, Department of Medicine, Surgery and Neuroscience, Azienda Ospedaliera Universitaria Senese, Policlinico Le Scotte, 53100 Siena, Italy; saracheleschi@hotmail.com (S.C.); sara_tenti@hotmail.it (S.T.); fioravanti7@virgilio.it (A.F.)

[2] Section of Orthopedics and Traumatology, Department of Medicine, Surgery and Neurosciences, University of Siena, Policlinico Le Scotte, 53100 Siena, Italy; stefano.giannotti@unisi.it

[3] Geriatric Unit, Department of Internal Medicine and Geriatrics, University of Palermo, Viale Scaduto, 90100 Palermo, Italy

[4] Department of Public Health, Epidemiology and Health Economics, University of Liège, Quartier Hôpital, Avenue Hippocrate 13, Bât. B23, 4000 Liège, Belgium; jyreginster@uliege.be

* Correspondence: nicola.veronese@unipa.it

Citation: Cheleschi, S.; Tenti, S.; Giannotti, S.; Veronese, N.; Reginster, J.-Y.; Fioravanti, A. A Combination of Celecoxib and Glucosamine Sulfate Has Anti-Inflammatory and Chondroprotective Effects: Results from an In Vitro Study on Human Osteoarthritic Chondrocytes. *Int. J. Mol. Sci.* **2021**, *22*, 8980. https://doi.org/10.3390/ijms22168980

Academic Editor: Yousef Abu-Amer

Received: 7 July 2021
Accepted: 17 August 2021
Published: 20 August 2021

Publisher's Note: MDPI stays neutral with regard to jurisdictional claims in published maps and institutional affiliations.

Abstract: This study investigated the possible anti-inflammatory and chondroprotective effects of a combination of celecoxib and prescription-grade glucosamine sulfate (GS) in human osteoarthritic (OA) chondrocytes and their possible mechanism of action. Chondrocytes were treated with celecoxib (1.85 µM) and GS (9 µM), alone or in combination with *IL-1β* (10 ng/mL) and a specific nuclear factor (NF)-κB inhibitor (BAY-11-7082, 1 µM). Gene expression and release of some pro-inflammatory mediators, metalloproteinases (*MMPs*), and type II collagen (Col2a1) were evaluated by qRT-PCR and ELISA; apoptosis and mitochondrial superoxide anion production were assessed by cytometry; B-cell lymphoma (BCL)2, antioxidant enzymes, and *p50* and *p65* NF-κB subunits were analyzed by qRT-PCR. Celecoxib and GS alone or co-incubated with *IL-1β* significantly reduced expression and release of cyclooxygenase (*COX*)-2, prostaglandin (*PG*)E2, IL-1β, IL-6, tumor necrosis factor (*TNF*)-α, and *MMPs*, while it increased Col2a1, compared to baseline or IL-1β. Both drugs reduced apoptosis and superoxide production; reduced the expression of superoxide dismutase, catalase, and nuclear factor erythroid; increased *BCL2*; and limited *p50* and *p65*. Celecoxib and GS combination demonstrated an increased inhibitory effect on *IL-1β* than that observed by each single treatment. Drugs effects were potentiated by pre-incubation with BAY-11-7082. Our results demonstrated the synergistic effect of celecoxib and GS on OA chondrocyte metabolism, apoptosis, and oxidative stress through the modulation of the NF-κB pathway, supporting their combined use for the treatment of OA.

Keywords: celecoxib; glucosamine sulfate; osteoarthritis; chondrocytes; inflammation; chondroprotection; oxidative stress; NF-κB

1. Introduction

Osteoarthritis (OA) is the most common degenerative musculoskeletal disorder that affects the entire joint. Its main symptoms are chronic pain, functional limitation, instability, and deformity, with a considerable reduction in quality of life; therefore, OA is considered the leading cause of disability and impairment in middle-aged and older people worldwide and represents a real burden to health care systems [1,2]. The pathogenesis of OA is complex and remains largely unknown; however, it is assumed that multiple factors including aging, gender, joint injury, obesity, and metabolic factors contribute to the onset and the progression of the disease [1]. Furthermore, the risk of developing OA is increased by physical inactivity and by a low-fiber diet rich in sugar and saturated fats. All these different factors are associated with an alteration of composition and function of the gut microbiota, causative of low-grade inflammation, which is an important contributor to joint damage in OA [3,4]. This microbial dysbiosis could represent the missing link between the different conditions contributing to OA pathogenesis, suggesting microbiota as a new pharmacological strategy for OA management [5,6].

Current strategies for the management of OA include a combination of pharmacological and/or non-pharmacological approaches. Among the pharmacological treatments, the updated European Society for Clinical and Economic Aspects of Osteoporosis and Osteoarthritis (ESCEO) algorithm recommends chronic symptomatic slow-acting drugs for OA (SYSADOAs), such as prescription-grade glucosamine sulfate (GS) or chondroitin sulfate (CS), as first-line long-term background treatment, and as-needed paracetamol as a short-term step to rescue analgesia only [7]. Topical nonsteroidal anti-inflammatory drugs (NSAIDs) may be added to the treatment regimen in step 1 if the patient is still symptomatic after establishing appropriate background pharmacological therapy with SYSADOAs, and rescue analgesia with paracetamol provides insufficient symptom relief. The use of oral NSAIDs (selective or non-selective) is proposed as second step, and short-term therapy, with selective COX-2 inhibitors (COXIBs) preferred in the case of increased gastro-intestinal risk [7]. Despite this protocol being endorsed by several groups of experts from around the world, the recommendation to use SYSADOAs as first-line background treatment for knee OA is not endorsed by other respected scientific societies [8–12]. Recently, the ESCEO working group reinforced the use of GS and CS as first-line long-term treatment for their activity on gut microbiota. Indeed, they have limited intestinal absorption and are predominantly utilized as substrates by the gut microbiota. They may have prebiotic properties and exert their therapeutic effects through gut bacterial pathways [5,13,14].

Traditionally, COXIBs have been widely used for their well-established analgesic and anti-inflammatory properties for the treatment of OA; in recent years, growing evidence raised the question of whether COXIBs can be viewed as disease-modifying OA drugs (DMOADs), able to reduce cartilage degradation and slow down OA disease progression [15–18]. Different in vivo and in vitro studies focused on the potential role of celecoxib as DMOADs [15,19–22]. In particular, this drug showed the ability to decrease the production of prostaglandin *(PG)E2*, interleukin *(IL)-1β*, tumor necrosis factor *(TNF)-α*, and nitric oxide (NO) release, and it increased the synthesis of proteoglycans and type II collagen (Col2a1) in human OA cartilage and chondrocytes [21–23]. Furthermore, celecoxib reduced the synthesis of metalloproteinases *(MMPs)*, apoptosis, and the activation of nuclear factor (NF)-κB and receptor activator of NF-κB ligand (RANKL) in OA chondrocytes, fibroblast-like synoviocytes, and subchondral bone osteoblasts [21,24,25].

GS is an amino-monosaccharide and a natural constituent of long-chain glycosaminoglycans present in human tissues, with the highest part in cartilage matrix. The high-quality prescription-grade crystalline GS formulation is widely used for the treatment of OA due to the demonstrated symptomatic effects as well as disease-modifying properties [26–31]. Furthermore, its specific role in cartilage and chondrocyte metabolism has been also demonstrated [30,32]. Indeed, different studies showed the effects of GS in reducing expression of *COX-2*, PGE2 production, and inhibiting activation of the NF-κB pathway in human OA chondrocytes and synoviocytes [33–35]. Furthermore, GS promoted chondrocyte proliferation and proteoglycan production, while it decreased the expression of inducible form of nitric oxide *(iNOS)*, *IL-6*, and *TNF-α* and matrix degrading factors [35–38].

The aim of the present study was to investigate the possible anti-inflammatory and chondroprotective effects of celecoxib and GS, tested alone or in combination, in human OA chondrocytes in the presence of *IL-1β*. In particular, matrix-degrading enzymes *(MMP-1, MMP-3, MMP-13)*, Col2a1, and cytokines *(COX-2, PGE2, IL-1β, IL-6, TNF-α)* were analyzed at their expression levels as well as at their release in the supernatant. Cell viability, the ratio of apoptosis, and the mRNA levels of the anti-apoptotic mediator B-cell lymphoma 2 (BCL)2 were also assessed. Furthermore, the production of mitochondrial superoxide anion and the gene levels of the main antioxidant enzymes—superoxide dismutase *(SOD)-2*, catalase *(CAT)*, glutathione peroxidase *(GPx)4*, and nuclear factor erythroid 2 like 2 *(NRF2)*—were evaluated. Finally, possible regulation of the NF-κB pathway was detected.

2. Results

2.1. Celecoxib and GS Attenuate Inflammation

Figures 1 and 2 show the effects of treatment with celecoxib (1.85 μM) and GS (9 μM), for 24 h and 48 h, on gene expression and supernatant release of the main pro-inflammatory mediators, in OA chondrocytes stimulated or not with *IL-1β*.

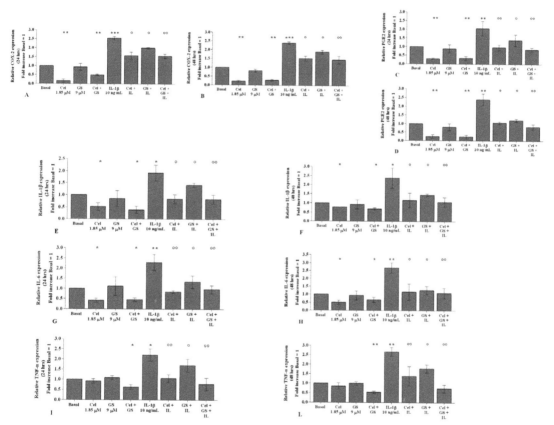

Figure 1. Celecoxib and GS reduce the expression of pro-inflammatory cytokines. Human osteoarthritic (OA) chondrocytes were incubated for 24 and 48 h with celecoxib (1.85 μM) and prescription-grade glucosamine sulfate (GS) (9 μM) (2 h of pre-treatment) in the presence of interleukin *(IL)-1β* (10 ng/mL). (**A–L**) Expression levels of cyclooxygenase *(COX)-2*, prostaglandin *(PG)E2*, *IL-1β*, *IL-6*, and tumor necrosis factor *(TNF)-α* analyzed by quantitative real-time PCR. The gene expression was referenced to the ratio of the value of interest and the value of the basal condition, reported equal to 1. Data were represented as mean ± SD of triplicate values. * $p < 0.05$, ** $p < 0.01$, *** $p < 0.001$ versus basal condition. ° $p < 0.05$, °° $p < 0.01$ versus *IL-1β*.

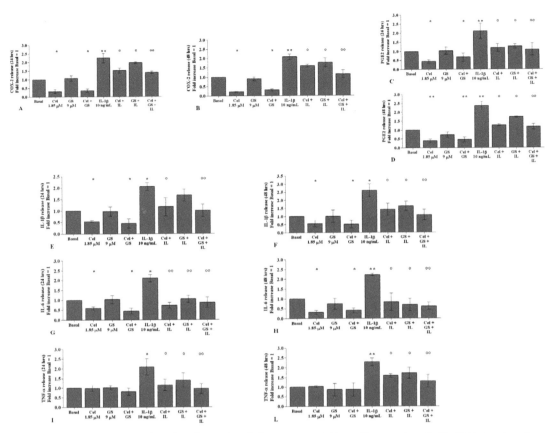

Figure 2. Celecoxib and GS reduce the release of pro-inflammatory cytokines. Human osteoarthritic (OA) chondrocytes were incubated for 24 and 48 h with celecoxib (1.85 μM) and prescription-grade glucosamine sulfate (GS) (9 μM) (2 h of pretreatment) in the presence of interleukin *(IL)-1β* (10 ng/mL). (**A–L**) Total amount of cyclooxygenase *(COX)-2*, prostaglandin *(PG)E2*, *IL-1β*, *IL-6*, and tumor necrosis factor *(TNF)-α*, released in the supernatant, analyzed by ELISA assay. The total amount was referenced to the ratio of the value of interest and the value of the basal condition, reported equal to 1. Data were represented as mean ± SD of triplicate values. * $p < 0.05$, ** $p < 0.01$ versus basal condition. ° $p < 0.05$, °° $p < 0.01$ versus *IL-1β*.

The treatment of OA chondrocytes with celecoxib, tested alone or in combination with GS, significantly reduced *COX-2*, *PGE2*, *IL-1β*, and *IL-6* gene expression and release in comparison to basal conditions ($p < 0.05$, $p < 0.01$), while no changes in TNF-α were observed (Figure 1A–L, Figure 2A–L). The incubation with GS alone did not show any detectable modification compared to baseline (Figure 1A–L, Figure 2A–L).

Stimulation of the cells with *IL-1β* caused a significant up-regulation of all analyzed genes ($p < 0.05$, $p < 0.01$). Pre-treatment of the cells with celecoxib or GS significantly limited the negative effect of *IL-1β*, in particular when the drugs were tested in combination, both at 24 and 48 h ($p < 0.05$, $p < 0.01$) (Figure 1A–L, Figure 2A–L).

2.2. Effects of Celecoxib and GS on Cellular Survival and Apoptosis

The incubation of chondrocytes with celecoxib or GS alone significantly increased the percentage of survival cells, reduced the apoptotic rate, and up-regulated the gene expression of the anti-apoptotic marker *BCL2* ($p < 0.05$), in comparison to basal conditions, at both analyzed time points (Figures S1 and S2, Figure 3A–F); this trend was maintained and enhanced when the compounds were tested in combination ($p < 0.05$, $p < 0.01$). On the contrary, the stimulus with *IL-1β* significantly reduced viability ($p < 0.01$) and induced apoptosis ($p < 0.01$), which were counteracted by the pre-incubation of the cells with celecoxib and GS alone and, especially, in combination ($p < 0.05$, $p < 0.01$) (Figure 3A–F).

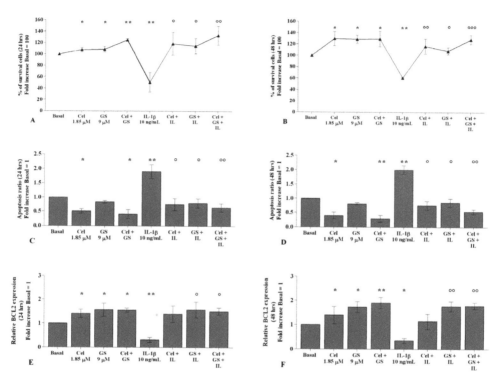

Figure 3. Celecoxib and GS regulate viability and apoptosis. Human osteoarthritic (OA) chondrocytes were incubated for 24 and 48 h with celecoxib (1.85 μM) and prescription-grade glucosamine sulfate (GS) (9 μM) (2 h of pre-treatment) in the presence of interleukin *(IL)-1β* (10 ng/mL). (**A,B**) Evaluation of cell viability by MTT assay. (**C,D**) Apoptosis detection performed by flow cytometry analysis and measured with Annexin Alexa fluor 488 assay. Data were expressed as the percentage of positive cells for Annexin-V and propidium iodide (PI) staining. (**E,F**) Expression levels of B-cell lymphoma (BCL2) analyzed by quantitative real-time PCR. The percentage of surviving cells, the ratio of apoptosis, and the gene expression were referenced to the ratio of the value of interest and the value of the basal condition, reported equal to 100 or 1. Data were represented as mean ± SD of triplicate values. * $p < 0.05$, ** $p < 0.01$ versus basal condition. ° $p < 0.05$, °° $p < 0.01$, °°° $p < 0.001$ versus *IL-1β*.

2.3. Celecoxib and GS Modulate the Oxidant/Antioxidant System

The potential role of celecoxib and GS in the regulation of oxidant/antioxidant balance in chondrocytes stimulated with *IL-1β* was reported in Figure S3 and Figure 4. Celecoxib and GS, analyzed alone or in combination, significantly reduced the production of mitochondrial superoxide anion and the gene expression of *SOD-2*, *CAT*, and *NRF2*, at 24 and 48 h, compared to baseline ($p < 0.05$, Figure 4A–H). Conversely, *IL-1β* stimulus induced mitochondrial ROS production and mRNA levels of the antioxidant enzymes ($p < 0.05$, $p < 0.01$); otherwise, pre-treatment with either celecoxib or GS limited the negative effect of *IL-1β* on redox balance, with an enhancement when the drugs were used in combination, both at 24 and 48 h ($p < 0.01$, $p < 0.001$) (Figure 4A–H).

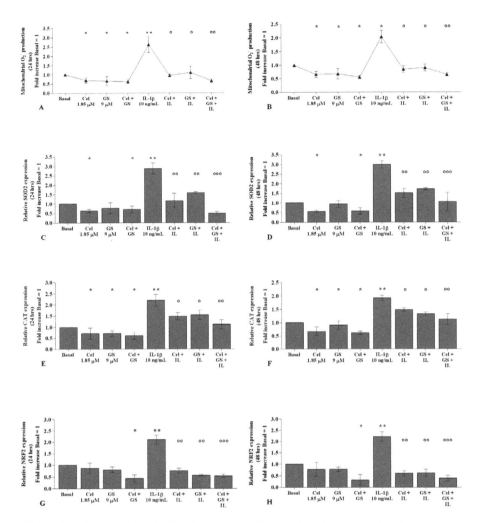

Figure 4. Celecoxib and GS regulate oxidative stress balance. Human osteoarthritic (OA) chondrocytes were incubated for 24 and 48 h with celecoxib (1.85 µM) and prescription-grade glucosamine sulfate (GS) (9 µM) (2 h of pre-treatment) in the presence of interleukin *(IL)-1β* (10 ng/mL). (**A,B**) Mitochondrial superoxide anion production evaluated by MitoSox Red staining at flow cytometry. (**C–H**) Expression levels of superoxide dismutase *(SOD)-2*, catalase *(CAT)*, and nuclear factor erythroid 2 like 2 *(NRF2)* analyzed by quantitative real-time PCR. The production of superoxide anion and the gene expression were referenced to the ratio of the value of interest and the value of basal condition, reported equal to 1. Data were represented as mean ± SD of triplicate values. * $p < 0.05$, ** $p < 0.01$ versus basal condition. ° $p < 0.05$, °° $p < 0.01$, °°° $p < 0.001$ versus *IL-1β*.

2.4. Celecoxib and GS Regulate Cartilage Turnover

As reported in Figures 5 and 6, the gene expression and supernatant release of the matrix-degrading enzymes—*MMP-1*, *MMP-3*, and *MMP-13*—did not show any significant change in OA chondrocytes incubated, for 24 and 48 h, with celecoxib or GS alone in comparison to basal conditions (Figure 5A–F, Figure 6A–F). GS significantly increased the expression and release of *Col2a1* ($p < 0.05$, $p < 0.01$) when tested alone or in combination with celecoxib (Figure 5G–H, Figure 6G–H).

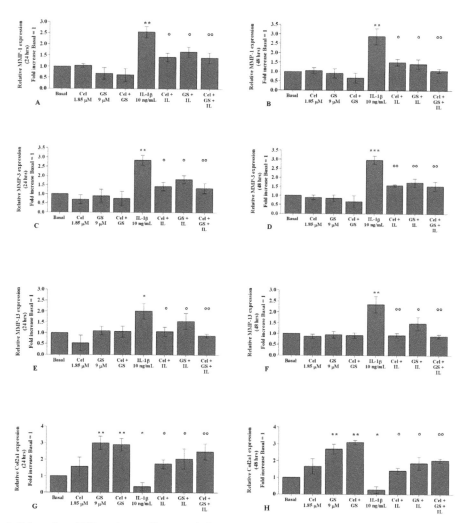

Figure 5. Celecoxib and GS regulate cartilage metabolism. Human osteoarthritic (OA) chondrocytes were incubated for 24 and 48 h with celecoxib (1.85 μM) and prescription-grade glucosamine sulfate (GS) (9 μM) (2 h of pre-treatment) in the presence of interleukin *(IL)-1β* (10 ng/mL). (**A–H**) Expression levels of metalloproteinase *(MMP)-1, -3, -13*, and type II collagen (*Col2a1*), analyzed by quantitative real-time PCR. The gene expression was referenced to the ratio of the value of interest and the value of basal condition, reported equal to 1. Data were represented as mean ± SD of triplicate values. * $p < 0.05$, ** $p < 0.01$, *** $p < 0.001$ versus basal condition. ° $p < 0.05$, °° $p < 0.01$ versus *IL-1β*.

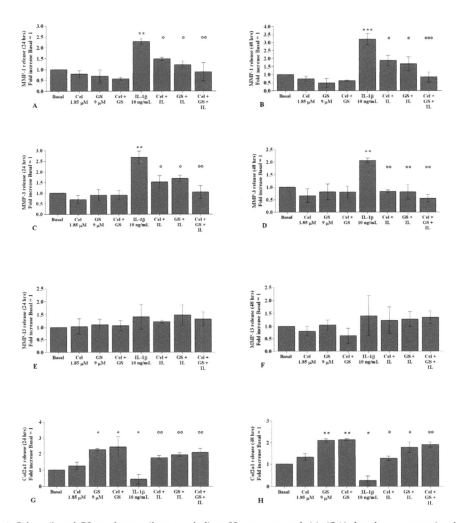

Figure 6. Celecoxib and GS regulate cartilage metabolism. Human osteoarthritic (OA) chondrocytes were incubated for 24 and 48 h with celecoxib (1.85 μM) and prescription-grade glucosamine sulfate (GS) (9 μM) (2 h of pre-treatment) in the presence of interleukin *(IL)-1β* (10 ng/mL). (**A–H**) Total amount of metalloproteinase *(MMP)-1, -3, -13*, and type II collagen (Col2a1) released in the supernatant, analyzed by ELISA assay. The total amount was referenced to the ratio of the value of interest and the value of the basal condition, reported equal to 1. Data were represented as mean ± SD of triplicate values. * $p < 0.05$, ** $p < 0.01$, *** $p < 0.001$ versus basal condition. ° $p < 0.05$, °° $p < 0.01$, °°° $p < 0.001$ versus *IL-1β*.

The statistically significant increase in *MMP-1*, *MMP-3*, and *MMP-13* and the down-regulation of *Col2a1* induced by *IL-1β* stimulus ($p < 0.05$, $p < 0.01$, $p < 0.001$) were partially inhibited by pre-treatment of the cells with celecoxib or GS. Co-incubation of OA chondrocytes with both drugs induced a more significant exacerbation by the combination of them, both at 24 and 48 h ($p < 0.05$, $p < 0.01$, $p < 0.001$) (Figure 5A–H, Figure 6A–H).

2.5. Celecoxib and GS Reduce NF-κB Signaling Pathway Activation

Figure 7 shows the effects of celecoxib and GS on NF-κB signaling pathway regulation. PCR real-time analysis reported no significant changes in OA chondrocytes incubated for 4 h with celecoxib or GS alone in comparison to baseline, except for the combination of them, which induced a significant reduction in *p65* and *p50* subunits gene expression ($p < 0.01$, $p < 0.05$, Figure 7A,B). As expected, the significant up-regulation of *p65* and *p50* gene expression induced by *IL-1β* stimulus ($p < 0.01$, $p < 0.05$) was partially counteracted by the pre-treatment of the cells with celecoxib or GS ($p < 0.05$) and, especially, when the drugs were tested in combination ($p < 0.01$) (Figure 7A,B).

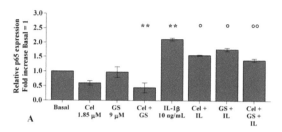

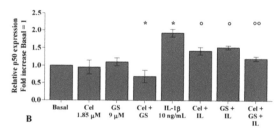

Figure 7. Celecoxib and GS modulate the NF-κB signaling pathway. Human osteoarthritic (OA) chondrocytes were incubated for 4 h with celecoxib (1.85 μM) and prescription-grade glucosamine sulfate (GS) (9 μM) (2 h of pre-treatment) in the presence of interleukin *(IL)-1β* (10 ng/mL). (**A,B**) Expression levels of *p65* and *p50* subunits were analyzed by quantitative real-time PCR. The gene expression was referenced to the ratio of the value of interest and the value of basal condition, reported equal to 1. Data were represented as mean ± SD of triplicate values. * $p < 0.05$, ** $p < 0.01$ versus basal condition. ° $p < 0.05$, °° $p < 0.01$ versus *IL-1β*.

2.6. NF-κB Inhibitor Enhances Celecoxib and GS-Induced Effects

To demonstrate the involvement of the NF-κB signaling pathway in mediating celecoxib and GS-induced effects on inflammatory, apoptotic, and oxidative stress mediators, OA chondrocytes were pre-incubated with a specific NF-κB inhibitor (BAY 11-7082, IKKα/β) (Figures 8–10).

The transcriptional levels of *COX-2*, *PGE2*, *IL-1β*, *IL-6*, *TNF-α* (Figure 8), *SOD-2*, *CAT*, *NRF2* (Figure 9), *MMP-1*, *MMP-3*, and *MMP-13* (Figure 10) were significantly reduced ($p < 0.01$, $p < 0.001$) in OA cells incubated with BAY 11-7082, while an up-regulation of *Col2a1* mRNA levels was observed ($p < 0.05$, Figure 10) in comparison to the basal condition and *IL-1β*.

The co-treatment of the cells with BAY 11-7082 and celecoxib or GS, alone or in combination, did not show any significant difference in target gene expression with respect to what was observed in OA chondrocytes incubated with BAY 11-7082 alone (Figures 8–10).

Furthermore, incubation of the NF-κB inhibitor with celecoxib and GS, in the presence of *IL-1β* stimulus, significantly reduced the expression levels of the analyzed genes beyond that caused by each treatment and, in particular, limited that induced by *IL-1β* (Figures 8–10).

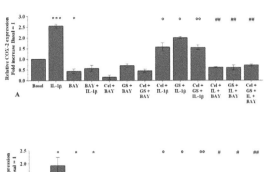
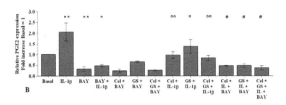
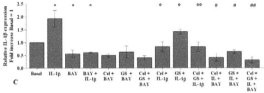
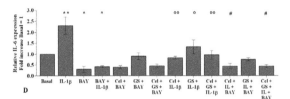
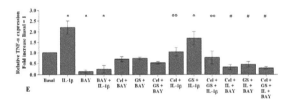

Figure 8. BAY 11-7082 influences celecoxib and GS effects on pro-inflammatory cytokines. Human osteoarthritic (OA) chondrocytes were incubated for 24 h with celecoxib (1.85 μM) and prescription-grade glucosamine sulfate (GS) (9 μM) (2 h of pre-treatment) in the presence of interleukin *(IL)-1β* (10 ng/mL) and BAY 11-7082 1 μM (NF-κB inhibitor, 2 h of pre-treatment). (**A–E**) Expression levels of cyclooxygenase *(COX)-2*, prostaglandin *(PG)E2*, *IL-1β*, *IL-6*, and tumor necrosis factor *(TNF)-α* analyzed by quantitative real-time PCR. The gene expression was referenced to the ratio of the value of interest and the value of basal condition, reported equal to 1. Data were represented as mean ± SD of triplicate values. * $p < 0.05$, ** $p < 0.01$, *** $p < 0.001$ versus basal condition. ° $p < 0.05$, °° $p < 0.01$ versus *IL-1β*. # $p < 0.05$, ## $p < 0.01$ versus celecoxib or GS plus BAY.

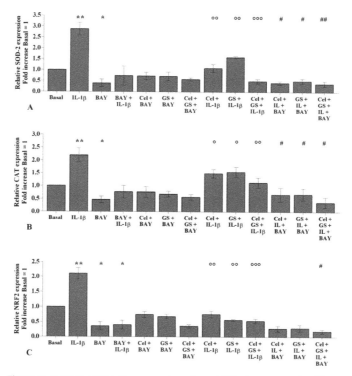

Figure 9. BAY 11-7082 influences celecoxib and GS effects on anti-oxidant enzymes expression. Human osteoarthritic (OA) chondrocytes were incubated for 24 h with celecoxib (1.85 μM) and prescription-grade glucosamine sulfate (GS) (9 μM) (2 h of pre-treatment) in the presence of interleukin *(IL)-1β* (10 ng/mL) and BAY 11-7082 1 μM (NF-κB inhibitor, 2 h of pre-treatment). (**A–C**) Expression levels of superoxide dismutase *(SOD)-2*, catalase *(CAT)*, and nuclear factor erythroid 2 like 2 *(NRF2)* analyzed by quantitative real-time PCR. The gene expression was referenced to the ratio of the value of interest and the value of basal condition, reported equal to 1. Data were represented as mean ± SD of triplicate values. * $p < 0.05$, ** $p < 0.01$ versus basal condition. ° $p < 0.05$, °° $p < 0.01$, °°° $p < 0.001$ versus *IL-1β*. # $p < 0.05$, ## $p < 0.01$ versus celecoxib or GS plus BAY.

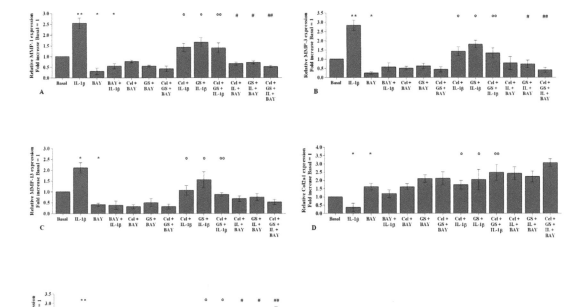

Figure 10. BAY 11-7082 enhances celecoxib and GS effects on cartilage metabolism. Human osteoarthritic (OA) chondrocytes were incubated for 24 h with celecoxib (1.85 μM) and prescription-grade glucosamine sulfate (GS) (9 μM) (2 h of pre-treatment) in the presence of interleukin *(IL)-1β* (10 ng/mL) and BAY 11-7082 1 μM (NF-κB inhibitor, 2 h of pre-treatment). (**A–E**) Expression levels of metalloproteinase (*MMP*)-1, -3, -13, type II collagen (*Col2a1*), and B-cell lymphoma (*BCL2*) analyzed by quantitative real-time PCR. The gene expression was referenced to the ratio of the value of interest and the value of basal condition, reported equal to 1. Data were represented as mean ± SD of triplicate values. * $p < 0.05$, ** $p < 0.01$ versus basal condition. ° $p < 0.05$, °° $p < 0.01$ versus *IL-1β*. # $p < 0.05$, ## $p < 0.01$ versus celecoxib or GS plus BAY.

3. Discussion

The goal of the present research was to examine the possible anti-inflammatory and chondroprotective effects of a combination of celecoxib and GS on inflammation, cartilage turnover, apoptosis, and oxidative stress in human OA chondrocyte cultures, and the potential mechanism of action underlying their favorable effects.

The concentrations of celecoxib and GS tested in the present study seem to be the most appropriate to reflect the mean plasma concentration of drugs reaching the systemic circulation, and they were chosen according to those used by other authors [39,40]. Furthermore, our chondrocytes were grown in culture medium containing low concentrations of glucose (DMEM with 25 mmol/L of glucose), to avoid any possible competition with GS for glucose transporters, thus impeding adequate GS uptake into the cells [35,41]. Finally, the cultures were stimulated with *IL-1β*, a potent pro-inflammatory cytokine generally used in in vitro models to mimic the circumstances driving to in vivo cartilage degradation and inflammatory status [35,42].

Our first result confirmed the significant increase in gene expression and supernatant release of the main pro-inflammatory cytokines, *IL-1β*, *IL-6*, *TNF-α*, and *PGE2*, the latter probably related to the increase in *COX-2*, in OA chondrocytes stimulated with *IL-1β*, as previously reported [22,35]. The incubation of the cells with celecoxib or GS counteracted the negative effects of *IL-1β* on these mediators, similarly to what was observed on OA chondrocytes and OA canine models by other authors [19,22,23,33,35]. Furthermore, we demonstrated, for the first time, a synergistic anti-inflammatory effect of celecoxib and GS, when tested in combination, in *IL-1β*-treated chondrocytes, with an activity retention until 48 h of treatment.

The regulation of chondrocytes survival is important for the maintenance of a proper cartilage structure and function. Indeed, morphological changes due to an increase in apoptosis are typical features of OA damage [43]. The analysis of viability and apoptosis carried out in the present study showed a reduction in survival and an increase in apoptotic chondrocytes in the presence of *IL-1β*, which appeared in agreement with previous research [22,44,45]. On the contrary, celecoxib and GS, tested alone or in combination, increased viability and decreased apoptosis, with a concomitant up-regulation of the anti-apoptotic marker *BCL2*; the anti-apoptotic effect of our drugs was also demonstrated in OA cells stimulated with *IL-1β*. These results are consistent with other authors who reported the ability of both compounds to promote proliferation and reduce the apoptosis rate of OA chondrocytes with or without the influence of the negative stimulus of *IL-1β* [21,22,38,46]. Furthermore, we firstly observed that the anti-apoptotic activity of celecoxib and GS was increased when *IL-1β*-stimulated chondrocytes were simultaneously incubated with the drugs, at both 24 and 48 h of treatment.

Accumulating evidence indicates ROS and reactive nitrogen species as important mediators of cartilage damage that occurs in OA; the failure in oxidant/antioxidant balance in OA chondrocytes induces an altered redox status, which promotes cartilage breakdown and makes cells more susceptible to oxidant-mediated apoptosis [2]. In the current study, the assessment of oxidative stress showed an increase in mitochondrial superoxide anion production and antioxidant enzymes expression, *SOD2, CAT*, and of the transcriptional factor *NRF2*, in OA chondrocytes exposed to *IL-1β*, in agreement with our previous findings [22]. Furthermore, we demonstrated the ability of celecoxib or GS to decrease ROS release and antioxidant enzyme gene levels, and their effect was also maintained following *IL-1β* stimulus, in line with the current literature. Indeed, some authors reported the reduction of superoxide anion production and SOD2 activity, caused by celecoxib, in OA chondrocytes stimulated with *IL-1β* [22,47]. Similarly, a decrease in superoxide anion and inducible nitric oxide synthase (iNOS) expression, induced by *IL-1β*, was found in human OA chondrocytes treated with GS [48–50]. Interestingly, our results further demonstrated that the activation of oxidative stress caused by *IL-1β* was strongly reversed by the simultaneous treatment of the cells with celecoxib and GS, indicating a more efficacious anti-oxidant effect of the studied drugs when used in combination.

The activation of different matrix-degrading enzymes, such as *MMP-1, MMP-3*, and *MMP-13*, and the consequent degradation of proteoglycans and Col2a1 represents one of main characteristics of OA and has been amply demonstrated in human OA articular cartilage and chondrocytes following *IL-1β* stimulus [9,17,18,41,45,46]. In agreement with these data, in the present paper, we observed a significant increase in *MMP-1, -3*, and *-13* and a reduction in *Col2a1* gene expression and supernatant release in *IL-1β*-stimulated OA chondrocytes. The incubation of our cultures with celecoxib or GS alone did not modify the studied *MMPs* and Col2a1, according to other findings [47,48], while it was able to counteract the negative effect of *IL-1β* on these factors, especially when the drugs were co-incubated, until 48 h of treatment, suggesting a possible anti-catabolic effect of the tested compounds. In a similar manner, other authors reported a reduction in *MMP-1, MMP-3, MMP-13*, aggrecanases, and a production of proteoglycans and *Col2a1* in *IL-1β*-stimulated OA chondrocytes treated with celecoxib or GS [16,22,35,36,51–56], while no data from the literature are available concerning the combination of celecoxib and GS on cartilage turnover.

Finally, our experience focused on a deeper investigation on the potential mechanism of action underlying favorable effects of celecoxib and GS combination on chondrocytes metabolism through analysis of the NF-κB signaling pathway.

It is known that NF-κB proteins constitute a family of ubiquitously expressed transcription factors triggering the expression of inflammatory mediators and matrix-degrading enzymes involved in detrimental processes occurring during OA [57].

A number of studies showed the protective role of GS on cartilage metabolism by inhibiting activation of the NF-κB signaling pathway, as well as its nuclear translocation, in human OA chondrocytes stimulated with *IL-1β* [33]; this effect was also observed when GS was used at a range of concentration similar to that found at plasma concentration, as established by pharmacokinetics studies [37,40].

Growing evidence suggests that celecoxib exerts a direct effect on cartilage metabolism by modulating pathways independent to *COX-2* activity and PGE2 inhibition, probably through the regulation of NF-kB signaling [15,47,58].

Our data are in line with the current literature demonstrating that the treatment of OA chondrocytes with celecoxib or GS reduced NF-kB signal activation as well as *p50* and *p65* subunits nuclear translocation induced by *IL-1β*; this effect was strongly enhanced when the drugs were tested in combination. We further demonstrated that the use of a specific NF-κB inhibitor, BAY11-7082, reduced the effect of *IL-1β* on inflammation, oxidative stress, apoptosis, and cartilage turnover, potentiating the activity of celecoxib and GS, as previously reported [54]. This allows us to speculate the hypothesis that celecoxib and GS could be effective in the regulation of chondrocyte metabolism through a direct inhibition of NF-κB signaling.

Different findings pointed out that GS seems to exert its effect on NF-κB-dependent transcription via an epigenetic mechanism, regulating the demethylation of specific CpG sites of DNA in the IL1β promoter, responsible for the aberrant expression of *MMPs*, *ADAMTS*, and *IL-1β* in human articular chondrocytes [37,54]. On the other hand, it is currently not completely defined how celecoxib mediates the activity of NF-κB, but it is possible to assume that it follows the PI3K/AKT/IKK/NF-kB pathway regulation, implicated in the regulation of apoptosis and cell proliferation, as demonstrated in different studies on cancer cell lines [59,60].

4. Materials and Methods

4.1. Sample Collection and Cell Cultures

Human OA articular cartilage was collected from femoral heads of five non-obese (body mass index ranging from 20 to 23 kg/m^2) and non-diabetic patients (two men and three women, age ranging from 65 to 75) with coxarthrosis according to ACR criteria [61], undergoing hip replacement surgery.

OA grade ranged from moderate to severe, and cartilage showed typical disease changes, as the presence of chondrocyte clusters, fibrillation, and loss of metachromasia (Mankin degree 3–7) [62]. The femoral heads were supplied by the Orthopaedic Surgery, University of Siena, Italy. The use of human articular samples was authorized by the Ethic Committee of Azienda Ospedaliera Universitaria Senese/Siena University Hospital (decision no. 13931/18) and the informed consent of the donor.

After surgery, cartilage fragments were aseptically dissected and processed by an enzymatic digestion, as previously described [63]. For growth and expansion, cells were cultured in Dulbecco's Modified Eagle Medium (DMEM) (Euroclone, Milan, Italy) with phenol red and 4 mM L-glutamine, supplemented with 10% fetal bovine serum (FBS) (Euroclone, Milan, Italy), 200 U/mL penicillin, and 200 μg/mL streptomycin (P/S) (Sigma-Aldrich, Milan, Italy). The medium was changed twice a week, and the cell morphology was examined daily with an inverted microscope (Olympus IMT-2, Tokyo, Japan). OA primary chondrocytes at the first passage were employed for the experiments [64]. For each single experiment a cell culture from a unique donor was used.

4.2. Pharmacological Treatment

Human OA chondrocytes were plated in 6-well dishes at a starting density of 1×10^5 cells/well until 85% confluence. Prescription-grade crystalline GS (Dona®) and celecoxib (Celebrex®) were supplied by Meda Pharma SpA (Viatris group). The powders of the substances were dissolved in the culture medium in phosphate-buffered saline (PBS) (Euroclone, Milan, Italy), according to the instructions, and directly diluted in the culture medium for the treatment to achieve the final concentrations required.

The cells were cultured in DMEM enriched with 0.5% FBS and 2% P/S, and they were treated for 24 and 48 h with celecoxib and GS, at the concentration of 1.85 μM and 9 μM, respectively, to better reproduce their therapeutic effect in vivo. The treatment was performed in the presence of *IL-1β* (10 n g/mL) (Sigma-Aldrich, Italy), added after 2 h of pre-incubation with the drugs; the experiments were also assessed analyzing the combination of both drugs at 24 and 48 h. Afterwards, the cells were recovered and immediately processed to carry out flow cytometry and quantitative real-time PCR, while the supernatant was collected and stored at −80 °C until ELISA assay.

Some cultures were pre-incubated for 2 h with BAY 11-7082 1 μM (NF-κB inhibitor, IKKα/β, Sigma–Aldrich, Milan, Italy) and then treated for 24 h with celecoxib and GS. Afterwards, the gene expression of the target genes (*COX-2, IL-1β, IL-6, TNF-α, MMP-1, MMP-3, MMP-13, Col2a1, BCL2, SOD-2, CAT,* and *NRF2*) was evaluated.

4.3. Cell Viability

The viability of the cells after pharmacological treatment was evaluated by MTT (3-[4,4-dimethylthiazol-2-yl]-2,5-diphenyl-tetrazoliumbromide) (Sigma-Aldrich, Milan, Italy) for each experimental condition, as previously described [65]. Timing of drug treatment was selected according to the percentage of surviving cells (Figure S1). The percentage of surviving cells was evaluated as (absorbance of considered sample)/(absorbance of control) $\times$ 100. Data were reported as OD units per 10^4 adherent cells.

4.4. RNA Isolation and Quantitative Real-Time PCR

OA chondrocyte were grown and maintained in 6-well dishes at a starting density of 1×10^5 cells/well until they became 85% confluent in DMEM supplemented with 10% FBS, before replacement with 0.5% FBS for the treatment. Then, cells were collected, and total RNA was extracted using TriPure Isolation Reagent (Euroclone, Milan, Italy) according to the manufacturer's instructions. Five hundred nanograms of RNA of target genes was reverse-transcribed by using the QuantiTect Reverse Transcription kit (Qiagen, Hilden, Germany), according to the manufacturer's instructions. Target genes were assessed by real-time PCR using the QuantiFast SYBR Green PCR kit (Qiagen, Hilden, Germany). Primers used for PCR reactions are listed in Table S1.

All qPCR reactions were achieved in glass capillaries by a LightCycler 1.0 (Roche Molecular Biochemicals, Mannheim, Germany) with LightCycler Software Version 3.5. The reaction procedure has been described in detail in our previous studies [63].

For the data analysis, the Ct values of each sample and the efficiency of the primer set were calculated by LinReg Software and converted into relative quantities [66,67]. The normalization was performed considering Actin Beta (*ACTB*) as a housekeeping gene for the analyzed target genes [68].

4.5. ELISA Assay

After the pharmacological treatment, the supernatant was collected and stored at −80 °C until analysis. PGE2 production, the release of *COX-2, IL-1β, IL-6, TNF-α, MMP-1, MMP-3, MMP-13,* and *Col2a1* were detected using ELISA kits (Boster Biological Technology, CA, USA).

IL-1β limit of detection was 250 pg/mL. Inter-assay and intra-assay coefficients of variation were 5.7–8.9%and 4.1–7.3%, respectively.

IL-6 limit of detection was 300 pg/mL. Inter-assay and intra-assay coefficients of variation were 7.2–8.6% and 6.2–7.4%, respectively.

TNF-α limit of detection was 1000 pg/mL. Inter-assay and intra-assay coefficients of variation were 5.4–6.4% and 4.8–7.4%, respectively.

MMP-1 limit of detection was 10,000 pg/mL. Inter-assay and intra-assay coefficients of variation were 7.6–8.3% and 5.8–6.5%, respectively.

MMP-3 limit of detection was 10000 pg/mL. Inter-assay and intra-assay coefficients of variation were 6.2–6.9% and 6.4–6.9%, respectively.

MMP-13 limit of detection was 10,000 pg/mL. Inter-assay and intra-assay coefficients of variation were 7.5–8.1% and 6.4–7.0%, respectively.

Col2a1 limit of detection was 20 ng/mL. Inter-assay and intra-assay coefficients of variation were <10% and <8%, respectively.

4.6. Apoptosis Detection

Apoptotic cells were measured by using the Annexin V-FITC and propidium iodide (PI) (ThermoFisher Scientific, Milan, Italy) kit. OA chondrocyte were seeded in 12-well plates (8×10^4 cells/well) for 24 h in DMEM with 10% FBS, before replacement with 0.5% FBS used for the treatment. The apoptosis assay was performed as previously described [69]. A total of 10,000 events (1×10^4 cells per assay) were measured by the instrument. The results were examined with Cell Quest software (Version 4.0, Becton Dickinson, San Jose, CA, USA). Cells simultaneously stained with Alexa Fluor 488 annexin-V and PI were considered for the evaluation of apoptosis (total apoptosis) [22]. The results were represented as percentage of positive cells to each dye.

4.7. Mitochondrial Superoxide Anion ($\bullet O_2^-$) Production

OA chondrocyte were seeded in 12 well-plates (8×10^4 cells/well) for 24 h in DMEM with 10% FCS, before replacement with 0.5% FBS for the treatment. The mitochondrial superoxide anion detection has been performed by MitoSOX Red staining as previously described [69]. A density of 1×10^4 cells per assay (a total of 10,000 events) was measured by flow cytometry, and data were analyzed with CellQuest software (Version 4.0, Becton Dickinson, San Jose, CA, USA). Results were collected as median of fluorescence (AU) and represented the mean of three independent experiments.

4.8. Statistical Analysis

Three independent experiments were carried out, and the results were expressed as the mean ± standard deviation (SD) of triplicate values for each experiment. Data normal distribution was evaluated by Shapiro–Wilk, D'Agostino and Pearson, and Kolmogorov–Smirnov tests. Flow cytometry, ELISA, and Western blot results were assessed by ANOVA with Bonferroni post hoc test. Quantitative real-time PCR was evaluated by one-way ANOVA with a Tukey's post hoc test using $2^{-\Delta\Delta CT}$ values for each sample. All analyses were performed through the SAS System (SAS Institute Inc., Cary, NC, USA) and GraphPad Prism 6.1. A *p*-value < 0.05 was considered as statistically significant.

5. Conclusions

In the present study we confirm the anti-inflammatory and anti-catabolic effects of the therapeutic dose of prescription-grade GS on human OA chondrocyte metabolism.

Furthermore, our results demonstrate the chondroprotective role of celecoxib in OA cells, reinforcing the evidence in favor of using this drug as potential DMOADs. In fact, in vitro studies showed the direct effects of celecoxib on cartilage, bone, and synoviocytes metabolism [15], raising the question of whether it is more than an anti-inflammatory and analgesic drug and, thus, has additional disease modifying effects.

A number of clinical studies reported that the combination of celecoxib and GS effectively modulate immune inflammatory response, oxidative stress damage, and joint pain and function in patients with knee OA [70–72]. Our results demonstrate, for the first time, the synergistic effect of celecoxib and GS on human OA chondrocyte metabolism. In particular, this combination treatment exerts a protective role on chondrocytes against the detrimental activities induced by *IL-1β* stimulus, reducing inflammation, apoptosis, oxidative stress, and regulating cartilage turnover, and this activity was effective through direct regulation of NF-κB signaling pathway activation.

Taken together, our in vitro findings suggest that the simultaneous treatment of celecoxib and GS seems to be more effective overall than each single treatment alone, for all the evaluated processes. This result may support the use of a combination therapy for the treatment of OA in clinical practice, since attenuating multiple pathways leading to inflammation and joint destruction can facilitate a safe and effective management of OA.

Our data provide indicative interesting results that deserve to be confirmed with further investigations.

Some limitations need to be mentioned. The same analyses on healthy primary chondrocytes are recommended, to better understand the effectiveness of celecoxib and GS on chondrocyte homeostasis and, in particular, their relevance in OA damage. Then, a deeper examination of the molecular mechanism responsible for the pharmacological effects may contribute to find out the exact role of celecoxib and GS in OA.

Supplementary Materials: The following are available online at https://www.mdpi.com/article/10.3390/ijms22168980/s1.

Author Contributions: Conceptualization, S.C., S.T. and A.F.; Data curation, S.C.; Investigation, S.C. and S.T.; Methodology, S.C. and S.G.; Supervision, A.F.; Validation, N.V.; Writing—original draft, S.C., J.-Y.R. and A.F.; Writing—review and editing, S.C., S.T., S.G., N.V., J.-Y.R. and A.F. All authors have read and agreed to the published version of the manuscript.

Funding: This research received no external funding.

Informed Consent Statement: Informed consent was obtained from all subjects involved in the study.

Conflicts of Interest: The authors declare no conflict of interest.

References

1. Ratneswaran, A.; Kapoor, M. Osteoarthritis year in review: Genetics, genomics, epigenetics. *Osteoarthr. Cartil.* **2021**, *29*, 151–160. [CrossRef] [PubMed]
2. Zheng, L.; Zhang, Z.; Sheng, P.; Mobasheri, A. The role of metabolism in chondrocyte dysfunction and the progression of osteoarthritis. *Ageing Res. Rev.* **2021**, *66*, 101249. [CrossRef]
3. Rizzoli, R. Microbiota and Bone Health: The Gut-Musculoskeletal Axis. *Calcif. Tissue Int.* **2018**, *102*, 385–386. [CrossRef] [PubMed]
4. Berenbaum, F.; Wallace, I.J.; Lieberman, D.E.; Felson, D.T. Modern-day environmental factors in the pathogenesis of osteoarthritis. *Nat. Rev. Rheumatol.* **2018**, *14*, 674–681. [CrossRef] [PubMed]
5. Biver, E.; Berenbaum, F.; Valdes, A.M.; de Carvalho, I.A.; Bindels, L.B.; Brandi, M.L.; Calder, P.C.; Castronovo, V.; Cavalier, E.; Cherubini, A.; et al. Gut microbiota and osteoarthritis management: An expert consensus of the European society for clinical and economic aspects of osteoporosis, osteoarthritis and musculoskeletal diseases (ESCEO). *Ageing Res. Rev.* **2019**, *55*, 100946. [CrossRef]
6. Wang, Z.; Zhu, H.; Jiang, Q.; Zhu, Y.Z. The gut microbiome as non-invasive biomarkers for identifying overweight people at risk for osteoarthritis. *Microb. Pathog.* **2021**, *157*, 104976. [CrossRef] [PubMed]
7. Bruyère, O.; Honvo, G.; Veronese, N.; Arden, N.K.; Branco, J.; Curtis, E.M.; Al-Daghri, N.M.; Herrero-Beaumont, G.; Martel-Pelletier, J.; Pelletier, J.P.; et al. An updated algorithm recommendation for the management of knee osteoarthritis from the European Society for Clinical and Economic Aspects of Osteoporosis, Osteoarthritis and Musculoskeletal Diseases (ESCEO). *Semin. Arthritis Rheum.* **2019**, *49*, 337–350. [CrossRef]
8. Bannuru, R.R.; Osani, M.C.; Vaysbrot, E.E.; Arden, N.K.; Bennell, K.; Bierma-Zeinstra, S.M.A.; Kraus, V.B.; Lohmander, L.S.; Abbott, J.H.; Bhandari, M.; et al. OARSI guidelines for the non-surgical management of knee, hip, and polyarticular osteoarthritis. *Osteoarthr. Cartil.* **2019**, *27*, 1578–1589. [CrossRef]
9. Kucharz, E.J.; Szántó, S.; Ivanova Goycheva, M.; Petronijević, M.; Šimnovec, K.; Domżalski, M.; Gallelli, L.; Kamenov, Z.; Konstantynowicz, J.; Radunović, G.; et al. Correction to: Endorsement by Central European experts of the revised ESCEO algorithm for the management of knee osteoarthritis. *Rheumatol. Int.* **2019**, *39*, 1661–1662, Erratum in: *Rheumatol. Int.* **2019**, *39*, 1117–1123. [CrossRef]

10. Kolasinski, S.L.; Neogi, T.; Hochberg, M.C.; Oatis, C.; Guyatt, G.; Block, J.; Callahan, L.; Copenhaver, C.; Dodge, C.; Felson, D.; et al. 2019 American College of Rheumatology/Arthritis Foundation Guideline for the Management of Osteoarthritis of the Hand, Hip, and Knee. *Arthritis Rheumatol.* **2020**, *72*, 220–233, Erratum in: *Arthritis Rheumatol.* **2021**, *73*, 799. [CrossRef]
11. Arden, N.K.; Perry, T.A.; Bannuru, R.R.; Bruyère, O.; Cooper, C.; Haugen, I.K.; Hochberg, M.C.; McAlindon, T.E.; Mobasheri, A.; Reginster, J.-Y. Non-surgical management of knee osteoarthritis: Comparison of ESCEO and OARSI 2019 guidelines. *Nat. Rev. Rheumatol.* **2021**, *17*, 59–66. [CrossRef] [PubMed]
12. Zhang, Z.; Huang, C.; Cao, Y.; Mu, R.; Zhang, M.C.; Xing, D.; Fan, D.; Ding, Y.; Guo, J.; Hou, Y.; et al. 2021 revised algorithm for the management of knee osteoarthritis-the Chinese viewpoint. *Aging Clin. Exp. Res.* **2021**, *33*, 2141–2147. [CrossRef]
13. Rani, A.; Baruah, R.; Goyal, A. Prebiotic Chondroitin Sulfate Disaccharide Isolated from Chicken Keel Bone Exhibiting Anticancer Potential Against Human Colon Cancer Cells. *Nutr. Cancer* **2019**, *71*, 825–839. [CrossRef] [PubMed]
14. Shmagel, A.; Demmer, R.; Knights, D.; Butler, M.; Langsetmo, L.; Lane, N.E.; Ensrud, K. The Effects of Glucosamine and Chondroitin Sulfate on Gut Microbial Composition: A Systematic Review of Evidence from Animal and Human Studies. *Nutrients* **2019**, *11*, 294. [CrossRef] [PubMed]
15. Zweers, M.C.; de Boer, T.N.; van Roon, J.; Bijlsma, J.W.; Lafeber, F.P.; Mastbergen, S.C. Celecoxib: Considerations regarding its potential disease-modifying properties in osteoarthritis. *Arthritis Res. Ther.* **2011**, *13*, 239. [CrossRef]
16. Fioravanti, A.; Tinti, L.; Pascarelli, N.A.; Di Capua, A.; Lamboglia, A.; Cappelli, A.; Biava, M.; Giordani, A.; Niccolini, S.; Galeazzi, M.; et al. In Vitro effects of VA441, a new selective cyclooxygenase-2 inhibitor, on human osteoarthritic chondrocytes exposed to IL-1β. *J. Pharmacol. Sci.* **2012**, *120*, 6–14. [CrossRef]
17. Nakata, K.; Hanai, T.; Take, Y.; Osada, T.; Tsuchiya, T.; Shima, D.; Fujimoto, Y. Disease-modifying effects of COX-2 selective inhibitors and non-selective NSAIDs in osteoarthritis: A systematic review. *Osteoarthr. Cartil.* **2018**, *26*, 1263–1273. [CrossRef]
18. Timur, U.T.; Caron, M.M.J.; Jeuken, R.M.; Bastiaansen-Jenniskens, Y.M.; Welting, T.J.M.; van Rhijn, L.W.; van Osch, G.J.V.M.; Emans, P.J. Chondroprotective Actions of Selective COX-2 Inhibitors In Vivo: A Systematic Review. *Int. J. Mol. Sci.* **2020**, *21*, 6962. [CrossRef] [PubMed]
19. Mastbergen, S.C.; Jansen, N.W.; Bijlsma, J.W.; Lafeber, F.P. Differential direct effects of cyclo-oxygenase-1/2 inhibition on proteoglycan turnover of human osteoarthritic cartilage: An in vitro study. *Arthritis Res. Ther.* **2006**, *8*, 1–9. [CrossRef]
20. Matsuda, K.; Nakamura, S.; Matsushita, T. Celecoxib inhibits nitric oxide production in chondrocytes of ligament-damaged osteoarthritic rat joints. *Rheumatol. Int.* **2006**, *26*, 991–995. [CrossRef]
21. Ou, Y.; Tan, C.; An, H.; Jiang, D.; Quan, Z.; Tang, K.; Luo, X. Selective COX-2 inhibitor ameliorates osteoarthritis by repressing apoptosis of chondrocyte. *Med. Sci. Monit.* **2012**, *18*, BR247–BR252. [CrossRef] [PubMed]
22. Cheleschi, S.; Calamia, V.; Fernandez-Moreno, M.; Biava, M.; Giordani, A.; Fioravanti, A.; Anzini, M.; Blanco, F. In vitro comprehensive analysis of VA692 a new chemical entity for the treatment of osteoarthritis. *Int. Immunopharmacol.* **2018**, *64*, 86–100. [CrossRef] [PubMed]
23. de Boer, T.N.; Huisman, A.M.; Polak, A.A.; Niehoff, A.G.; van Rinsum, A.C.; Saris, D.; Bijlsma, J.W.; Lafeber, F.J.; Mastbergen, S.C. The chondroprotective effect of selective COX-2 inhibition in osteoarthritis: Ex vivo evaluation of human cartilage tissue after in vivo treatment. *Osteoarthr. Cartil.* **2009**, *17*, 482–488. [CrossRef] [PubMed]
24. Cha, H.S.; Ahn, K.S.; Jeon, C.H.; Kim, J.; Koh, E.M. Inhibitory effect of cyclo-oxygenase-2 inhibitor on the production of matrix metalloproteinases in rheumatoid fibroblast-like synoviocytes. *Rheumatol. Int.* **2004**, *24*, 207–211. [CrossRef]
25. Tat, S.K.; Pelletier, J.P.; Lajeunesse, D.; Fahmi, H.; Duval, N.; Martel-Pelletier, J. Differential modulation of RANKL isoforms by human osteoarthritic subchondral bone osteoblasts: Influence of osteotropic factors. *Bone* **2008**, *43*, 284–291. [CrossRef]
26. Reginster, J.Y.; Deroisy, R.; Rovati, L.C.; Lee, R.L.; Lejeune, E.; Bruyere, O.; Giacovelli, G.; Henrotin, Y.; Dacre, J.E.; Gossett, C. Long-term effects of glucosamine sulphate on osteoarthritis progression: A randomised, placebo-controlled clinical trial. *Lancet* **2001**, *357*, 251–256. [CrossRef]
27. Pavelká, K.; Gatterová, J.; Olejarová, M.; Machacek, S.; Giacovelli, G.; Rovati, L.C. Glucosamine sulfate use and delay of progression of knee osteoarthritis: A 3-year, randomized, placebo-controlled, double-blind study. *Arch. Intern. Med.* **2002**, *162*, 2113–2123. [CrossRef]
28. Giordano, N.; Fioravanti, A.; Papakostas, P.; Montella, A.; Giorgi, G.; Nuti, R. The efficacy and tolerability of glucosamine sulfate in the treatment of knee osteoarthritis: A randomized, double-blind, placebo-controlled trial. *Curr. Ther. Res. Clin. Exp.* **2009**, *70*, 185–196. [CrossRef]
29. Tenti, S.; Giordano, N.; Mondanelli, N.; Giannotti, S.; Maheu, E.; Fioravanti, A. A retrospective observational study of glucosamine sulfate in addition to conventional therapy in hand osteoarthritis patients compared to conventional treatment alone. *Aging Clin. Exp. Res.* **2020**, *32*, 1161–1172. [CrossRef]
30. Veronese, N.; Demurtas, J.; Smith, L.; Reginster, J.Y.; Bruyère, O.; Beaudart, C.; Honvo, G.; Maggi, S.; on behalf of the European Geriatric Medicine Society Special Interest Groups in Systematic Reviews and Meta-Analyses and Arthritis. Glucosamine sulphate: An umbrella review of health outcomes. *Ther. Adv. Musculoskelet. Dis.* **2020**, *12*. [CrossRef]
31. Beaudart, C.; Lengelé, L.; Leclercq, V.; Geerinck, A.; Sanchez-Rodriguez, D.; Bruyère, O.; Reginster, J.Y. Symptomatic Efficacy of Pharmacological Treatments for Knee Osteoarthritis: A Systematic Review and a Network Meta-Analysis with a 6-Month Time Horizon. *Drugs* **2020**, *80*, 1947–1959. [CrossRef] [PubMed]
32. Rovati, L.C.; Girolami, F.; Persiani, S. Crystalline glucosamine sulfate in the management of knee osteoarthritis: Efficacy, safety, and pharmacokinetic properties. *Ther. Adv. Musculoskelet. Dis.* **2012**, *4*, 167–180. [CrossRef]

33. Largo, R.; Alvarez-Soria, M.A.; Díez-Ortego, I.; Calvo, E.; Sánchez-Pernaute, O.; Egido, J.; Herrero-Beaumont, G. Glucosamine inhibits IL-1beta-induced NFkappaB activation in human osteoarthritic chondrocytes. *Osteoarthr. Cartil.* **2003**, *11*, 290–298. [CrossRef]

34. Chan, P.S.; Caron, J.P.; Rosa, G.J.; Orth, M.W. Glucosamine and chondroitin sulfate regulate gene expression and synthesis of nitric oxide and prostaglandin E(2) in articular cartilage explants. *Osteoarthr. Cartil.* **2005**, *13*, 387–394. [CrossRef]

35. Chiusaroli, R.; Piepoli, T.; Zanelli, T.; Ballanti, P.; Lanza, M.; Rovati, L.C.; Caselli, G. Experimental pharmacology of glucosamine sulfate. *Int. J. Rheumatol.* **2011**, *2011*, 939265. [CrossRef]

36. Bassleer, C.; Rovati, L.; Franchimont, P. Stimulation of proteoglycan production by glucosamine sulfate in chondrocytes isolated from human osteoarthritic articular cartilage in vitro. *Osteoarthr. Cartil.* **1998**, *6*, 427–434. [CrossRef]

37. Kucharz, E.J.; Kovalenko, V.; Szántó, S.; Bruyère, O.; Cooper, C.; Reginster, J.Y. A review of glucosamine for knee osteoarthritis: Why patented crystalline glucosamine sulfate should be differentiated from other glucosamines to maximize clinical outcomes. *Curr. Med. Res. Opin.* **2016**, *32*, 997–1004. [CrossRef]

38. Ma, Y.; Zheng, W.; Chen, H.; Shao, X.; Lin, P.; Liu, X.; Li, X.; Ye, H. Glucosamine promotes chondrocyte proliferation via the Wnt/β catenin signaling pathway. *Int. J. Mol. Med.* **2018**, *42*, 61–70. [CrossRef] [PubMed]

39. Walter, M.F.; Jacob, R.F.; Day, C.A.; Dahlborg, R.; Weng, Y.; Mason, R.P. Sulfone COX-2 inhibitors increase susceptibility of human LDL and plasma to oxidative modification: Comparison to sulfonamide COX-2 inhibitors and NSAIDs. *Atherosclerosis* **2004**, *177*, 235–243. [CrossRef]

40. Persiani, S.; Roda, E.; Rovati, L.C.; Locatelli, M.; Giacovelli, G.; Roda, A. Glucosamine oral bioavailability and plasma pharmacokinetics after increasing doses of crystalline glucosamine sulfate in man. *Osteoarthr. Cartil.* **2005**, *13*, 1041–1049. [CrossRef]

41. Calamia, V.; Mateos, J.; Fernández-Puente, P.; Lourido, L.; Rocha, B.; Fernández-Costa, C.; Montell, E.; Vergés, J.; Ruiz-Romero, C.; Blanco, F.J. A pharmacoproteomic study confirms the synergistic effect of chondroitin sulfate and glucosamine. *Sci. Rep.* **2014**, *4*, 5069. [CrossRef] [PubMed]

42. Goldring, S.R.; Goldring, M.B. The role of cytokines in cartilage matrix degeneration in osteoarthritis. *Clin. Orthop. Relat. Res.* **2004**, *427*, S27–S36. [CrossRef]

43. Hwang, H.S.; Kim, H.A. Chondrocyte Apoptosis in the Pathogenesis of Osteoarthritis. *Int. J. Mol. Sci.* **2015**, *16*, 26035–26054. [CrossRef]

44. Héraud, F.; Héraud, A.; Harmand, M.F. Apoptosis in normal and osteoarthritic human articular cartilage. *Ann. Rheum. Dis.* **2000**, *59*, 959–965. [CrossRef]

45. Cheleschi, S.; Fioravanti, A.; De Palma, A.; Corallo, C.; Franci, D.; Volpi, N.; Bedogni, G.; Giannotti, S.; Giordano, N. Methylsulfonylmethane and mobilee prevent negative effect of IL-1β in human chondrocyte cultures via NF-κB signaling pathway. *Int. Immunopharmacol.* **2018**, *65*, 129–139, Erratum in: *Int Immunopharmacol.* **2019**, *74*, 105775. [CrossRef] [PubMed]

46. Luo, M.; Xu, F.; Wang, Q.; Luo, W. The inhibiting effect of glucosamine sulfate combined with loxoprofen sodium on chondrocyte apoptosis in rats with knee osteoarthritis. *J. Musculoskelet. Neuronal Interact.* **2021**, *21*, 113–120. [PubMed]

47. Tsutsumi, R.; Ito, H.; Hiramitsu, T.; Nishitani, K.; Akiyoshi, M.; Kitaori, T.; Yasuda, T.; Nakamura, T. Celecoxib inhibits production of MMP and NO via down-regulation of NF-kappaB and JNK in a PGE2 independent manner in human articular chondrocytes. *Rheumatol. Int.* **2008**, *28*, 727–736. [CrossRef]

48. Alvarez-Soria, M.A.; Herrero-Beaumont, G.; Moreno-Rubio, J.; Calvo, E.; Santillana, J.; Egido, J.; Largo, R. Long-term NSAID treatment directly decreases COX-2 and mPGES-1 production in the articular cartilage of patients with osteoarthritis. *Osteoarthr. Cartil.* **2008**, *16*, 1484–1493. [CrossRef]

49. Mendis, E.; Kim, M.M.; Rajapakse, N.; Kim, S.K. Sulfated glucosamine inhibits oxidation of biomolecules in cells via a mechanism involving intracellular free radical scavenging. *Eur. J. Pharmacol.* **2008**, *579*, 74–85. [CrossRef] [PubMed]

50. Valvason, C.; Musacchio, E.; Pozzuoli, A.; Ramonda, R.; Aldegheri, R.; Punzi, L. Influence of glucosamine sulphate on oxidative stress in human osteoarthritic chondrocytes: Effects on HO-1, p22(Phox) and iNOS expression. *Rheumatol. (Oxf.)* **2008**, *47*, 31–35. [CrossRef]

51. Cho, H.; Walker, A.; Williams, J.; Hasty, K.A. Study of osteoarthritis treatment with anti-inflammatory drugs: Cyclooxygenase-2 inhibitor and steroids. *BioMed Res. Int.* **2015**, *2015*, 595273. [CrossRef]

52. Cheleschi, S.; Pascarelli, N.A.; Valacchi, G.; Di Capua, A.; Biava, M.; Belmonte, G.; Giordani, A.; Sticozzi, C.; Anzini, M.; Fioravanti, A. Chondroprotective effect of three different classes of anti-inflammatory agents on human osteoarthritic chondrocytes exposed to IL-1β. *Int. Immunopharmacol.* **2015**, *28*, 794–801. [CrossRef]

53. Sanchez, C.; Mateus, M.M.; Defresne, M.P.; Crielaard, J.M.; Reginster, J.Y.; Henrotin, Y.E. Metabolism of human articular chondrocytes cultured in alginate beads. Longterm effects of interleukin 1beta and nonsteroidal antiinflammatory drugs. *J. Rheumatol.* **2002**, *29*, 772–782.

54. Imagawa, K.; de Andrés, M.C.; Hashimoto, K.; Pitt, D.; Itoi, E.; Goldring, M.B.; Roach, H.I.; Oreffo, R.O. The epigenetic effect of glucosamine and a nuclear factor-kappa B (NF-kB) inhibitor on primary human chondrocytes–implications for osteoarthritis. *Biochem. Biophys. Res. Commun.* **2011**, *405*, 362–367. [CrossRef] [PubMed]

55. Su, S.C.; Tanimoto, K.; Tanne, Y.; Kunimatsu, R.; Hirose, N.; Mitsuyoshi, T.; Okamoto, Y.; Tanne, K. Celecoxib exerts protective effects on extracellular matrix metabolism of mandibular condylar chondrocytes under excessive mechanical stress. *Osteoarthr. Cartil.* **2014**, *22*, 845–851. [CrossRef] [PubMed]

56. Sanches, M.; Assis, L.; Criniti, C.; Fernandes, D.; Tim, C.; Renno, A.C.M. Chondroitin sulfate and glucosamine sulfate associated to photobiomodulation prevents degenerative morphological changes in an experimental model of osteoarthritis in rats. *Lasers Med. Sci.* **2018**, *33*, 549–557. [CrossRef]

57. Rigoglou, S.; Papavassiliou, A.G. The NF-κB signalling pathway in osteoarthritis. *Int. J. Biochem. Cell Biol.* **2013**, *45*, 2580–2584. [CrossRef]

58. Tegeder, I.; Niederberger, E.; Israr, E.; Gühring, H.; Brune, K.; Euchenhofer, C.; Grösch, S.; Geisslinger, G. Inhibition of NF-kappaB and AP-1 activation by R- and S-flurbiprofen. *FASEB J.* **2001**, *15*, 2–4. [CrossRef] [PubMed]

59. Cai, F.; Chen, M.; Zha, D.; Zhang, P.; Zhang, X.; Cao, N.; Wang, J.; He, Y.; Fan, X.; Zhang, W.; et al. Curcumol potentiates celecoxib-induced growth inhibition and apoptosis in human non-small cell lung cancer. *Oncotarget* **2017**, *8*, 115526–115545. [CrossRef] [PubMed]

60. Tudor, D.V.; Bâldea, I.; Olteanu, D.E.; Fischer-Fodor, E.; Piroska, V.; Lupu, M.; Călinici, T.; Decea, R.M.; Filip, G.A. Celecoxib as a Valuable Adjuvant in Cutaneous Melanoma Treated with Trametinib. *Int. J. Mol. Sci.* **2021**, *22*, 4387. [CrossRef]

61. Altman, R.; Alarcón, G.; Appelrouth, D.; Bloch, D.; Borenstein, D.; Brandt, K.; Brown, C.; Cooke, T.D.; Daniel, W.; Feldman, D.; et al. The American College of Rheumatology criteria for the classification and reporting of osteoarthritis of the hip. *Arthritis Rheum.* **1991**, *34*, 505–514. [CrossRef]

62. Mankin, H.J.; Dorfman, H.; Lippiello, L.; Zarins, A. Biochemical and metabolic abnormalities in articular cartilage from osteoarthritic human hips. II. Correlation of morphology with biochemical and metabolic data. *J. Bone Joint Surg. Am.* **1971**, *53*, 523–537. [CrossRef]

63. Cheleschi, S.; Tenti, S.; Mondanelli, N.; Corallo, C.; Barbarino, M.; Giannotti, S.; Gallo, I.; Giordano, A.; Fioravanti, A. MicroRNA-34a and MicroRNA-181a Mediate Visfatin-Induced Apoptosis and Oxidative Stress via NF-κB Pathway in Human Osteoarthritic Chondrocytes. *Cells* **2019**, *8*, 874. [CrossRef]

64. Francin, P.J.; Guillaume, C.; Humbert, A.C.; Pottie, P.; Netter, P.; Mainard, D.; Presle, N. Association between the chondrocyte phenotype and the expression of adipokines and their receptors: Evidence for a role of leptin but not adiponectin in the expression of cartilage-specific markers. *J. Cell Physiol.* **2011**, *226*, 2790–2797. [CrossRef]

65. Cheleschi, S.; Tenti, S.; Barbarino, M.; Giannotti, S.; Bellisai, F.; Frati, E.; Fioravanti, A. Exploring the Crosstalk between Hydrostatic Pressure and Adipokines: An In vitro Study on Human Osteoarthritic Chondrocytes. *Int. J. Mol. Sci.* **2021**, *22*, 2745. [CrossRef]

66. Pfaffl, M.W. A new mathematical model for relative quantification in real-time RT-PCR. *Nucleic Acids Res.* **2001**, *29*, e45. [CrossRef]

67. Ramakers, C.; Ruijter, J.M.; Deprez, R.H.; Moorman, A.F. Assumption-free analysis of quantitative real-time polymerase chain reaction (PCR) data. *Neurosci. Lett.* **2003**, *339*, 62–66. [CrossRef]

68. Vandesompele, J.; De Preter, K.; Pattyn, F.; Poppe, B.; Van Roy, N.; De Paepe, A.; Speleman, F. Accurate normalization of real-time quantitative RT-PCR data by geometric averaging of multiple internal control genes. *Genome Biol.* **2002**, *3*, 1–12. [CrossRef]

69. Cheleschi, S.; Barbarino, M.; Gallo, I.; Tenti, S.; Bottaro, M.; Frati, E.; Giannotti, S.; Fioravanti, A. Hydrostatic Pressure Regulates Oxidative Stress through microRNA in Human Osteoarthritic Chondrocytes. *Int. J. Mol. Sci.* **2020**, *21*, 3653. [CrossRef] [PubMed]

70. Selvan, T.; Rajiah, K.; Nainar, M.S.; Mathew, E.M. A clinical study on glucosamine sulfate versus combination of glucosamine sulfate and NSAIDs in mild to moderate knee osteoarthritis. *Sci. World J.* **2012**, *2012*, 902676. [CrossRef] [PubMed]

71. Amuzadeh, F.; Kazemian, G.; Rasi, A.M.; Khazanchin, A.; Khazanchin, A.; Kazemi, P. Comparison of the efficacy of combination of glucosamine sulfate and celecoxib versus celecoxib alone for the pain, morning stiffness, function relief of females with osteoarthritis grade 1&2 of the knee (a comparative study). *Indian J. Fundam. Appl. Life Sci.* **2015**, *5*, 129–136.

72. Deng, G.; Chen, X.; Yang, K.; Wu, A.; Zeng, G. Combined effect of celecoxib and glucosamine sulfate on inflammatory factors and oxidative stress indicators in patients with knee osteoarthritis. *Trop. J. Pharm. Res.* **2019**, *18*, 397–402. [CrossRef]

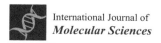

International Journal of
Molecular Sciences

MDPI

Brief Report

Proteomic Analysis of the Meniscus Cartilage in Osteoarthritis

Jisook Park [1], Hyun-Seung Lee [2], Eun-Bi Go [1], Ju Yeon Lee [3], Jin Young Kim [3], Soo-Youn Lee [2,4,5,*]
and Dae-Hee Lee [6,*]

1   Samsung Biomedical Research Institute, Samsung Medical Center, Sungkyunkwan University School
    of Medicine, Seoul 06351, Korea; js944837@hanmail.net (J.P.); geb926@naver.com (E.-B.G.)
2   Department of Laboratory Medicine and Genetics, Samsung Medical Center, Sungkyunkwan University
    School of Medicine, Seoul 06351, Korea; hyunseung1011.lee@samsung.com
3   Research Center for Bioconvergence Analysis, Korea Basic Science Institute, Cheongju 28119, Korea;
    jylee@kbsi.re.kr (J.Y.L.); jinyoung@kbsi.re.kr (J.Y.K.)
4   Department of Clinical Pharmacology and Therapeutics, Samsung Medical Center, Seoul 06351, Korea
5   Department of Health Science and Technology, Samsung Advanced Institute of Health Science
    and Technology, Sungkyunkwan University, Seoul 06351, Korea
6   Department of Orthopedic Surgery, Samsung Medical Center, Sungkyunkwan University School of Medicine,
    Seoul 06351, Korea
*   Correspondence: suddenbz@skku.edu (S.-Y.L.); eoak22.lee@samsung.com (D.-H.L.)

Citation: Park, J.; Lee, H.-S.; Go, E.-B.; Lee, J.Y.; Kim, J.Y.; Lee, S.-Y.; Lee, D.-H. Proteomic Analysis of the Meniscus Cartilage in Osteoarthritis. *Int. J. Mol. Sci.* **2021**, *22*, 8181. https://doi.org/10.3390/ijms22158181

Academic Editor: Nicola Veronese

Received: 2 June 2021
Accepted: 27 July 2021
Published: 30 July 2021

Abstract: The distribution of differential extracellular matrix (ECM) in the lateral and medial menisci can contribute to knee instability, and changes in the meniscus tissue can lead to joint disease. Thus, deep proteomic identification of the lateral and medial meniscus cartilage is expected to provide important information for treatment and diagnosis of various knee joint diseases. We investigated the proteomic profiles of 12 lateral/medial meniscus pairs obtained from excess tissue of osteoarthritis patients who underwent knee arthroscopy surgery using mass spectrometry-based techniques and measured 75 ECM protein levels in the lesions using a multiple reaction monitoring (MRM) assay we developed. A total of 906 meniscus proteins with a 1% false discovery rate (FDR) was identified through a tandem mass tag (TMT) analysis showing that the lateral and medial menisci had similar protein expression profiles. A total of 131 ECM-related proteins was included in meniscus tissues such as collagen, fibronectin, and laminin. Our data showed that 14 ECM protein levels were differentially expressed in lateral and medial lesions ($p < 0.05$). We present the proteomic characterization of meniscal tissue with mass spectrometry-based comparative proteomic analysis and developed an MRM-based assay of ECM proteins correlated with tissue regeneration. The mass spectrometry dataset has been deposited to the MassIVE repository with the dataset identifier MSV000087753.

Keywords: meniscus; proteomics; MRM; ECM

1. Introduction

The knee is the largest hinge joint associated with weight-bearing and movement in the human body. The meniscus is at type of fibrocartilage, has properties similar to those of bone, and serves many important biomechanical functions such as stabilizing joints and absorbing damage. The knee contains medial and lateral menisci; the medial meniscus tends to experience more frequent damage than the lateral meniscus due to its anatomical structure and articular mechanism [1]. Such damage includes a tear, which occurs when placing excessive pressure on or twisting the knee joint. Meniscal degeneration and surgically removed meniscus are risk factors for osteoarthritis [2], while aging of the meniscus results in molecular and cellular changes. Thus, an understanding of the proteomic changes in the medial and lateral meniscal tissues will contribute to uncovering the cause of knee-related degenerative disease.

The extracellular matrix (ECM) plays an essential role in many processes, including cell-cell adhesion, signaling, and tissue repair. The meniscal ECM consists of water, fibrillar protein, proteoglycans, and adhesive glycoproteins, the activities of which are not fully understood.

To date, meniscus proteomics studies are rare, although information on hyaline cartilage protein has been reported [3–5]. Recently, global proteomic investigations have been performed on medial meniscal tissues to analyze the global protein expression profiles in radial zones using mass spectrometric technologies. Pairwise comparisons of the medial/lateral meniscus is a potentially unique model for the study of cartilage proteomics in osteoarthritis genesis and progression, because the anatomical structure and biomechanical configuration of the knee is typically associated with much more severe cartilage loss on the predominantly weight-bearing medial compartment. Also, pairwise comparisons of the lateral/medial meniscus have advantages independent of heterogeneous factors such as age, sex, osteoarthritis severity, underlying disease, and individual variability.

Deep proteomics might be a powerful tool in characterization of meniscal tissues [6,7]. Therefore, we investigated the proteome profile of meniscal tissue of lateral and medial lesions and characterized the extracellular matrix proteins. Herein, we provide extracellular matrix data and use multiple reaction monitoring (ECM-MRM) assays to compare expression levels in two lesion types.

2. Results

2.1. Proteomic Analysis of Meniscal Tissues

Semi-quantitative analysis was performed on meniscal tissues to compare the protein compositions of lateral and medial lesions using six plex-tandem mass tag (TMT) labeling. A total of 7876 unique peptides representing 906 proteins (903 genes) were identified in the meniscal tissues. Here, we found that the lateral and medial menisci have similar protein expression profiles. Most proteins showed similar concentrations in the lateral and medial lesions. Cartilage oligomeric matrix protein (COMP), cartilage intermediate layer protein (CILP), aggrecan (CAN), and 7 types of collagens (collagen type I, III, VI, XII, XIV, XV, and XVIII) were dominantly identified in both groups (Supplementary Table S1). A total of 24 proteins showed more than a two-fold concentration difference between the two lesions on TMT analysis. Of them, eleven proteins were ECM proteins (46% of the total), and further verified using MRM assay (Supplementary Table S2).

2.2. Characterization of ECM Proteins in the Meniscus

Among 906 proteins identified, 131 ECM or ECM-associated proteins were identified in meniscal tissues by MatrisomeDB 2.0 (http://www.pepchem.org/matrisomedb accessed on 31 May 2021) that integrated experimental proteomic data on the ECM composition of meniscal tissues (Supplementary Figure S1A). These proteins were categorized into 41 ECM glycoproteins, 14 proteoglycans, 11 collagen isoforms, 34 ECM regulators, 16 ECM affiliated proteins, and 15 secreted factors (Supplementary Figure S1B). To identify their biological function, we conducted functional enrichment analysis of the 131 proteins (130 genes) using Funrich software (Supplementary Figure S1C). Cell growth and/or maintenance (37.7% of genes) and protein metabolism (23.1%) were enriched according to the biological process. Extracellular matrix (82%) and ECM-related (38.3%) genes were dominantly enriched in the cellular component. According to molecular function, 34.6% of genes were categorized in the extracellular matrix structural constituent. These genes were highly involved in biological pathways such as the epithelial to mesenchymal transition (34%) and beta3 integrin cell surface interaction (20%). Interestingly, the structural constituents of cytoskeleton, ribosome, and extracellular matrix were dominantly enriched in both meniscal tissues by functional analysis.

2.3. Development of the MRM Method for ECM Proteins

ECM played a structural role and contributed to the mechanical properties of cartilage tissues. Thus, we focused on 131 ECM-related proteins (130 genes) identified in meniscal tissues by LC-MS/MS analysis. A number of the 131 proteins assigned to ECM proteins was analyzed by the MRM method. Herein, 3024 MRM transitions were generated using Skyline software against 474 peptides from 131 ECM proteins of interest. These MRM transitions were experimentally refined in protein extracts obtained from pooled meniscal tissues. Of them, MRM assays of 119 proteins were established (Supplementary Table S3).

2.4. Differentially Expressed ECM Proteins Identified in the Meniscus by MRM Assay

To identify ECM proteins differentially expressed in lateral and medial meniscus, we measured 75 ECM proteins of interest in 12 lateral/medial pairs obtained from meniscus tissues from osteoarthritis patients during total knee arthroscopy using MRM assay. Herein, we showed that 14 proteins were different in the two lesions using the Wilcoxon test ($p < 0.05$) (Supplementary Table S4, Figure 1). Nine proteins consisting of collagen alpha-1(XVIII) chain (COL18A1), Cystatin-B (CSTB), Cathepsin D (CTSD), Cathepsin Z (CTSZ), Protein ERGIC-53 (LMAN1), Protein S100-A13 (S100A13), Adiponectin (ADIPOQ), Alpha-1-antichymotrypsin (SERPINA3), and SPARC-related modular calcium-binding protein 2 (SMOC2) had greater expression in the medial lesion compared to the lateral (Figure 1A). In contrast, expression of the five proteins Kininogen-1 (KNG1), Secreted frizzled-related protein 3 (FRZB), Plasminogen (PLG), Protein S100-A1 (S100A1), and Protein S100-A10 (S100A10) decreased in the medial lesions (Figure 1B). Interestingly, among these proteins, the MRM results of SMOC2 and FRZB are consistent with those of the TMT experiment, where SMOC2 increased 2.3-fold and FRZB decreased 2-fold in medial lesions.

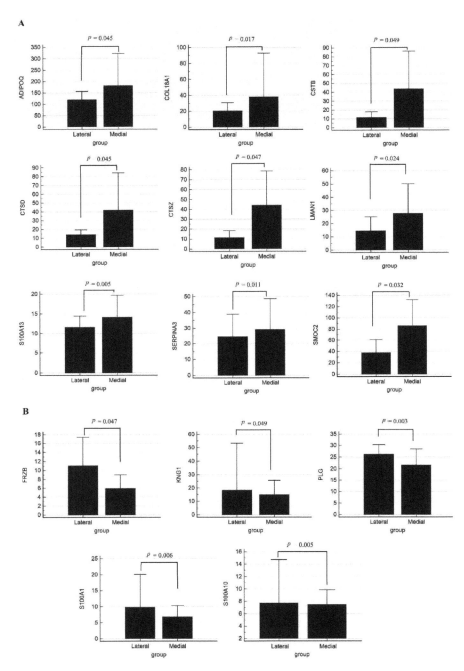

Figure 1. MRM results of meniscal tissues. (**A**) Increased proteins in medial lesions, (**B**) Decreased proteins in medial lesions by the Wilcoxon test. A *p*-value < 0.05 is statistically significant.

3. Discussion

To investigate the type and distribution of ECM proteins in meniscal tissue is very important in cartilage tissue engineering as well as in identifying related disease etiologies, including osteoarthritis. Several studies have profiled the proteome of articular cartilage and medial meniscus tissue, but the ECM profile in these tissues is not sufficiently covered and quantified [8,9]. Thus, in this study, we characterized the proteomic profile of meniscal tissues consisting of medial and lateral lesions from osteoarthritis patients, which are still uncovered their protein composition but also quantified. We focused on meniscal ECM proteins, which contribute to repair and regenerate tissues and reported that ECM composition and expression levels in both lesions using both TMT analysis and MRM-MS. Herein we first provided the characterization of osteoarthritic meniscus using quantitative-based proteomic analysis, although there was few concentration change for major cartilage proteins such as COMP, CILP, CAN and collagens in the protein expression profile between lateral and medial meniscus.

Recently only a few pairwise comparisons of the lateral and medial osteoarthritis knee have been conducted (Supplementary Table S5). Moreover, only one study was performed for the proteomic comparison between osteoarthritis menisci. Our study was conducted as a preliminary study to help us understand the mechanisms of osteoarthritis by comparing protein composition within lateral and medial from an expanded number of osteoarthritis subjects. We think it is important to analyze ECM proteins and to discover biomarkers that are definitely lacking in this field.

Osteoarthritis is caused by failure of chondrocytes to maintain homeostasis between synthesis and degradation of ECM components, such as polypeptide, growth factors and cytokines. Recent studies reported that the Wnt/β-catenin pathway plays an important role in the pathophysiology of osteoarthritis [10]. We found that these differentially expressed ECM proteins were increased in regulation of peptidase activity, biological extracellular matrix processes, and ECM modulation. Among these ECM proteins, FRZB showed lower expression in the medial meniscus than lateral meniscus, whereas SMOC2, CSTB, CTSD, and CTSZ showed higher expression in the medial than lateral meniscus. FRZB acts as the WNT inhibitor, and loss of function of FRZB results from excessive WNT activation and increases susceptibility to osteoarthritis [10]. SMOC2 is a member of the secreted protein acidic and rich in cysteine (SPARC) family and is associated with adult wound healing and age-dependent bone loss. Lu et al. recently demonstrated that SMOC2 directly interacted with WNT receptors and activated the WNT/β-catenin pathway in endometrial carcinoma [11]. Furthermore, inflammation modulators (such as CSTB, CTSD, and CTSZ), which have been reported to contribute to osteoarthritis, were more highly expressed in the medial than lateral meniscus [12]. These proteins might play an important role in regulation of chondrocyte growth and proliferation compared to cartilage proteins, which have a slow turnover rate. Therefore, alteration of these proteins can affect ECM regeneration, leading to promotion of osteoarthritis.

Our study has some limitations. First, we could not perform comparisons between osteoarthritis patients and healthy controls, because it is difficult to obtain intact meniscus samples from healthy subjects. Also, it is unclear whether the differences in protein expression levels of ECM in lateral and medial menisci from osteoarthritis patients directly correlate with tissue damage. Further study should be conducted to elucidate the relationship between the patterns of protein expression in meniscus and tissue damage in osteoarthritis.

Despite these limitations, the results of this study would be expected to provide important information in the treatment and diagnosis of various joint diseases as well as osteoarthritis in the future.

4. Methods

4.1. Clinical Samples

This study enrolled 12 osteoarthritis patients who received knee arthroscopy surgery at Samsung Medical Center. All 12 patients were female and had a mean age of 72.9 years (range 65–82 year). Tissue from lateral/medial menisci pairs was obtained during surgery, and the mean weight of the tissues was 2260 mg (range 950–4100 mg). Written informed consent was obtained from all enrolled patients. This study was approved by the Institutional Review Board (IRB) of Samsung Medical Center (Seoul, Korea) (IRB file No. 2015-12-166).

4.2. Preparation of Tissues

About 200–300 mg of cartilage tissue was cut from each sample and pulverized in liquid nitrogen using a ball grinder. RIPA buffer (150 mM sodium chloride, 1% Triton X-100, 1% sodium deoxycholate, 0.1% SDS, 50 mM Tris-HCl pH 7.5, 2 mM EDTA, sterile solution, protease inhibitor) was added to the pulverized tissue and sonicated four times for 15 s each. A total of 500 µg of protein extract was subjected to FASP [13]. Trypsin digestion was performed in a microwave at 450 W and 55 °C for one hour using a Rapid Enzyme Digestion system (Asta, Seoul, Korea). Desalting and concentration of the samples were performed using a StrataTM-X 33 um (Phenomenex Inc., Torrance, CA, USA) according to manufacturer instructions. These protein extracts were subjected to further mass spectrometry-based comparative proteomic analysis and an MRM assay (Figure 2).

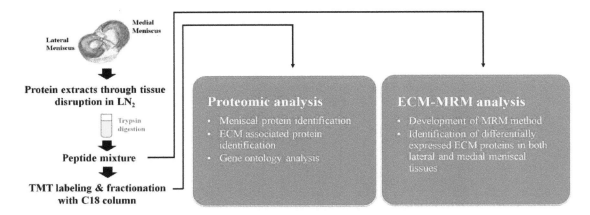

Figure 2. Summary of the experimental design.

4.3. LC-MS/MS Analysis

In-solution digestion with trypsin, followed by 6-plex TMT treatment were performed according to the manufacturer's instructions (Thermo Fisher Scientific, Waltham, MA, USA). After pooling each disease group, labeled peptide mixtures were separated via reverse phase HPLC into 12 fractions and were analyzed using an Orbitrap Elite mass spectrometer (Thermo Finnigan, San Jose, CA, USA) equipped with a nano-electrospray ion source.

The TMT-labeled peptide mixtures were analyzed using an Orbitrap Elite mass spectrometer equipped with a nano-electrospray ion source. The mobile phase consisted of buffer A (0.1% formic acid in water) and buffer B (0.1% formic acid in ACN). After injecting a sample onto the analytical column (75 um × 50 cm packed C18, 2 um particles, 100 Å pores) (Thermo Finnigan, CA, USA), a 90-min gradient method was used to separate the peptide mixture. Sample loading onto the analytical column was conducted at 3% buffer B, the mobile phase was held at 4% buffer B for 1 min, followed by a linear gradient to 32%

buffer B over 91 min, followed by a linear gradient to 80% buffer B over 8 min at a flow rate of 300 nL/min.

4.4. MRM Assay for ECM Protein Determination

To develop the MRM assay, ECM MatrisomeDB 2.0 depository (http://www.matrisomedb. org/) (accessed on 20 September 2018) was used to extract ECM-related proteins from the identified meniscal tissue profile. Those peptides and MRM transitions were generated using Skyline 4.1.011796 (MacCoss Lab Software, Seattle, WA, USA) and employed for further refinement of the selected peptides. At least three transitions from one proteotypic peptide were generated; 2 or 3 peptide charge states containing 8–30 amino acids, no post-translational modification (PTM), and non-specific cleavage were not allowed. Therefore, a total of 3024 MRM transitions was generated against 131 ECM proteins and 474 peptides. These MRM transitions were refined experimentally in protein extracts obtained from pooled meniscal tissues. A minimum of 3 MRM transitions per peptide should match the same retention times with $S/N > 10$. MRM was performed in positive mode using a QTRAP 5500 hybrid triple quadrupole/linear ion trap mass spectrometer (Sciex, Framingham, MA, USA) interfaced with a nano-electrospray ion source.

4.5. Data Annotation

All MS/MS spectra were searched against the UniProt Human protein database (8 August 2016, Reviewed 20197proteins) using the Integrated Proteomics Pipeline v.3 (IP2) search algorithm for peptide identification. The search parameters were as follows: specific to trypsin with two missed cleavages, variable modification of methionine oxidation, fixed modification of carbamidomethyl cysteine, ± 10 ppm precursor-ion tolerance, ± 600 ppm fragment-ion tolerance, and ± 10 reporter ion tolerance.

Peak area ratio (PAR) was calculated to compare expression profiles among meniscal tissues. The peak area of each peptide transition was divided by the peak area of the corresponding transition from the isotope-labeled peptide. The concentration of these proteins was calculated as the product of PAR.

Gene Ontology (GO) analysis was performed using Funrich software (Version 3.1.3) and the web-based browser STRING (https://string-db.org) (accessed on 19 November 2019) to classify the cellular components, biological process, and molecular function.

4.6. Statistics

Data acquired from MRM experiments were analyzed using the SPSS statistical package (IBM Corporation, Somers, NY, USA) ver 21.0 and MedCalc software ver 19.0.7 (Mariakerke, Belgium). Non-parametric tests were used for all proteomic markers. The proteomic differences in expression of markers between lateral and medial menisci groups were assessed with the Wilcoxon test. A p-value ≤ 0.05 was considered statistically significant.

Supplementary Materials: The following are available online at https://www.mdpi.com/article/10.3390/ijms22158181/s1.

Author Contributions: Conception and design, J.P.; analysis and interpretation of the data, J.P., J.Y.L., J.Y.K. and E.-B.G.; drafting of the article, J.P. and H.-S.L.; critical revision of the article for important intellectual content, S.-Y.L.; final approval of the article, S.-Y.L. and D.-H.L.; provision of study materials or patients, D.-H.L.; collection and assembly of data, J.P. and E.-B.G. All authors have read and agreed to the published version of the manuscript.

Funding: This work was supported by the National Research Foundation of Korea (NRF) grant funded by the Korea government (MSIT) (2021R1A2C1006409).

Institutional Review Board Statement: This study was approved by the Institutional Review Board (IRB) of Samsung Medical Center (Seoul, Korea) (IRB file No. 2015-12-166).

Informed Consent Statement: Informed consent was obtained from all subjects involved in the study.

Data Availability Statement: The data presented in this study are openly available in the MassIVE at https://massive.ucsd.edu, (accessed on 19 November 2019), reference number [MSV000087753].

Conflicts of Interest: The authors declare no conflict of interest.

References

1. Makris, E.A.; Hadidi, P.; Athanasiou, K.A. The knee meniscus: Structure-function, pathophysiology, current repair techniques, and prospects for regeneration. *Biomaterials* **2011**, *32*, 7411–7431. [CrossRef] [PubMed]
2. Poulsen, E.; Goncalves, G.H.; Bricca, A.; Roos, E.M.; Thorlund, J.B.; Juhl, C.B. Knee osteoarthritis risk is increased 4-6 fold after knee injury—A systematic review and meta-analysis. *Br. J. Sports Med.* **2019**, *53*, 1454–1463. [CrossRef] [PubMed]
3. Hsueh, M.F.; Khabut, A.; Kjellstrom, S.; Onnerfjord, P.; Kraus, V.B. Elucidating the Molecular Composition of Cartilage by Proteomics. *J. Proteome Res.* **2016**, *15*, 374–388. [CrossRef] [PubMed]
4. Bell, P.A.; Wagener, R.; Zaucke, F.; Koch, M.; Selley, J.; Warwood, S.; Knight, D.; Boot-Handford, R.P.; Thornton, D.J.; Briggs, M.D. Analysis of the cartilage proteome from three different mouse models of genetic skeletal diseases reveals common and discrete disease signatures. *Biol. Open* **2013**, *2*, 802–811. [CrossRef] [PubMed]
5. Ribitsch, I.; Mayer, R.L.; Egerbacher, M.; Gabner, S.; Kandula, M.M.; Rosser, J.; Haltmayer, E.; Auer, U.; Gultekin, S.; Huber, J.; et al. Fetal articular cartilage regeneration versus adult fibrocartilaginous repair: Secretome proteomics unravels molecular mechanisms in an ovine model. *Dis. Model. Mech.* **2018**, *11*, dmm033092. [CrossRef] [PubMed]
6. Liu, S.; Zhang, W.; Zhang, F.; Roepstorff, P.; Yang, F.; Lu, Z.; Ding, W. TMT-Based Quantitative Proteomics Analysis Reveals Airborne PM2.5-Induced Pulmonary Fibrosis. *Int. J. Environ. Res. Public Health* **2018**, *16*, 98. [CrossRef]
7. Svala, E.; Lofgren, M.; Sihlbom, C.; Ruetschi, U.; Lindahl, A.; Ekman, S.; Skioldebrand, E. An inflammatory equine model demonstrates dynamic changes of immune response and cartilage matrix molecule degradation in vitro. *Connect. Tissue Res.* **2015**, *56*, 315–325. [CrossRef] [PubMed]
8. Folkesson, E.; Turkiewicz, A.; Ryden, M.; Hughes, H.V.; Ali, N.; Tjornstrand, J.; Onnerfjord, P.; Englund, M. Proteomic characterization of the normal human medial meniscus body using data-independent acquisition mass spectrometry. *J. Orthop. Res.* **2020**, *38*, 1735–1745. [CrossRef] [PubMed]
9. Folkesson, E.; Turkiewicz, A.; Englund, M.; Onnerfjord, P. Differential protein expression in human knee articular cartilage and medial meniscus using two different proteomic methods: A pilot analysis. *BMC Musculoskelet. Disord.* **2018**, *19*, 416. [CrossRef] [PubMed]
10. Wang, Y.; Fan, X.; Xing, L.; Tian, F. Wnt signaling: A promising target for osteoarthritis therapy. *Cell Commun. Signal.* **2019**, *17*, 97. [CrossRef] [PubMed]
11. Lu, H.; Ju, D.D.; Yang, G.D.; Zhu, L.Y.; Yang, X.M.; Li, J.; Song, W.W.; Wang, J.H.; Zhang, C.C.; Zhang, Z.G.; et al. Targeting cancer stem cell signature gene SMOC-2 Overcomes chemoresistance and inhibits cell proliferation of endometrial carcinoma. *EBioMedicine* **2019**, *40*, 276–289. [CrossRef] [PubMed]
12. Ben-Aderet, L.; Merquiol, E.; Fahham, D.; Kumar, A.; Reich, E.; Ben-Nun, Y.; Kandel, L.; Haze, A.; Liebergall, M.; Kosińska, M.K.; et al. Detecting cathepsin activity in human osteoarthritis via activity-based probes. *Arthritis Res. Ther.* **2015**, *17*, 69. [CrossRef] [PubMed]
13. Wisniewski, J.R.; Zougman, A.; Nagaraj, N.; Mann, M. Universal sample preparation method for proteome analysis. *Nat. Methods* **2009**, *6*, 359–362. [CrossRef] [PubMed]

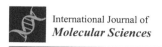

International Journal of
Molecular Sciences

MDPI

Article

Osteoarthritis-Related Inflammation Blocks TGF-β's Protective Effect on Chondrocyte Hypertrophy via (de)Phosphorylation of the SMAD2/3 Linker Region

Nathalie Thielen [1], Margot Neefjes [1], Renske Wiegertjes [1], Guus van den Akker [2], Elly Vitters [1], Henk van Beuningen [1], Esmeralda Blaney Davidson [1], Marije Koenders [1], Peter van Lent [1], Fons van de Loo [1], Arjan van Caam [1] and Peter van der Kraan [1,*]

1   Department of Experimental Rheumatology, Radboud University Medical Center, 6500 MD Nijmegen, The Netherlands; Nathalie.Thielen@radboudumc.nl (N.T.); Margot.Neefjes@radboudumc.nl (M.N.); Renske.Wiegertjes@radboudumc.nl (R.W.); Elly.Vitters@radboudumc.nl (E.V.); Henk.vanBeuningen@radboudumc.nl (H.v.B.); Esmeralda.BlaneyDavidson@radboudumc.nl (E.B.D.); Marije.Koenders@radboudumc.nl (M.K.); Peter.vanLent@radboudumc.nl (P.v.L.); Fons.vandeLoo@radboudumc.nl (F.v.d.L.); Arjan.vanCaam@radboudumc.nl (A.v.C.)
2   Department of Orthopedic Surgery, Maastricht University, 6200 MD Maastricht, The Netherlands; g.vandenakker@maastrichtuniversity.nl
*   Correspondence: Peter.vanderKraan@radboudumc.nl

Citation: Thielen, N.; Neefjes, M.; Wiegertjes, R.; van den Akker, G.; Vitters, E.; van Beuningen, H.; Blaney Davidson, E.; Koenders, M.; van Lent, P.; van de Loo, F.; et al. Osteoarthritis-Related Inflammation Blocks TGF-β's Protective Effect on Chondrocyte Hypertrophy via (de)Phosphorylation of the SMAD2/3 Linker Region. *Int. J. Mol. Sci.* **2021**, *22*, 8124. https://doi.org/10.3390/ijms22158124

Academic Editor: Alfonso Baldi

Received: 30 June 2021
Accepted: 26 July 2021
Published: 29 July 2021

Abstract: Osteoarthritis (OA) is a degenerative joint disease characterized by irreversible cartilage damage, inflammation and altered chondrocyte phenotype. Transforming growth factor-β (TGF-β) signaling via SMAD2/3 is crucial for blocking hypertrophy. The post-translational modifications of these SMAD proteins in the linker domain regulate their function and these can be triggered by inflammation through the activation of kinases or phosphatases. Therefore, we investigated if OA-related inflammation affects TGF-β signaling via SMAD2/3 linker-modifications in chondrocytes. We found that both Interleukin (IL)-1β and OA-synovium conditioned medium negated SMAD2/3 transcriptional activity in chondrocytes. This inhibition of TGF-β signaling was enhanced if SMAD3 could not be phosphorylated on Ser213 in the linker region and the inhibition by IL-1β was less if the SMAD3 linker could not be phosphorylated at Ser204. Our study shows evidence that inflammation inhibits SMAD2/3 signaling in chondrocytes via SMAD linker (de)-phosphorylation. The involvement of linker region modifications may represent a new therapeutic target for OA.

Keywords: TGF-β; osteoarthritis; cartilage; SMAD2/3 signaling; linker modifications; inflammation

1. Introduction

Osteoarthritis (OA) is characterized by irreversible cartilage breakdown and regarded as a multifactorial disease in which inflammation is involved [1,2]. Synovitis is present in osteoarthritic joints and the production of inflammatory cytokines and chemokines is increased [3–6]. These pro-inflammatory cytokines, such as Interleukin (IL)-1β can have a direct (negative) effect on cartilage homeostasis [7,8], but can also modulate the transforming growth factor-β (TGF-β) signaling [9,10].

TGF-β is a crucial growth factor for articular cartilage maintenance [11]. Via intracellular activation of the transcription factors SMAD2 and SMAD3, TGF-β inhibits chondrocyte hypertrophy and MMP13 expression [12]. On the other hand, signaling via its alternative SMAD1/5/9 signaling route promotes these detrimental processes. A disturbed balance between the two SMAD signaling routes has been proposed as a cause for OA pathology [13,14]. TGF-β signaling disruption can occur at different stages in its signaling cascade. For instance, inflammatory mediators can regulate the TGF-β receptor expression and increase the expression of inhibitory SMAD7 [15]. Alternatively, inflammatory pathways can induce post-translational modification of the linker region of SMAD proteins to modulate their function [16,17]. This linker domain connects the N-terminal MH1 domain, which is important for DNA binding and nuclear transport, to their C-terminal MH2 domain, which is responsible for the SMAD receptor and SMAD–SMAD interactions and gene transcription activation [18–21]. Importantly, the linker region can be phosphorylated on specific serine and threonine residues, and this regulates nuclear entry, SMAD–protein interactions, and SMAD turnover, thereby greatly affecting SMAD function [16,22,23]. Still, the relative importance of these SMAD linker modifications in cartilage biology and OA pathogenesis has not been investigated and is poorly understood.

In this study we explored whether OA-related inflammation dysregulates TGF-β signaling in chondrocytes via inflammation-driven SMAD2/3 protein linker-modifications.

2. Results

2.1. IL-1β and OAS-cm Negate the Anti-Hypertrophic Function of TGF-β in Bovine Cartilage Explants

Hypertrophy-like changes in chondrocytes play a role in OA progression [24]. To study whether inflammation modulates such changes, a model for hypertrophy was set-up. For this, we cultured bovine cartilage tissue explants for 2 weeks ex vivo which, both with and without the addition of FCS in the culture medium, induced hypertrophy-like differentiation, as confirmed by a ~97-fold increase in *COL10A1* expression ($2^{6.6 \, \Delta Ct}$, $p < 0.0001$) (Figure 1A). To demonstrate the anti-hypertrophic function of the TGF-β ex vivo, recombinant human (rh), TGF-β1 was added to culture medium (without FCS) every 3rd day. *COL10A1* expression was dose-dependently inhibited by TGF-β, with an EC_{50} of 0.1 ng/mL and 85% inhibition at 1.0 ng/mL TGF-β ($2^{5.6 \, \Delta Ct}$, $p = 0.0002$) (Figure 1A). Co-incubation with the ALK-5 kinase activity inhibitor SB-505124 fully blocked TGF-β's effect on *COL10A1* expression with a 74-fold difference compared with the vehicle (DMSO) ($2^{6.2 \, \Delta Ct}$, $p = 0.0021$) (Figure 1B). To study the interaction between TGF-β and inflammatory mediators in this model of hypertrophy, explants were exposed to 0.1 ng/mL TGF-β combined with 0.1 ng/mL IL-1β or 0.5% OA synovium-conditioned medium (OAS-cm). Importantly, we first established that these concentrations did not modulate *COL10A1* expression themselves (Appendix A). Pre-incubation of explants for 1 h with IL-1β prior to the addition of TGF-β negated anti-hypertrophic TGF-β signaling with ~2.2 fold difference ($2^{1.2 \, \Delta Ct}$, $p = 0.0144$) (Figure 1C). The addition of OAS-cm prior to TGF-β strikingly negated anti-hypertrophic TGF-β signaling with a 7.0-fold difference. ($2^{2.8 \, \Delta Ct}$, $p = 0.0113$) (Figure 1D).

2.2. IL-1β and OAS-cm Inhibit TGF-β Transcriptional Activity in Different Chondrocyte Cell Lines

Hereafter, we used three different human chondrocyte-like cell lines (G6, H11, SW1353) to identify the cause of this interaction between functional TGF-β signaling and inflammatory mediators. We chose to use cell lines because it is difficult to efficiently genetically modify primary chondrocytes in explants culture. First, we established that a similar inhibitory effect occurs in these cell lines as in cartilage explants on TGF-β transcriptional activity. To perform this, we made use of a SBE-pNL1.2 luciferase reporter assay, which is SMAD2/3 and SMAD4-dependent (Appendix B). In all three cell lines, the luciferase signal was induced by TGF-β stimulation alone and this effect was significantly inhibited when pre-incubated for either 1 or 16 h with 0.1 ng/mL IL-1β or 0.5% OAS-cm (Figure 2A and Appendix B). This inhibition was further investigated in SW1353 cells (Figure 2B,C). Pre-incubation with 0.001 ng/mL IL-1β (area under the curve (AUC) = 86, $p = 0.95$) and 0.01 ng/mL IL-1β (AUC = 70, $p = 0.12$) did not inhibit TGF-β transcriptional activity (AUC = 92). However, 0.1 ng/mL IL-1β (AUC = 48, $p = 0.0018$), 1 ng/mL IL-1β (AUC = 40, $p = 0.0004$) and 10 ng/mL IL-1β (AUC = 33, $p = 0.0002$), pre-incubated for 1 h did significantly inhibit TGF-β transcriptional activity (Figure 2B). Pre-incubation with OAS-cm for 1 h inhibited TGF-β transcriptional activity (AUC = 85) from 35% inhibition with 1% OAS-cm (AUC = 54, $p = 0.0063$) up to 83% inhibition with 10% OAS-cm (AUC = 13, $p < 0.0001$)

(Figure 2C). Combining these data supports the conclusion that OA-related inflammation has an inhibitory effect on TGF-β signaling in chondrocytes.

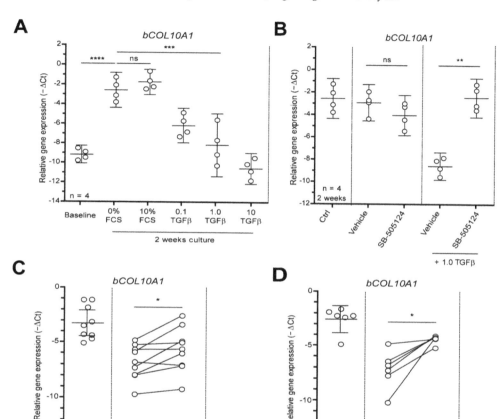

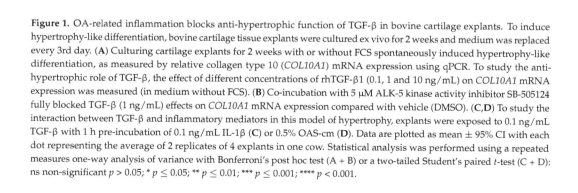

Figure 1. OA-related inflammation blocks anti-hypertrophic function of TGF-β in bovine cartilage explants. To induce hypertrophy-like differentiation, bovine cartilage tissue explants were cultured ex vivo for 2 weeks and medium was replaced every 3rd day. (**A**) Culturing cartilage explants for 2 weeks with or without FCS spontaneously induced hypertrophy-like differentiation, as measured by relative collagen type 10 (*COL10A1*) mRNA expression using qPCR. To study the anti-hypertrophic role of TGF-β, the effect of different concentrations of rhTGF-β1 (0.1, 1 and 10 ng/mL) on *COL10A1* mRNA expression was measured (in medium without FCS). (**B**) Co-incubation with 5 μM ALK-5 kinase activity inhibitor SB-505124 fully blocked TGF-β (1 ng/mL) effects on *COL10A1* mRNA expression compared with vehicle (DMSO). (**C,D**) To study the interaction between TGF-β and inflammatory mediators in this model of hypertrophy, explants were exposed to 0.1 ng/mL TGF-β with 1 h pre-incubation of 0.1 ng/mL IL-1β (**C**) or 0.5% OAS-cm (**D**). Data are plotted as mean ± 95% CI with each dot representing the average of 2 replicates of 4 explants in one cow. Statistical analysis was performed using a repeated measures one-way analysis of variance with Bonferroni's post hoc test (A + B) or a two-tailed Student's paired *t*-test (C + D): ns non-significant $p > 0.05$; * $p \leq 0.05$; ** $p \leq 0.01$; *** $p \leq 0.001$; **** $p < 0.001$.

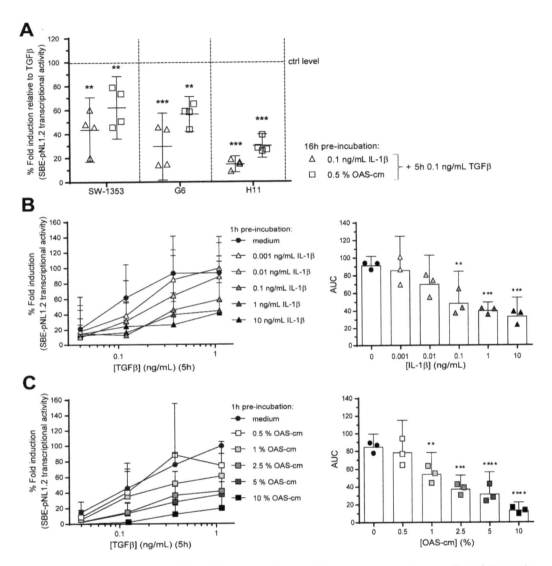

Figure 2. OA-related inflammation inhibits TGF-β transcriptional activity in particular chondrocytes. To study interaction between OA-related inflammation and functional TGF-β signaling, three chondrocyte-like cell lines (SW1353, G6 and H11) were transfected with a SMAD2/3 transcriptional reporter construct (SBE-pNL1.2). (**A**) After transfection, cells were re-plated, pre-incubated overnight (16 h) with medium, 0.1 ng/mL IL-1β or 0.5% OAS-cm and, thereafter, stimulated for 5 h with 0.1 ng/mL TGF-β. Luciferase activity was measured relative to experimental condition stimulated with TGF-β, as set at 100% (ctrl level). Data represent mean ± 95% CI of four independent experiments performed in quadruple. (**B,C**) In SW1353 cells, this was investigated further, but now with 1 h pre-incubation with a concentration series of (**B**) IL-1β (0.001–10 ng/mL) or (**C**) OAS-cm (0.5–10%) before stimulation with increasing concentrations of TGF-β for 5 h. Data represent mean ± 95% CI of three independent experiments performed in quadruple. Per experiment the area under the curve (AUC) was calculated and displayed. Statistical analysis was performed using a one-way ANOVA with Dunnett's multiple comparison test comparing the mean to the mean of the condition stimulated with solely TGF-β: ** $p \leq 0.01$; *** $p \leq 0.001$; **** $p < 0.001$.

2.3. IL-1β and OAS-cm Do Not Inhibit C-Terminal Phosphorylation of SMAD2/3 and Do Not Regulate Receptor Level Expression

Upon TGF-β binding to the receptor, R-SMAD transcription factors become activated by phosphorylation of serine residues on their carboxy (C)-terminus, which causes them to form a complex with co-SMAD4, translocate to the nucleus and regulate gene transcription [25]. In search of an explanation for the strong inhibition of OA-related inflammatory factors on TGF-β signaling, we first investigated if IL-1β and OAS-cm influence C-terminal SMAD phosphorylation. As expected, TGF-β supplementation strongly increased pSMAD2/3C in both primary bovine chondrocytes and SW1353 cells, whereas IL-1β or OAS-cm did not (Figure 3A). However, pSMAD2/3C was not decreased by either 1, 6 or 24 h pre-incubation with IL-1β or OAS-cm (Figure 3A, upper panels), which excluded a direct effect on C-terminal SMAD phosphorylation. Another underlying cause for the disturbed TGF-β signaling could be a shifted balance from protective pSMAD2/3 to deleterious pSMAD1/5 [26,27]. However, in both primary chondrocytes and SW1353 cells, we observed that pSMAD1/5C was also not affected by 1, 6 or 24 h pre-incubation of IL-1β or OAS-cm (Figure 3A, middle panels). Together, these observations strongly indicate that the TGF-β-receptor complexes were unaffected. In support of this, we did not find changes in the receptor expression at the mRNA level. The stimulation of both primary chondrocytes and SW1353 cells with 0.1 ng/mL IL-1β or 5% OAS-cm for 1 h did not alter *TGFBR2* or *ALK5* receptor levels (Figure 3C), nor did stimulation for 6 h with IL-1β. Note that, in SW1353 6 h stimulation with 0.1 ng/mL, IL-1β did induce (and not reduce) *TGFBR2* ($p = 0.0426$) and did not change *ALK5* expression.

The duration and intensity of the SMAD depends on the abundance and availability of ligands and their inhibitors [28]. We also confirmed that the signal duration was not affected. In primary bovine chondrocytes, TGF-β-induced pSMAD2/3C lasted up to at least 3 h after stimulation, whereas pSMAD1/5C already disappeared after 3 h TGF-β stimulation. In both cell types, the length of the pSMAD signal was not affected by addition of IL-1β or OAS-cm (Figure 3B). Together, these data indicate that the inhibitory effect that we found on TGF-β signaling, was caused downstream of receptor-mediated SMAD activation. One such mechanism is through the induction of inhibitory SMAD7; however, in our experiments, *SMAD7* expression levels were not increased by inflammatory stimuli (Figure 3C). The exception was the 1 h stimulation with 5% OAS-cm, which did increase *SMAD7* expression in bovine chondrocytes but not in SW1353 cells.

2.4. IL-1β and OAS-cm Inhibit TGF-β via (de-)Phosphorylation of the SMAD2/3 Linker Region

Aside from C-terminal phosphorylation, SMAD proteins can also be post-translationally phosphorylated at serine and threonine residues within the linker region: SMAD2 at threonine (T) 220 and serines (S) 245, 250, 255 and SMAD3 at the corresponding T179, S204, S208 and S213 [17] (Figure 4A). TGF-β-induced transcriptional activity is regulated by SMAD linker modifications in several cell types [29–32]; therefore, we hypothesized that SMAD2/3 linker modifications are responsible for the effect of IL-1β and OAS-cm on TGF-β signaling in chondrocytes. We studied linker phosphorylation at those specific linker threonine and serine residues by Western blotting. SMAD2 and SMAD3 linker threonine and serine modifications were detectable within 1 h following IL-1β or OAS-cm stimulation (Figure 4B,C). Concentrations of 0.1, 1 and 10 ng/mL IL-1β induced phosphorylation of SMAD2L serines and SMAD3L S204 ($p = 0.0256$), but did not change pSMAD3L S208 ($p = 0.1333$) or S213 ($p = 0.7633$). Additionally, OAS-cm did induce pSMAD2L serines and pSMAD3L S204 ($p = 0.0232$), but not pSMAD3L S208 ($p = 0.0973$) and it significantly decreased the phosphorylation of SMAD3L S213 ($p = 0.0047$). The phosphorylation of SMAD2L T220 was not induced by IL-1β, but only by OAS-cm, whereas SMAD3L T179 was not regulated by either stimulus. These data suggest a role for especially serine linker modifications in regulating TGF-β signaling in chondrocytes.

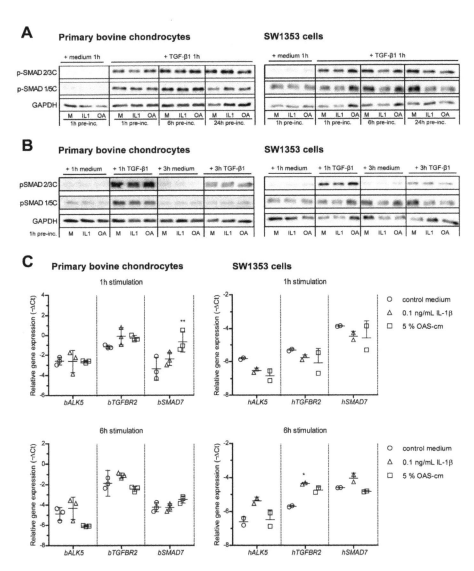

Figure 3. IL-1β and OAS-cm do not alter C-terminal phosphorylation of SMAD transcription factors and do not regulate receptor level expression. In search of an explanation for the inhibition of OA-related inflammatory factors on functional TGF-β signaling, we investigated if IL-1β and OAS-cm influence C-terminal SMAD2/3 and SMAD1/5 phosphorylation in bovine chondrocytes cultured in monolayer and in SW1353 chondrosarcoma cells using Western blot (**A**,**B**). Pre-incubation for different time periods (1, 6 and 24 h) with 0.1 ng/mL IL-1β (IL1) or 2.5% OAS-cm (OA) did not alter p-SMADC activation with 1 ng/mL TGF-β (**A**) and also signal duration was not affected (**B**). GAPDH was included as loading control. (**C**) Relative gene expression of TGF-β receptors ALK5 and TGFBR2 and inhibitory SMAD7 in bovine chondrocytes and SW1353 cells 1 h and 6 h after stimulation with medium supplemented with 0.1 ng/mL IL-1β or 5% OAS-cm. Data are plotted as mean ± SD with each dot representing the average of 2 replicates of 4 explants in one cow (*n* = 3), or in case of the SW1353 cells of two independent experiments performed in duplicate. Statistical analysis was performed using a one-way ANOVA with Bonferroni's post hoc test: * $p \leq 0.05$; ** $p \leq 0.01$.

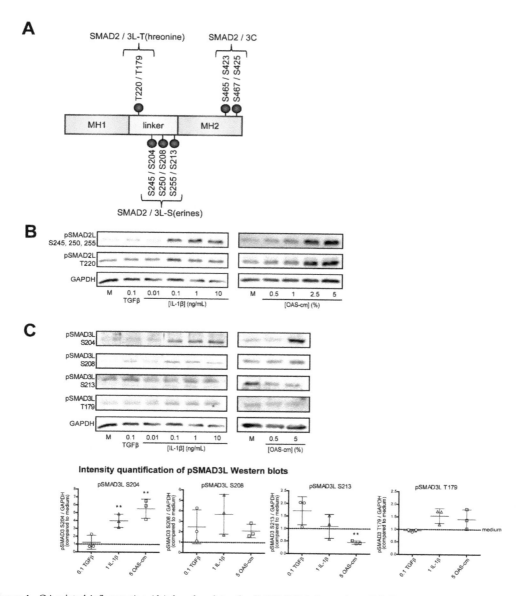

Figure 4. OA-related inflammation (de)phosphorylates the SMAD 2/3 linker region. SMAD proteins can also be post-translationally phosphorylated at serine and threonine residues within their linker (L) region: SMAD2 at threonine (T) 220 and serines (S) 245, 250, 255 and SMAD3 at the corresponding T179, S204, S208 and S213. (**A**) Schematic illustration of the SMAD2 and SMAD3 proteins and their phospho-epitopes in the linker (L) region and C-terminus. (**B,C**) Chondrocytes were treated for 1 h with 0.1 ng/mL TGF-β or with different concentrations of IL-1β (0.01–10 ng/mL) or OAS-cm (0.5–5%) and subsequently phosphorylation at the different phospho-sites in the linker region of SMAD2 (**B**) and SMAD3 (**C**) were visualized on Western blot. Quantification of the Western blots was performed with ImageJ. Data are presented as dot plots with mean ± SD, with each dot representing one donor, *n* = 3. GAPDH was used as loading control. Statistics were performed using two-tailed Student's paired *t*-test: ** *p* ≤ 0.01.

To further explore the importance of SMAD linker modifications, we used five different SMAD3 variants, which cannot be phosphorylated at specific sites in the linker domain due to mutations from the linker serines to alanines and the linker threonine to a valine (Figure 5A). Equal over-expression of the different SMAD linker variants was checked with flow cytometry (Appendix C). In all conditions, over 90% of the cells were positively stained for FLAG and the geometric mean of this over-expression was not different, demonstrating that all SMAD3 variants were overexpressed equally to facilitate a fair comparison between conditions.

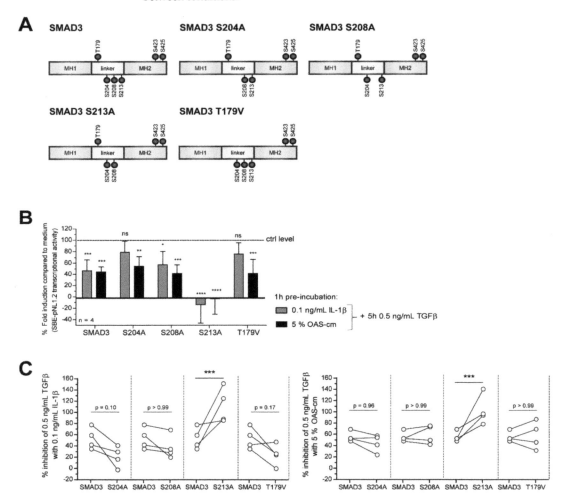

Figure 5. *Cont.*

Figure 5. When the SMAD3 linker could not be modified, TGFβ transcriptional activity was differently regulated by OA-related inflammation. To study the role of the SMAD3 linker phospho-sites in regulating TGF-β signaling, we made use of individual SMAD3 linker variants. (**A**) Schematic illustration of the different SMAD3 variants which cannot be phosphorylated on specific sites in their linker domain due to mutations from the serines (S) to alanines (A) (S204A, S208A, S213A) and the threonine (T) to a valine (V) (T179V). (**B,C**) SW1353 cells were transfected with the SBE-pNL1.2 construct, re-plated afterwards and transduced with the different SMAD variants. After a 48 h transduction and after overnight serum-starvation, we pre-incubated 1 h with 0.1 ng/mL IL-1β or 5% OAS-cm and then stimulated with 0.5 ng/mL TGF-β, after which luciferase signal was measured. (**B**) Percentage fold induction compared to medium was depicted, relative to experimental condition stimulated with 0.5 ng/mL TGF-β set at 100% (ctrl level). Data represent mean ± SD of four independent experiments performed in quadruple. (**C**) The percentage inhibition of 0.5 ng/mL TGF-β with 0.1 ng/mL IL-1β or with 5% OAS-cm was calculated and compared between the normal SMAD3 transduced cells and the conditions transduced with the SMAD linker mutants. Every dot represents one independent experiment performed in quadruple. Statistical analysis was performed using a one-way ANOVA with Dunnett's multiple comparison test. ns— non-significant; * $p \leq 0.05$; ** $p \leq 0.01$; *** $p \leq 0.001$; **** $p < 0.001$. (**D**) Summarized findings regarding the effect of inflammation-induced dephosphorylation of SMAD3L S213 on SMAD2/3 transcriptional activity and the hypothetical role of IL-1β-induced S204 linker modification. Green arrows represent activation and red "T" shapes represent inhibition.

We pre-incubated 1 h with 0.1 ng/mL IL-1-β or 5% OAS-cm and then stimulated cells for 5 h with 0.5 ng/mL TGF-β after which luciferase signal was measured. Similarly to before, in the condition with normal SMAD3 variant, results indicated inhibition of SMAD2/3 transcriptional activity with 0.1 ng/mL IL-1-β or 5% OAS-cm. However, in chondrocytes over-expressing SMAD3 S204A or T179V mutant inhibition with IL-1-β was no longer statistically significant (Figure 5B). We compared the percentage inhibition of 0.5 ng/mL TGF-β with these inflammatory stimuli between the normal SMAD3 transduced cells and the conditions with the SMAD linker mutants (Figure 5C). When we overexpressed a SMAD mutant which could not be phosphorylated at the S204, we observed the trend that TGF-β signaling was less inhibited by IL-1β by an average of 32% ($p = 0.10$) in four separate experiments. We did not observe this with OAS-cm ($p = 0.96$). Remarkably, the inhibiting effect of both IL-1β and OAS-cm was significantly stronger when serine 213 could not be phosphorylated with 59% ($p = 0.001$) and 46% ($p = 0.0003$), respectively (Figure 5C). In Figure 5D, we summarized our findings regarding the effect of OA-related inflammation-induced dephosphorylation of SMAD3L S213 on SMAD2/3 transcriptional activity and of IL-1β-induced SMAD3L S204 modification.

3. Discussion

In this study, we showed that there is a link between OA-related inflammation and disturbed TGF-β signaling in chondrocytes. Our results indicate that IL-1β and OAS-cm can stimulate hypertrophy-like differentiation by decreasing TGF-β transcriptional activity. In addition, we demonstrate that the inhibition of TGF-β signaling was significantly enhanced when the SMAD3 linker phosphorylation on S213 cannot take place, while inhibition is possibly less pronounced when S204 cannot be phosphorylated. These observations indicate an important role for these modifications in regulating SMAD2/3 signaling in chondrocytes.

OA is a complex and multifactorial disease and it is recognized that both systemic and local inflammation disturb homeostasis of cartilage in the osteoarthritic joint [1,2].

The enhanced expression of IL-1β and its receptor (IL1R1) are found in chondrocytes and synovial membranes of OA patients [33,34], although its role in OA is still under debate [8,35–38]. OA can certainly not only be attributed solely to the effect of IL-1β and other pro-inflammatory cytokines contribute to OA pathogenesis [39–44]. For instance, IL-8, TNF-α and H_2O_2 also stimulate chondrocyte hypertrophy [45–47]. In this study, both IL-1β and patient-derived OAS-cm, containing an unknown mix of cytokines, chemokines and growth factors [48], were used as models of OA-related inflammation.

A crucial role for TGF-β in chondrocytes is controlling hypertrophy and blocking chondrocyte terminal differentiation through SMAD2/3 signaling [11,49]. In this study, we support this anti-hypertrophic effect of TGF-β, since it blocks *COL10A1* upregulation, the most evaluated hypertrophy marker in bovine cartilage explants. Importantly, we also showed that the pre-incubation of 0.1 ng/mL IL-1β or 0.5% OAS-cm before the addition of TGF-β clearly negated this inhibitory effect. These inflammatory stimuli also blocked SMAD2/3 transcriptional activity in three different human chondrocyte-like cell lines—G6, H11 and SW1353. This effect was quite strong and rapid, since only 1 h pre-incubation with 0.1 ng/mL IL-1β or 5% OAS-cm was sufficient to inhibit SMAD2/3 transcriptional activity for 47 and 64%, respectively, in SW1353 cells. Together, these results support the findings that OA-related inflammation blocks protective TGF-β signaling in chondrocytes. Previous studies reported similar interactions between pro-inflammatory stimuli and TGF-β signaling in chondrocytes [10,50]. For instance, Roman-Blas et al. reported that IL-1β treatment resulted in the suppression of the DNA-binding activity of SMAD3/4 and suppression of SMAD2/3 phosphorylation in chondrocytes [10] and Madej et al. showed that both IL-1β and OAS-cm impair the mechanical activation of SMAD2/3 signaling in bovine cartilage explants [50].

One way how inflammatory cytokines can modulate TGF-β induced pSMAD2/3 signaling is via a reduction in ALK5 or TGFBR2 receptor signaling [15,51]. In our experimental set-up, this is unlikely the explanation of the observed inflammation-induced inhibiting effect on SMAD2/3 transcriptional activity. Namely, our findings show that IL-1β or OAS-cm, in both primary bovine chondrocytes and SW1353 cells, did not affect C-terminal SMAD2/3 and SMAD1/5/8 phosphorylation. In support, no *ALK5* and *TGFBR2* mRNA downregulation was measured with IL-1β or OAS-cm stimulation. In SW1353 cells, *TGFBR2* was even induced (and not reduced) 6 h after IL-1β stimulation. Based on these results, we infer that the inhibitory effect, which we found on TGF-β signaling, is downstream of the receptor-mediated SMAD activation. Madej et al. also reported no effect of IL-1β or OAS-cm on their own on *ALK5* and *TGFBR2* receptor expression in bovine cartilage explants, while these inflammatory conditions partly suppressed the mechanically mediated SMAD2/3 signaling [50]. On the other hand, Baugé et al. showed that pro-inflammatory mediators such as IL-1β can reduce *TGFBR2* expression in human OA monolayer chondrocytes [15]. This might be due to the fact that they used OA chondrocytes for their study, which might react differently on cytokines than non-OA chondrocytes, which we used in our studies. Other than the modulation of receptor expression, IL-1β can increase the expression of inhibitory SMAD7 via NF-κB the activation in chondrocytes, which inhibits SMAD2/3 signaling [9]. However, in our study, short-time periods of 1 and 6 h with IL-1β did not result in increased *SMAD7* mRNA levels in primary bovine chondrocytes and SW1353 cells. Additionally, Roman-Blas et al. reported that SMAD7 is not involved in the suppression of TGF-β signaling induced by IL-1β [10]. Stimulation with OAS-cm for 1 h induced SMAD7 in bovine chondrocytes, but this effect disappeared 6 h after stimulation. This could possibly be explained by the TGF-β presence in OAS-cm, which also increased the expression of inhibitory *SMAD7* itself [27], since it was not shown for IL-1β.

Next, we investigated if IL-1β and OAS-cm interact with SMAD-dependent signaling through the modification of the SMAD2/3 linker region. Previous studies showed that the phosphorylation of the specific serine and threonine residues in the regulatory linker region control SMAD2/3 function. Mutations in the SMAD3 linker strongly enhanced TGF-β-induced responses in breast cancer cells and increased tumorigenesis in the liver [30,52]. SMAD2 linker phosphorylation elevated mRNA levels of glycosaminoglycan synthesizing enzymes in vascular smooth muscle cells [53] and also the phosphorylation of the SMAD2 linker mediates synthesis of extracellular matrix proteins, such as collagens and proteoglycans [31,32,54]. The phosphorylation and dephosphorylation of the serine and threonine residues in the linker domain is dependent on kinases (e.g., MAPK) and phosphatases (e.g., DUSP1) [17,22,23,55,56]. Particularly, these are also induced by OA-related inflammatory stimuli [57–59], which led us to hypothesize that inflammation-induced kinases or phosphatases also affect the SMAD linker region in chondrocytes. We reported earlier that IL-1β induces SMAD2L serine phosphorylation in stem cells [60]. In the current study, we also reported that in chondrocytes phosphorylation of the SMAD2L serines and SMAD3L S204 were observed within 1 h following IL-1β or OAS-cm stimulation. Notably, OAS-cm also significantly decreased pSMAD3L S213. pSMAD3L S208 and T179 were not regulated by IL-1β or OAS-cm, suggesting a less pronounced role of these linker modifications in blocking protective TGF-β effects in chondrocytes. In our study, we did not only show which SMAD linker residues were (de-)phosphorylated by inflammatory stimuli, but also examined whether these specific inflammation-induced linker modifications explain the observed inhibiting effects of inflammation on TGF-β signaling by using individual SMAD3 phospho-mutants. Most other studies make use of a SMAD2/3 EPSM mutant, which cannot be phosphorylated in the linker region on any phospho-site [29,61,62]. Using individual SMAD3 linker phospho-mutants, we investigated the effect of every single SMAD linker modification separately.

To further study the role of the inflammation-induced pSMAD3L S204, we made use of a SMAD3 mutant which could not be phosphorylated at the serine 204 site (S204A). The inhibition of the SMAD2/3 transcriptional activity was not significantly inhibited anymore with IL-1β when SMAD3 S204A was over-expressed, while this was the case when normal SMAD3 was over-expressed. However, the average effect of 32% less inhibition with IL-1β was not significant ($p = 0.10$) compared to the inhibiting effect in the condition using normal SMAD3. A high variation between samples could explain this non-significance. For this study, the unstable nature of the SBE-pNL1.2 luciferase construct was chosen for its high sensitivity and large detection window compared to other stable luciferases [63]. Since the direction of the effect observed with the SMAD3 S204 mutant was constant across four separate experiments, we carefully propose that SMAD3L S204 phosphorylation mediates the effect of IL-1β on SMAD2/3 signaling (summarized in Figure 5D). Linker modifications are able to regulate the nuclear localization of the SMADs and this could be the possible explanation why in our study SMAD3 S204 was essential for the blocking effect of IL-1β on SMAD2/3 transcriptional activity. Kretzschmar et al. reported that in a mouse mammary epithelial cell line, Ras-activated ERK-induced pSMAD3 S204 resulted in cytoplasmic retention and the consequent repression of canonical TGF-β signaling [61]. Additionally, in epithelial cells, excessive Ras signaling demonstrated lower pSMAD3C tumor suppression [64,65]. A similar process could take place in chondrocytes and explain our results. On the other hand, contradictory findings were reported in different cell types. For instance, it was reported that in fibroblasts and mesangial cells, ERK-induced pSMAD3L S204 enhanced SMAD3-mediated COL1A2 promotor activity [66] and glycogen synthase kinase 3 (GSK3)-induced pSMAD3L S204 was strengthening SMAD3 transcriptional activity by enhancing its affinity to CREB-binding protein [23]. SMAD signaling could also be regulated via binding to ubiquitin ligases, such as Smurf2 or NEDD4L, resulting in SMAD degradation [67,68], but SMAD3 S204 phosphorylation has not been reported to regulate SMAD3 stability [67,69,70]. Another explanation could be the binding of pSMAD3L S204 to the phosphatase PPM1A/PP2Cα, which is known to dephosphorylate the SMAD2/3 C-terminus, and thereby regulate TGF-β signaling [71,72]. However, such interaction has not yet been investigated and further research into why SMAD3 S204 phosphorylation is essential for the inhibitory effect of IL-1β in chondrocytes is required.

The effect of OAS-cm on TGF-β signaling was not inhibited using the SMAD3 S204A mutant, while OAS-cm stimulation induced the phosphorylation of S204 on Western blot. This suggests that the inhibition by OAS-cm is regulated differently than with IL-1β, and S204 phosphorylation is not required to allow the OAS-cm-induced inhibition of SMAD2/3 transcriptional activity. OAS-cm is a mixture of cytokines which all have diverse roles on the SMAD3 linker and follow different kinetics of (de-)phosphorylation. The functional outcome of the SMAD2/3 linker phosphorylation for SMAD2/3 transcriptional activity depends on the combination of phosphorylation sites in linker and C-terminal regions, which brings some levels of complexity. This could explain why we did find S204 phosphorylation with OAS-cm on Western blot when looking at it as a single object, but did not observe an effect on the OAS-cm-induced inhibition of SMAD2/3 transcriptional activity when this phosphorylation could not occur anymore.

Interestingly, Browne et al. found an opposing role for SMAD3L S213 compared to S204 phosphorylation on COL1A2 promotor binding [66]. This is consistent with our study where we also showed contradictory results for SMAD3L S204 and S213 phosphorylation. Namely, the inhibiting effect of both IL-1β or OAS-cm was significantly enhanced when SMAD3L S213 could not be phosphorylated with 59% and 46%, respectively. This suggests that the phosphorylation of SMAD3L S213 protected against the inhibiting effect of IL-1β and OAS-cm on transcriptional SMAD2/3 signaling (summarized in Figure 5D). In literature, several lines of evidence report that SMAD3L S213 phosphorylation, induced by the Ras/JNK pathway, results in the transport of SMAD3 to the nucleus [16,64]. This would suggest that with the dephosphorylation of the S213 site SMAD2/3 remains in the cytoplasm and thereby prevents transcriptional activity. We found that OAS-cm significantly decreased the phosphorylation of SMAD3L S213, and thereby OAS-cm contributed itself to the inhibition on SMAD2/3 transcriptional activity. We reported earlier that combined IL-1β and TGF-β treatment in stem cells resulted in more linker-modified SMAD2 in the cytoplasm and less nuclear pSMAD2C [60]. Other studies showed that IL-1β-induced TAK activity resulted in cytoplasmic retention of the SMADs [73,74]. In future studies, the effect of linker modifications on the cellular localization of the SMAD complexes should, therefore, be examined.

The phosphorylation of SMAD3 S213 is protective against OA-related inflammation in chondrocytes. As a therapeutic strategy, it would be possible to activate kinases that are known to phosphorylate S213 in chondrocytes. Ras/JNK, CDK2, CDK4, SKI and integrin all have been reported to enhance pSMAD3L S213 phosphorylation in different cell types [70,75–77]. Another option is to inhibit phosphatases which catalyze the removal of phosphate groups. Small C-terminal domain phosphatases (SCPs) are known to dephosphorylate pSMAD3L S213 in the nucleus, resulting in the dissociation from SMAD4 and the export of SMAD3 to the cytoplasm [56,71,78,79]. SCP, therefore, could be an interesting therapeutic target. Blocking it could enhance the protective TGF-β signaling through the inhibition of dephosphorylation of the SMAD3 S213 linker phosphor-site by inflammation, resulting eventually in more SMAD3 in the nucleus. The identification of an inhibitor for SCP1 is ongoing [80,81]. For future in vivo studies, one must careful use these SCP inhibitors, since the phosphorylation of SMAD3 S213 results in cell-type specific effects. Namely, the nuclear retention of pSMAD3L S213 is reported to enhance pro-oncogenic signaling in cancer cells, by facilitating mitogenic signaling via the upregulation of the transcription factor c-Myc [64,70,75–77,82]. This shows that the phosphorylation of SMAD3L S213 can be malicious in cancer cells, while in chondrocytes S213 phosphorylation seems to be protective against OA-related inflammation. The discrepancy between these observations in different cell-types warns us to extract these results and more cell-specific research on the function of SMAD linker modifications is needed.

It is a limitation of this study that we were not able to transfect primary chondrocyte explants with the SMAD3 linker variants. Therefore, we could not test if the linker region was important in regulating the hypertrophic differentiation of chondrocytes in our hypertrophy model. Future studies are needed for the identification of interacting proteins of the

SMAD2/3 linker domain. For example, it would be of great interest to study the difference in the interaction of normal SMAD3 versus SMAD3 S204 or S213 linker mutants with RUNX2/3 and MEF2C, which are important transcription factors in driving chondrocyte hypertrophy [83,84].

In conclusion, the SMAD2/3 linker region is critical for the regulation of TGF-β signaling. The relevance of SMAD linker modifications in fibrosis, cancer and cardiovascular disease was described earlier but not in joint diseases. In this study, also the relevance for chondrocytes was established. Joint inflammation during OA development will result in kinase and phosphatase activation that could (de-)phosphorylate the SMAD linker region independent of the C-terminal phosphorylation, including the S204 and S213 site [85]. We showed that the (de)-phosphorylation of these linker sites led to a disturbance of the TGF-β signaling pathway in cartilage, which is of great importance for chondrocyte homeostasis maintenance. An additional investigation in chondrocytes is needed to identify the specific kinases and phosphatases for the individual SMAD linker phospho-sites, the impact of these modifications on the cellular location of the SMAD-complexes and the functional consequences for the cartilage. Inhibition studies of relevant kinases and phosphates may result in new therapeutic targets for OA.

4. Materials and Methods

4.1. Primary Cell Culture

Articular cartilage was obtained from metacarpophalangeal joints (MCP) of skeletally mature cows (>3 years old) post mortem. Full cartilage thickness explants were isolated with 3 mm diameter biopsy punches (Kai Medical Seki, Japan) and randomly distributed over the different conditions (two times four explants per cow per condition). Explants were equilibrated overnight before start of experiments in DMEM/F12 medium, supplemented with 100 mg/l sodium pyruvate, 100 U/mL penicillin and 100 µg/mL streptomycin at 37 °C and 5% CO_2. To obtain chondrocytes to culture in monolayer, cartilage slices were digested overnight with 1.5 mg/mL collagenase B (Roche Diagnostics, Basel, Switzerland) in DMEM/F12 at 37 °C. The next day, chondrocyte suspension was spun down at $300 \times g$ for 10 min, washed three times using saline and resuspended in DMEM/F12 containing 10% fetal calf serum (FCS), 100 mg/L sodium pyruvate, 100 U/mL penicillin and 100 µg/mL streptomycin (complete DMEM/F12). Chondrocytes were plated at a density of 8×10^4 cells/cm^2 and cultured for 1 week at 37 °C and 5% CO_2 to form a monolayer. Medium was refreshed every three days. Before start of experiments, chondrocytes were serum-starved (0% FCS) overnight. Each experiment was conducted three times in multiple donors and conditions were always tested in technical duplicate.

4.2. Chondrocyte Cell Line Culture

SW1353 human chondrosarcoma cells were cultured in complete DMEM/F12 at 37 °C and 5% CO_2. For experiments, cells were plated at a density of 3×10^4 cells/cm^2. Human G6 and H11 adult articular chondrocytes were derived from femoral head cartilage of an anonymous donor, transduced with a temperature-dependent SV40 large oncogene, resulting in proliferation at 32 °C, but not at 37 °C [86]. G6 and H11 chondrocytes were cultured at 32 °C with complete DMEM/F12 except with 5% FCS. For experiments G6 and H11, cells were plated at a density of 8×10^4 cells/cm^2. Chondrocytes were serum-starved overnight in DMEM/F12 medium supplemented with 0.1% FCS (SW1353) or 0.5% FCS (G6 and H11) before start of experiments.

4.3. Chondrocyte Stimulation

Chondrocytes were stimulated with recombinant human (rh) TGF-β1 (BioLegend, San Diego, CA, USA), rhIL-1β (R&D Systems, Minneapolis, MN, USA), OA synovium-conditioned medium (OAS-cm), or a combination of these mediators, for time periods and dosages indicated in Figure legends. OAS-cm was obtained by culturing synovium from OA patients for 24 h, whereafter debris was removed by centrifugation at $300 \times g$ and medium was stored in aliquots at −20 °C until further use [48]. To inhibit ALK5 kinase activity, 5 μM SB-505124 (Sigma-Aldrich, Burlington, MA, USA) was used, dissolved in dimethyl sulfoxide (DMSO).

4.4. Plasmid DNA, Adenoviral Production and Transduction

To study SMAD2/3 transcriptional activity, a luciferase reporter assay (SBE-pNL1.2) was produced, where a SMAD binding element (SBE) (three times AGTATGTCTAGACTGA) with spacer (CTCGAGGATATCAAGATCTGGCCTCGGCGGCCTAGATGAGACACT) and minimal promotor (AGAGGGTATATAATGGAAGCTCGACTTCCAG) (GeneCust, Boynes, France) was cloned into a NanoLuc luciferase with a protein destabilization domain (pNL1.2) (Promega, Madison, WI, USA) [63]. Sequences were verified by Sanger sequencing. Knock-out of SMAD2, SMAD3 or SMAD4 prevented luciferase induction with TGF-β, suggesting the reporter assay is SMAD2/3-dependent (Appendix B). Plasmid transduction was optimized for the different cell lines by analysis of fluorescent (GFP) protein expressing cells with FACS. G6 and H11 chondrocytes were seeded in a cell density of 8×10^4 cells/cm^2 and transfected with Lipofectamine 2000 Transfection Reagent (Invitrogen, Waltham, MA, USA) according to manufacturer's protocol. SW1353 were seeded in a density of 2.6×10^4 cells/cm^2 and transfected with FuGENE6 Transfection Reagent (Promega, Madison, WI, USA) according to manufacturer's protocol. SMAD3 linker mutant expression plasmids, containing an N-terminal FLAG-tag, were bought from Addgene (Watertown, MA, USA) (SMAD3, #14052; SMAD3 T179V, #26997; SMAD3 S204A, #27114; SMAD3 S208A, #27115; SMAD3 S213A, #27116; SMAD3 EPSM, #14963). All SMAD inserts were directionally cloned into the adenoviral vector pShuttle and verified by Sanger sequencing. Adenovirus was produced with the AdEasy Adenoviral Vector System (Agilent, Santa Clara, CA, USA) in the N52E6 adenovirus producer cell line. SW1353, already transfected with SBE-pNL1.2, was transduced with adenovirus of the different SMAD3 linker mutants. To compare equal over-expression of the different mutants, flow cytometry was used to quantify FLAG-tag expression with PE anti-FLAG tag Antibody (clone L5, Biolegend, San Diego, CA, USA) using a Gallios flow cytometry analyzer and analyzed using Kaluza software version 2.1 (both from Beckman Coulter, Brea, CA, USA).

4.5. SMAD-Luciferase Transcriptional Reporter Assay

After transfection with 1.0 μg SBE-pNL1.2 per 100,000 cells, cells were detached by trypsinization and seeded in white polystyrene 96-well plates at a density of 3×10^4 cells/cm^2 for the SW1353 and 8×10^4 cells/cm^2 for the G6 and H11 chondrocytes. Cells were serum-starved overnight, 1 h pre-incubated with DMEM/F12 (control), rhIL-1β (R&D Systems, Minneapolis, MN, USA) or OAS-cm and then stimulated with rhTGF-β1 (Biolegend, San Diego, CA, USA) for 5 h. Cells were lysed 5 h post-stimulation using 30 μL ultra-pure water. An equal amount of Nano-Glo luciferase reagent (Promega, Madison, WI, USA) was added and luminescence was determined at 470–480 nm (Clariostar, BMG Labtech, Ortenberg, Germany). Each condition was performed in quadruple and the mean per experiment was depicted.

4.6. Protein Isolation and Western Blot

Chondrocytes were lysed in lysis buffer (Cell Signaling, Danvers, MA, USA) containing complete protease inhibitor cocktail (Roche Diagnostics, Basel, Switzerland). Samples were sonicated on ice, using a Bioruptor (Diagenode, Liege, Belgium; 10 cycles of 30 s sonication and 30 s rest). Protein concentration was determined with a BCA-assay (Thermo Scientific, Waltham, MA, USA) and normalized. Reducing Laemmli Sample buffer (2% SDS, 10% glycerol, 100 mM Tris HCl, pH 6.8, 100 mM DTT and Bromophenol bleu) were added and samples were boiled at 95 °C for 5 min. Protein samples were separated on a 10% bis-acrylamide SDS-PAGE gel and transferred to 0.45 μm pore nitrocellulose membrane using wet transfer (Towbin buffer, 2 h, 275 mA at 4 °C). Non-specific antibody binding was blocked for 1 h with 5% non-fat dry milk (Friesland Campina, Amersfoort, The Netherlands) or 5% BSA in TBS-T (15 mM Tris-HCl, pH 7.4, 0.1% Tween). Cells were incubated overnight at 4 °C with primary antibodies directed against pSMAD2/3C-Ser463/467 (1:1000, CST 3101), pSMAD1/5C-Ser426/428 (1:1000, CST 9511), pSMAD2L-Ser245/250/255 (1:1000, CST 3104), pSMAD2L-Thr220 (1:1000, NBP 1-004982), pSMAD3L-Ser204 (1:1000, Abcam 63402), pSMAD3L-Ser208 (1:1000, Abcam 138659), pSMAD3L-Ser213 (1:1000, Abcam 63403), pSMAD3L-Thr179 (1:1000, Abcam 74062) or anti-FLAG (1:10,000, Sigma-Aldrich 3165). Afterwards, membranes were incubated with polyclonal Goat anti-Rabbit or Rabbit anti-Mouse coupled to horseradish peroxidase (1:1500, Dako) for 1 h at RT. Signal was detected using enhanced chemiluminescence (ECL) prime kit (GE Healthcare, Chicago, IL, USA) on an ImageQuant LAS4000 (Leica, Wetzlar, Germany). As loading control, GAPDH (1:10,000, Sigma-Aldrich 1403850) was used and ImageJ (Fiji 1.51n) was used for quantification.

4.7. RNA Isolation and Quantitative Real-Time PCR

Cartilage explants were homogenized using a micro-dismembrator (B. Braun, Oss, The Netherlands) for 1 min at 1500 rpm. Subsequently, total messenger RNA (mRNA) was isolated using RNeasy Fibrous tissues kit (Qiagen, Hilden, Germany) according to manufacturer's protocol. From cell lines and primary chondrocytes cultured in monolayer, mRNA was isolated using 500 μL TRIzol (Sigma-Aldrich, Burlington, MA, USA), according to manufacturer's protocol. After isolation, a maximum of 1 μg of mRNA was treated with 1 μL DNAse (Life Technologies, Carlsbad, CA, USA) for 15 min at room temperature to remove possible genomic DNA, followed by 10 min inactivation by incubation at 65 °C with 1 μL 25 mM EDTA (Life Technologies). mRNA was reverse transcribed to complementary DNA using 1.9 μL ultrapure water, 2.4 μL 10x DNAse buffer, 2.0 μL 0.1 M dithiothreitol, 0.8 μL 25 mM dNTP, 0.4 μg oligo dT primer, 200 U M-MLV reverse transcriptase (all Life Technologies, Carlsbad, CA, USA) and 0.5 μL 40 U/mL RNAsin (Promega, Madison, WI, USA) and incubated for 5 min at 25 °C, 60 min at 39 °C, and 5 min at 95 °C using a thermocycler. Gene expression was measured using SYBR Green Master Mix (Applied Biosystems, Waltham, MA, USA) and 0.25 mM primers (Biolegio, Nijmegen, the Neterlands) (Table 1) with a StepOnePlus real-time PCR system (Applied Biosystems, Waltham, MA, USA). The amplification protocol was 10 min at 95 °C, followed by 40 cycles of 15 s at 95 °C and 1 min at 60 °C. Melting curves were analyzed to confirm product specificity. To calculate the relative gene expression ($-\Delta Ct$), the average of three reference genes was used: *bGAPDH*, *bRPL22* and *bRPS14* for bovine chondrocytes or *hGAPDH*, *hRPL22* and *hRPS27A* for human chondrocyte cell lines.

4.8. Statistical Analysis

Quantitative data of gene expression analysis were expressed as column scatter graphs and displayed mean values of a technical duplicate sample per donor (primary chondrocytes) or separate experiments (SW1353 cells) with corresponding 95% confidence interval (CI) or standard deviations (SD) (see Figure legends). For SBE-pNL1.2 transcriptional assays, conditions were investigated in quadruplo and expressed as mean per experiment with corresponding 95% confidence interval (CI). Area under the curve (AUC) was calculated for three separate experiments. Differences were tested using displayed means with analysis of variance (ANOVA) followed by Dunnett's or Bonferroni's post-test to take multiple comparisons into account (see Figure legends). Differences in pSMAD2 and pSMAD3L protein were tested using an unpaired two-tailed *t*-test and displayed as mean ± SD. Statistical differences were considered as significant if the *p*-value was below 0.05. All analyses were performed using Graph Pad Prism version 7.0 (GraphPad Software, San Diego, CA, USA).

Int. J. Mol. Sci. **2021**, *22*, 8124

Table 1. Primer sequences as used in this study.

Gene and Species	Forward Sequence (5′ → 3′)	Reverse Sequence (5′ → 3′)
bGAPDH	CACCCACGGCAAGTTCAAC	TCTCGCTCCTGGAAGATGGT
bRPS14	CATCACTGCCCTCCACATCA	TTCCAATCCGCCCAATCTTCA
bRPL22	GTTCGCTCACCTCCCTTTCTG	GCAGCATCCATGATTCCATCT
bCOL10A1	CCATCCAACACCAAGACACAGT	TGCTCTCCTCTCAGTGATACACCTT
bMMP3	AAACTCACCTCACGTACAGAATTG	TCCCAGACCGTCAGAGCTTT
bSMAD7	GGGCTTTCAGATTCCCAACTT	CTCCCAGTATGCCACCACG
bTGFBR2	GGCTGTCTGGAGGAAGAATGA	GTCTCTCCGGACCCCTTTCT
bALK5	CAGGACCACTGCAATAAAATAGAACTT	TGCCAGTTCAACAGGACCAA
hGAPDH	ATCTTCTTTTGCGTCGCCAG	TTCCCCATGGTGTCTGAGC
hRPL22	TCGCTCACCTCCCTTTCTAA	TCACGGTGATCTTGCTCTTG
hRPS27A	TGGCTGTCCTGAAATATTATAAGGT	CCCCAGCACCACATTCATCA
hSMAD7	CCTTAGCCGACTCTGCGAACTA	CCAGATAATTCGTTCCCCCTGT
hTGFBR2	CTGGTGCTCTGGGAAATGACA	TCGCCCTCGATCTCTCAACA
hALK5	CGACGGCGTTACAGTGTTTCT	CCCATCTGTCACACAAGTAAA

Author Contributions: Conception and design, N.T., G.v.d.A., E.B.D., A.v.C. and P.v.d.K.; Collection and acquisition of data, N.T., M.N., R.W., G.v.d.A., E.V., H.v.B. and A.v.C.; Analysis and interpretation of data, N.T., M.N., R.W., G.v.d.A., E.V., H.v.B., E.B.D., P.v.L., F.v.d.L., M.K., A.v.C. and P.v.d.K.; Drafting of the manuscript, N.T., A.v.C. and P.v.d.K.; Critical revision, N.T., M.N., R.W., G.v.d.A., E.V., H.v.B., E.B.D., P.v.L., F.v.d.L., M.K., A.v.C. and P.v.d.K.; Final approval of the article: N.T., M.N., R.W., G.v.d.A., E.V., H.v.B., E.B.D., P.v.L., F.v.d.L., M.K., A.v.C. and P.v.d.K. All authors have read and agreed to the published version of the manuscript.

Funding: This study was supported by a grant from the Dutch Arthritis Foundation (ReumaNederland), with grant number 16-1-40.

Institutional Review Board Statement: Not applicable.

Informed Consent Statement: Not applicable.

Conflicts of Interest: The authors have nothing to disclose; there is no conflict of interest.

Appendix A

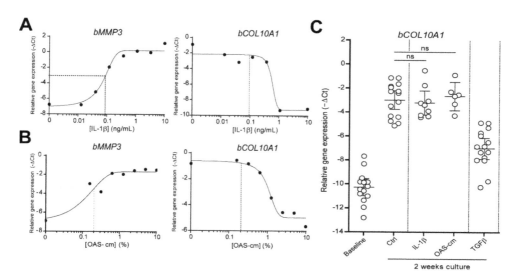

Scheme A1. Dose response curves for IL-1β and OAS-cm and the effect of these stimuli on collagen type 10 expression.
To calculate which concentrations of IL-β and OAS-cm we should use in our hypertrophy-model we performed a dose response curve with IL-1β (**A**) and with OAS-cm (**B**) in bovine cartilage explants. Explants were cultured in the presence of IL-1β or OAS-cm as indicated on the X-axis for 2 weeks, and medium was refreshed every 3rd day. Relative gene expression of the read-out gene matrix metalloproteinase 3 (*MMP3*) and of collagen type 10 (*COL10A1*) was measured using qPCR. The concentrations of 0.1 ng/mL IL-1β and 0.5% OAS-cm were chosen for further experiments since these match the EC-50 in inducing *MMP3* expression. (**C**) Interaction of these inflammatory stimuli with TGF-β in regulating hypertrophic differentiation, as calculated with measuring gene expression *COL10A1* was investigated in several cow donors. It was established that the concentrations of 0.1 ng/mL IL-1β and 0.5% OAS-cm did not modulate *COL10A1* expression themselves. Data are plotted as mean ± 95 % CI with each dot representing the average of 2 replicates of 4 explants in one cow. Statistical analysis was performed using a repeated measures one-way analysis of variance with Bonferroni's post-hoc test: ns = non-significant.

Appendix B

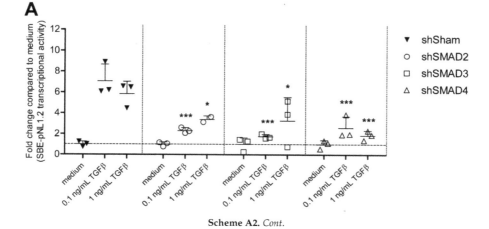

Scheme A2. *Cont.*

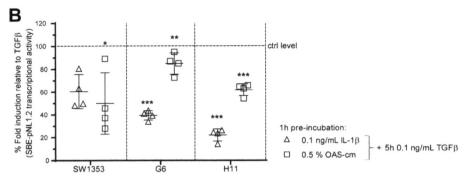

Scheme A2. The SBE-pNL1.2 luciferase reporter assay is SMAD2, SMAD3 and SMAD4 dependent. (**A**) SW1353 cells were transfected with the SBE-pNL1.2 luciferase construct, where after they were transfected with short hairpin (sh) lentivirus to knockout SMAD2 (shSMAD2), SMAD3 (shSMAD3) or SMAD4 (shSMAD4) or control (shSham). At 48 h after transduction, SW1353 cells were stimulated with 0.1 or 1 ng/mL TGF-β and after 5h SMAD2/3 transcriptional activity was determined. Data is expressed as fold change with TGF-β relative to medium control and plotted as mean ± SD of a technical triplicate. (**B**) To study interaction between OA-related inflammation and functional TGF-β signaling three chondrocyte-like cell lines (SW1353, G6 and H11) were transfected with the SBE-pNL1.2 construct. After transfection, cells were re-plated, pre-incubated for 1 hour with medium, 0.1 ng/mL IL-1β or 0.5 % OAS-cm and thereafter stimulated for 5h with 0.1 ng/mL TGF-β. Luciferase activity was measured relative to experimental condition stimulated with TGF-β, as set at 100% (ctrl level). Data represents mean ± 95 % CI of four independent experiments performed in quadruple. Statistical analysis was performed using (**A**) Two-way ANOVA with Bonferroni's post-hoc test or (**B**) a one-way ANOVA with Dunnett's multiple comparison test comparing the mean to the mean of the condition stimulated with solely TGF-β: * $p \leq 0.05$; ** $p \leq 0.01$; *** $p \leq 0.001$.

Appendix C

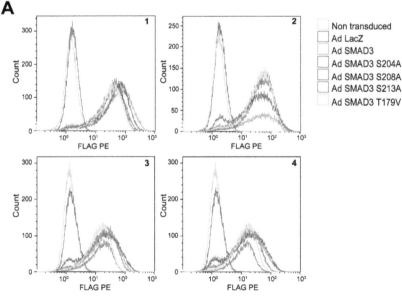

Scheme A3. *Cont.*

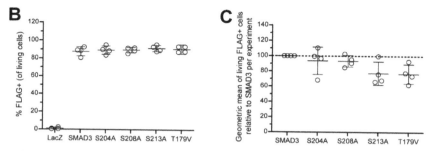

Scheme A3. High and equal over-expression between SMAD variants. To compare conditions between the SMAD3 linker mutants and normal SMAD3 equal over-expression is required. SW1353 cells were transfected with the SBE-pNL1.2 construct, re-plated afterwards and transduced with adenoviral vectors (Ad) with the different SMAD variants, a control virus (LacZ) or left untreated (non transduced). (**A**) Flow cytometry was used to quantify FLAG-tag expression with PE anti-FLAG Tag Antibody. First, debris was excluded based on forward and side scatter, followed by the selection of single and viable (stained with eFLuor780 viability dye) cells. Afterwards, FLAG-positive cells were gated based on the autofluorescence of unlabeled cells. Histograms of the FLAG-PE stainings of four individual experiments were displayed. (**B**) Flow cytometric analysis showed that with adenoviral transduction in all conditions with the SMAD variants over 90% of all living cells were positively stained for FLAG and (**C**) the geometric mean of this over-expression was not different between conditions with normal SMAD3 and the SMAD3 linker mutants, meaning that all SMAD3 variants were overexpressed equally. Therefore, we were able to fairly compare conditions. Data is represented as dot plots with every dot representing an individual experiment and is plotted as mean ± SD and statistical analysis was performed using one-way ANOVA with Dunett's post-hoc test compared to the condition transduced with normal SMAD3. No significant results compared to normal SMAD3 condition were measured.

References

1. Chow, Y.Y.; Chin, K.Y. The Role of Inflammation in the Pathogenesis of Osteoarthritis. *Mediat. Inflamm.* **2020**, *2020*. [CrossRef] [PubMed]
2. Van den Bosch, M.H.J.; van Lent, P.; van der Kraan, P.M. Identifying effector molecules, cells, and cytokines of innate immunity in OA. *Osteoarthr. Cartil.* **2020**, *28*, 532–543. [CrossRef] [PubMed]
3. Scanzello, C.R.; Goldring, S.R. The role of synovitis in osteoarthritis pathogenesis. *Bone* **2012**, *51*, 249–257. [CrossRef]
4. D'Agostino1, M.A.; Conaghan, P.; le Bars, M.; Baron, G.; Grassi, W.; Martin-Mola, E.; Wakefield, R.; Brasseur, J.-L.; So, A.; Backhaus, M.; et al. EULAR report on the use of ultrasonography in painful knee osteoarthritis. Part 1: Prevalence of inflammation in osteoarthritis. *Ann. Rheum. Dis* **2005**, *64*, 1703–1709. [CrossRef] [PubMed]
5. Roemer, F.W.; Guermazi, A.; Felson, D.T.; Niu, J.; Nevitt, M.C.; Crema, M.D.; Lynch, J.A.; Lewis, C.E.; Torner, J.; Zhalng, Y. Presence of MRI-detected joint effusion and synovitis increases the risk of cartilage loss in knees without osteoarthritis at 30-month follow-up: The MOST study. *Ann. Rheum. Dis.* **2011**, *70*, 1804–1809. [CrossRef]
6. Kortekaas, M.C.; Kwok, W.Y.; Reijnierse, M.; Stijnen, T.; Kloppenburg, M. Brief Report: Association of Inflammation With Development of Erosions in Patients With Hand Osteoarthritis: A Prospective Ultrasonography Study. *Arthritis Rheumatol.* **2016**, *68*, 392–397. [CrossRef]
7. Vincenti, M.P.; Brinckerhoff, C.E. Transcriptional regulation of collagenase (MMP-1, MMP-13) genes in arthritis: Integration of complex signaling pathways for the recruitment of gene-specific transcription factors. *Arthritis Res.* **2002**, *4*, 157–164. [CrossRef]
8. Cortial, D.; Gouttenoire, J.; Rousseau, C.F.; Ronzieère, M.-C.; Piccardi, N.; Msika, P.; Herbage, D.; Malletin-Gerin, F.; Freyria, A.l.-M. Activation by IL-1 of bovine articular chondrocytes in culture within a 3D collagen-based scaffold. An in vitro model to address the effect of compounds with therapeutic potential in osteoarthritis. *Osteoarthr. Cartil.* **2006**, *14*, 631–640. [CrossRef]
9. Bauge, C.; Attia, J.; Leclercq, S.; Pujol, J.P.; Galera, P.; Boumediene, K. Interleukin-1beta up-regulation of Smad7 via NF-kappaB activation in human chondrocytes. *Arthritis Rheum.* **2008**, *58*, 221–226. [CrossRef]
10. Roman-Blas, J.A.; Stokes, D.G.; Jimenez, S.A. Modulation of TGF-beta signaling by proinflammatory cytokines in articular chondrocytes. *Osteoarthr. Cartil.* **2007**, *15*, 1367–1377. [CrossRef] [PubMed]
11. Thielen, N.G.M.; van der Kraan, P.M.; van Caam, A.P.M. TGFbeta/BMP Signaling Pathway in Cartilage Homeostasis. *Cells* **2019**, *8*, 969. [CrossRef]
12. Chen, C.G.; Thuillier, D.; Chin, E.N.; Alliston, T. Chondrocyte-intrinsic Smad3 represses Runx2-inducible matrix metalloproteinase 13 expression to maintain articular cartilage and prevent osteoarthritis. *Arthritis Rheum.* **2012**, *64*, 3278–3289. [CrossRef]
13. Van der Kraan, P.M.; Blaney Davidson, E.N.; Blom, A.; van den Berg, W.B. TGF-beta signaling in chondrocyte terminal differentiation and osteoarthritis: Modulation and integration of signaling pathways through receptor-Smads. *Osteoarthr. Cartil.* **2009**, *17*, 1539–1545. [CrossRef] [PubMed]

14. Van der Kraan, P.M.; Blaney Davidson, E.N.; van den Berg, W.B. A role for age-related changes in TGFbeta signaling in aberrant chondrocyte differentiation and osteoarthritis. *Arthritis Res. Ther.* **2010**, *12*, 201. [CrossRef] [PubMed]
15. Bauge, C.; Legendre, F.; Leclercq, S.; Elissalde, J.M.; Pujol, J.P.; Galera, P.; Boumediene, K. Interleukin-1beta impairment of transforming growth factor beta1 signaling by down-regulation of transforming growth factor beta receptor type II and up-regulation of Smad7 in human articular chondrocytes. *Arthritis Rheum.* **2007**, *56*, 3020–3032. [CrossRef]
16. Matsuzaki, K. Smad phospho-isoforms direct context-dependent TGF-beta signaling. *Cytokine Growth Factor Rev.* **2013**, *24*, 385–399. [CrossRef] [PubMed]
17. Kamato, D.; Burch, M.L.; Piva, T.J.; Rezaei, H.B.; Rostam, M.A.; Xu, S.; Zheng, W.; Little, P.J.; Osman, N. Transforming growth factor-beta signalling: Role and consequences of Smad linker region phosphorylation. *Cell. Signal.* **2013**, *25*, 2017–2024. [CrossRef] [PubMed]
18. Massague, J. TGF-beta signal transduction. *Annu. Rev. Biochem.* **1998**, *67*, 753–791. [CrossRef] [PubMed]
19. Shi, Y. Structural insights on Smad function in TGFbeta signaling. *Bioessays* **2001**, *23*, 223–232. [CrossRef]
20. Hill, C.S. Nucleocytoplasmic shuttling of Smad proteins. *Cell Res.* **2009**, *19*, 36–46. [CrossRef]
21. Sapkota, G.; Knockaert, M.; Alarcon, C.; Montalvo, E.; Brivanlou, A.H.; Massague, J. Dephosphorylation of the linker regions of Smad1 and Smad2/3 by small C-terminal domain phosphatases has distinct outcomes for bone morphogenetic protein and transforming growth factor-beta pathways. *J. Biol. Chem.* **2006**, *281*, 40412–40419. [CrossRef]
22. Matsuzaki, K. Smad phosphoisoform signaling specificity: The right place at the right time. *Carcinogenesis* **2011**, *32*, 1578–1588. [CrossRef]
23. Millet, C.; Yamashita, M.; Heller, M.; Yu, L.R.; Veenstra, T.D.; Zhang, Y.E. A negative feedback control of transforming growth factor-beta signaling by glycogen synthase kinase 3-mediated Smad3 linker phosphorylation at Ser-204. *J. Biol. Chem.* **2009**, *284*, 19808–19816. [CrossRef] [PubMed]
24. Van der Kraan, P.M.; van den Berg, W.B. Chondrocyte hypertrophy and osteoarthritis: Role in initiation and progression of cartilage degeneration? *Osteoarthr. Cartil.* **2012**, *20*, 223–232. [CrossRef]
25. Li, T.F.; O'Keefe, R.J.; Chen, D. TGF-beta signaling in chondrocytes. *Front. Biosci.* **2005**, *10*, 681–688. [CrossRef]
26. Zhao, W.; Wang, T.; Luo, Q.; Chen, Y.; Leung, V.Y.L.; Wen, C.; Shah, M.F.; Pan, H.; Chiu, K.; Cao, X.; et al. Cartilage degeneration and excessive subchondral bone formation in spontaneous osteoarthritis involves altered TGF-beta signaling. *J. Orthop. Res.* **2016**, *34*, 763–770. [CrossRef]
27. Van Caam, A.; Madej, W.; Thijssen, E.; Garcia de Vinuesa, A.; van den Berg, W.; Goumans, M.J.; ten Diike, P.; Davidson, E.B.; van der Kraan, P.M. Expression of TGFbeta-family signalling components in ageing cartilage: Age-related loss of TGFbeta and BMP receptors. *Osteoarthr. Cartil.* **2016**, *24*, 1235–1245. [CrossRef] [PubMed]
28. Hata, A.; Chen, Y.G. TGF-beta Signaling from Receptors to Smads. *Cold Spring Harb. Perspect. Biol.* **2016**, *8*, a022061. [CrossRef] [PubMed]
29. Bae, E.; Kim, S.J.; Hong, S.; Liu, F.; Ooshima, A. Smad3 linker phosphorylation attenuates Smad3 transcriptional activity and TGF-beta1/Smad3-induced epithelial-mesenchymal transition in renal epithelial cells. *Biochem. Biophys. Res. Commun.* **2012**, *427*, 593–599. [CrossRef] [PubMed]
30. Bae, E.; Sato, M.; Kim, R.-J.; Kwak, M.-K.; Naka, K.; Gim, J.; Kadota, M.; Tang, B.; Flanders, K.C.; Kim, T.-A.; et al. Definition of smad3 phosphorylation events that affect malignant and metastatic behaviors in breast cancer cells. *Cancer Res.* **2014**, *74*, 6139–6149. [CrossRef] [PubMed]
31. Burch, M.L.; Zheng, W.; Little, P.J. Smad linker region phosphorylation in the regulation of extracellular matrix synthesis. *Cell. Mol. Life Sci.* **2011**, *68*, 97–107. [CrossRef]
32. Li, F.; Zeng, B.; Chai, Y.; Cai, P.; Fan, C.; Cheng, T. The linker region of Smad2 mediates TGF-beta-dependent ERK2-induced collagen synthesis. *Biochem. Biophys. Res. Commun.* **2009**, *386*, 289–293. [CrossRef]
33. Melchiorri, C.; Meliconi, R.; Frizziero, L.; Silvestri, T.; Pulsatelli, L.; Mazzetti, I.; Borzì, R.M.; Uguccioni, M.; Facchini, A. Enhanced and coordinated in vivo expression of inflammatory cytokines and nitric oxide synthase by chondrocytes from patients with osteoarthritis. *Arthritis Rheum.* **1998**, *41*, 2165–2174. [CrossRef]
34. Martel-Pelletier, J.; McCollum, R.; DiBattista, J.; Faure, M.P.; Chin, J.A.; Fournier, S.; Sarfati, M.; Pelletier, J.P. The interleukin-1 receptor in normal and osteoarthritic human articular chondrocytes. Identification as the type I receptor and analysis of binding kinetics and biologic function. *Arthritis Rheum.* **1992**, *35*, 530–540. [CrossRef] [PubMed]
35. Radons, J.; Bosserhoff, A.K.; Grassel, S.; Falk, W.; Schubert, T.E. p38MAPK mediates IL-1-induced down-regulation of aggrecan gene expression in human chondrocytes. *Int. J. Mol. Med.* **2006**, *17*, 661–668. [CrossRef] [PubMed]
36. Fernandes, J.C.; Martel-Pelletier, J.; Pelletier, J.P. The role of cytokines in osteoarthritis pathophysiology. *Biorheology* **2002**, *39*, 237–246. [PubMed]
37. Nasi, S.; Ea, H.K.; So, A.; Busso, N. Revisiting the Role of Interleukin-1 Pathway in Osteoarthritis: Interleukin-1alpha and -1beta, and NLRP3 Inflammasome Are Not Involved in the Pathological Features of the Murine Meniscectomy Model of Osteoarthritis. *Front. Pharmacol.* **2017**, *8*, 282. [CrossRef] [PubMed]
38. Van Dalen, S.C.; Blom, A.B.; Sloetjes, A.W.; Helsen, M.M.; Roth, J.; Vogl, T.; van de Loo, F.A.J.; Koenders, M.I.; van der Kraan, P.M.; van den Berg, W.B.; et al. Interleukin-1 is not involved in synovial inflammation and cartilage destruction in collagenase-induced osteoarthritis. *Osteoarthr. Cartil.* **2017**, *25*, 385–396. [CrossRef] [PubMed]

39. Kapoor, M.; Martel-Pelletier, J.; Lajeunesse, D.; Pelletier, J.P.; Fahmi, H. Role of proinflammatory cytokines in the pathophysiology of osteoarthritis. *Nat. Rev. Rheumatol.* **2011**, *7*, 33–42. [CrossRef] [PubMed]

40. Liacini, A.; Sylvester, J.; Li, W.Q.; Huang, W.; Dehnade, F.; Ahmad, M.; Zafarullah, M. Induction of matrix metalloproteinase-13 gene expression by TNF-alpha is mediated by MAP kinases, AP-1, and NF-kappaB transcription factors in articular chondrocytes. *Exp. Cell Res.* **2003**, *288*, 208–217. [CrossRef]

41. Laavola, M.; Leppanen, T.; Hamalainen, M.; Vuolteenaho, K.; Moilanen, T.; Nieminen, R.; Moilanen, E. IL-6 in Osteoarthritis: Effects of Pine Stilbenoids. *Molecules* **2018**, *24*, 109. [CrossRef]

42. Van Lent, P.L.; Blom, A.B.; Schelbergen, R.F.; Sloetjes, A.; Lafeber, F.P.; Lems, W.F.; Cats, H.; Vogl, T.; Roth, J.; van den Berg, W.B. Active involvement of alarmins S100A8 and S100A9 in the regulation of synovial activation and joint destruction during mouse and human osteoarthritis. *Arthritis Rheum.* **2012**, *64*, 1466–1476. [CrossRef] [PubMed]

43. Hulin-Curtis, S.L.; Bidwell, J.L.; Perry, M.J. Association between CCL2 haplotypes and knee osteoarthritis. *Int. J. Immunogenet.* **2013**, *40*, 280–283. [CrossRef]

44. Heldens, G.T.; Blaney Davidson, E.N.; Vitters, E.L.; Schreurs, B.W.; Piek, E.; van den Berg, W.B.; van der Kraan, P.M. Catabolic factors and osteoarthritis-conditioned medium inhibit chondrogenesis of human mesenchymal stem cells. *Tissue Eng. Part A* **2012**, *18*, 45–54. [CrossRef]

45. Cecil, D.L.; Johnson, K.; Rediske, J.; Lotz, M.; Schmidt, A.M.; Terkeltaub, R. Inflammation-induced chondrocyte hypertrophy is driven by receptor for advanced glycation end products. *J. Immunol.* **2005**, *175*, 8296–8302. [CrossRef]

46. Merz, D.; Liu, R.; Johnson, K.; Terkeltaub, R. IL-8/CXCL8 and growth-related oncogene alpha/CXCL1 induce chondrocyte hypertrophic differentiation. *J. Immunol.* **2003**, *171*, 4406–4415. [CrossRef]

47. Morita, K.; Miyamoto, T.; Fujita, N.; Kubota, Y.; Ito, K.; Takubo, K.; Miyamoto, K.; Ninomiya, K.; Suzuki, T.; Iwasaki, R.; et al. Reactive oxygen species induce chondrocyte hypertrophy in endochondral ossification. *J. Exp. Med.* **2007**, *204*, 1613–1623. [CrossRef]

48. Van Beuningen, H.M.; de Vries-van Melle, M.L.; Vitters, E.L.; Schreurs, W.; van den Berg, W.B.; van Osch, G.J.; van der Kraan, P.M. Inhibition of TAK1 and/or JAK can rescue impaired chondrogenic differentiation of human mesenchymal stem cells in osteoarthritis-like conditions. *Tissue Eng. Part A* **2014**, *20*, 2243–2252. [CrossRef]

49. Van der Kraan, P.M. Differential Role of Transforming Growth Factor-beta in an Osteoarthritic or a Healthy Joint. *J. Bone Metab.* **2018**, *25*, 65–72. [CrossRef]

50. Madej, W.; Buma, P.; van der Kraan, P. Inflammatory conditions partly impair the mechanically mediated activation of Smad2/3 signaling in articular cartilage. *Arthritis Res. Ther.* **2016**, *18*, 146. [CrossRef]

51. Elshaier, A.M.; Hakimiyan, A.A.; Rappoport, L.; Rueger, D.C.; Chubinskaya, S. Effect of interleukin-1beta on osteogenic protein 1-induced signaling in adult human articular chondrocytes. *Arthritis Rheum.* **2009**, *60*, 143–154. [CrossRef]

52. Murata, M.; Yoshida, K.; Yamaguchi, T.; Matsuzaki, K. Linker phosphorylation of Smad3 promotes fibro-carcinogenesis in chronic viral hepatitis of hepatocellular carcinoma. *World J. Gastroenterol.* **2014**, *20*, 15018–15027. [CrossRef] [PubMed]

53. Rostam, M.A.; Kamato, D.; Piva, T.J.; Zheng, W.; Little, P.J.; Osman, N. The role of specific Smad linker region phosphorylation in TGF-beta mediated expression of glycosaminoglycan synthesizing enzymes in vascular smooth muscle. *Cell. Signal.* **2016**, *28*, 956–966. [CrossRef]

54. Burch, M.L.; Yang, S.N.; Ballinger, M.L.; Getachew, R.; Osman, N.; Little, P.J. TGF-beta stimulates biglycan synthesis via p38 and ERK phosphorylation of the linker region of Smad2. *Cell. Mol. Life Sci.* **2010**, *67*, 2077–2090. [CrossRef]

55. Yu, J.S.; Ramasamy, T.S.; Murphy, N.; Holt, M.K.; Czapiewski, R.; Wei, S.K.; Cui, W. PI3K/mTORC2 regulates TGF-beta/Activin signalling by modulating Smad2/3 activity via linker phosphorylation. *Nat. Commun.* **2015**, *6*, 7212. [CrossRef]

56. Bruce, D.L.; Sapkota, G.P. Phosphatases in SMAD regulation. *FEBS Lett.* **2012**, *586*, 1897–1905. [CrossRef]

57. Djouad, F.; Rackwitz, L.; Song, Y.; Janjanin, S.; Tuan, R.S. ERK1/2 activation induced by inflammatory cytokines compromises effective host tissue integration of engineered cartilage. *Tissue Eng. Part A* **2009**, *15*, 2825–2835. [CrossRef] [PubMed]

58. Geng, Y.; Valbracht, J.; Lotz, M. Selective activation of the mitogen-activated protein kinase subgroups c-Jun NH2 terminal kinase and p38 by IL-1 and TNF in human articular chondrocytes. *J. Clin. Investig.* **1996**, *98*, 2425–2430. [CrossRef] [PubMed]

59. Manley, G.C.A.; Stokes, C.A.; Marsh, E.K.; Sabroe, I.; Parker, L.C. DUSP10 Negatively Regulates the Inflammatory Response to Rhinovirus through Interleukin-1beta Signaling. *J. Virol.* **2019**, *93*, e01659-18. [CrossRef]

60. Van den Akker, G.G.; van Beuningen, H.M.; Vitters, E.L.; Koenders, M.I.; van de Loo, F.A.; van Lent, P.L.; Davidson, E.N.B.; van der Kraan, P.M. Interleukin 1 beta-induced SMAD2/3 linker modifications are TAK1 dependent and delay TGFbeta signaling in primary human mesenchymal stem cells. *Cell. Signal.* **2017**, *40*, 190–199. [CrossRef] [PubMed]

61. Kretzschmar, M.; Doody, J.; Timokhina, I.; Massague, J. A mechanism of repression of TGFbeta/ Smad signaling by oncogenic Ras. *Genes Dev.* **1999**, *13*, 804–816. [CrossRef]

62. Park, S.; Yang, K.M.; Park, Y.; Hong, E.; Hong, C.P.; Park, J.; Pang, K.; Lee, J.; Park, B.; Lee, S. Identification of Epithelial-Mesenchymal Transition-related Target Genes Induced by the Mutation of Smad3 Linker Phosphorylation. *J. Cancer Prev.* **2018**, *23*, 1–9. [CrossRef]

63. Neefjes, M.; Housmans, B.A.C.; van den Akker, G.G.H.; van Rhijn, L.W.; Welting, T.J.M.; van der Kraan, P.M. Reporter gene comparison demonstrates interference of complex body fluids with secreted luciferase activity. *Sci. Rep.* **2021**, *11*, 1359. [CrossRef]

64. Sekimoto, G.; Matsuzaki, K.; Yoshida, K.; Mori, S.; Murata, M.; Seki, T.; Matsui, H.; Fujisawa, J.; Okazaki, K. Reversible Smad-dependent signaling between tumor suppression and oncogenesis. *Cancer Res.* **2007**, *67*, 5090–5096. [CrossRef]

65. Tarasewicz, E.; Jeruss, J.S. Phospho-specific Smad3 signaling: Impact on breast oncogenesis. *Cell Cycle* **2012**, *11*, 2443–2451. [CrossRef] [PubMed]

66. Browne, J.A.; Liu, X.; Schnaper, H.W.; Hayashida, T. Serine-204 in the linker region of Smad3 mediates the collagen-I response to TGF-beta in a cell phenotype-specific manner. *Exp. Cell Res.* **2013**, *319*, 2928–2937. [CrossRef] [PubMed]

67. Gao, S.; Alarcon, C.; Sapkota, G.; Rahman, S.; Chen, P.Y.; Goerner, N.; Macias, M.J.; Erdjument-Bromage, H.; Tempst, P.; Massagué, J. Ubiquitin ligase Nedd4L targets activated Smad2/3 to limit TGF-beta signaling. *Mol. Cell.* **2009**, *36*, 457–468. [CrossRef] [PubMed]

68. Heldin, C.H.; Moustakas, A. Role of Smads in TGFbeta signaling. *Cell Tissue Res.* **2012**, *347*, 21–36. [CrossRef]

69. Kamaraju, A.K.; Roberts, A.B. Role of Rho/ROCK and p38 MAP kinase pathways in transforming growth factor-beta-mediated Smad-dependent growth inhibition of human breast carcinoma cells in vivo. *J. Biol. Chem.* **2005**, *280*, 1024–1036. [CrossRef]

70. Matsuura, I.; Denissova, N.G.; Wang, G.; He, D.; Long, J.; Liu, F. Cyclin-dependent kinases regulate the antiproliferative function of Smads. *Nature* **2004**, *430*, 226–231. [CrossRef]

71. Wrighton, K.H.; Willis, D.; Long, J.; Liu, F.; Lin, X.; Feng, X.H. Small C-terminal domain phosphatases dephosphorylate the regulatory linker regions of Smad2 and Smad3 to enhance transforming growth factor-beta signaling. *J. Biol. Chem.* **2006**, *281*, 38365–38375. [CrossRef] [PubMed]

72. Wrighton, K.H.; Lin, X.; Feng, X.H. Phospho-control of TGF-beta superfamily signaling. *Cell Res.* **2009**, *19*, 8–20. [CrossRef] [PubMed]

73. Hoffmann, A.; Preobrazhenska, O.; Wodarczyk, C.; Medler, Y.; Winkel, A.; Shahab, S.; Huylebroeck, D.; Gross, G.; Verschueren, K. Transforming growth factor-beta-activated kinase-1 (TAK1), a MAP3K, interacts with Smad proteins and interferes with osteogenesis in murine mesenchymal progenitors. *J. Biol. Chem.* **2005**, *280*, 27271–27283. [CrossRef]

74. Benus, G.F.J.D.; Wierenga, A.T.J.; de Gorter, D.J.J.; Schuringa, J.J.; van Bennekum, A.M.; Drenth-Diephuis, L.; Vellenga, E.; Eggen, B.J.L. Inhibition of the transforming growth factor beta (TGFbeta) pathway by interleukin-1beta is mediated through TGFbeta-activated kinase 1 phosphorylation of SMAD3. *Mol. Biol. Cell* **2005**, *16*, 3501–3510. [CrossRef]

75. Nagata, H.; Hatano, E.; Tada, M.; Murata, M.; Kitamura, K.; Asechi, H.; Narita, M.; Yanagida, A.; Tamaki, N.; Yagi, S.; et al. Inhibition of c-Jun NH2-terminal kinase switches Smad3 signaling from oncogenesis to tumor- suppression in rat hepatocellular carcinoma. *Hepatology* **2009**, *49*, 1944–1953. [CrossRef]

76. Chen, D.; Lin, Q.; Box, N.; Roop, D.; Ishii, S.; Matsuzaki, K.; Fan, T.; Hornyak, T.J.; Reed, J.A.; Stavnezer, E.; et al. SKI knockdown inhibits human melanoma tumor growth in vivo. *Pigment Cell Melanoma Res.* **2009**, *22*, 761–772. [CrossRef] [PubMed]

77. Hamajima, H.; Ozaki, I.; Zhang, H.; Iwane, S.; Kawaguchi, Y.; Eguchi, Y.; Matsuhashi, S.; Mizuta, T.; Matsuzaki, K.; Fujimoto, K. Modulation of the transforming growth factor-beta1-induced Smad phosphorylation by the extracellular matrix receptor beta1-integrin. *Int. J. Oncol.* **2009**, *35*, 1441–1447. [PubMed]

78. Liu, T.; Feng, X.H. Regulation of TGF-beta signalling by protein phosphatases. *Biochem. J.* **2010**, *430*, 191–198. [CrossRef]

79. Knockaert, M.; Sapkota, G.; Alarcon, C.; Massague, J.; Brivanlou, A.H. Unique players in the BMP pathway: Small C-terminal domain phosphatases dephosphorylate Smad1 to attenuate BMP signaling. *Proc. Natl. Acad. Sci. USA* **2006**, *103*, 11940–11945. [CrossRef]

80. Zhang, M.; Cho, E.J.; Burstein, G.; Siegel, D.; Zhang, Y. Selective inactivation of a human neuronal silencing phosphatase by a small molecule inhibitor. *ACS Chem. Biol.* **2011**, *6*, 511–519. [CrossRef] [PubMed]

81. Otsubo, K.; Yoneda, T.; Kaneko, A.; Yagi, S.; Furukawa, K.; Chuman, Y. Development of a Substrate Identification Method for Human Scp1 Phosphatase Using Phosphorylation Mimic Phage Display. *Protein Pept. Lett.* **2018**, *25*, 76–83. [CrossRef] [PubMed]

82. Mori, S.; Matsuzaki, K.; Yoshida, K.; Furukawa, F.; Tahashi, Y.; Yamagata, H.; Sekimoto, G.; Seki, T.; Matsui, H.; Nishizawa, M.; et al. TGF-beta and HGF transmit the signals through JNK-dependent Smad2/3 phosphorylation at the linker regions. *Oncogene* **2004**, *23*, 7416–7429. [CrossRef] [PubMed]

83. Neefjes, M.; van Caam, A.P.M.; van der Kraan, P.M. Transcription Factors in Cartilage Homeostasis and Osteoarthritis. *Biology* **2020**, *9*, 290. [CrossRef]

84. Dreher, S.I.; Fischer, J.; Walker, T.; Diederichs, S.; Richter, W. Significance of MEF2C and RUNX3 Regulation for Endochondral Differentiation of Human Mesenchymal Progenitor Cells. *Front. Cell Dev. Biol.* **2020**, *8*, 81. [CrossRef] [PubMed]

85. Kamato, D.; Do, B.H.; Osman, N.; Ross, B.P.; Mohamed, R.; Xu, S.; Little, P.J. Smad linker region phosphorylation is a signalling pathway in its own right and not only a modulator of canonical TGF-beta signalling. *Cell. Mol. Life Sci.* **2020**, *77*, 243–251. [CrossRef]

86. Van de Loo, F.A.; Veenbergen, S.; van den Brand, B.; Bennink, M.B.; Blaney-Davidson, E.; Arntz, O.J.; van Beuningen, H.M.; van der Kraan, P.M.; van den Berg, W.B. Enhanced suppressor of cytokine signaling 3 in arthritic cartilage dysregulates human chondrocyte function. *Arthritis Rheum.* **2012**, *64*, 3313–3323. [CrossRef]

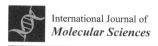

International Journal of
Molecular Sciences

MDPI

Article

Males and Females Have Distinct Molecular Events in the Articular Cartilage during Knee Osteoarthritis

Chenshuang Li [1] and Zhong Zheng [2,3,*]

1   Department of Orthodontics, School of Dental Medicine, University of Pennsylvania, Philadelphia, PA 19104, USA; lichens@upenn.edu
2   Division of Growth and Development, Section of Orthodontics, School of Dentistry, University of California, Los Angeles, CA 90095, USA
3   Department of Surgery, David Geffen School of Medicine, University of California, Los Angeles, CA 90095, USA
*   Correspondence: zzheng@dentistry.ucla.edu; Tel.: +1-(310)-206-5646

Abstract: Osteoarthritis (OA) is a major public health challenge that imposes a remarkable burden on the affected individuals and the healthcare system. Based on the clinical observation, males and females have different prevalence rates and severity levels of OA. Thus, sex-based differences may play essential roles in OA's prognosis and treatment outcomes. To date, the comprehensive understanding of the relationship between sex and OA is still largely lacking. In the current study, we analyzed a published transcriptome dataset of knee articular cartilage (GSE114007) from 18 healthy (five females, 13 males) and 20 OA (11 females, nine males) donors to provide a slight insight into this important but complex issue. First, comparing female healthy cartilage samples with those of males revealed 36 differential expression genes (DEGs), indicating the fundamental sex-related differences at the molecular level. Meanwhile, 923 DEGs were distinguished between OA and healthy female cartilage, which can be enriched to 15 Reactome pathways. On the other hand, when comparing OA and healthy male cartilage, there are only 419 DEGs were identified, and only six pathways were enriched against the Reactome database. The different signaling response to OA in the male and female cartilage was further enforced by recognizing 50 genes with significantly different OA-responsive expression fold changes in males and females. Particularly, 14 Reactome pathways, such as "Extracellular matrix organization", "Collagen biosynthesis and modifying enzymes", "Dissolution of fibrin clot", and "Platelet Aggregation (Plug formation)", can be noted from these 50 sex-dependent OA-responsive genes. Overall, the current study explores the Sex as a Biological Variable (SABV) at the transcriptomic level in the knee articular cartilage in both healthy status and OA event, which could help predict the differential OA prognosis and treatment outcome of males and female patients.

Keywords: sex as a biological variable; osteoarthritis; cartilage; whole transcriptome sequencing; molecules

Citation: Li, C.; Zheng, Z. Males and Females Have Distinct Molecular Events in the Articular Cartilage during Knee Osteoarthritis. *Int. J. Mol. Sci.* **2021**, *22*, 7876. https://doi.org/10.3390/ijms22157876

Academic Editors: Nicola Veronese and Alfonso Baldi

Received: 26 May 2021
Accepted: 21 July 2021
Published: 23 July 2021

Publisher's Note: MDPI stays neutral with regard to jurisdictional claims in published maps and institutional affiliations.

1. Introduction

As the most common form of arthritis, osteoarthritis (OA) is a series of pathology that causes persistent pain, swelling, and reduced motion in the affected joints. For years, OA was identified as an age-related pathology; thus, it has been called "wear and tear" arthritis. During the past few years, OA is increasingly recognized as a highly heterogeneous group of diseases characterized by variable clinical phenotypes, which may contribute to the inconsistency of clinical prognosis and treatment response [1].

With the growing recognition of Sex as a Biological Variable (SABV) in the pathophysiology of a diversity of diseases [2], the impact the sex on OA has also attracted more and more attention. To date, it is well known that OA has a higher prevalence in women than men, as 62% of OA patients are women [3]. Indeed, women have a consistently higher OA prevalence rate than men in all age groups between the 30s to 95 plus [4]. Worldwide estimates are that 9.6% of men and 18% of women aged over 60 have symptomatic OA [5]. Moreover, disability and loss of function associated with OA are higher in women [6,7]. Besides, the US Medical Expenditure Panel Survey data for the years 1996 to 2005 found that OA-related out-of-pocket (OOP) costs incurred by women were greater than those by men [8], and more women than men were hospitalized for OA [9]. In the US, OA increased annual per capita absenteeism costs of $5.5 billion for female workers verse $4.8 billion for male workers [8].

Clinically, the incidence of OA increases dramatically in women around the time of menopause [10]; therefore, the modulating role of sex hormones on OA was proposed [11]. For example, estrogen is one of the most deeply investigated sex hormones in OA [12]. Although estrogen is considered to have protective potency against OA, the effects of estrogen replacement therapy and selective estrogen receptor modulators in preserving and/or restoring joint tissue in OA are controversial among currently published reports [13,14]. Besides estrogen, sex hormone-binding globulin [15], follicle-stimulating hormone [16], dehydroepiandrosterone [17], progesterone [18], and testosterone [19] may all influence OA progression. However, none of these sex hormones can completely explain all differences observed between male and female OA patients [20]. For instance, at a macro level, males and females have different thicknesses of cartilage [21], subchondral bone density [22], and muscle strength [23]; while at a micro level, tissue and cells from females have different, or even distinct, responses in comparison with those from males [20]. Recently, Kim et al. [24] found that OA-related studies were largely performed in male subjects and animals, although females face more OA risk and more server symptoms [4–7]. Undoubtedly, fully considering SABV will set the fundamental to understanding the distinguished clinical complaints between males and females and is an essential step for effective therapy development, which, unfortunately, is still largely lacking.

Although synovium and subchondral bone are known to involve in OA recently, articular cartilage is still the major target of OA-related investigations. Articular cartilage is hyaline cartilage that does not have blood vessels, nerves, or lymphatics [25]. It is composed of a dense extracellular matrix (ECM) with a sparse distribution of chondrocytes. The major components of the ECM are water, collagen, and proteoglycans, which are critical to maintaining the mechanical property of the cartilage [25]. In a healthy microenvironment, the balance between cartilage synthesis and degradation is strictly regulated [26]. In the OA scenario, chondrocytes express more catabolic molecules, such as matrix metallopeptidase 13 (MMP-13), and less anabolic matrix, such as type II collagen [27,28], and thus matrix remodeling, inappropriate hypertrophy-like maturation, and cartilage calcification appear [29]. A net loss of proteoglycan content is also one of the hallmarks of all stages of OA cartilage degeneration [26]. In addition to the well-known anabolic and catabolic components, increasingly more biological factors have been noted to participate in OA's molecular events. For instance, nerve growth factor (NGF), which was primarily discovered for its roles in sensory neuron proliferation and sensitization, is recently reported to regulate articular chondrocytes' calcification [30]. Another example is C1q and TNF related 1 (C1QTNF1), whose modulating effects on chondrocyte proliferation and maturation is revealed recently, belongs to a newly discovered family of highly conserved adiponectin paralog proteins [31]. Therefore, a more detailed dissection of the molecular events in the OA cartilage is needed to assist the understanding of SABV in OA pathophysiology.

2. Results

2.1. Male and Female Cartilage Are Not Molecularly Identical in the Healthy Status

We first compare the mRNA sequencing data from the male and female healthy cartilage to investigate if the transcriptomic profiles are the same for both genders. Within the 23,714 identified genes, the expression of the commonly used cartilage anabolic markers, such as *Collagen Type II Alpha 1 Chain (COL2A1)*, *Aggrecan (ACAN)*, *cartilage oligomeric matrix protein (COMP)*, and *SRY-box 9 (SOX9)*, and catabolic markers, such as *Runt-related transcription factor2 (Runx2)*, *MMP13*, *ADAM metallopeptidase with thrombospondin type 1 motif 4 (ADAMTS4)*, and *ADAMTS5*, are not significantly different between the healthy male and female cartilage (Supplemental Table S1).

On the other hand, we identify 10 DEGs with a *p*-value less than 0.05 that are highly expressed in healthy female cartilage than their male counterparts, and 26 DEGs with a *p*-value less than 0.05 whose expression level is lower in females (Figure 1). For all these 36 DEGs, only *TSIX transcript, XIST antisense RNA (TSIX)* has an adjusted *p*-value less than 0.05 (Figure 1C and Supplemental Table S1, highlighted in red). Among the latter 26 genes whose expression levels are lower in females, 15 genes are Y-chromosome linked (Figure 1C), demonstrating the reliability of the current study. Thus, the different expression levels of non-Y-chromosome-linked genes between males and females may present the SABV at a molecular level (Figure 1).

Pathway enrichment was used to uncover the potential functional interaction among these 36 DEGs, while only 14 genes could be recognized by the Reactome knowledgebase. DEGs that were not recognized by the current Reactome database are summarized in Supplemental Table S2. The Reactome recognized genes were clustered into "chromatin organization", "hemostasis", "disease", "metabolism", "transport of small molecules", "metabolism of proteins", and "extracellular matrix organization." Among them, nine identified pathways have a *p*-value less than 0.05, but none of them qualified as a significant enrichment that should have an FDR smaller than 0.05 (Table 1 and Supplemental Table S3).

Table 1. The pathway enrichment result of the significant male-vs.-female DEGs in healthy cartilage against the Reactome knowledgebase (*p* < 0.05). Note: no pathways have an FDR value less than 0.05.

Pathway Identifier	Pathway Name	#Entities Found	#Entities Total	Entities Ratio	Entities *p*-Value	Entities FDR	Submitted Entities Found
R-HSA-3214842	HDMs demethylate histones	2	31	2.11×10^{-3}	2.96×10^{-3}	2.46×10^{-1}	KDM5D; UTY
R-HSA-76009	Platelet Aggregation (Plug Formation)	2	53	3.60×10^{-3}	8.36×10^{-3}	2.46×10^{-1}	APBB1IP; COL1A2
R-HSA-9673163	Oleoyl-phe metabolism	1	5	3.40×10^{-4}	1.28×10^{-2}	2.46×10^{-1}	PM20D1
R-HSA-430116	GP1b-IX-V activation signaling	1	12	8.15×10^{-4}	3.05×10^{-2}	2.46×10^{-1}	COL1A2
R-HSA-2214320	Anchoring fibril formation	1	15	1.02×10^{-3}	3.80×10^{-2}	2.46×10^{-1}	COL1A2
R-HSA-75892	Platelet Adhesion to exposed collagen	1	16	1.09×10^{-3}	4.05×10^{-2}	2.46×10^{-1}	COL1A2
R-HSA-1247673	Erythrocytes take up oxygen and release carbon dioxide	1	16	1.09×10^{-3}	4.05×10^{-2}	2.46×10^{-1}	AQP1
R-HSA-381426	Regulation of Insulin-like Growth Factor (IGF) transport and uptake by Insulin-like Growth Factor Binding Proteins (IGFBPs)	2	127	8.63×10^{-3}	4.26×10^{-2}	2.46×10^{-1}	IGFBP4; IGFALS
R-HSA-166187	Mitochondrial Uncoupling	1	18	1.22×10^{-3}	4.54×10^{-2}	2.46×10^{-1}	PM20D1

2.2. ECM Organization Is the Major Event in OA Cartilage of Females, But Not That of Males

We then analyzed the cartilage gene expression changes during OA of males and females separately. First, in the female cartilage, there were 923 DEGs in total, among which 382 were downregulated and 541 were upregulated during OA (Figure 2 and Supplemental Table S4). Among these genes, 30 significantly downregulated DEGs and 45 upregulated ones were identified with an adjusted *p*-value less than 0.05 (Supplemental Table S4, highlighted in red). Ranking based on the *p*-values, the top 15 significantly downregulated genes were summarized in Figure 2C, while the top 15 significantly upregulated in Figure 2D.

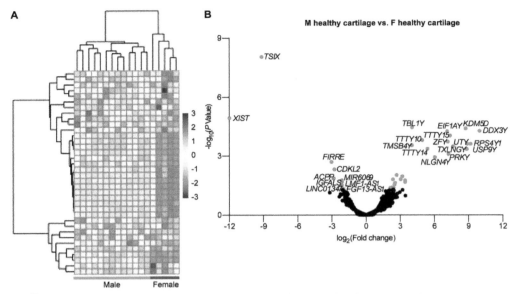

SYMBOL	GENENAME	log₂FC	p-Value	Adjusted p-Value	

The list of genes significantly differently expressed in healthy cartilage from different genders (M vs. F)

SYMBOL	GENENAME	$\log_2$FC	p-Value	Adjusted p-Value	
XIST	X inactive specific transcript	−11.9826179	1.13×10^{-5}	0.13	Genes significantly higher in female healthy cartilage
TSIX	TSIX transcript, XIST antisense RNA	−9.15195022	8.52×10^{-9}	2.02×10^{-4}	
FIRRE	firre intergenic repeating RNA element	−3.0236161	1.97×10^{-3}	1.00	
ACPP	acid phosphatase, prostate	−2.8343501	1.34×10^{-2}	1.00	
CDKL2	cyclin dependent kinase like 2	−2.76016588	4.72×10^{-3}	1.00	
MIR6069	microRNA 6069	−2.12906384	1.69×10^{-2}	1.00	
LMF1-AS1	LMF1 antisense RNA 1	−2.12138647	2.97×10^{-2}	1.00	
IGFALS	insulin like growth factor binding protein acid labile subunit	−2.11149761	2.02×10^{-2}	1.00	
LINC01347	long intergenic non-protein coding RNA 1347	−2.05139248	4.76×10^{-2}	1.00	
FGF13-AS1	FGF13 antisense RNA 1	−2.03696841	4.53×10^{-2}	1.00	
HPDL	4-hydroxyphenylpyruvate dioxygenase like	2.141954189	4.15×10^{-2}	1.00	
EPYC	epiphycan	2.25652128	4.02×10^{-2}	1.00	
MIR4435-2HG	MIR4435-2 host gene	2.372374666	1.52×10^{-2}	1.00	
AQP1	aquaporin 1 (Colton blood group)	2.403948864	3.96×10^{-2}	1.00	
PM20D1	peptidase M20 domain containing 1	2.50036009	2.76×10^{-2}	1.00	
IGFBP4	insulin like growth factor binding protein 4	2.551571643	2.27×10^{-2}	1.00	
COL1A2	collagen type I alpha 2 chain	2.681158922	9.04×10^{-3}	1.00	
MXRA5	matrix remodeling associated 5	3.045579134	1.48×10^{-2}	1.00	
APBB1IP	amyloid beta precursor protein binding family B member 1 interacting protein	3.186944768	1.05×10^{-2}	1.00	
PDLIM1	PDZ and LIM domain 1	3.433347223	1.72×10^{-2}	1.00	
THY1	Thy-1 cell surface antigen	3.434138186	2.07×10^{-2}	1.00	
TMSB4Y	thymosin beta 4 Y-linked	4.030472407	2.86×10^{-4}	0.57	Genes significantly higher in male healthy cartilage
TBL1Y	transducin beta like 1 Y-linked	4.049034132	3.46×10^{-5}	0.22	
TTTY10	testis-specific transcript, Y-linked 10	4.923022484	1.57×10^{-4}	0.46	
TTTY14	testis-specific transcript, Y-linked 14	5.394276193	4.30×10^{-4}	0.70	
NLGN4Y	neuroligin 4 Y-linked	6.039451083	1.15×10^{-3}	1.00	
EIF1AY	eukaryotic translation initiation factor 1A Y-linked	7.12549032	5.48×10^{-4}	0.22	
ZFY	zinc finger protein Y-linked	7.179194709	1.87×10^{-4}	0.49	
PRKY	protein kinase Y-linked (pseudogene)	7.232816432	7.76×10^{-4}	1.00	
TTTY15	testis-specific transcript, Y-linked 15	7.383590476	9.14×10^{-4}	0.31	
TXLNGY	taxilin gamma pseudogene, Y-linked	7.628499066	3.29×10^{-4}	0.60	
KDM5D	lysine demethylase 5D	8.755006507	3.92×10^{-5}	0.22	
USP9Y	ubiquitin specific peptidase 9 Y-linked	8.841066229	4.42×10^{-4}	0.70	
UTY	ubiquitously transcribed tetratricopeptide repeat containing, Y-linked	8.890363257	2.42×10^{-4}	0.52	
RPS4Y1	ribosomal protein S4 Y-linked 1	9.18414167	2.40×10^{-4}	0.52	
DDX3Y	DEAD-box helicase 3 Y-linked	9.972184804	5.24×10^{-5}	0.22	

Figure 1. The differential expressed genes (DEGs) detected between male and female healthy knee cartilage samples. (**A**) Heatmap and (**B**) volcano diagrams for DEG visualization. DEGs with a p-value less than 0.05 are highlighted in red. (**C**) The list of genes that are significantly differentially expressed in healthy male and female cartilage. DEGs with a statistically significant higher level in females have a negative $\log_2$FC value, while those highly expressed in males have a positive $\log_2$FC value. The gene with an adjusted p-value less than 0.05 is highlighted in red. The Y-chromosome linked genes are highlighted in blue font.

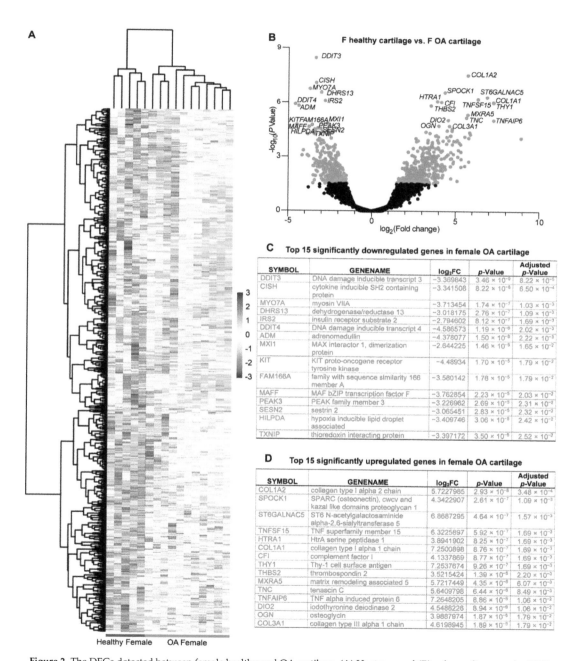

Figure 2. The DEGs detected between female healthy and OA cartilage. (**A**) Heatmap and (**B**) volcano diagrams for DEG visualization. DEGs with a *p*-value less than 0.05 are highlighted in red. (**C**) Top 15 genes significantly downregulated in female cartilage in response to OA. (**D**) Top 15 genes significantly upregulated in female cartilage in response to OA. DEGs with an adjusted *p*-value less than 0.05 are highlighted in red.

In the Reactome knowledgebase, 424 of the 923 DEGs could not be matched (Supplemental Table S5); thus, the pathways were enriched based on the other 499 DEGs. Overall, there were 68 pathways with a $p < 0.05$, among which 15 pathways with an FDR less than 0.05 (Table 2 and Supplemental Table S6). Nine of the 15 pathways are related to ECM organization (Table 2). For the other six pathways, "FOXO-mediated transcription of cell cycle genes", "FOXO-mediated transcription", and "RUNX3 regulated immune response and cell migration" belong to the event "gene expression (transcription)", "Response of EIF2AK1 (HRI) to heme deficiency" belongs to the event "cellular responses to external stimuli", "Interleukin-4 and Interleukin-13 signaling" belongs to the event "immune system", and "Gap junction assembly" belongs to the event "vesicle-mediated transport" (Table 2). In particular, 55 of 499 identified DEGs were enriched in "extracellular matrix organization", which is the most significant event in the female cartilage in response to OA.

Table 2. The top 15 pathways enriched from the OA-responsive DEGs in female cartilage. Note: all pathways in the list have an FDR value less than 0.05.

Pathway Identifier	Pathway Name	#Entities Found	#Entities Total	Entities Ratio	Entities *p*-Value	Entities FDR	Submitted Entities Found
R-HSA-1474244	Extracellular matrix organization	55	330	2.24×10^{-2}	7.42×10^{-8}	1.06×10^{-4}	COL18A1; SPARC; ITGAM; ELN; SERPINE1; ITGB2; TNC; HAPLN1; ADAMTS5; ADAMTS2; EFEMP1; TNN; CTSK; TNR; ITGB8; MME; ITGA4; COL25A1; PCOLCE; ASPN; VCAN; COL2A1; MMP13; OPTC; COL6A1; ADAM12; PECAM1; COL8A1; MMP19; LAMA5; COL15A1; COL13A1; HTRA1; FBLN1; LTBP2; FBLN5; ADAMTS14; SPP1; NCAM1; COL26A1; LAMB3; LUM; FN1; GDF5; COL1A1; COL3A1; CAPN12; BMP1; COL1A2; COL5A1; P4HA3; COL5A2; TLL1
R-HSA-9617828	FOXO-mediated transcription of cell cycle genes	12	27	1.83×10^{-3}	1.50×10^{-6}	8.48×10^{-4}	NOTCH3; CDKN1A; CDKN1B; GADD45A; CCNG2; FOXO3; KLF4
R-HSA-9614085	FOXO-mediated transcription	25	110	7.47×10^{-3}	1.79×10^{-6}	8.48×10^{-4}	IGFBP1; NOTCH3; CDKN1A; CDKN1B; GADD45A; CITED2; FOXO6; FOXO3; KLF4; FBXO32; BCL6; CCNG2; DDIT3; TXNIP; PLXNA4
R-HSA-3000178	ECM proteoglycans	20	79	5.37×10^{-3}	4.01×10^{-6}	1.42×10^{-3}	LAMA5; ITGAM; SPARC; LUM; SERPINE1; FN1; TNC; HAPLN1; ASPN; COL1A1; VCAN; COL3A1; COL2A1; COL1A2; COL5A1; TNN; COL6A1; COL5A2; TNR; NCAM1
R-HSA-1650814	Collagen biosynthesis and modifying enzymes	19	76	5.16×10^{-3}	8.23×10^{-6}	2.34×10^{-3}	COL18A1; COL26A1; COL15A1; COL13A1; COL25A1; PCOLCE; COL1A1; ADAMTS2; ADAMTS14; COL3A1; COL2A1; BMP1; COL1A2; COL5A1; P4HA3; COL6A1; COL5A2; COL8A1; TLL1
R-HSA-1474228	Degradation of the extracellular matrix	28	148	1.01×10^{-3}	1.32×10^{-5}	3.08×10^{-3}	COL18A1; LAMA5; COL15A1; COL13A1; ELN; HTRA1; ADAMTS5; CTSK; SPP1; COL26A1; LAMB3; MME; COL25A1; FN1; COL1A1; COL3A1; MMP13; COL2A1; COL1A2; CAPN12; BMP1; COL5A1; OPTC; COL6A1; COL5A2; COL8A1; MMP19; TLL1
R-HSA-216083	Integrin cell surface interactions	20	87	5.91×10^{-3}	1.59×10^{-5}	3.08×10^{-3}	COL18A1; ITGAM; COL13A1; ITGA4; LUM; ITGB2; FN1; TNC; COL1A1; COL3A1; COL2A1; COL1A2; COL5A1; COL6A1; COL5A2; SPP1; PECAM1; COL8A1; ITGB8
R-HSA-9648895	Response of EIF2AK1 (HRI) to heme deficiency	11	29	1.97×10^{-3}	1.74×10^{-5}	3.08×10^{-3}	PPP1R15A; DDIT3; CEBPG; TNR; TRIB3; ATF3

Table 2. *Cont.*

Pathway Identifier	Pathway Name	#Entities Found	#Entities Total	Entities Ratio	Entities *p*-Value	Entities FDR	Submitted Entities Found
R-HSA-1442490	Collagen degradation	17	69	4.69×10^{-3}	2.88×10^{-5}	4.22×10^{-3}	COL18A1; COL26A1; COL15A1; COL13A1; MME; COL25A1; COL1A1; COL3A1; MMP13; COL2A1; COL1A2; COL5A1; CTSK; COL6A1; COL5A2; MMP19; COL8A1
R-HSA-6785807	Interleukin-4 and Interleukin-13 signaling	35	216	1.47×10^{-2}	2.97×10^{-5}	4.22×10^{-3}	NOTCH3; LAMA5; CDKN1A; ITGAM; ITGB2; FN1; RORC; TWIST1; FOXO3; VEGFA; COL1A2; SOCS1; CCND1; BCL6; IRF4; BIRC5; IL6R; FAN1
R-HSA-8948216	Collagen chain trimerization	13	44	2.99×10^{-3}	4.11×10^{-5}	5.30×10^{-3}	COL18A1; COL26A1; COL15A1; COL13A1; COL25A1; COL1A1; COL3A1; COL2A1; COL1A2; COL5A1; COL6A1; COL5A2; COL8A1
R-HSA-1474290	Collagen formation	21	104	7.06×10^{-3}	6.24×10^{-5}	7.36×10^{-3}	COL18A1; COL26A1; COL15A1; COL13A1; LAMB3; COL25A1; PCOLCE; COL1A1; ADAMTS2; ADAMTS14; COL3A1; MMP13; COL2A1; BMP1; COL1A2; COL5A1; P4HA3; COL6A1; COL5A2; COL8A1; TLL1
R-HSA-8949275	RUNX3 Regulates Immune Response and Cell Migration	6	10	6.79×10^{-4}	1.30×10^{-4}	1.41×10^{-2}	ITGA4; SPP1; RORC
R-HSA-2022090	Assembly of collagen fibrils and other multimeric structures	15	67	4.55×10^{-3}	2.30×10^{-4}	2.33×10^{-2}	COL18A1; COL15A1; LAMB3; PCOLCE; COL1A1; COL3A1; MMP13; COL2A1; BMP1; COL1A2; COL5A1; COL6A1; COL5A2; COL8A1; TLL1
R-HSA-190861	Gap junction assembly	11	41	2.79×10^{-3}	3.52×10^{-4}	3.31×10^{-2}	GJC1; PLK4; GJB2; TUBB3; TUBB4B; TUBA4A; TUBA8

Second, we analyzed the male cartilage in the same way. Male samples have much less OA-responsive DEGs compared with female samples. There were 419 DEGs in total, 186 upregulated and 233 downregulated, among which 18 downregulated and four upregulated DEGs have an adjusted *p*-value less than 0.05 (Figure 3 and Supplemental Table S7, highlighted in red). In addition, the top 15 significant upregulated and downregulated genes based on *p*-value in male cartilage during OA were not as same as those in female cartilage. The top 15 significantly downregulated genes in male cartilage were listed in Figure 3C, while the top 15 significantly upregulated genes in Figure 3D.

In the Reactome knowledgebase, 202 of the 419 DEGs could not be matched (Supplemental Table S8). Thus, the pathways enrichment based on the other 217 DEGs dispersed the molecular events including "immune system", "signal transduction", "neuronal system", "hemostasis", "gene expression (transcription)", "metabolism", "DNA replication", "transport of small molecules", "disease", "metabolism of proteins", "cell cycle", "autophagy", "vesicle-mediated transport", "cellular responses to external stimuli", and "extracellular matrix organization". There are 79 pathways that have a *p*-value less than 0.05, among which six have an FDR less than 0.05 (Table 3 and Supplemental Table S9). Here, "Response of EIF2AK1 (HRI) to heme deficiency" belongs to the event "cellular responses to external stimuli", "ATF4 activates genes in response to endoplasmic reticulum stress" and "PERK regulates gene expression" belong to the event "metabolism of proteins", "NGF-stimulated transcription" and "Nuclear Events (kinase and transcription factor activation)" belong to the event "signal transduction", and "MECP2 regulates neuronal receptors and channels" belongs to the event "gene expression (transcription)". None of these six pathways are categorized in the event of "extracellular matrix organization".

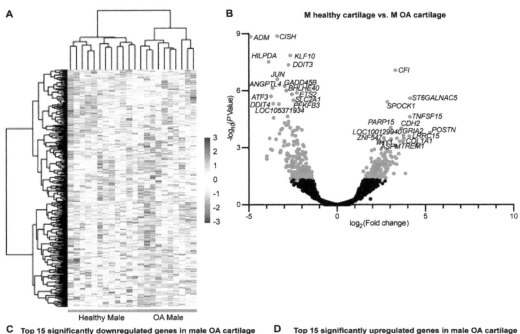

Figure 3. The DEGs detected between male healthy and OA cartilage. (**A**) Heatmap and (**B**) volcano diagrams for DEG visualization. DEGs with a *p*-value less than 0.05 are highlighted in red. (**C**) Top 15 genes significantly downregulated in male cartilage in response to OA. (**D**) Top 15 genes significantly upregulated in male cartilage in response to OA. DEGs with an adjusted *p*-value less than 0.05 are highlighted in red.

2.3. Male and Female Cartilage Have Significant Different Alteration Genes during OA

To confirm the differences between male and female cartilage in response to OA as observed above, we also compared the gene expression fold change in both sexes and identified 63 DEGs with a $p < 0.05$ (Supplemental Table S10). By referencing the single-sex OA—healthy cartilage comparison results, genes that do not have OA-responsive alteration(s) in either gender were excluded to eliminate the false positive result and lead to the identification of 50 DEGs (Table 4). Note that none of these genes were detected with an adjusted *p*-value less than 0.05, while 23 of these 50 DEGs could not be recognized by Reactome (Supplemental Table S11). Based on the 27 Reactome-recognized genes, 60 pathways were enriched ($p < 0.05$; Supplemental Table S12). Among them, 14 pathways have an FDR less than 0.05, which could be clustered in the events of "Extracellular matrix organization" (including "Extracellular matrix organization", "Collagen biosynthesis and modifying enzymes", "Collagen chain trimerization", "Collagen formation", "Assembly of collagen fibrils and other multimeric structures", "Collagen degradation", "ECM proteoglycans", "Integrin cell surface interactions", and "Anchoring fibril formation"), "Hemostasis" (including "Dissolution of Fibrin Clot", "GP1b-IX-V activation signaling", "Platelet Aggregation (Plug Formation)", and "Platelet Adhesion to exposed collagen"), and "Disease" (including "Diseases of glycosylation") (Table 5). These results further validate male and female cartilage differences at the molecular event level in response to OA.

Table 3. The top 15 pathways enriched from the OA-responsive DEGs in male cartilage. Pathways with an FDR less than 0.05 are highlighted in red.

Pathway Identifier	Pathway Name	#Entities Found	#Entities Total	Entities Ratio	Entities *p*-Value	Entities FDR	Submitted Entities Found
R-HSA-9648895	Response of EIF2AK1 (HRI) to heme deficiency	10	29	1.97×10^{-3}	1.32×10^{-7}	1.43×10^{-4}	PPP1R15A; DDIT3; CEBPG; TNR; CHAC1; ATF3
R-HSA-380994	ATF4 activates genes in response to endoplasmic reticulum stress	9	34	2.31×10^{-3}	4.71×10^{-6}	2.56×10^{-3}	IGFBP1; DDIT3; CEBPG; ATF3; HERPUD1
R-HSA-9031628	NGF-stimulated transcription	11	56	3.80×10^{-3}	7.12×10^{-6}	2.58×10^{-3}	FOSL1; EGR1; ARC; EGR3; FOSB; FOS; TRIB1; JUNB
R-HSA-9022699	MECP2 regulates neuronal receptors and channels	8	32	2.17×10^{-3}	2.37×10^{-5}	5.35×10^{-3}	GRIA2; GRIN2A; OPRK1; SLC2A3
R-HSA-381042	PERK regulates gene expression	9	42	2.85×10^{-3}	2.46×10^{-5}	5.35×10^{-3}	IGFBP1; DDIT3; CEBPG; ATF3; HERPUD1
R-HSA-198725	Nuclear Events (kinase and transcription factor activation)	11	80	5.43×10^{-3}	1.70×10^{-4}	3.07×10^{-2}	FOSL1; EGR1; ARC; EGR3; FOSB; FOS; TRIB1; JUNB
R-HSA-6791312	TP53 Regulates Transcription of Cell Cycle Genes	9	65	4.42×10^{-3}	6.18×10^{-4}	9.58×10^{-2}	CCNA2; NOTCH3; BTG2; CDKN1A; PLK2; CDK1
R-HSA-6785807	Interleukin-4 and Interleukin-13 signaling	18	216	1.47×10^{-2}	8.82×10^{-4}	1.19×10^{-1}	NOTCH3; CDKN1A; COL1A2; IRF4; ITGB2; LIF; FOS; TNFRSF1B; JUNB; VEGFA
R-HSA-6804757	Regulation of TP53 Degradation	7	43	2.92×10^{-3}	9.81×10^{-4}	1.19×10^{-1}	CCNA2; USP2; UBC; CDK1; PDK1
R-HSA-69895	Transcriptional activation of cell cycle inhibitor p21	3	6	4.08×10^{-4}	1.36×10^{-3}	1.29×10^{-1}	NOTCH3; CDKN1A
R-HSA-69560	Transcriptional activation of p53 responsive genes	3	6	4.08×10^{-4}	1.36×10^{-3}	1.29×10^{-1}	NOTCH3; CDKN1A
R-HSA-6806003	Regulation of TP53 Expression and Degradation	7	46	3.12×10^{-3}	1.44×10^{-3}	1.29×10^{-1}	CCNA2; USP2; UBC; CDK1; PDK1
R-HSA-1538133	G0 and Early G1	6	38	2.58×10^{-3}	2.59×10^{-3}	2.07×10^{-1}	TOP2A; CCNA2; CDK1
R-HSA-9617828	FOXO-mediated transcription of cell cycle genes	5	27	1.83×10^{-3}	2.99×10^{-3}	2.07×10^{-1}	NOTCH3; CDKN1A; KLF4
R-HSA-194313	VEGF ligand-receptor interactions	3	8	5.43×10^{-4}	3.05×10^{-3}	2.07×10^{-1}	PGF; VEGFA

Table 4. OA-responsive DEGs that have significantly different expression fold changes between males and females, and significantly ($p < 0.05$) altered in at least one gender. DEGs significantly upregulated in response to OA are highlighted in red, and those significantly downregulated in blue.

SYMBOL	OM-HM		OF-HF		OM-HM vs. OF-HF	
	log₂FC	*p*-Value	log₂FC	*p*-Value	log₂FC	*p*-Value
ADAMTS2	1.036311	4.73×10^{-1}	4.245269	1.24×10^{-4}	−3.208959	1.37×10^{-2}
AKR1C2	0.716720	7.69×10^{-1}	2.893709	2.96×10^{-4}	−2.176989	3.56×10^{-2}
APBB1IP	1.029711	4.80×10^{-1}	4.594870	1.20×10^{-4}	−3.565158	9.94×10^{-3}
AQP1	0.781688	6.57×10^{-1}	3.956589	2.86×10^{-4}	−3.174901	1.43×10^{-2}
ARMS2	−0.356654	9.08×10^{-1}	2.345976	1.51×10^{-2}	−2.702631	1.64×10^{-2}
BAALC	0.980694	5.17×10^{-1}	3.404522	5.70×10^{-4}	−2.423828	4.66×10^{-2}
C1QTNF1	0.619342	8.09×10^{-1}	2.996843	2.75×10^{-3}	−2.377501	4.77×10^{-2}
CAVIN4	0.237081	9.28×10^{-1}	2.976823	3.48×10^{-3}	−2.739743	2.87×10^{-2}
CCDC163	0.768465	7.15×10^{-1}	−2.087867	1.36×10^{-2}	2.856332	2.44×10^{-3}
CDCA2	0.439866	8.37×10^{-1}	3.382528	1.19×10^{-3}	−2.942662	2.26×10^{-2}
CDKL2	0.651973	7.13×10^{-1}	−2.454556	1.72×10^{-3}	3.106529	1.36×10^{-2}
COL15A1	0.397324	9.18×10^{-1}	2.601580	2.23×10^{-3}	−2.204256	4.27×10^{-2}
COL18A1	0.108196	9.90×10^{-1}	2.571811	5.21×10^{-3}	−2.463615	2.16×10^{-2}
COL1A1	3.791243	3.33×10^{-4}	7.250090	8.76×10^{-7}	−3.458847	3.88×10^{-2}
COL1A2	2.206448	2.20×10^{-2}	5.722798	2.93×10^{-8}	−3.516351	4.58×10^{-3}
CYBB	1.286525	3.93×10^{-1}	5.141565	9.37×10^{-4}	−3.855040	3.95×10^{-2}

Table 4. *Cont.*

SYMBOL	OM-HM		OF-HF		OM-HM vs. OF-HF	
	log₂FC	*p*-Value	log₂FC	*p*-Value	log₂FC	*p*-Value
DKK3	0.654166	7.59×10^{-1}	3.287993	5.43×10^{-4}	−2.633827	2.58×10^{-2}
DPT	0.826854	6.55×10^{-1}	3.052945	3.79×10^{-4}	−2.226091	4.61×10^{-2}
EMB	0.540007	7.61×10^{-1}	3.865787	9.00×10^{-4}	−3.325780	2.08×10^{-2}
EMX2OS	−0.745100	6.41×10^{-1}	3.025770	3.24×10^{-2}	−3.770870	2.35×10^{-2}
EPYC	0.082818	9.87×10^{-1}	2.941842	4.25×10^{-3}	−2.859024	1.52×10^{-2}
FAN1	0.487189	7.97×10^{-1}	−2.529764	4.07×10^{-2}	3.016953	3.39×10^{-2}
FBLN5	0.820198	6.62×10^{-1}	3.185592	1.17×10^{-3}	−2.365394	4.72×10^{-2}
GAP43	1.465410	2.56×10^{-1}	4.712171	6.43×10^{-5}	−3.246761	2.64×10^{-2}
HMGB4	0.067476	9.82×10^{-1}	2.557579	1.19×10^{-2}	−2.490102	4.46×10^{-2}
HPDL	−0.057707	9.88×10^{-1}	2.475639	1.40×10^{-2}	−2.533346	3.20×10^{-2}
IFI44L	0.012213	9.96×10^{-1}	3.090819	1.51×10^{-2}	−3.078605	3.65×10^{-2}
IGFBP4	0.764578	6.78×10^{-1}	3.556192	8.62×10^{-4}	−2.791614	2.86×10^{-2}
LINC02447	0.377013	8.91×10^{-1}	−2.237060	2.63×10^{-5}	2.614072	2.53×10^{-2}
LOC100507250	0.452652	8.45×10^{-1}	−2.527564	1.12×10^{-2}	2.980216	1.19×10^{-2}
LOC101929122	0.056037	9.84×10^{-1}	2.846396	5.90×10^{-3}	−2.790359	2.55×10^{-2}
MIR4435-2HG	0.335817	9.45×10^{-1}	3.246292	3.10×10^{-4}	−2.910474	6.24×10^{-3}
MXRA5	2.179711	4.13×10^{-2}	5.721745	4.35×10^{-6}	−3.542034	1.59×10^{-3}
NEURL1B	−0.431259	8.20×10^{-1}	2.888588	1.59×10^{-2}	−3.319847	1.87×10^{-2}
NGF	1.338201	3.52×10^{-1}	5.880944	5.41×10^{-5}	−4.542743	8.71×10^{-3}
OGN	1.571206	1.44×10^{-1}	3.988797	1.87×10^{-5}	−2.417591	4.88×10^{-2}
PALM2	0.305307	9.84×10^{-1}	2.300331	4.37×10^{-3}	−1.995024	4.34×10^{-2}
PDLIM1	0.824352	6.02×10^{-1}	5.213650	1.57×10^{-4}	−4.389298	6.60×10^{-3}
PECAM1	−0.523163	7.50×10^{-1}	3.413773	3.56×10^{-2}	−3.936936	3.52×10^{-2}
PLAU	1.131386	4.51×10^{-1}	4.754242	1.15×10^{-3}	−3.622856	4.01×10^{-2}
PLK4	0.921031	5.52×10^{-1}	3.702119	5.00×10^{-4}	−2.781088	3.84×10^{-2}
RCAN1	0.462142	8.79×10^{-1}	2.998940	8.88×10^{-4}	−2.536799	2.38×10^{-2}
S100A4	1.739908	8.02×10^{-2}	4.787812	2.72×10^{-5}	−3.047904	2.23×10^{-2}
SERPINE1	−0.128314	9.57×10^{-1}	3.610779	1.52×10^{-3}	−3.739093	5.28×10^{-3}
SERPINE2	1.067892	4.41×10^{-1}	3.350974	1.14×10^{-4}	−2.283082	4.46×10^{-2}
SGIP1	−0.199640	9.58×10^{-1}	2.341629	3.22×10^{-2}	−2.541269	3.86×10^{-2}
THY1	3.064184	3.65×10^{-4}	7.253767	9.26×10^{-7}	−4.189584	7.67×10^{-3}
TNFAIP6	3.028402	1.71×10^{-3}	7.264821	8.86×10^{-6}	−4.236418	1.56×10^{-2}
TSIX	1.327472	4.64×10^{-1}	−3.508086	3.20×10^{-2}	4.835558	1.38×10^{-2}
VCAN	−0.392235	8.76×10^{-1}	2.248223	3.39×10^{-2}	−2.640458	3.07×10^{-2}

Table 5. The top 15 pathways enriched from the DEGs that differently altered in response to OA in male and female cartilage. Pathways with an FDR less than 0.05 are highlighted in red.

Pathway Identifier	Pathway Name	#Entities Found	#Entities Total	Entities Ratio	Entities *p*-Value	Entities FDR	Submitted Entities Found
R-HSA-1474244	Extracellular matrix organization	10	330	2.24×10^{-2}	8.68×10^{-7}	2.38×10^{-4}	COL1A1; COL18A1; VCAN; COL15A1; ADAMTS2; COL1A2; SERPINE1; PECAM1; FBLN5
R-HSA-1650814	Collagen biosynthesis and modifying enzymes	5	76	5.16×10^{-3}	1.58×10^{-5}	2.17×10^{-3}	COL1A1; COL18A1; COL15A1; ADAMTS2; COL1A2
R-HSA-75205	Dissolution of Fibrin Clot	3	14	9.51×10^{-4}	2.83×10^{-5}	2.32×10^{-3}	SERPINE2; PLAU; SERPINE1
R-HSA-8948216	Collagen chain trimerization	4	44	2.99×10^{-3}	3.41×10^{-5}	2.32×10^{-3}	COL1A1; COL18A1; COL15A1; COL1A2
R-HSA-1474290	Collagen formation	5	104	7.07×10^{-3}	6.96×10^{-5}	3.76×10^{-3}	COL1A1; COL18A1; COL15A1; ADAMTS2; COL1A2
R-HSA-2022090	Assembly of collagen fibrils and other multimeric structures	4	67	4.55×10^{-3}	1.71×10^{-4}	7.45×10^{-3}	COL1A1; COL18A1; COL15A1; COL1A2
R-HSA-1442490	Collagen degradation	4	69	4.69×10^{-3}	1.91×10^{-4}	7.45×10^{-3}	COL1A1; COL18A1; COL15A1; COL1A2
R-HSA-3000178	ECM proteoglycans	4	79	5.37×10^{-3}	3.18×10^{-4}	1.08×10^{-2}	COL1A1; VCAN; COL1A2; SERPINE1
R-HSA-216083	Integrin cell surface interactions	4	87	5.91×10^{-3}	4.57×10^{-4}	1.37×10^{-2}	COL1A1; COL18A1; COL1A2; PECAM1
R-HSA-430116	GP1b-IX-V activation signaling	2	12	8.15×10^{-4}	1.14×10^{-3}	3.08×10^{-2}	COL1A1; COL1A2
R-HSA-76009	Platelet Aggregation (Plug Formation)	3	53	3.60×10^{-3}	1.37×10^{-3}	3.13×10^{-2}	COL1A1; APBB1IP; COL1A2

Table 5. *Cont.*

Pathway Identifier	Pathway Name	#Entities Found	#Entities Total	Entities Ratio	Entities *p*-Value	Entities FDR	Submitted Entities Found
R-HSA-3781865	Diseases of glycosylation	5	202	1.37×10^{-2}	1.42×10^{-3}	3.13×10^{-2}	VCAN; ADAMTS2; SERPINE2; OGN; BAALC
R-HSA-2214320	Anchoring fibril formation	2	15	1.02×10^{-3}	1.77×10^{-3}	3.71×10^{-2}	COL1A1; COL1A2
R-HSA-75892	Platelet Adhesion to exposed collagen	2	16	1.09×10^{-3}	2.01×10^{-3}	3.81×10^{-2}	COL1A1; COL1A2
R-HSA-1474228	Degradation of the extracellular matrix	4	148	1.01×10^{-2}	3.18×10^{-3}	5.73×10^{-2}	COL1A1; COL18A1; COL15A1; COL1A2

3. Discussion

It is broadly accepted that exploring the OA-responsive biomarkers shared by both genders will pave the path for developing the therapeutics that benefit both male and female OA patients [32]. On the other hand, the distinguished clinical appearance between male and female patients warrants the mechanistic investigation at the molecule level. In the current study, the global gene expression profiles of knee joint articular cartilage from male and female donors of a well-accepted dataset [33–42], GSE114007, were comprehensively compared to gain insight into the understanding of the SABV not only in the healthy status, but also in the response of OA stimulation.

Firstly, the 36 identified male-vs.-female DEGs in healthy cartilage confirmed the hypothesis that the SABV is not limited to the thickness and articular surface areas [21,43] but extended to the static transcriptomic level. In particular, besides the 15 Y-chromosome-linked genes, several genes among the 36 male-vs.-female DEGs in healthy cartilage have been correlated with OA development and progression. For example, as an intensively investigated long non-coding RNA (lncRNA), *XIST* is highly expressed in OA cartilage tissue and IL-1β-treated chondrocytes [44] and has anti-apoptosis and chondroprotective effects [45]. On the other hand, another lncRNA, *MIR4435-2HG*, is downregulated in OA [46] and may have inhibition effects on the progression of OA [47]. Regarding the ECM components, a small leucine-rich proteoglycan (SLRP), epiphycan, plays an important role in maintaining joint integrity, and *epiphycan*-deficient mice spontaneously develop OA with age [48]; *Col1A2* is one of the typical markers for fibrocartilage [49] and *MXRA5* is highly expressed in the synovial fluid of OA patients [50]. Some other DEGs identified in our current studies have also been associated with OA in previous investigations. For instance, *PDLIM1* is downregulated in IL-1β-treated chondrocytes [51], *THY1* is highly expressed in OA cartilage and could be induced by IL-1β [52], and *EIF1AY* has been identified as one of the 9 OA diagnostic biomarkers [53]. In addition, AQP1 promotes caspase-3 activation and thereby contributes to chondrocyte apoptosis [54], and thus the activation of AQP1 induced by OA process can be used to control the tissue degeneration [55].

In addition, *IGFBP4* has been identified as the late response gene of parathyroid hormone-related protein (PTHrP) in chondrocytes [56]. It functions as an IGF-1 inhibitor and participates in the inflammatory response [57]. Meanwhile, *IGFALS* encodes a serum protein that binds IGFs to increase their half-life and vascular distribution [58]. As the male healthy articular cartilage has a lower expression level of *IGFALS* and higher expression level of *IGFBP4* than female cartilage, we infer that IGF-1 signaling is less activated in male cartilage than their female counterpart.

Note that among these 36 DEGs, only *TSIX* has an adjusted *p*-value less than 0.05, indicating the significance of TSIX for gender-dependent biological differences in the articular cartilage. However, the detailed function of TSIX in cartilage remains blank. In addition, the limited available sample could lead to only one DEG identified with an adjusted *p*-value less than 0.05 identified, while more DEGs with a *p*-value less than 0.05 (36 DEGs) were recognized. Thus, further studies are undoubtedly encouraged to fully understand the SABV in healthy knee articular cartilage at the molecular level, which warrants a worldwide collaboration for more database collection in a diverse of populations.

Interestingly, when we profile OA-responsive transcriptional changes in male and female cartilage separately, the amount of OA-responsive DEGs with an adjusted *p*-value less than 0.05 in female cartilage is triple that in male cartilage, indicating more intense OA-induced molecular changes in female cartilage than that in male counterparts. This transcriptomic difference could be correlated with the clinical observation that women experience more severe OA symptoms than men [59,60]. Considering the different total amounts of OA-responsive DEGs, it is no surprise to find that the top 15 OA-responsive upregulated and downregulated DEGs are not identical in male and female cartilage. In fact, male and female cartilage do share some top OA-responsive DEGs with an adjusted *p*-value less than 0.05, such as *CISH, ADM, HLPDA, DDIT3, DDIT4, CFI, ST6GALNAC5, SPOCK1,* and *TNFSF15*. Regarding the Reactome-enriched pathways, "response of EIF2AK1 (HRI) to heme deficiency" is the common significant pathway with adjusted *p*-value less than 0.05 in response to OA stimulation shared by male and female cartilage. These shared genes and pathways could be considered as potential targets for OA diagnosis and treatment, which can benefit both genders.

The OA-responsive molecular events in female cartilage are tightly clustered in the "extracellular matrix organization", which could explain the reason that female patients have more severe OA-related cartilage defects than males [60,61]. Meanwhile, "FOXO-mediated transcription", "RUNX3-regulated immune response and cell migration", and "Interleukin-4 and Interleukin-13 signaling", the pathways with FDR less than 0.05, might be additional key pathways to regulate OA in females. In fact, recent studies demonstrate that FOXO transcription factors modulate autophagy and proteoglycan 4 in cartilage, and conditional knockout FOXOs could induce OA-like changes in the mice [62,63]. On the other hand, ECM degradation does not present as the leading OA-responsive event in the male cartilage. Instead, "ATF4 activates genes in response to endoplasmic reticulum stress", "NGF-stimulated transcription", "MECP2 regulates neuronal receptors and channels", "PERK regulates gene expression", and "Nuclear Events (kinase and transcription factor activation)" were enriched from the OA-responsive DEGs in male cartilage with FDR less than 0.05, indicating a distinct molecular response to OA between male and female cartilage. The activation of the PERK-ATF4-CHOP axis is especially known to mediate impaired cartilage function [64]; however, the effects of these male-specific OA-responsive pathways in arthritis are still unknown.

SABV of cartilage in response to OA was further evaluated by comparing the OA-response DEGs from both genders directly, by which 50 genes with significantly different expression fold changes were identified, but none of the genes has an adjusted *p*-value less than 0.05. As expected, "Extracellular matrix organization" is the major sex-relative differential event harboring 9 of the 14 enriched pathways. There are also differences in "Hemostasis" and "Diseases of glycosylation" events. Note that several genes clustered in the event "Hemostasis" (including pathways "Dissolution of Fibrin Clot", "GP1b-IX-V activation signaling", "Platelet Aggregation (Plug Formation)", and "Platelet Adhesion to exposed collagen") have also been investigated in OA-related area. For example, *SER-PINE1* has been identified as one of the OA-specific genes in human joint fibroblast-like synoviocytes [65]. While *SERPINE2*, a contributor for both "Hemostasis" and "Diseases of glycosylation" events, upregulated by IL-1α stimulation in human chondrocytes, and recombinant SERPINE2 may protect chondrocytes by inhibiting MMP-13 expression [66]. Besides, high platelet counts within the normal range are significantly associated with knee and hip OA in women aged above 50 [67].

Considering aging may be an important indicator of OA, it is not a surprise that the donors of the OA groups are older than the healthy group when the dataset was built [33]. Interestingly, specifically grouping the samples in the same dataset GSE114007 by donor age, Chen et al. concluded that age is not a dependent variable for differentially expressed gene identification [41]. Here, as demonstrated in Table 6, no difference regarding donor age between males and females was found in healthy cartilages nor OA samples. Thus, the age contribution on OA-responsive differentially expressed genes, if any, has already been considered in parallel for both genders. Note that comparing healthy cartilage of different age stages for each gender would be an interesting and important topic for gaining more insight on the molecular events in senescence, particularly in a gender-dependent manner. Besides, an inter-cohort validation should be conducted in the future to verify the genes and pathways discovered in the current study. Last but not least, it is the first time that multiple genes and pathways mentioned above are associated with chondrogenic differentiation, maintenance, and pathology. The underlying mechanistic and functional details are largely unknown. No doubt, a huge amount of effort should be devoted on a global base to transferring the discovery here to the real world.

Table 6. The sample size and age information for each group.

Group	Sample Size	Age Range (years)	Mean Age	OA Score Range	Mean OA Score
Healthy Female	5	27–57	42 yrs	1–1	1
Healthy Male	13	18–61	34.5 yrs	1–1	1
OA Female	11	52–82	66.3 yrs	4–4	4
OA Male	9	51–71	64.9 yrs	4–4	4

4. Materials and Methods

By using the keywords "osteoarthritis" and "cartilage" in the NCBI GEO DataSets website [68] with the selection of "*Homo sapiens*" under the column of "Top Organisms" and "Expression profiling by high throughput sequencing" under the column of "study type", 31 series were identified. After reviewing all these datasets to check if they provided the sex information of the donors, one series (GSE114007) containing transcriptome data of human knee cartilage samples was included in the current study [33]. In this dataset, there were samples from 5 healthy female donors (age 27–57, mean 42), 13 healthy male donors (age 18–61, mean 34.5), 11 OA female donors (age 52–82, mean 66.3), and 9 OA male donors (age 51–71, mean 64.9) (Table 6 and Supplemental Table S13). According to the original study of this dataset, there is no significant difference between healthy and OA samples in other factors, such as the health condition of the donors, tissue sampling location, and body mass index [33,41]. SRA data of all the samples were downloaded from NCBI SRA website [69]. Following comparisons were conducted: (1) male healthy (HM) cartilage with female healthy (HF) cartilage to explore the baseline molecular differences in the articular cartilage between genders, (2) male OA (OM) cartilage with HM cartilage to detect the molecular changes in response to OA in males, (3) female OA (OF) cartilage with HF cartilage to detect the molecular changes in response to OA in females, and (4) OA-responsive DEGs in males (OM-HM) with that in females (OF-HF) to find the genes altered significantly different between genders during OA (OM-HM vs. OF-HF). Data analyses were performed on the Galaxy platform (UseGalaxy.org; [70]) with an established, broadly validated protocol [71–73]. Briefly, the FASTQC RNA-seq reads were aligned to the human genome (GRCh38) using HISAT2 aligner (Galaxy Version 2.1.0+galaxy 5) with default parameters [74]. Raw counts of sequencing read for the feature of genes were extracted by featureCounts (Galaxy Version 1.6.4+galaxy1) [75]. Then, the limma package (Galaxy version 3.38.3 + galaxy3) was used to identify DEGs with its *voom* method [76,77]. Expressed genes were selected as their counts per million (CPM), value not less than 1 in at least two samples across the entire experiment, while lowly expressed genes were removed for the flowing analyses. The parameters were set as 1 for minimum $\log_2$ Fold change and 0.05 for *p*-value adjustment threshold. As our current investigation is an explorative study, Benjamini–Hochberg correction was employed in the limma-voom analysis for *p* value adjustment [78], which is highly recommandated by the limma user guide [79]. To provide FDR control, the limma Test significance relative to a fold-change threshold (TREAT) function was applied to select genes that are more likely to be biologically significant [80], accompanied by the Robust Setting to protect against outlier genes [81]. A trimmed mean of M values (TMM) method was used for normalization among RNA samples. Quasi-likelihood F-tests (ANOVA-like analysis) were achieved to identify DEGs [82]. Genes with fold change (FC) more than 2 and p value less than 0.05 were assigned as DEGs. Heatmap diagrams were conducted in R (version 3.6.3) [83] with packages *pheatmap* (version 1.0.12), while volcano plots were generated by GraphPad Prism (version 8.2.1; GraphPad Software, Inc., San Diego, CA, USA). Pathway enrichment of identified DEGs was performed against the Reactome knowledgebase [84]. The enriched pathways with a false discovery rate (FDR) less than 0.05 were considered significantly meaningful.

5. Conclusions

In summary, our current study confirmed SABV in the knee cartilage at the transcriptomic level in both healthy and OA statuses. This study, at least partially, explains the clinical observed sex-relative differences of OA outcomes. Due to the lack of knowledge about some of the identified DEGs, further worldwide collaboration is necessary to comprehensively uncover the sex-relative differences of knee articular cartilage health and disease.

Supplementary Materials: The following are available online at https://www.mdpi.com/article/10.3390/ijms22157876/s1.

Author Contributions: Conceptualization, C.L.; methodology, C.L. and Z.Z.; validation, C.L. and Z.Z.; formal analysis, Z.Z.; writing—original draft preparation, C.L.; writing—review and editing, Z.Z. Both authors have read and agreed to the published version of the manuscript.

Funding: This study was supported by the American Association of Orthodontists Foundation (AAOF) Orthodontic Faculty Development Fellowship Award, American Association of Orthodontists (AAO) Full-Time Faculty Fellowship Award, and University of Pennsylvania School of Dental Medicine Joseph and Josephine Rabinowitz Award for Excellence in Research for Chenshuang Li.

Institutional Review Board Statement: Not applicable.

Informed Consent Statement: Not applicable.

Data Availability Statement: The data presented in this study are contained within this article and Supplementary Materials.

Conflicts of Interest: The authors declare no conflict of interest.

References

1. Kriegova, E.; Manukyan, G.; Mikulkova, Z.; Gabcova, G.; Kudelka, M.; Gajdos, P.; Gallo, J. Gender-related differences observed among immune cells in synovial fluid in knee osteoarthritis. *Osteoarthr. Cartil.* **2018**, *26*, 1247–1256. [CrossRef] [PubMed]
2. Regitz-Zagrosek, V. Sex and gender differences in health. Science & Society Series on Sex and Science. *EMBO Rep.* **2012**, *13*, 596–603. [CrossRef] [PubMed]
3. Yelin, E.; Weinstein, S.; King, T. The burden of musculoskeletal diseases in the United States. *Semin. Arthritis Rheum.* **2016**, *46*, 259–260. [CrossRef]
4. Safiri, S.; Kolahi, A.A.; Smith, E.; Hill, C.; Bettampadi, D.; Mansournia, M.A.; Hoy, D.; Ashrafi-Asgarabad, A.; Sepidarkish, M.; Almasi-Hashiani, A.; et al. Global, regional and national burden of osteoarthritis 1990-2017: A systematic analysis of the Global Burden of Disease Study 2017. *Ann. Rheum. Dis.* **2020**, *79*, 819–828. [CrossRef]
5. World Health Organization. Chronic Diseases and Health Promotion—Chronic Rheumatic Conditions. Available online: https://www.who.int/chp/topics/rheumatic/en/#:~{}:text=Worldwide%20estimates%20are%20that%209.6,major%20daily%20activities%20of%20life (accessed on 23 December 2020).
6. Parmelee, P.A.; Harralson, T.L.; McPherron, J.A.; DeCoster, J.; Schumacher, H.R. Pain, disability, and depression in osteoarthritis: Effects of race and sex. *J. Aging Health* **2012**, *24*, 168–187. [CrossRef]
7. Keefe, F.J.; Lefebvre, J.C.; Egert, J.R.; Affleck, G.; Sullivan, M.J.; Caldwell, D.S. The relationship of gender to pain, pain behavior, and disability in osteoarthritis patients: The role of catastrophizing. *Pain* **2000**, *87*, 325–334. [CrossRef]
8. International, O.R.S. Osteoarthritis: A Serious Disease, Submitted to the U.S. Food and Drug Administration. Available online: https://oarsi.org/sites/default/files/docs/2016/oarsi_white_paper_oa_serious_disease_121416_1.pdf (accessed on 19 December 2019).
9. Helmick, C.G.; Watkins-Castillo, S.I. The Burden of Musculoskeletal Diseases in the United States—Hospitalization. Available online: https://www.boneandjointburden.org/2014-report/ivc10/hospitalization (accessed on 19 December 2020).
10. Phinyomark, A.; Osis, S.T.; Hettinga, B.A.; Kobsar, D.; Ferber, R. Gender differences in gait kinematics for patients with knee osteoarthritis. *BMC Musculoskelet Disord* **2016**, *17*, 157. [CrossRef]

11. Boyan, B.D.; Hart, D.A.; Enoka, R.M.; Nicolella, D.P.; Resnick, E.; Berkley, K.J.; Sluka, K.A.; Kwoh, C.K.; Tosi, L.L.; O'Connor, M.I.; et al. Hormonal modulation of connective tissue homeostasis and sex differences in risk for osteoarthritis of the knee. *Biol. Sex. Differ.* **2013**, *4*, 3. [CrossRef] [PubMed]

12. Rosner, I.A.; Goldberg, V.M.; Getzy, L.; Moskowitz, R.W. Effects of estrogen on cartilage and experimentally induced osteoarthritis. *Arthritis Rheum.* **1979**, *22*, 52–58. [CrossRef] [PubMed]

13. Roman-Blas, J.A.; Castaneda, S.; Largo, R.; Herrero-Beaumont, G. Osteoarthritis associated with estrogen deficiency. *Arthritis Res. Ther.* **2009**, *11*, 241. [CrossRef]

14. Ganova, P.; Zhivkova, R.; Kolarov, A.; Ivanovska, N. Influence of estradiol treatment on bone marrow cell differentiation in collagenase-induced arthritis. *Inflamm. Res.* **2020**, *69*, 533–543. [CrossRef]

15. Qu, Z.; Huang, J.; Yang, F.; Hong, J.; Wang, W.; Yan, S. Sex hormone-binding globulin and arthritis: A Mendelian randomization study. *Arthritis Res. Ther.* **2020**, *22*, 118. [CrossRef] [PubMed]

16. Wang, Y.; Zhang, M.; Huan, Z.; Shao, S.; Zhang, X.; Kong, D.; Xu, J. FSH directly regulates chondrocyte dedifferentiation and cartilage development. *J. Endocrinol.* **2020**. [CrossRef]

17. Huang, K.; Wu, L.D. Dehydroepiandrosterone: Molecular mechanisms and therapeutic implications in osteoarthritis. *J. Steroid Biochem. Mol. Biol.* **2018**, *183*, 27–38. [CrossRef]

18. Wardhana, S.E.; Datau, E.A.; Ongkowijaya, J.; Karema-Kaparang, A.M. Transdermal bio-identical progesterone cream as hormonal treatment for osteoarthritis. *Acta Med. Indones.* **2013**, *45*, 224–232. [PubMed]

19. Jin, X.; Wang, B.H.; Wang, X.; Antony, B.; Zhu, Z.; Han, W.; Cicuttini, F.; Wluka, A.E.; Winzenberg, T.; Blizzard, L.; et al. Associations between endogenous sex hormones and MRI structural changes in patients with symptomatic knee osteoarthritis. *Osteoarthr. Cartil.* **2017**, *25*, 1100–1106. [CrossRef]

20. Contartese, D.; Tschon, M.; De Mattei, M.; Fini, M. Sex Specific Determinants in Osteoarthritis: A Systematic Review of Preclinical Studies. *Int. J. Mol. Sci.* **2020**, *21*, 3696. [CrossRef]

21. Otterness, I.G.; Eckstein, F. Women have thinner cartilage and smaller joint surfaces than men after adjustment for body height and weight. *Osteoarthr. Cartil.* **2007**, *15*, 666–672. [CrossRef]

22. Dequeker, J.; Mokassa, L.; Aerssens, J. Bone density and osteoarthritis. *J. Rheumatol. Suppl.* **1995**, *43*, 98–100. [PubMed]

23. Miller, A.E.; MacDougall, J.D.; Tarnopolsky, M.A.; Sale, D.G. Gender differences in strength and muscle fiber characteristics. *Eur. J. Appl. Physiol. Occup. Physiol.* **1993**, *66*, 254–262. [CrossRef] [PubMed]

24. Kim, J.R.; Kim, H.A. Molecular Mechanisms of Sex-Related Differences in Arthritis and Associated Pain. *Int. J. Mol. Sci.* **2020**, *21*, 7938. [CrossRef]

25. Sophia Fox, A.J.; Bedi, A.; Rodeo, S.A. The basic science of articular cartilage: Structure, composition, and function. *Sports Health* **2009**, *1*, 461–468. [CrossRef]

26. Sandell, L.J.; Aigner, T. Articular cartilage and changes in arthritis. An introduction: Cell biology of osteoarthritis. *Arthritis Res.* **2001**, *3*, 107–113. [CrossRef] [PubMed]

27. Li, C.S.; Zhang, X.; Peault, B.; Jiang, J.; Ting, K.; Soo, C.; Zhou, Y.H. Accelerated Chondrogenic Differentiation of Human Perivascular Stem Cells with NELL-1. *Tissue Eng. Part A* **2016**, *22*, 272–285. [CrossRef] [PubMed]

28. Li, C.; Zheng, Z.; Ha, P.; Jiang, W.; Berthiaume, E.A.; Lee, S.; Mills, Z.; Pan, H.; Chen, E.C.; Jiang, J.; et al. Neural EGFL like 1 as a potential pro-chondrogenic, anti-inflammatory dual-functional disease-modifying osteoarthritis drug. *Biomaterials* **2020**, *226*, 119541. [CrossRef] [PubMed]

29. Houard, X.; Goldring, M.B.; Berenbaum, F. Homeostatic mechanisms in articular cartilage and role of inflammation in osteoarthritis. *Curr. Rheumatol. Rep.* **2013**, *15*, 375. [CrossRef]

30. Jiang, Y.; Tuan, R.S. Role of NGF-TrkA signaling in calcification of articular chondrocytes. *FASEB J.* **2019**, *33*, 10231–10239. [CrossRef]

31. Janowska, J.D. C1q/TNF-related Protein 1, a Multifunctional Adipokine: An Overview of Current Data. *Am. J. Med. Sci.* **2020**, *360*, 222–228. [CrossRef]

32. Li, C.; Zheng, Z. Cartilage Targets of Knee Osteoarthritis Shared by Both Genders. *Int. J. Mol. Sci.* **2021**, *22*, 569. [CrossRef]

33. Fisch, K.M.; Gamini, R.; Alvarez-Garcia, O.; Akagi, R.; Saito, M.; Muramatsu, Y.; Sasho, T.; Koziol, J.A.; Su, A.I.; Lotz, M.K. Identification of transcription factors responsible for dysregulated networks in human osteoarthritis cartilage by global gene expression analysis. *Osteoarthr. Cartil.* **2018**, *26*, 1531–1538. [CrossRef]

34. Yi, P.; Xu, X.; Yao, J.; Qiu, B. Effect of DNA methylation on gene transcription is associated with the distribution of methylation sites across the genome in osteoarthritis. *Exp. Ther. Med.* **2021**, *22*, 719. [CrossRef]

35. Yi, P.; Xu, X.; Yao, J.; Qiu, B. Analysis of mRNA Expression and DNA Methylation Datasets According to the Genomic Distribution of CpG Sites in Osteoarthritis. *Front. Genet.* **2021**, *12*, 618803. [CrossRef]

36. Yuan, W.H.; Xie, Q.Q.; Wang, K.P.; Shen, W.; Feng, X.F.; Liu, Z.; Shi, J.T.; Zhang, X.B.; Zhang, K.; Deng, Y.J.; et al. Screening of osteoarthritis diagnostic markers based on immune-related genes and immune infiltration. *Sci. Rep.* **2021**, *11*, 7032. [CrossRef]

37. Li, X.; Liao, Z.; Deng, Z.; Chen, N.; Zhao, L. Combining bulk and single-cell RNA-sequencing data to reveal gene expression pattern of chondrocytes in the osteoarthritic knee. *Bioengineered* **2021**, *12*, 997–1007. [CrossRef]

38. Xu, J.; Zeng, Y.; Si, H.; Liu, Y.; Li, M.; Zeng, J.; Shen, B. Integrating transcriptome-wide association study and mRNA expression profile identified candidate genes related to hand osteoarthritis. *Arthritis Res. Ther.* **2021**, *23*, 81. [CrossRef] [PubMed]

39. Jiang, L.; Zhou, Y.; Shen, J.; Chen, Y.; Ma, Z.; Yu, Y.; Chu, M.; Qian, Q.; Zhuang, X.; Xia, S. RNA Sequencing Reveals LINC00167 as a Potential Diagnosis Biomarker for Primary Osteoarthritis: A Multi-Stage Study. *Front. Genet.* **2020**, *11*, 539489. [CrossRef] [PubMed]

40. Zheng, L.; Chen, W.; Xian, G.; Pan, B.; Ye, Y.; Gu, M.; Ma, Y.; Zhang, Z.; Sheng, P. Identification of abnormally methylated-differentially expressed genes and pathways in osteoarthritis: A comprehensive bioinformatic study. *Clin. Rheumatol.* **2021**. [CrossRef]

41. Chen, H.; Chen, L. An integrated analysis of the competing endogenous RNA network and co-expression network revealed seven hub long non-coding RNAs in osteoarthritis. *Bone Joint Res.* **2020**, *9*, 90–98. [CrossRef] [PubMed]

42. Gao, X.; Sun, Y.; Li, X. Identification of key gene modules and transcription factors for human osteoarthritis by weighted gene co-expression network analysis. *Exp. Ther. Med.* **2019**, *18*, 2479–2490. [CrossRef] [PubMed]

43. Faber, S.C.; Eckstein, F.; Lukasz, S.; Muhlbauer, R.; Hohe, J.; Englmeier, K.H.; Reiser, M. Gender differences in knee joint cartilage thickness, volume and articular surface areas: Assessment with quantitative three-dimensional MR imaging. *Skeletal Radiol.* **2001**, *30*, 144–150. [CrossRef] [PubMed]

44. Liu, Y.; Liu, K.; Tang, C.; Shi, Z.; Jing, K.; Zheng, J. Long non-coding RNA XIST contributes to osteoarthritis progression via miR-149-5p/DNMT3A axis. *Biomed. Pharmacother.* **2020**, *128*, 110349. [CrossRef] [PubMed]

45. Lian, L.P.; Xi, X.Y. Long non-coding RNA XIST protects chondrocytes ATDC5 and CHON-001 from IL-1beta-induced injury via regulating miR-653-5p/SIRT1 axis. *J. Biol. Regul Homeost. Agents* **2020**, *34*, 379–391. [CrossRef] [PubMed]

46. Xiao, Y.; Bao, Y.; Tang, L.; Wang, L. LncRNA MIR4435-2HG is downregulated in osteoarthritis and regulates chondrocyte cell proliferation and apoptosis. *J. Orthop. Surg. Res.* **2019**, *14*, 247. [CrossRef] [PubMed]

47. Liu, Y.; Yang, Y.; Ding, L.; Jia, Y.; Ji, Y. LncRNA MIR4435-2HG inhibits the progression of osteoarthritis through miR-510-3p sponging. *Exp. Ther. Med.* **2020**, *20*, 1693–1701. [CrossRef]

48. Nuka, S.; Zhou, W.; Henry, S.P.; Gendron, C.M.; Schultz, J.B.; Shinomura, T.; Johnson, J.; Wang, Y.; Keene, D.R.; Ramirez-Solis, R.; et al. Phenotypic characterization of epiphycan-deficient and epiphycan/biglycan double-deficient mice. *Osteoarthr. Cartil.* **2010**, *18*, 88–96. [CrossRef] [PubMed]

49. Fernandes, A.M.; Herlofsen, S.R.; Karlsen, T.A.; Kuchler, A.M.; Floisand, Y.; Brinchmann, J.E. Similar properties of chondrocytes from osteoarthritis joints and mesenchymal stem cells from healthy donors for tissue engineering of articular cartilage. *PLoS ONE* **2013**, *8*, e62994. [CrossRef]

50. Balakrishnan, L.; Nirujogi, R.S.; Ahmad, S.; Bhattacharjee, M.; Manda, S.S.; Renuse, S.; Kelkar, D.S.; Subbannayya, Y.; Raju, R.; Goel, R.; et al. Proteomic analysis of human osteoarthritis synovial fluid. *Clin. Proteomics* **2014**, *11*, 6. [CrossRef]

51. Joos, H.; Albrecht, W.; Laufer, S.; Reichel, H.; Brenner, R.E. IL-1beta regulates FHL2 and other cytoskeleton-related genes in human chondrocytes. *Mol. Med.* **2008**, *14*, 150–159. [CrossRef]

52. Chanmee, T.; Phothacharoen, P.; Thongboonkerd, V.; Kasinrerk, W.; Kongtawelert, P. Characterization of monoclonal antibodies against a human chondrocyte surface antigen. *Monoclon Antib. Immunodiagn. Immunother.* **2013**, *32*, 180–186. [CrossRef]

53. Wang, X.; Yu, Y.; Huang, Y.; Zhu, M.; Chen, R.; Liao, Z.; Yang, S. Identification of potential diagnostic gene biomarkers in patients with osteoarthritis. *Sci. Rep.* **2020**, *10*, 13591. [CrossRef]

54. Gao, H.; Gui, J.; Wang, L.; Xu, Y.; Jiang, Y.; Xiong, M.; Cui, Y. Aquaporin 1 contributes to chondrocyte apoptosis in a rat model of osteoarthritis. *Int. J. Mol. Med.* **2016**, *38*, 1752–1758. [CrossRef]

55. Musumeci, G.; Leonardi, R.; Carnazza, M.L.; Cardile, V.; Pichler, K.; Weinberg, A.M.; Loreto, C. Aquaporin 1 (AQP1) expression in experimentally induced osteoarthritic knee menisci: An in vivo and in vitro study. *Tissue Cell* **2013**, *45*, 145–152. [CrossRef] [PubMed]

56. Hoogendam, J.; Farih-Sips, H.; van Beek, E.; Lowik, C.W.; Wit, J.M.; Karperien, M. Novel late response genes of PTHrP in chondrocytes. *Horm. Res.* **2007**, *67*, 159–170. [CrossRef] [PubMed]

57. Miyagawa, I.; Nakayamada, S.; Nakano, K.; Yamagata, K.; Sakata, K.; Yamaoka, K.; Tanaka, Y. Induction of Regulatory T Cells and Its Regulation with Insulin-like Growth Factor/Insulin-like Growth Factor Binding Protein-4 by Human Mesenchymal Stem Cells. *J. Immunol.* **2017**, *199*, 1616–1625. [CrossRef] [PubMed]

58. Domene, S.; Domene, H.M. The role of acid-labile subunit (ALS) in the modulation of GH-IGF-I action. *Mol. Cell Endocrinol.* **2020**, *518*, 111006. [CrossRef] [PubMed]

59. Srikanth, V.K.; Fryer, J.L.; Zhai, G.; Winzenberg, T.M.; Hosmer, D.; Jones, G. A meta-analysis of sex differences prevalence, incidence and severity of osteoarthritis. *Osteoarthr. Cartil.* **2005**, *13*, 769–781. [CrossRef]

60. Hame, S.L.; Alexander, R.A. Knee osteoarthritis in women. *Curr. Rev. Musculoskelet. Med.* **2013**, *6*, 182–187. [CrossRef]

61. Hanna, F.S.; Teichtahl, A.J.; Wluka, A.E.; Wang, Y.; Urquhart, D.M.; English, D.R.; Giles, G.G.; Cicuttini, F.M. Women have increased rates of cartilage loss and progression of cartilage defects at the knee than men: A gender study of adults without clinical knee osteoarthritis. *Menopause* **2009**, *16*, 666–670. [CrossRef]

62. Matsuzaki, T.; Alvarez-Garcia, O.; Mokuda, S.; Nagira, K.; Olmer, M.; Gamini, R.; Miyata, K.; Akasaki, Y.; Su, A.I.; Asahara, H.; et al. FoxO transcription factors modulate autophagy and proteoglycan 4 in cartilage homeostasis and osteoarthritis. *Sci. Transl. Med.* **2018**, *10*. [CrossRef]

63. Lee, K.I.; Choi, S.; Matsuzaki, T.; Alvarez-Garcia, O.; Olmer, M.; Grogan, S.P.; D'Lima, D.D.; Lotz, M.K. FOXO1 and FOXO3 transcription factors have unique functions in meniscus development and homeostasis during aging and osteoarthritis. *Proc. Natl. Acad. Sci. USA* **2020**, *117*, 3135–3143. [CrossRef]

64. Kang, X.; Yang, W.; Feng, D.; Jin, X.; Ma, Z.; Qian, Z.; Xie, T.; Li, H.; Liu, J.; Wang, R.; et al. Cartilage-Specific Autophagy Deficiency Promotes ER Stress and Impairs Chondrogenesis in PERK-ATF4-CHOP-Dependent Manner. *J. Bone Miner. Res.* **2017**, *32*, 2128–2141. [CrossRef]

65. Cai, P.; Jiang, T.; Li, B.; Qin, X.; Lu, Z.; Le, Y.; Shen, C.; Yang, Y.; Zheng, L.; Zhao, J. Comparison of rheumatoid arthritis (RA) and osteoarthritis (OA) based on microarray profiles of human joint fibroblast-like synoviocytes. *Cell Biochem. Funct.* **2019**, *37*, 31–41. [CrossRef]

66. Santoro, A.; Conde, J.; Scotece, M.; Abella, V.; Lois, A.; Lopez, V.; Pino, J.; Gomez, R.; Gomez-Reino, J.J.; Gualillo, O. SERPINE2 Inhibits IL-1alpha-Induced MMP-13 Expression in Human Chondrocytes: Involvement of ERK/NF-kappaB/AP-1 Pathways. *PLoS ONE* **2015**, *10*, e0135979. [CrossRef] [PubMed]

67. Kwon, Y.J.; Koh, I.H.; Chung, K.; Lee, Y.J.; Kim, H.S. Association between platelet count and osteoarthritis in women older than 50 years. *Ther. Adv. Musculoskelet. Dis.* **2020**, *12*, 1759720X20912861. [CrossRef] [PubMed]

68. NCBI. GEO DataSets. Available online: https://www.ncbi.nlm.nih.gov/gds (accessed on 22 July 2021).

69. NCBI. SRA. Available online: https://www.ncbi.nlm.nih.gov/sra (accessed on 22 July 2021).

70. Afgan, E.; Baker, D.; Batut, B.; van den Beek, M.; Bouvier, D.; Cech, M.; Chilton, J.; Clements, D.; Coraor, N.; Gruning, B.A.; et al. The Galaxy platform for accessible, reproducible and collaborative biomedical analyses: 2018 update. *Nucleic Acids Res.* **2018**, *46*, W537–W544. [CrossRef] [PubMed]

71. Batut, B.; Hiltemann, S.; Bagnacani, A.; Baker, D.; Bhardwaj, V.; Blank, C.; Bretaudeau, A.; Brillet-Gueguen, L.; Cech, M.; Chilton, J.; et al. Community-Driven Data Analysis Training for Biology. *Cell Syst.* **2018**, *6*, 752–758.e751. [CrossRef]

72. Doyle, M.; Phipson, B.; Maksimovic, J.; Trigos, A.; Ritchie, M.; Dashnow, H.; Su, S.; Law, C. 2: RNA-seq Counts to Genes (Galaxy Training Materials). Available online: https://training.galaxyproject.org/training-material/topics/transcriptomics/tutorials/rna-seq-counts-to-genes/tutorial.html (accessed on 6 July 2021).

73. Doyle, M.; Phipson, B.; Dashnow, H. 1: RNA-Seq Reads to Counts (Galaxy Training Materials). Available online: https://training.galaxyproject.org/training-material/topics/transcriptomics/tutorials/rna-seq-reads-to-counts/tutorial.html (accessed on 6 July 2021).

74. Kim, D.; Langmead, B.; Salzberg, S.L. HISAT: A fast spliced aligner with low memory requirements. *Nat. Methods* **2015**, *12*, 357–360. [CrossRef]

75. Liao, Y.; Smyth, G.K.; Shi, W. featureCounts: An efficient general purpose program for assigning sequence reads to genomic features. *Bioinformatics* **2014**, *30*, 923–930. [CrossRef]

76. Smyth, G.K. LIMMA: Linear Models for Microarray Data. In *Bioinformatics and Computational Biology Solutions Using R and Bioconductor. Statistics for Biology and Health*; Gentleman, R.C.V.J., Huber, W., Irizarry, R.A., Dudoit, S., Eds.; Springer: New York, NY, USA, 2005. [CrossRef]

77. Law, C.W.; Chen, Y.; Shi, W.; Smyth, G.K. voom: Precision weights unlock linear model analysis tools for RNA-seq read counts. *Genome Biol.* **2014**, *15*, R29. [CrossRef]

78. Benjamini, Y.; Hochberg, Y. Controlling the False Discovery Rate: A Practical and Powerful Approach to Multiple Testing. *J. R. Stat. Soc. Ser. B Methodol.* **1995**, *57*, 289–300. [CrossRef]

79. Smyth, G.K.; Ritchie, M.; Thorne, N.; Wettenhall, J.; Shi, W.; Hu, Y. limma: Linear Models for Microarray and RNA-Seq Data User's Guide. Available online: https://www.bioconductor.org/packages/devel/bioc/vignettes/limma/inst/docf/usersguide.pdf (accessed on 14 July 2021).

80. McCarthy, D.J.; Smyth, G.K. Testing significance relative to a fold-change threshold is a TREAT. *Bioinformatics* **2009**, *25*, 765–771. [CrossRef] [PubMed]

81. Phipson, B.; Lee, S.; Majewski, I.J.; Alexander, W.S.; Smyth, G.K. Robust Hyperparameter Estimation Protects against Hypervariable Genes and Improves Power to Detect Differential Expression. *Ann. Appl. Stat.* **2016**, *10*, 946–963. [CrossRef] [PubMed]

82. Lun, A.T.; Chen, Y.; Smyth, G.K. It's DE-licious: A Recipe for Differential Expression Analyses of RNA-seq Experiments Using Quasi-Likelihood Methods in edgeR. *Methods Mol. Biol.* **2016**, *1418*, 391–416. [CrossRef]

83. Team, R.C. R: A Language and Environment for Statistical Computing. Available online: http://www.R-project.org/. (accessed on 6 July 2021).

84. Jassal, B.; Matthews, L.; Viteri, G.; Gong, C.; Lorente, P.; Fabregat, A.; Sidiropoulos, K.; Cook, J.; Gillespie, M.; Haw, R.; et al. The reactome pathway knowledgebase. *Nucleic Acids Res.* **2020**, *48*, D498–D503. [CrossRef] [PubMed]

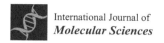

International Journal of
Molecular Sciences

MDPI

Article

The Hexosamine Biosynthetic Pathway as a Therapeutic Target after Cartilage Trauma: Modification of Chondrocyte Survival and Metabolism by Glucosamine Derivatives and PUGNAc in an Ex Vivo Model

Jana Riegger [1], Julia Baumert [1], Frank Zaucke [2] and Rolf E. Brenner [1,*]

[1] Division for Biochemistry of Joint and Connective Tissue Diseases, Department of Orthopedics, University of Ulm, 89081 Ulm, Germany; jana.riegger@uni-ulm.de (J.R.); julia.baumert@uni-ulm.de (J.B.)
[2] Dr. Rolf M. Schwiete Research Unit for Osteoarthritis, Department of Orthopaedics (Friedrichsheim), University Hospital Frankfurt, Goethe University, 60528 Frankfurt/Main, Germany; Frank.Zaucke@kgu.de
* Correspondence: rolf.brenner@uni-ulm.de; Tel.: +49-731-500-63280

Abstract: The hexosamine biosynthetic pathway (HBP) is essential for the production of uridine diphosphate N-acetylglucosamine (UDP-GlcNAc), the building block of glycosaminoglycans, thus playing a crucial role in cartilage anabolism. Although O-GlcNAcylation represents a protective regulatory mechanism in cellular processes, it has been associated with degenerative diseases, including osteoarthritis (OA). The present study focuses on HBP-related processes as potential therapeutic targets after cartilage trauma. Human cartilage explants were traumatized and treated with GlcNAc or glucosamine sulfate (GS); PUGNAc, an inhibitor of O-GlcNAcase; or azaserine (AZA), an inhibitor of GFAT-1. After 7 days, cell viability and gene expression analysis of anabolic and catabolic markers, as well as HBP-related enzymes, were performed. Moreover, expression of catabolic enzymes and type II collagen (COL2) biosynthesis were determined. Proteoglycan content was assessed after 14 days. Cartilage trauma led to a dysbalanced expression of different HBP-related enzymes, comparable to the situation in highly degenerated tissue. While GlcNAc and PUGNAc resulted in significant cell protection after trauma, only PUGNAc increased COL2 biosynthesis. Moreover, PUGNAc and both glucosamine derivatives had anti-catabolic effects. In contrast, AZA increased catabolic processes. Overall, "fueling" the HBP by means of glucosamine derivatives or inhibition of deglycosylation turned out as cells and chondroprotectives after cartilage trauma.

Keywords: hexosamine biosynthetic pathway; cartilage trauma; post-traumatic osteoarthritis; chondrocytes; O-GlcNAcylation; glucosamine; cell death; therapy

Citation: Riegger, J.; Baumert, J.; Zaucke, F.; Brenner, R.E. The Hexosamine Biosynthetic Pathway as a Therapeutic Target after Cartilage Trauma: Modification of Chondrocyte Survival and Metabolism by Glucosamine Derivatives and PUGNAc in an Ex Vivo Model. *Int. J. Mol. Sci.* **2021**, *22*, 7247. https://doi.org/10.3390/ijms22147247

Academic Editor: Nicola Veronese

Received: 23 June 2021
Accepted: 2 July 2021
Published: 6 July 2021

Publisher's Note: MDPI stays neutral with regard to jurisdictional claims in published maps and institutional affiliations.

1. Introduction

As the most common joint disease in the elderly population and one of the leading causes of disability in age, osteoarthritis (OA) has a high impact on today's society [1]. Preceding injuries are considered a major risk factor in joint degeneration, causing a special form called post-traumatic OA (PTOA), which can also affect the younger population and accounts for about 10% of the total incidence of knee OA [2].

The pathogenesis of PTOA is induced by a traumatic impact causing a sudden increase of cell death and subsequent synovial inflammation. The surviving chondrocytes secrete excessive amounts of catabolic enzymes, such as matrix metalloproteinases (MMPs) and proteases of the ADAMTS (a disintegrin and metalloproteinase with thrombospondin motifs) family, which contribute to the breakdown of the main cartilage components type II collagen and aggrecan [3]. These catabolic processes can persist over years, driving progressive cartilage degeneration.

Despite huge scientific efforts, the development of efficient drugs, preventing or delaying the onset of PTOA, remains difficult, in particular due to the complex pathomechanisms involved. Most therapeutic approaches, such as non-steroidal anti-inflammatory drugs (NSAIDs), focus on symptomatic relief and represent just a temporary solution [4]. Besides NSAIDs, which can also be considered rapid-acting symptom modifying osteoarthritis drugs (SMOADS), there are slow-acting drugs, also referred to as symptomatic slow acting drugs for osteoarthritis (SYSADOA), including cytokine modulators, such as diacerein, glucosamine, and chondroitin as precursors of matrix components, as well as hyaluronan (also known as hyaluronic acid) [5,6].

These matrix precursors and hyaluronan have one thing in common; they contribute to or are derived from the hexosamine biosynthetic pathway (HBP), which plays a substantial role in cartilage homeostasis [7]. In principle, the HBP is a branch of glycolysis, although it is not involved in energy generation but production of uridine diphosphate N-acetylglucosamine (UDP-GlcNAc). The rate-limiting enzyme, glutamine fructose-6-phosphate amidotransferase (GFAT-1), converts fructose-6-phosphate into glucosamine 6-phosphate, the precursor of GlcNAc (Figure 1). GlcNAc is the essential building block for the biosynthesis of glycosaminoglycans (GAGs), such as keratan sulfate, chondroitin sulfate, and hyaluronan, which represent about 90% of the total mass of aggrecan, the most abundant proteoglycan (PG) in articular cartilage [8]. The transfer of GlcNAc to proteins represents a special form of glycosylation (O-GlcNAcylation) and requires energy, enabled by coupling the monosaccharide with the nucleotide UDP. O-GlcNAcylation is not only essential for PG synthesis but also functions as a regulatory mechanism for various cellular processes [9,10]. This post-transcriptional modification is controlled by two enzymes: O-GlcNAc transferase (OGT), which drives the addition of UDP-GlcNAc to proteins, and the N-acetylglucosaminidase (OGA or O-GlcNAcase), which reverses the reaction. O-GlcNAcylation is highly responsive towards different stimuli, including trauma and cytokines [11], and has been found to be dysregulated in OA and other age-related degenerative diseases [11–13].

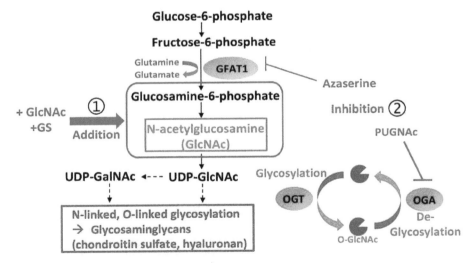

Figure 1. Schematic illustration of the hexosamine biosynthetic pathway (HBP), its role in glycosaminoglycan synthesis and potential therapeutic targeting. In the present study, the HBP is targeted in different ways: (1) glucosamine derivatives (N-acetylglucosamine (GlcNAc) or glucosamine sulfate (GS)) were added at different concentrations to enhance the bioavailability of the substrate for uridine diphosphate GlcNAc (UDP-GlcNAc) generation; (2) the rate-limiting enzyme, glutamine fructose-6-phosphate amidotransferase (GFAT1), was inhibited by means of Azaserine, while hydrolysis of O-GlcNAc residues (de-glycosylation) was suppressed using PUGNAc, a specific inhibitor of OGA. GalNAc = N-Acetylgalactosamine, OGA = N-acetylglucosaminidase, OGT = O-GlcNAc transferase, PUGNAc = O-(2-acetamido-2deoxy-D-glucopyranosylidene)amino-N-phenylcarbamate.

Concerning the fundamental importance of the HBP for the biosynthesis of matrix components, it might be rational to increase the substrate availability via glucosamine supplementation as a therapeutic approach in OA. In fact, there are various promising in vitro studies reporting anabolic, antioxidative, anti-catabolic (chondroprotective), pro-mitotic, and anti-inflammatory effects of glucosamines on chondrocytes [14–17]. However, the overall efficacy of glucosamines in OA therapy remains controversially discussed due to contradictory results, especially with regard to clinical trials [4,18–20].

Despite the central role of the HBP and protein O-GlcNAcylation in cartilage, the influence of a traumatic single impact as a potential trigger or suppressor of HBP-related processes in cartilage tissue has not been taken into account so far. Therefore, this study will not directly focus on potential therapeutic effects of the glucosamine derivatives GlcNAc and glucosamine sulfate (GS) but rather considers the HBP as a whole to investigate its possible involvement in post-traumatic processes and its relevance as a therapeutic target after cartilage trauma in particular.

2. Results

2.1. Gene Expression of HBP-Related Enzymes Is Altered after Cartilage Trauma and in Highly Degenerated Tissue

Human cartilage tissue explants were subjected to a single impact load of 0.59 J using a drop-tower model, as previously described [21]. This trauma suppressed gene expression levels of OGT by 25%, while increasing that of OGA by 35% (Figure 2A,B), thus significantly changing the ratio of OGA to OGT ([vs. C] 2-fold; Figure 2C). This alteration was markedly reduced by GlcNAc, PUGNAc, and AZA; however, the attenuating effect was only significant in the case of 10 mM GlcNAc. Despite increased gene expression of OGA in presence of its inhibitor PUGNAc, mRNA levels of OGT were likewise enhanced, resulting in an overall alleviated ratio of OGA to OGT, which was comparable to the control level. While trauma and subsequent treatment had no significant effect on mRNA levels of GFAT-1 in macroscopically intact cartilage (Figure 2D), gene expression analysis of highly degenerated cartilage tissue (ICRS score $\geq$ 3) revealed a significant reduction in GFAT-1 expression of about 50% compared to macroscopically intact tissue (ICRS score $\leq$ 1) (Figure 2E). Moreover, the ICRS score $\geq$ 3 tissue exhibited an about 1.8-fold increased ratio of OGA to OGT (Figure 2F).

2.2. GlcNAc and PUGNAc Exert Cell Protective Effects after Cartilage Trauma

To investigate potential involvement of the HBP in the regulation of cell death and survival after cartilage trauma, cell viability was assessed by means of a live/dead staining (Figure 3C). 7 days after trauma, the cell viability was significantly decreased by about 20% ([vs. C] Figure 3A: −16.8%, Figure 3B: −25%). While treatment with GlcNAc revealed significant cell protective effects ([vs. T] 2.5 mM: +11.3%; 5 mM: +13.6%; 10 mM: +14.6%), no improvement, except further reduction of the cell viability, was observed in the case of high-dose GS administration (Figure 3A). Due to the cell toxic effects observed for high concentrations (5 and 10 mM) of GS, these conditions were only exemplarily tested ($n = 3$).

While the addition of GFAT-inhibitor AZA had no significant effect on the percentage of living cells after cartilage trauma, inhibition of OGA by PUGNAc significantly promoted the survival of chondrocytes ([vs. T] 0.1 mM: +14.4%; 0.15 mM: +15.7%; Figure 3B).

2.3. While PUGNAc Revealed Chondroanabolic Effects, Glucosamine Derivatives GlcNAc and GS Suppressed Type II Collagen Synthesis after Cartilage Trauma

Possible involvement of the HBP in chondroanabolic effects after cartilage trauma was addressed by gene expression analysis of COL2A1, hyaluronan synthase 2 (HAS2), and aggrecan, as well as quantification of CPII, which reflects the actual biosynthesis of type II collagen (Figure 4).

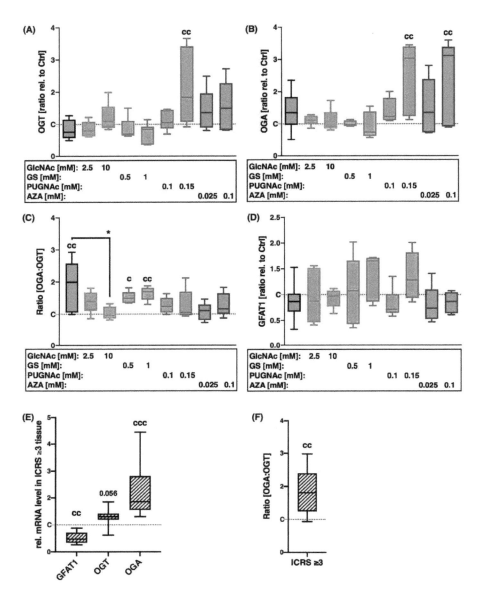

Figure 2. Gene expression levels of HBP-related enzymes 7 days after trauma and in highly degenerated tissue. Gene expression of HBP-related enzymes was evaluated in (**A,B,D**), impacted and subsequently treated cartilage explants, as well as (**E**) highly degenerated cartilage tissue (ICRS grade ≥ 3). Moreover, the ratio of OGA to OGT was calculated for (**C**) impacted and subsequent treated cartilage explants, as well as (**F**) OA cartilage. Statistical analysis: (**A,B,D**) one-way ANOVA, (**C**) the Kruskal–Wallis test, (**E**) multiple *t*-tests, (**F**) unpaired two-tailed *t*-test. Significant differences between groups were depicted as: [versus T] * = $p < 0.05$; [versus C] c = $p < 0.05$, cc = $p < 0.01$; all data sets $n \geq 5$; ICRS grade ≥ 3 tissue $n \geq 6$. Shaded boxes = traumatized cartilage explants (T), striped boxes = highly degenerated cartilage tissue (ICRS grade ≥ 3).

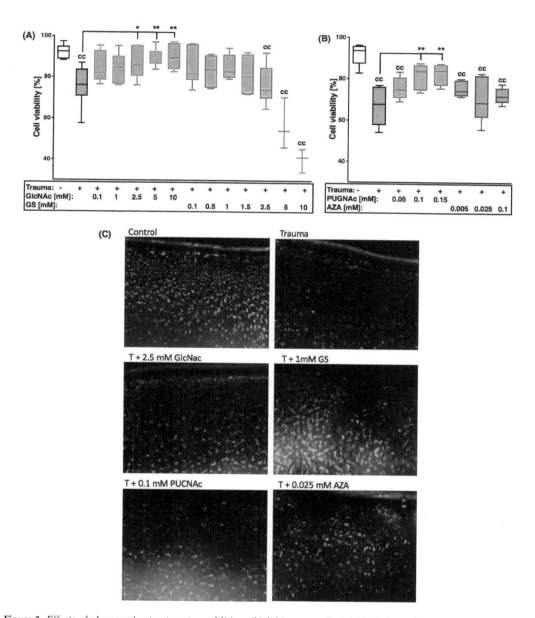

Figure 3. Effects of glucosamine treatment or addition of inhibitors on cell viability 7 days after cartilage trauma. Impacted cartilage explants were treated with different concentrations of (**A**) glucosamine derivatives GlcNAc or GS or (**B**) OGA-inhibitor PUGNAc and GFAT-1-Inhibitor AZA, respectively, for 7 days. (**C**) Exemplary fluorescence images of live/dead staining. Statistical analysis: (**A,B**) one-way ANOVA. Significant differences between groups were depicted as: [versus T] * = $p < 0.05$, ** = $p < 0.01$; [versus C] cc = $p < 0.01$; all data sets $n \geq 5$, except for 5 mM and 10 mM GS, $n = 3$. Blank box = unimpacted control (C), shaded boxes = traumatized cartilage explants (T).

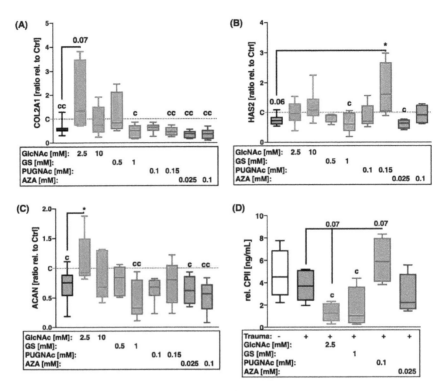

Figure 4. Effects of glucosamine, PUGNAc, and AZA on chondroanabolic processes 7 days after cartilage trauma. Chondroanabolism was evaluated by means of gene expression analysis of (**A**) COL2A1, (**B**) HAS2, and (**C**) ACAN, as well as by (**D**) quantification of CPII release. Statistical analysis: (**A,B**) Kruskal–Wallis test, (**C,D**) one-way ANOVA. Significant differences between groups were depicted as: [versus T] * = $p < 0.05$; [versus C] c = $p < 0.05$, cc = $p < 0.01$; all data sets $n \geq 5$. Blank box = unimpacted control (C), shaded boxes = traumatized cartilage explants (T).

Compared to the unimpacted cartilage, chondroanabolic gene expression was significantly reduced after trauma (Figure 4A–C). Although, treatment with 2.5 mM GlcNAc enhanced the gene expression of COL2A1 ([vs. T] 2.4-fold) and ACAN ([vs. T] 1.6-fold), both glucosamine derivatives suppressed the biosynthesis of type II collagen ([vs. C] GlcNAc: -3.5 ng/mL; GS: -3 ng/mL; Figure 4D). Moreover, 1 mM GS further reduced gene expression of ACAN.

While AZA had rather anti-anabolic effects, as demonstrated by reduced biosynthesis of type II collagen ([vs. C] -2.3 ng/mL), PUGNAc significantly induced both gene expression of HAS2 ([vs. T] 2.4-fold) and the release of CPII ([vs. T] +2.2 ng/mL), despite unchanged mRNA levels of COL2A1.

2.4. Trauma-Induced Expression of MMPs and Subsequent Type II Collagen Degradation Are Markedly Decreased after Treatment with Glucosamines or PUGNAc

Possible influence of the HBP on trauma-induced expression of MMPs and subsequent breakdown of type II collagen was evaluated by gene expression analysis of MMP-1 and -13 (Figure 5A,B), quantification of secreted MMP-2 (zymographical detection; Figure 6 and MMP-13 (Figure 5C), as well as the degradation product of type II collagen (C2C), generated by MMP-1, -8, and -13 (Figure 5D).

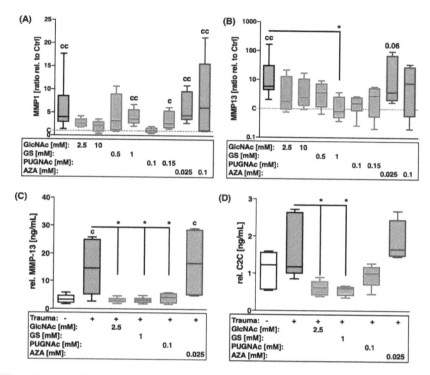

Figure 5. Effects of glucosamine treatment or addition of inhibitors on trauma-induced expression of collagenases and COL2A breakdown 7 days after trauma. Catabolic processes were assessed by the means of gene expression analysis of (**A**) MMP-1 and (**B**) MMP-13, as well as (**C**) quantification of MMP-13 release and (**D**) type II collagen breakdown product C2C. Statistical analysis: (**A,B**) Kruskal–Wallis test, (**C,D**) one-way ANOVA. Significant differences between groups were depicted as: [versus T] * = $p < 0.05$; [versus C] c = $p < 0.05$, cc = $p < 0.01$; all data sets $n \geq 5$. Blank box = unimpacted control (C), shaded boxes = traumatized cartilage explants (T).

Cartilage trauma resulted in excessive gene expression of ECM-degrading MMPs ([vs. C] MMP1: 4-fold; MMP13: 5.8-fold), though concentration of C2C was not significantly enhanced compared to the unimpacted control. Both glucosamine derivatives exhibited anti-catabolic effects to varying degrees. While GlcNAc had stronger suppressive effects, with respect to the gene expression of MMP-1 (Figure 5A), GS revealed higher efficacy in the case of MMP-13 (Figure 5B). However, GlcNAc and GS demonstrated equal anti-catabolic and chondroprotective effects, respectively, concerning the secretion of MMP-13 ([vs. T] GlcNAc: −11.54 ng/mL; GS: −11.8 ng/mL; Figure 5C) and subsequent degradation of type II collagen ([vs. T] both −0.97 ng/mL; Figure 5D). Moreover, GlcNAc significantly reduced the conversion of pro-MMP-2 to active MMP-2 by 2.9-fold (Figure 6C).

Although, comparable anti-catabolic effects were found after inhibition of OGA by means of PUGNAc, as demonstrated by decreased secretion of MMP-13 ([vs. T] −11 ng/mL), the reduction of the degradation product C2C was less pronounced ([vs. T] −0.57 ng/mL). While no significant changes could be observed for the secretion of pro-MMP2 (Figure 6A), the addition of AZA increased the zymographically detectable amount of active MMP-2 ([vs. C] 4-fold; [vs. T] 3-fold; Figure 6B) and the generation of C2C ([vs. T] +0.5 ng/mL) after cartilage trauma.

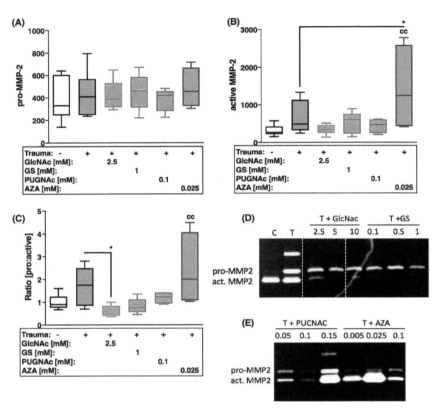

Figure 6. Effects of glucosamine treatment or addition of inhibitors on trauma-induced secretion and activation of MMP-2 7 days after trauma. Release of (**A**) pro-MMP-2 and (**B**) active MMP-2 was measured by means of gelatin zymography, as exemplarily demonstrated in (**D,E**). (**C**) Ratio of zymographically detectable pro-MMP-2 to active MMP-2. Statistical analysis: (**A–C**) one-way ANOVA. Significant differences between groups were depicted as: [versus T] * = $p < 0.05$; [versus C] cc = $p < 0.01$; all data sets $n \geq 5$. Blank box = unimpacted control (C), shaded boxes = traumatized cartilage explants (T).

2.5. Trauma-Induced Expression of Aggrecanases and Subsequent Aggrecan Degradation Are Largely Decreased after Treatment with Glucosamines or PUGNAc

Influence of the HBP on trauma-induced expression and proteolytic activity of aggrecanases was determined by the gene expression analysis of ADAMTS4 and 5, estimation of the aggrecanase activity, and the histological assessment of PG by means of Safranin-O staining.

After cartilage trauma, gene expression levels of ADAMTS-4 and -5 were significantly enhanced ([vs. C] ADAMTS4: 7.4-fold; ADAMTS5: 3-fold; Figure 7A,B). This was reflected in increased aggrecanase activity ([vs. C] 2.9-fold; Figure 7C), which can be considered proportional to the total aggrecanase amount. Additionally, histological assessment of PG by means of Saf-O staining confirmed the increased loss of PG in traumatized cartilage explants (Figure 7D). Treatment with glucosamines or PUGNAc significantly suppressed trauma-induced gene expression of aggrecanases, as well as aggrecanase activity ([vs. T] GlcNAc: −4.8-fold; GS: −3.5-fold; PUGNAc: −4.9-fold). These anti-catabolic effects and the subsequent preservation of PG could be confirmed in the corresponding Saf-O staining of GlcNAc and PUGNAc treated cartilage 14 days after trauma. In contrast, AZA had no additional effect on the expression levels of aggrecanases after trauma, though resulted in strong PG depletion, as demonstrated in the severe de-staining of the cartilage matrix.

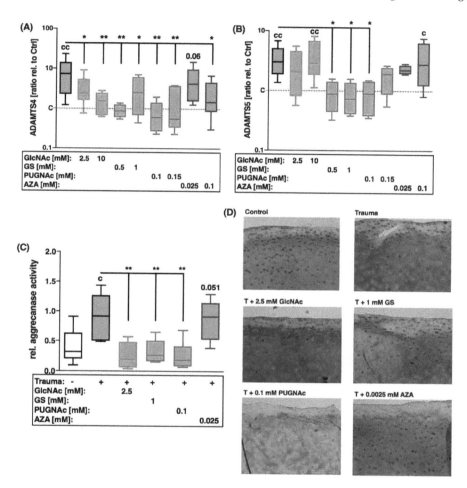

Figure 7. Effects of glucosamine treatment or addition of inhibitors on trauma-induced expression of aggrecanases and PG breakdown 7 days and 14 days after trauma. Catabolic processes were assessed by means of gene expression analysis of (**A**) ADAMTS-4 and (**B**) ADAMTS-5, as well as (**C**) quantification of relative aggrecanase activity (7 days after trauma). Moreover, (**D**) PG content in cartilage explants 14 days after trauma and corresponding treatments were evaluated by means of exemplary images of cartilage after Saf-O staining. Statistical analysis: (**A–C**) one-way ANOVA. Significant differences between groups were depicted as: [versus T] * = $p < 0.05$, ** = $p < 0.01$; [versus C] c = $p < 0.05$, cc = $p < 0.01$; all data sets $n \geq 5$. Blank box = unimpacted control (C), shaded boxes = traumatized cartilage explants (T).

3. Discussion

The HBP is essentially responsible for the generation of UDP-GlcNAc, the building block for posttranscriptional O-GlcNAcylation, which is not only involved in the biosynthesis of PG but also in the regulation of various metabolic processes [9,10]. Despite its crucial role in cartilage homeostasis, the actual implication of the HBP during OA development and, in particular, after traumatic cartilage injury remains largely unknown.

In the present study, we investigated the impact of targeted manipulation of the HBP in various ways. First, we added two different glucosamine derivatives, GS and GlcNAc, in order to increase the substrate availability and potentially boost HBP activity. Second, we inhibited the enzymatic activity of OGA via PUGNAc, thus impairing reversibility of O-GlcNAcylation and causing accumulation of O-glycosylated proteins. Third, we directly inhibited the rate-limiting enzyme of the HBP, GFAT-1, by means of AZA in order to suppress the generation of UDP-GlcNAc and therefore reducing subsequent O-GlcNAcylation. Unlike previous studies, which mainly focus on glucosamine administration as a therapeutic approach against advanced and symptomatic OA, this is the first study evaluating targeted modulation of the HBP after a singular cartilage impact using a human ex vivo trauma model. The experimental design allows investigation of HBP-related processes as a possible therapeutic target after mechanical injury and subsequent cartilage degeneration on cellular and molecular level, which in vivo might promote the development of a PTOA.

Some years ago, glucosamines, and in particular GS, have been propagated to be an ideal therapeutic approach in OA treatment, combining both pain relief and cartilage regeneration. Accordingly, glucosamine application was highly recommended in the guidelines of the European League Against Rheumatism (EULAR) for the management of knee OA in 2003 [21]. In fact, different reviews and meta-analyses between 2003 and 2008 summarized the outcomes of various clinical trials on GS and concluded that it was effective in pain reduction, improvement of the joint functionality, as well as the overall reduction of OA progression and subsequent risk of joint replacement [22]. About 10 years later, the Osteoarthritis Research Society (OARSI) guidelines stated the recommendation about glucosamine treatment as "uncertain" in case of symptom relief and "not appropriate" for disease modification [4]. Taken together, therapeutic efficacy of glucosamines in OA disease remains controversial, especially because of the inconsistency between study reports deriving from industry-sponsored and independent trials, as well as a generally large heterogeneity among studies [4]. Nevertheless, as mentioned above, we investigated a novel aspect in glucosamine administration and therapeutic targeting of the HBP, respectively, with a focus on attenuation of trauma-induced pathomechanisms and thus prevention of PTOA development. In our study, GlcNAc exhibited cell protective effects after cartilage trauma; however, this could not be confirmed in the case of GS, which led to enhanced cell death in doses higher than 1.5 mM. In fact, both cell protective and as cytotoxic effects of glucosamines have been previously reported. On the one hand, glucosamine has been found to induce autophagy in chondrocytes, which is considered to facilitate cell survival and protect against cartilage degeneration [20,23–25]. On the other hand, long-term exposure and high glucosamine concentrations were found to promote mitochondrial and peroxisomal dysfunction, as well as accumulation of very long chain fatty acids (VLCFA) [20]. Therefore, glucosamines might act as inducers and suppressors of autophagic and apoptotic processes at the same time, possibly depending on the respective experimental conditions. Interestingly, cytotoxic effects have been reported for glucosamines (i.e., glucosamine hydrochloride (GlcN-HCl)), [20,26,27] but not in case of GlcNAc. In contrast to GlcNAc, glucosamine has been found to be actively internalized by chondrocytes via glucose transporters (GLUTs), thus inhibiting glucose uptake and leading to depleted intracellular ATP stores [28]. Shikhman et al. supposed that GlcNAc interacts with GLUTs, although positively affecting their affinity for glucose, the main source for energy supply and precursor of GAG synthesis in chondrocytes [28].

In line with Uitterlinden et al., who reported both anti-catabolic and anti-anabolic effects of GS and GlcN-HCl in OA cartilage [16], we found significant chondroprotective effects for GlcNAc and GS after cartilage trauma, but also observed an unexpected decline in CPII. On first sight, this finding contradicts the general opinion that glucosamine enhances the ECM synthesis in cartilage; however, post-translational modification of type II collagen does not depend upon the HBP or UDP-GlcNAc, respectively [29]. Therefore, the suppressive effects of glucosamines clearly deserve further investigation. While GS suppressed the gene expression of ACAN and HAS2, GlcNAc increased the corresponding mRNA levels to some extent, depending on the concentration. In accordance with this, GlcNAc has previously been found to accelerate the expression of HAS2 and subsequent synthesis of hyaluronan, while glucosamine resulted in opposite effects [16,28]. The differential impact of GlcNAc and GS on chondroanabolism might also account for divergent findings concerning the PG content, as demonstrated by Saf-O staining. Despite similar suppression of aggrecanases and MMPs found for both glucosamine derivatives, higher PG decline was found in GS treated cartilage explants compared to GlcNAc treated explants.

Anti-catabolic effects of glucosamines have been previously reported, though mainly addressing interleukin 1b (IL-1b)-mediated MMP and ADAMTS expression [14,30,31]. Nevertheless, similar to cytokine-induced catabolism, the therapeutic effects of glucosamine administration after cartilage trauma might result from the inhibition of OA-associated mitogen-activated protein kinase (MAPK) pathways, including c-Jun N-terminal kinase and p38, as shown for GS [32]. However, inhibition of IL-1b-induced catabolism by GlcNAc has not been found to have any effect on ERK, JNK, or p38 MAPK pathways [33]. Moreover, spontaneous (i.e., age-dependent) and induced (i.e., via OGA-inhibitor thiamet-G) accumulation of O-GlcNAcylated proteins has even been associated with enhanced MAPK phosphorylation [34,35]. This activation correspondingly induced both MMP expression and chondrogenic differentiation of ATDC5 cells at the same time [34]. These contradictory observations imply a dual effect of O-GlcNAcylation on MAPK signaling, which clearly deserves further investigation with regard to cartilage trauma and OA development.

In our study, PUGNAc administration resulted not only in cell and chondroprotective effects but also in chondroanabolic effects after cartilage trauma, implying a positive effect by OGA-inhibition and subsequent accumulation of O-glycosylated proteins. In line with this, inhibition of GFAT-1 by means of AZA was found to result in opposite effects. Hence, we concluded that HBP functionality and O-GlcNAcylation, respectively, is essential for cartilage homeostasis and provides protection against trauma-induced pathomechanisms. Accordingly, expression of OGT and O-GlcNAcylation is thought to be responsive to cellular stress, comprising oxidative stress, ER stress, ischemia reperfusion injury, and more; however, only little is known about regulation of OGA in injured cells [36,37]. Stress-induced upregulation of OGT leads to enhanced O-GlcNAc levels and can be considered a pro-survival signaling program, while, in contrast, reduced O-GlcNAcylation increases susceptibility of cells and tissues to injury [36,38,39]. Surprisingly, cartilage trauma did not induce the gene expression of OGT but OGA, which was also observed in highly degenerated tissue (ICRS score $\geq$ 3). Comparable findings were described by Tardio et al., who determined a similar alteration of the OGA to OGT ratio in cartilage of OA patients, as well as after IL-1b stimulation of isolated OA chondrocytes [13]. It might be possible that the responsiveness of this pro-survival signaling program decreases with age. In fact, aging has a high impact on protein O-GlcNAcylation and vice-versa. Accumulation of O-GlcNAc modified proteins has been associated with development and progression of various age-related diseases and was found in OA cartilage tissue, despite enhanced OGA levels [12,13]. Comparable accumulation of O-GlcNAc modified proteins has also been described in aged retina; however, though, the addition of PUGNAc or UDP-GlcNAc and subsequent enhancement of O-GlcNAcylation reduced intracellular oxidative stress levels [35], which corroborates our findings.

Direct inhibition of GFAT-1 by AZA, and thus attenuation of all HBP-associated processes, resulted in enhanced expression of catabolic enzymes and subsequent ECM destruction after cartilage trauma. This was demonstrated by increased concentrations of type II collagen breakdown product C2C and severe PG depletion in Saf-O stained cartilage explants. However, loss of PG in AZA-treated cartilage explants might also be a result of both enhancement of protease activity and decrease of ECM synthesis, as shown in reduced gene expression of COL2A1, HAS2, and ACAN, as well as type II collagen synthesis. There is only little known about the impact of GFAT-1 inhibition by AZA or any other component in cartilage; however, Honda et al. reported significant impairment in the synthesis of cartilage-characteristic PG-H in chicken embryos exposed to AZA [40].

4. Materials and Methods

4.1. Specimen Preparation and Cultivation Conditions

Overall, macroscopically intact tissue samples (International Cartilage Repair Society (ICRS) score $\leq$ 1) from femoral condyles of 15 patients (mean age 63 years; 8 male and 7 female patients) were included in the study. Human cartilage was obtained from donors undergoing total knee joint replacement due to OA. Informed consent was obtained from all patients according to the terms of the Ethics Committee of the University of Ulm. Full-thickness cartilage explants ($\varnothing$ = 6 mm) were harvested, weighed, and cultivated in serum-containing medium (1:1 DMEM/Ham's F12 supplemented with 10% fetal bovine serum, 0.5% penicillin/streptomycin (PAA Laboratories, Pasching, Austria), 0.5% L-glutamine, and 10 µg/mL 2-phospho-L-ascorbic acid trisodium salt) for 24 h in an incubator (37 °C, 5% CO_2, 95% humidity). Afterwards, the explants were traumatized and cultivated for 7 days and 14 days (only for histological assessment), respectively, in serum-free medium (DMEM supplemented with 1% sodium pyruvate, 0.5% L-glutamine, 1% non-essential amino acids, 0.5% penicillin/streptomycin, 10 µg/mL 2-phospho-L-ascorbic acid trisodium salt, and 0.1% insulin-transferrin-sodium selenite (Sigma-Aldrich, Taufkirchen, Germany)). All chemicals were purchased from Biochrom (Berlin, Germany), unless specified otherwise. Additionally, highly degenerated (ICRS score $\geq$ 3) and corresponding macroscopically intact tissue samples (ICRS grade $\leq$ 1) of 7 patients (mean age 67 years) were immediately snap frozen for RNA isolation to evaluate degeneration-associated changes in gene expression.

4.2. Impact Loading and Subsequent Treatment

The cartilage explants were subjected to a single impact load of 0.59 J using a drop-tower model, as previously described [41], and further cultivated under serum-free conditions (described above). Unloaded explants served as controls. Impacted cartilage explants were treated with the following additives (Sigma-Aldrich) for 7 and 14 days, respectively: GlcNAc or GS (each 0.1–10 mM), an inhibitor of O-GlcNAcase (PUGNAc (O-(2-acetamido-2deoxy-D-glucopyranosylidene)amino-N-phenylcarbamate): 0.05–0.15 mM) or the GFAT1-inhibitor azaserine (AZA: 0.005–0.1 mM) (Figure 1). Fresh additives were added concomitantly with medium change every 2–3 days.

4.3. Live/Dead Cell Cytotoxicity Assay

To determine the percentage of viable cells 7 days after trauma, a live/dead viability/cytotoxicity assay (Molecular Probes, Invitrogen) was performed, as previously described [42]. In short, unfixed tissue sections (0.5 mm thickness) were stained with 1 µM calcein AM and 2 µM ethidium homodimer-1 for 30 min. After washing in PBS, they were microscopically analyzed by means of a z-stack module (software AxioVision, Carl Zeiss, Jena, Germany). Three pictures were made from each tissue section. All cells on the picture were counted manually (Image J software version 1.42q). The average count per picture was about 2000 cells.

4.4. mRNA Isolation and cDNA Synthesis

For total RNA isolation 7 days after trauma, cryopreserved cartilage explants were pulverized with a microdismembrator S (B. Braun Biotech, Melsungen, Germany). Subsequently, RNA was isolated using the Lipid Tissue Mini Kit (Qiagen, Hilden, Germany). RNA was reverse transcribed with the Omniscript RT Kit (Qiagen) and used for quantitative real-time PCR analysis (StepOne-PlusTM Real-Time PCR System, Applied Biosystems, Darmstadt, Germany).

4.5. Quantitative Real-Time Polymerase Chain Reaction (qRT-PCR)

Determination of the relative expression levels was performed by means of qRT-PCR analysis using the $\Delta\Delta$ Ct method. To detect desired sequences, a TaqManTM Gene Expression Master Mix for TaqMan Gene Expression Assay (both Applied Biosystems) was used for the following probes: Hs00192708_m1 (ADAMTS4), Hs00199841_m1 (ADAMTS5), Hs00264051_m1 (COL2A1), Hs00899865_m1 (GFAT-1), Hs00193435_m1 (HAS2), Hs02800695_m1 (HPRT1), Hs00899658 (MMP-1), Hs00233992_m1 (MMP-13), Hs01028844_m1 (OGA/MGEA5), and Hs00269228_m1 (OGT). Power SYBR Green PCR Master Mix (Applied Biosystems) was used for 18S rRNA, 5′- CGCAGCTAGGAATAATGGAATAGG-3′ (forward), 5′ -CATGGCCT CAGTT CCGAAA-3′ (reverse), and Platinum SYBR Green qPCR SuperMix-UDG (Invitrogen, Darmstadt, Germany) for GAPDH, 5′-TGGTATCGTGGAAGGAC TCATG-3′ (forward), and 5′-TCTTCTGGGTGGCAGTGATG-3′ (reverse). mRNA expression was determined by normalizing the expression levels separately to the endogenous controls (18S rRNA, GAPDH, and HPRT1) and subsequently calculating the ratio mean values in relation to the gene expression level of the untreated, unimpacted control.

4.6. Culture Media Analysis by Means of Commercial ELISA Kits

Biomarker release into culture media (7 days after trauma) was evaluated by means of enzyme-linked immunosorbent assays (ELISAs): secreted MMP-13 was determined using the Human Quantikine ELISA kit (Ray-Biotech, Norcross, GA, USA). Evaluation of type II collagen synthesis was performed using a CPII ELISA (Ibex, Québec, QC, Canada). The assay quantified type II collagen carboxy propeptide (CP II) cleaved from pro-collagen II after its release into the matrix and directly correlated with newly synthetized type II collagen. Degradation of type II collagen was measured using a C2C ELISA (Ibex), detecting a neoepitope generated during collagenase-mediated breakdown of type II collagen. Aggrecanase activity was measured using the Sensitive Aggrecanase Activity Assay from Biotez (Berlin, Germany) for serum-free cell culture supernatants. The kit consists of two modules. First, the substrate (modified aggrecan interglobular domain) is proteolytically cleaved by sample-derived aggrecanases, releasing a peptide with a N-terminal ARGSVIL sequence. This peptide can then be quantified via the specific ELISA module. In principle, the assay quantifies the total aggrecanase activity, comprising that of ADAMTS-1, -4, and -5.

The total amounts of MMP-13, C2C, and CP II, as well as the aggrecanase activity, were relativized on the weight multiplied by cell viability of the corresponding cartilage explant [41,42].

4.7. Gelatin Zymography

Quantification of pro-MMP-2 and active MMP-2 was performed by gelatin zymography, as previously described [41]. In short, culture media (7 days after trauma) were mixed 1:2 with nonreducing zymogram sample buffer (Bio-Rad, Munich, Germany), loaded onto 10% polyacrylamide gels (Carl Roth, Karlsruhe, Germany) containing 2 mg/mL gelatin (Merck, Darmstadt, Deutschland). After electrophoresis (Mini-PROTEAN Tetra Cell System, Bio-Rad), the gels were washed in zymogram renaturation buffer twice for 15 min and incubated in zymogram development buffer for 20 h at 37 °C (both Bio-Rad). Staining with Coomassie solution and subsequent destaining revealed clear bands originating from MMP activity. Band intensities (INT*mm^2) were quantified with the Geldoc XR system (Bio-Rad) and relativized on tissue weight and cell viability, as mentioned above. An internal standard (positive control) was run on each gel and used to reduce the inter assay variance.

4.8. Safranin-O Staining

To evaluate the content of PG within the cartilage tissue, appropriate histological analysis was performed exemplarily ($n = 1$) 14 days after trauma. In short, explants were fixed (4% paraformaldehyde) and embedded in paraffin. Dewaxed and rehydrated sections (3.5 µm) were stained with SafO (Thermo Fisher Scientific, Schwerte, Germany) and Fast Green (Sigma-Aldrich), followed by a final staining of the cell nuclei by Gill's hematoxylin No. 3 (Sigma-Aldrich) and documentation with an Axioskop 2 mot plus (Zeiss, Oberkochen, Germany).

4.9. Statistical Analysis

Experiments were analyzed using GraphPad Prism8 (GraphPad Software Inc., La Jolla, CA, USA). Each data point represented an individual donor (biological replicate); technical replicates from the same donor were not performed. Data sets with $n \geq 5$ were tested for outliers by means of the Grubbs outlier test. Outliers were not included in statistical analyses. For parametric data sets, a one-way analysis of variance (ANOVA) with the Sidak post-test was used. Nonparametric data sets were analyzed by means of a Kruskal–Wallis test with Dunn's post-test. For data sets derived from highly degenerated tissue (ICRS grade $\geq$ 3), an unpaired two-tailed t-test was performed. The significant level was set to a = 0.05. Values in diagrams are given as boxplots (median; whiskers: min to max).

5. Conclusions

In conclusion, our results demonstrate the overall importance of the HBP in cartilage homeostasis and degeneration processes, which could be significantly influenced by targeted modification. In this context, we observed predominately chondroprotective and chondroanabolic effects associated with O-GlcNAcylation and the HBP after ex vivo cartilage trauma, implying that alteration of the glycosylation profile might have a detrimental impact on cartilage homeostasis. However, it cannot be excluded that excessive accumulation of O-GlcNAc modified proteins in age might negatively affect cartilage homeostasis in the same manner as its decline, as confirmed by the alteration in the gene expression of HBP-related enzymes in ex vivo traumatized macroscopically intact and in vivo highly degenerated OA cartilage. So far, it is not known whether this reflects a primary pathogenic event or an insufficient protective mechanism in aging and OA, respectively. With respect to various studies reporting contradictory effects of enhanced O-GlcNAcylation in aging, we conclude that this post-transcriptional modification might be a two-edged sword, in particular regarding degenerative diseases. However, in the early post-traumatic situation, the HBP may represent a promising therapeutic target.

Author Contributions: Conceptualization, R.E.B. and J.R.; validation, J.R. and J.B.; investigation, J.R. and J.B.; writing—original draft preparation, J.R.; writing—review and editing, R.E.B., J.B., J.R. and F.Z.; visualization, J.R.; project administration, R.E.B. and J.R.; funding acquisition, R.E.B., J.R. and F.Z. All authors have read and agreed to the published version of the manuscript.

Funding: This research study was funded by the Deutsche Initiative Arthroseforschung of the German Society of Orthopedics and Orthopedic Surgery (DGOOC). Moreover, this project was supported by the European Social Fund and by the Ministry of Science, Research and Arts Baden-Württemberg.

Institutional Review Board Statement: The study was conducted according to the guidelines of the Declaration of Helsinki and approved by the Ethical Committee of the University of Ulm, Germany (ethical approval number 353/18).

Informed Consent Statement: Informed consent was obtained from all subjects involved in the study.

Data Availability Statement: Data are contained within the article.

Conflicts of Interest: The authors declare no conflict of interest. The funders had no role in the design of the study; in the collection, analyses, or interpretation of data; in the writing of the manuscript, or in the decision to publish the results.

References

1. Hunter, D.J.; Schofield, D.; Callander, E. The individual and socioeconomic impact of osteoarthritis. *Nat. Rev. Rheumatol.* **2014**, *10*, 437–441. [CrossRef]
2. Thomas, A.C.; Hubbard-Turner, T.; Wikstrom, E.A.; Palmieri-Smith, R.M. Epidemiology of Posttraumatic Osteoarthritis. *J. Athl. Train.* **2017**, *52*, 491–496. [CrossRef]
3. Riegger, J.; Brenner, R.E. Pathomechanisms of Posttraumatic Osteoarthritis: Chondrocyte Behavior and Fate in a Precarious Environment. *Int. J. Mol. Sci.* **2020**, *21*, 1560. [CrossRef] [PubMed]
4. Bannuru, R.R.; Osani, M.C.; Vaysbrot, E.E.; Arden, N.K.; Bennell, K.; Bierma-Zeinstra, S.M.A. OARSI guidelines for the non-surgical management of knee, hip, and polyarticular osteoarthritis. *Osteoarthr. Cartil.* **2019**, *27*, 1578–1589. [CrossRef] [PubMed]

5. Bruyère, O.; Burlet, N.; Delmas, P.D.; Rizzoli, R.; Cooper, C.; Reginster, J.Y. Evaluation of symptomatic slow-acting drugs in osteoarthritis using the GRADE system. *BMC Musculoskelet. Disord.* **2008**, *9*, 165. [CrossRef] [PubMed]

6. Salazar, J.; Bello, L.; Chávez, M.; Añez, R.; Rojas, J.; Bermúdez, V. Glucosamine for Osteoarthritis: Biological Effects, Clinical Efficacy, and Safety on Glucose Metabolism. *Arthritis* **2014**, 1–13. [CrossRef] [PubMed]

7. Sun, C.; Shang, J.; Yao, Y.; Yin, X.; Liu, M.; Liu, H.; Zhou, Y. O-GlcNAcylation: A bridge between glucose and cell differentiation. *J. Cell. Mol. Med.* **2016**, *20*, 769–781. [CrossRef]

8. Kiani, C.; Chen, L.; Wu, Y.J.; Yee, A.J.; Yang, B.B. Structure and function of aggrecan. *Cell Res.* **2002**, *12*, 19–32. [CrossRef] [PubMed]

9. Chatham, J.C.; Nöt, L.G.; Fülöp, N.; Marchase, R.B. Hexosamine biosynthesis and protein O-glycosylation: The first line of defense against stress, ischemia, and trauma. *Shock* **2008**, *29*, 431–440. [CrossRef]

10. Hart, G.W.; Slawson, C.; Ramirez-Correa, G.; Lagerlof, O. Cross Talk Between O-GlcNAcylation and Phosphorylation: Roles in Signaling, Transcription, and Chronic Disease. *Annu. Rev. Biochem.* **2011**, *80*, 825–858. [CrossRef]

11. Tardio, L.; Andres, J.; Herrero-Beaumont, G.; Largo, R. Protein o-linked n-acetylglucosamine levels in the cartilage of patients with knee osteoarthritis. *Ann. Rheum. Dis.* **2011**, *70*, A86. [CrossRef]

12. Banerjee, P.S.; Lagerlöf, O.; Hart, G.W. Roles of O-GlcNAc in chronic diseases of aging. *Mol. Aspects Med.* **2016**, *51*, 1–15. [CrossRef]

13. Tardio, L.; Andrés-Bergós, J.; Zachara, N.E.; Larrañaga-Vera, A.; Rodriguez-Villar, C.; Herrero-Beaumont, G. O-linked N-acetylglucosamine (O-GlcNAc) protein modification is increased in the cartilage of patients with knee osteoarthritis. *Osteoarthr. Cartil.* **2014**, *22*, 259–263. [CrossRef]

14. Derfoul, A.; Miyoshi, A.D.; Freeman, D.E.; Tuan, R.S. Glucosamine promotes chondrogenic phenotype in both chondrocytes and mesenchymal stem cells and inhibits MMP-13 expression and matrix degradation. *Osteoarthr. Cartil.* **2007**, *15*, 646–655. [CrossRef] [PubMed]

15. Ma, Y.; Zheng, W.; Chen, H.; Shao, X.; Lin, P.; Liu, X.; Ye, H. Glucosamine promotes chondrocyte proliferation via the Wnt/β-catenin signaling pathway. *Int. J. Mol. Med.* **2018**. [CrossRef] [PubMed]

16. Uitterlinden, E.J.; Jahr, H.; Koevoet, J.L.M.; Jenniskens, Y.M.; Bierma-Zeinstra, S.M.A.; DeGroot, J.; Van Osch, G.J.V.M. Glucosamine decreases expression of anabolic and catabolic genes in human osteoarthritic cartilage explants. *Osteoarthr. Cartil.* **2006**, *14*, 250–257. [CrossRef] [PubMed]

17. Valvason, C.; Musacchio, E.; Pozzuoli, A.; Ramonda, R.; Aldegheri, R.; Punzi, L. Influence of glucosamine sulphate on oxidative stress in human osteoarthritic chondrocytes: Effects on HO-1, p22Phox and iNOS expression. *Rheumatology* **2008**, *47*, 31–35. [CrossRef]

18. Altman, R.D.; Abramson, S.; Bruyere, O.; Clegg, D.; Herrero-Beaumont, G.; Maheu, E.; Reginster, J.Y. Commentary: Osteoarthritis of the knee and glucosamine. *Osteoarthr. Cartil.* **2006**, *14*, 963–966. [CrossRef]

19. Fransen, M.; Agaliotis, M.; Nairn, L.; Votrubec, M.; Bridgett, L.; Su, S.; Day, R. Glucosamine and chondroitin for knee osteoarthritis: A double-blind randomised placebo-controlled clinical trial evaluating single and combination regimens. *Ann. Rheum. Dis.* **2015**, *74*, 851–858. [CrossRef]

20. Kang, Y.-H.; Park, S.; Ahn, C.; Song, J.; Kim, D.; Jin, E.-J. Beneficial reward-to-risk action of glucosamine during pathogenesis of osteoarthritis. *Eur. J. Med. Res.* **2015**, *20*, 89. [CrossRef]

21. Jordan, K.M. EULAR Recommendations 2003: An evidence based approach to the management of knee osteoarthritis: Report of a Task Force of the Standing Committee for International Clinical Studies Including Therapeutic Trials (ESCISIT). *Ann. Rheum. Dis.* **2003**, *62*, 1145–1155. [CrossRef]

22. Jerosch, J. Effects of Glucosamine and Chondroitin Sulfate on Cartilage Metabolism in OA: Outlook on Other Nutrient Partners Especially Omega-3 Fatty Acids. *Int. J. Rheumatol.* **2011**, 1–17. [CrossRef]

23. Caramés, B.; Taniguchi, N.; Otsuki, S.; Blanco, F.J.; Lotz, M. Autophagy is a protective mechanism in normal cartilage, and its aging-related loss is linked with cell death and osteoarthritis. *Arthritis Rheum.* **2010**, *62*, 791–801. [CrossRef]

24. Caramés, B.; Taniguchi, N.; Seino, D.; Blanco, F.J.; D'Lima, D.; Lotz, M. Mechanical injury suppresses autophagy regulators and pharmacologic activation of autophagy results in chondroprotection. *Arthritis Rheum.* **2012**, *64*, 1182–1192. [CrossRef]

25. Caramés, B.; Kiosses, W.B.; Akasaki, Y.; Brinson, D.C.; Eap, W.; Koziol, J.; Lotz, M.K. Glucosamine Activates Autophagy In Vitro and In Vivo: Glucosamine-Induced Activation of Autophagy. *Arthritis Rheum.* **2013**, *65*, 1843–1852. [CrossRef]

26. de Mattei, M.; Pellati, A.; Pasello, M.; de Terlizzi, F.; Massari, L.; Gemmati, D.; Caruso, A. High doses of glucosamine-HCl have detrimental effects on bovine articular cartilage explants cultured in vitro. *Osteoarthr. Cartil.* **2002**, *10*, 816–825. [CrossRef] [PubMed]

27. Lv, C.; Wang, L.; Zhu, X.; Lin, W.; Chen, X.; Huang, Z.; Yang, S. Glucosamine promotes osteoblast proliferation by modulating autophagy via the mammalian target of rapamycin pathway. *Biomed. Pharm.* **2018**, *99*, 271–277. [CrossRef] [PubMed]

28. Shikhman, A.R.; Brinson, D.C.; Valbracht, J.; Lotz, M.K. Differential metabolic effects of glucosamine and N-acetylglucosamine in human articular chondrocytes. *Osteoarthr. Cartil.* **2009**, *17*, 1022–1028. [CrossRef] [PubMed]

29. Schegg, B.; Hülsmeier, A.J.; Rutschmann, C.; Maag, C.; Hennet, T. Core Glycosylation of Collagen Is Initiated by Two β(1-O)Galactosyltransferases. *Mol. Cell. Biol.* **2009**, *29*, 943–952. [CrossRef]

30. Gouze, J.-N.; Gouze, E.; Popp, M.P.; Bush, M.L.; Dacanay, E.A.; Kay, J.D.; Ghivizzani, S.C. Exogenous glucosamine globally protects chondrocytes from the arthritogenic effects of IL-1beta. *Arthritis Res. Ther.* **2006**, *8*, R173. [CrossRef] [PubMed]

31. Sandy, J.D.; Gamett, D.; Thompson, V.; Verscharen, C. Chondrocyte-mediated catabolism of aggrecan: Aggrecanase-dependent cleavage induced by interleukin-1 or retinoic acid can be inhibited by glucosamine. *Biochem. J.* **1998**, *335*, 59–66. [CrossRef]
32. d'Abusco, S.A.; Calamia, V.; Cicione, C.; Grigolo, B.; Politi, L.; Scandurra, R. Glucosamine affects intracellular signalling through inhibition of mitogen-activated protein kinase phosphorylation in human chondrocytes. *Arthritis Res. Ther.* **2007**, *9*, R104. [CrossRef]
33. Shikhman, A.R.; Kuhn, K.; Alaaeddine, N.; Lotz, M. N-Acetylglucosamine prevents IL-1β-mediated activation of human chondrocytes. *J. Immunol.* **2001**, *166*, 5155–5160. [CrossRef]
34. Andrés-Bergós, J.; Tardio, L.; Larranaga-Vera, A.; Gómez, R.; Herrero-Beaumont, G.; Largo, R. The increase in O-linked N-acetylglucosamine protein modification stimulates chondrogenic differentiation both in vitro and in vivo. *J. Biol. Chem.* **2012**, *287*, 33615–33628. [CrossRef] [PubMed]
35. Zhao, L.; Feng, Z.; Zou, X.; Cao, K.; Xu, J.; Liu, J. Aging leads to elevation of O-GlcNAcylation and disruption of mitochondrial homeostasis in retina. *Oxid. Med. Cell. Longev.* **2014**, 1–11. [CrossRef] [PubMed]
36. Groves, J.A.; Lee, A.; Yildirir, G.; Zachara, N.E. Dynamic O-GlcNAcylation and its roles in the cellular stress response and homeostasis. *Cell Stress Chaperones* **2013**, *18*, 535–558. [CrossRef]
37. Martinez, M.R.; Dias, T.B.; Natov, P.S.; Zachara, N.E. Stress-induced O-GlcNAcylation: An adaptive process of injured cells. *Biochem. Soc. Trans.* **2017**, *45*, 237–249. [CrossRef]
38. Champattanachai, V.; Marchase, R.B.; Chatham, J.C. Glucosamine protects neonatal cardiomyocytes from ischemia-reperfusion injury via increased protein-associated O-GlcNAc. *Am. J. Physiol. Cell Physiol.* **2007**, *292*, C178–C187. [CrossRef]
39. Ngoh, G.A.; Facundo, H.T.; Hamid, T.; Dillmann, W.; Zachara, N.E.; Jones, S.P. Unique Hexosaminidase Reduces Metabolic Survival Signal and Sensitizes Cardiac Myocytes to Hypoxia/Reoxygenation Injury. *Circ. Res.* **2009**, *104*, 41–49. [CrossRef]
40. Honda, A.; Tsuboi, I.; Kimata, K.; Hirabayashi, Y.; Yamada, K.; Mori, Y. Abnormal synthesis of cartilage-characteristic proteoglycan in azaserine-induced micromelial limbs. *Biochem. J.* **1989**, *261*, 627–635. [CrossRef]
41. Riegger, J.; Joos, H.; Palm, H.-G.; Friemert, B.; Reichel, H.; Ignatius, A.; Brenner, R.E. Antioxidative therapy in an ex vivo human cartilage trauma-model: Attenuation of trauma-induced cell loss and ECM-destructive enzymes by N-acetyl cysteine. *Osteoarthr. Cartil.* **2016**, *24*, 2171–2180. [CrossRef] [PubMed]
42. Riegger, J.; Joos, H.; Palm, H.-G.; Friemert, B.; Reichel, H.; Ignatius, A.; Brenner, R.E. Striking a new path in reducing cartilage breakdown: Combination of antioxidative therapy and chondroanabolic stimulation after blunt cartilage trauma. *J. Cell. Mol. Med.* **2018**, *22*, 77–88. [CrossRef] [PubMed]

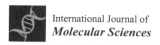

International Journal of
Molecular Sciences

MDPI

Article

A Novel Method Facilitating the Simple and Low-Cost Preparation of Human Osteochondral Slice Explants for Large-Scale Native Tissue Analysis

Jacob Spinnen [1,*], Lennard K. Shopperly [1], Carsten Rendenbach [2], Anja A. Kühl [3], Ufuk Sentürk [4], Daniel Kendoff [5], Shabnam Hemmati-Sadeghi [1], Michael Sittinger [1] and Tilo Dehne [1]

1   Department of Rheumatology, Charité-Universitätsmedizin Berlin, Corporate Member of Freie Universität Berlin, Humboldt Universität zu Berlin, and Berlin Institute of Health, 10117 Berlin, Germany; lennard.shopperly@charite.de (L.K.S.); shabnam.hemmati-sadeghi@charite.de (S.H.-S.); michael.sittinger@charite.de (M.S.); tilo.dehne@charite.de (T.D.)
2   Department of Oral and Maxillofacial Surgery, Charité-Universitätsmedizin Berlin, Corporate Member of Freie Universität Berlin, Humboldt Universität zu Berlin, and Berlin Institute of Health, 13353 Berlin, Germany; carsten.rendenbach@charite.de
3   iPATH Histopathology Core Unit, Charité-Universitätsmedizin Berlin, Corporate Member of Freie Universität Berlin, Humboldt Universität zu Berlin, and Berlin Institute of Health, 13353 Berlin, Germany; anja.kuehl@charite.de
4   Department of Orthopedics, Charité-Universitätsmedizin Berlin, Corporate Member of Freie Universität Berlin, Humboldt Universität zu Berlin, and Berlin Institute of Health, 13353 Berlin, Germany; ufuk.sentuerk@charite.de
5   Department of Orthopaedic Surgery, Helios Klinikum Berlin-Buch, 13125 Berlin, Germany; daniel.kendoff@helios-gesundheit.de
*   Correspondence: jacob.spinnen@charite.de

Citation: Spinnen, J.; Shopperly, L.K.; Rendenbach, C.; Kühl, A.A.; Sentürk, U.; Kendoff, D.; Hemmati-Sadeghi, S.; Sittinger, M.; Dehne, T. A Novel Method Facilitating the Simple and Low-Cost Preparation of Human Osteochondral Slice Explants for Large-Scale Native Tissue Analysis. *Int. J. Mol. Sci.* **2021**, *22*, 6394. https://doi.org/10.3390/ijms22126394

Academic Editor: Lih Kuo

Received: 25 May 2021
Accepted: 9 June 2021
Published: 15 June 2021

Abstract: For in vitro modeling of human joints, osteochondral explants represent an acceptable compromise between conventional cell culture and animal models. However, the scarcity of native human joint tissue poses a challenge for experiments requiring high numbers of samples and makes the method rather unsuitable for toxicity analyses and dosing studies. To scale their application, we developed a novel method that allows the preparation of up to 100 explant cultures from a single human sample with a simple setup. Explants were cultured for 21 days, stimulated with TNF-α or TGF-β3, and analyzed for cell viability, gene expression and histological changes. Tissue cell viability remained stable at >90% for three weeks. Proteoglycan levels and gene expression of *COL2A1*, *ACAN* and *COMP* were maintained for 14 days before decreasing. TNF-α and TGF-β3 caused dose-dependent changes in cartilage marker gene expression as early as 7 days. Histologically, cultures under TNF-α stimulation showed a 32% reduction in proteoglycans, detachment of collagen fibers and cell swelling after 7 days. In conclusion, thin osteochondral slice cultures behaved analogously to conventional punch explants despite cell stress exerted during fabrication. In pharmacological testing, both the shorter diffusion distance and the lack of need for serum in the culture suggest a positive effect on sensitivity. The ease of fabrication and the scalability of the sample number make this manufacturing method a promising platform for large-scale preclinical testing in joint research.

Keywords: osteoarthritis; osteochondral explant culture; joint modelling; pharmacological assay; native tissue analysis

1. Introduction

Osteoarthritis (OA) is a condition involving the degeneration of articular cartilage, sclerosis of subchondral bone and chronic inflammation of the synovial membrane. To date, it is the main cause of physical disability worldwide [1,2]. Both the underlying pathomechanisms of OA as well as the mechanisms of physiological reorganization of cartilage tissue are poorly understood. Due to this lack of understanding, the treatment of such defects remains challenging. However, research in recent years has provided increasing evidence that cartilage cells have the general ability to regenerate if stimulated correctly. Limited traumatic cartilage defects can now be successfully treated and regenerated by autologous chondrocyte transplantation and specific cell-modulating substances. The emergence of growth factors as therapeutic agents is expected to further enable the regeneration of osteochondral tissue [3–5], increasing the need for an adequate platform to assess cartilage (repair) treatment strategies.

Traditionally, two-dimensional chondrocyte cultures in monolayer and OA animal models have been the main tools available for preclinical testing of the efficacy and side effects (ADME (absorption, distribution, metabolism, excretion) screening) of such substances. Unfortunately, the former often leads to limited insights due to the lack of representation of the complex tissue composition of the joint, while the latter, in addition to ethical aspects, entails high costs and time expenditure and is therefore usually only applied when a basic efficacy already seems very likely [6,7]. Recently, this spectrum has been expanded to include sophisticated 3D cultures and organ-on-chip applications. However, 3D cultures are either effortful to maintain or, in the case of joint-on-a-chip, not yet commercially available. Therefore, rapid, agile research and development of regenerative therapeutics for cartilage regeneration is limited to a certain extent [8–10].

A sustainable middle ground in joint modelling is the use of tissue explants. Explants are living, native and functional parts from organs, which are obtained from donor tissues or cadavers. Explants can accurately represent part of the tissue composition and architecture. Specifically, the tissue cells remain in their native extracellular matrix (ECM) configuration and questions regarding their response to biological stimuli can be answered much more reliably in the native situation than, for example, with monolayer cultures of only one cell type [11–13]. However, this modelling technique is severely limited by the availability of donor tissue. Employing the frequently used technique of vertical punching of the tissue and subsequential production of osteochondral punchings with diameters of at least 3 mm, only a very small number of explants can be produced from a tissue sample, depending on the tissue properties. Furthermore, the diffusion of nutrients and potentially interacting proteins is severely impeded by the amount of glycosaminoglycans in the tissue [14]. Hence, the explant thickness negatively correlates with information that can be obtained about the behavior of cells located deeper in the tissue.

To address this issue, we have developed a low-cost and uncomplex method to produce explant cultures using a thin-section approach. Similar to the live-slice technology known from neurophysiology, the method allows the production of vital tissue slices with a thickness of 500–800 μm [15]. This allows the production of up to 100 slice cultures from a single tissue sample for subsequential analysis of many different substances and concentrations. Furthermore, the thin tissue architecture is suitable for easy-to-maintain semi-static culture conditions, as the perfusion distance is sufficiently short to reliably guide both nutrients and any therapeutic agents through the tissue to the target cells.

This study aimed to analyze the suitability of osteochondral slices for osteochondral tissue modelling and pharmacological screening of biologically active substances. For this purpose, we obtained a large number of human slice cultures from surgically explanted tibial plateaus and analyzed the behavior of the tissue over 21 days at the histological, metabolic and transcriptional levels. Furthermore, we examined the reactivity of the embedded chondrocytes to the factors TNF-α and TGF-β3, known to affect cartilage matrix synthesis, to determine whether the tissue is in a sufficiently close state to that of the native situation to be used as a testing device [16,17].

2. Results

To develop a physiological model for osteochondral tissue which allows for quick handling and high-throughput applications with limited donor material at hand, we developed a method for the manufacturing of native osteochondral live slice cultures from human joint tissue. 500–800 μm thick osteochondral slice cultures were prepared from 23 different surgically explanted tibial plateaus using a custom-made microtome insert and then cultured in hanging inserts of 24-well plates. In this study, we assessed whether the explanted live slice cultures maintain their physiological properties such as long-term cell viability, gene expression, extracellular matrix and responsiveness towards biological stimuli.

2.1. Suitability for Slicing Varies with the Degree of Subchondral Bone Sclerosis

23 of 25 donors were suitable for the production of slice explants. The extent of subchondral sclerosis of the bone proved to be a decisive factor for the suitability of slice culture production. The brittleness of the bone increases sharply with the degree of sclerosis, leading to the subchondral cancellous bone not being cut smoothly by the impact of the blade but instead being crushed. Three punch cylinders were easily obtained from all other donors, from each of which 30–36 slice cultures could be safely produced. For reasons of logistical feasibility, we only cultivated the slice cultures from one punch at a time-from a technical perspective, the cultivation of 90–100 slice cultures per donor would have been possible.

2.2. Confocal Laser Scanning Microscopy Shows Highly Conserved Spatial Cell Order

To validate the use of the resazurin assay and to evaluate the spatial distribution of living and dead cells, additional live/dead determination via CLSM was performed on 13 slices of two donors (7 and 8) after three weeks of culture. The slice explant cultures were thin enough to penetrate deep into the tissue layers with confocal laser microscopy and produce a three-dimensional image of the cell distribution- and vitality (3D rendered video in supplemental files). The analysis revealed >90% viability in non-heated slices, roughly 50% viability in slices that were heated for 30 min at 60 °C, and <10% chondrocyte viability after 60 min of heating (Figure 1a). Chondrocytes remained localized in their cartilage-typical, spatial alignment (column-like deep zone; pearl-bead structure in the mid-zone; tightly packed cells in the superficial zone, Figure 1a). No cell culture effects due to nutrition gradients were observed (e.g., no elongated cells in the peripheral tissue).

2.3. Resazurin Assay Correlates with Optically Determined Viability

To ensure that the resazurin assay sufficiently reflects viability and is not obstructed by the dense osteochondral ECM, samples of varying viability (obtained by heating at 60 °C) were analyzed with the resazurin metabolic assay and by live/dead determination via PI/FDA staining and CLSM analysis. The results of both methods were correlated, as shown by the correlation coefficient of $R^2 = 80$–84.5% (Figure 1b). We regarded this as sufficient to assess the general viability state of the tissue culture. Further viability analyses of tissue cultures were therefore performed using the resazurin assay since it allows for progredient viability analysis of the same tissue slice in a non-destructible manner.

2.4. Cell Viability Is Maintained in F^- and Increased in F^+ Groups over 21 Days

After 7 days, F^- cultured slices of the cytokine-stimulated groups exhibited either a slight increase or maintenance of viability as determined by the resazurin assay. Stimulation with TNF-α resulted in $101 \pm 23\%$ (10 ng/mL) and $106 \pm 31\%$ (40 ng/mL) compared to control, while TGF-β3 stimulated slices exhibited an increase to $113 \pm 26\%$. Unstimulated slices showed a slight decrease to $91 \pm 34\%$. No significant differences in viability from day 0 to day 7 as well as between the four different cytokine stimulation groups were observed. Addition of FBS to the culture medium resulted in significantly increased viability values in all stimulated groups (TNF-α: $214 \pm 58\%$ (low), $227 \pm 84\%$ (high); TGF-β3: $218 \pm 48\%$) and the control ($231 \pm 50\%$) (Figure 1c(i)). During three-week culture without FBS viability values of 114 ± 43, $108 \pm 52\%$ and $113 \pm 55\%$ were observed after 7, 14 and 21 days, respectively. Statistical analysis revealed no significant differences in viability between the timepoints (Figure 1c(ii)).

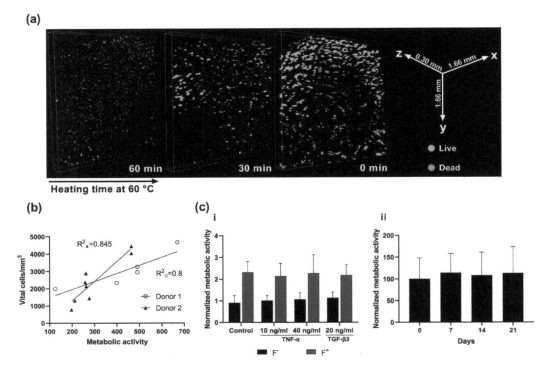

Figure 1. Viability analysis of osteochondral live slices. (**a**) Confocal laser scanning microscopy of slices at three weeks of culture following heating at 60 °C for 0, 30 or 60 min and live/dead staining with PI/FDA. Vital cells appear green, while dead cells appear red. (**b**) Correlation analysis of vital cell count as determined by CLSM and metabolic activity as determined by AlamarBlue resazurin assay. Two donors and a total of 13 slices with varying viability were analyzed and revealed correlation coefficients of 0.8 and 0.845. (**c**) Resazurin assay results with and without additional stimulation. i: Viability of slices on day 7 relative to day 0. Slices were stimulated with 10 or 40 ng/mL TNF-α or with 20 ng/mL TGF-β3, and either with or without FBS. ii: Viability of slices without FBS or other stimulating factors over 21 days, relative to day 0.

2.5. Expression of Cartilage-Typical Markers ACAN and COL2A1 Is Maintained for 14 Days in Unstimulated Slice Culture

Expression of cartilage-relevant genes *COL2A1* and *ACAN* remained stable relative to their day 0 value for 14 days and declined significantly by day 21 in unstimulated slice cultures (no stimulating factors, no FBS) (*COL2A1*: $32 \pm 23\%$, $p < 0.001$; *ACAN*: $51 \pm 64\%$, $p < 0.05$; Figure 2a). Cartilage remodeling marker *COL1A1* showed a short increase after 7 days but returned to levels comparable to day 0 by day 21. Expression of *COMP* decreased sooner and significantly to $45 \pm 30\%$ after 7 days and further to $27 \pm 21\%$ and $14 \pm 12\%$ after 14 and 21 days (all *p*-values < 0.001).

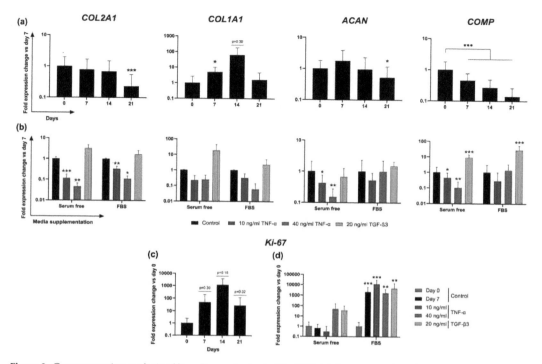

Figure 2. Gene expression analysis of live slice explants via RT-qPCR. (**a**) Gene expression of cartilage-typical markers *COL2A1, COL1A1, ACAN* and *COMP* in F^- cultured slices over three weeks (*n* = 12) relative to the day 0 value. (**b**) Gene expression of the same cartilage-typical markers as in A, after 7 days of stimulation with TNF-α or TGF-β3 and with or without FBS (*n* = 6) relative to the control on day 7. (**c**) Expression of proliferation marker *Ki-67* in F^- cultured slices over three weeks (*n* = 12) relative to the day 0 value and (**d**) after 7 days of stimulation with TNF-α or TGF-β3 and with or without FBS (*n* = 6), relative to the day 0 control to show the larger increase in the F^+ group. Statistically significant differences denoted as * $p < 0.05$, ** $p < 0.01$, *** $p < 0.001$.

2.6. Transcription of ECM Proteins Remains Highly Reactive to External Stimuli in F^- Culture

To test cell reactivity to external stimuli, we intended to induce measurable changes in chondrocyte gene expression. Slices were stimulated with TNF-α and TGF-β3 to either suppress or induce the expression of cartilage-relevant gene markers. Gene expression analysis showed differing results in the F^- and F^+ stimulation groups. In the F^- group, stimulation with TNF-α resulted in significant and dose-dependent reductions of *COL2A1, ACAN* and *COMP* expression. Compared to the day 7 control, *COL2A1* expression exhibited levels of 11 ± 7% and 5 ± 5% in low and high dose TNF-α stimulations, respectively. *ACAN* expression also was significantly lower at 42 ± 33% and 15 ± 12%, while *COMP* expression dropped to 44 ± 48% and 10 ± 14%. Stimulation with TGF-β3 resulted in a 19 ± 25-fold higher *COL1A1* expression and 9 ± 5-fold higher *COMP* expression (Figure 2b). Expression of *MMP13* did not change significantly after incubation with TNF-α but was significantly lower after stimulation with TGF-β3 (6 ± 6%, Supplemental Figure S1). In the F^+ group, stimulation with TNF-α resulted in a reduced *COL2A1* expression of 33 ± 11% in the lower concentration and 11 ± 4% in the high concentration compared to the control. Mean expression levels of *ACAN* and *COMP* in F^+ also decreased after TNF-α exposure, although no coherent dose-dependent or significant effects could be observed. TGF-β3 stimulation resulted in a 29 ± 25-fold higher expression of *COMP* and a 2.4 ± 2.7-fold higher *COL1A1* expression (Figure 2b), as well as a decrease to 42 ± 40% of *MMP13* expression (Supplemental Figure S1).

2.7. Addition of FBS to Culture Media Causes Dominant Effects on Proliferation Marker Ki-67 Expression

Expression of *Ki-67* as a marker for cell proliferation in serum-free culture varied strongly over three weeks and between donors, as shown by the very high standard deviations and surge to a >1000-fold increase on day 14 before it returned to a 28 ± 90-fold higher level compared to day 0 on day 21 (Figure 2c). Even though the average increase in *Ki-67* expression from day 0 to 7 was substantial, presumably because of the low absolute initial expression of *Ki-67* at day 0, very high variability between donors was observed and led to statistically insignificant results. Stimulation with low concentration TNF-α in F$^-$ groups led to 31 ± 65% of day 0 expression, while unexpectedly higher concentrated TNF-α resulted in a 50 ± 112-fold increase. TGF-β3 stimulation revealed a 37 ± 60-fold increase in expression after 7 days compared to day 0 control ($p = 0.06$). In the F$^+$ group, however, all 3 stimulation groups and the control exhibited statistically significant changes between day 0 and 7, reaching fold-changes compared to day 0 of 12,045 ± 17,483 (TNF-α low), 1686 ± 2180 (TNF-α high) and 4889 ± 9110 (TGF-β3). No statistically significant differences were detected among the F$^+$ cultured stimulation groups or between either of the groups and the day 7 negative control (Figure 2d).

2.8. Tissue Slices React to TNF-α Stimulation with Observable Remodeling of ECM and Cellular Swelling

To analyze whether native slice cultures retain their tissue-specific histological composition or whether they can respond to molecular stimuli with remodeling of the ECM, the slices of long-term culture and those of TNF-α-stimulated cultures were stained with Safranin-O, because TNF-α is an important inducer of matrix degeneration processes in cartilage. The proteoglycan contents of non-stimulated, F$^-$ cultured slices on days 0, 7, 14 and 21 (Figure 3a), as well as TNF-α-stimulated slices and negative controls on days 0 and 7 (Figure 3b), were quantified histomorphometrically. Even though a statistically significant decrease in proteoglycan content ($p < 0.05$) compared to day 0 was observed on day 7 in the long-term setup (Figure 3a(ii)), the mean proteoglycan content overall was maintained, as on days 14 and 21 it did not significantly differ from day 0. Proteoglycan content in the TNF-α-treated group was significantly lower than in the untreated control on day 7 (68 ± 24%; $p < 0.05$; Figure 3b(ii)). Corresponding to the changes in gene expression, TNF-α-stimulated slices exhibited a strongly altered histomorphology. Intra-cartilage fibers appeared less dense, while chondrocyte diameter and apparent volume increased (Figure 3c).

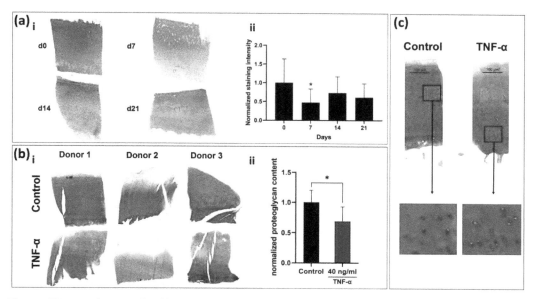

Figure 3. Histomorphometrical and histological analysis of live slices. (**a**) Safranin-O-stained slices of one donor (i) and histomorphometrical analysis (ii) over three weeks. (**b**) Comparison of staining intensity in TNF-α-stimulated and non-stimulated slices. Stimulated slices (three exemplary donors shown in (i)) show a mean reduction in red intensity of 32% (ii, *n* = 6). (**c**) Representative picture of TNF-α-treated slice and control. TNF-α-treated slices show less intense Safranin-O staining, loosened matrix structure and swollen cells in the mid-zone of the cartilage. Statistically significant differences denoted as * $p < 0.05$.

3. Discussion

The herein presented cost- and time-effective setup of surgical punch, 3D-printed microtome insert and rotary microtome is a reliable method to produce up to 100 explant cultures from a single human tissue sample. Critical to the usability of these thin osteo-chondral slice cultures is the long-term preservation of native tissue configuration and cell vitality despite thermal and mechanical stress development during preparation on the microtome and exposure of cells to atmospheric oxygen levels. CLSM analysis showed high cell vitality in both superficial and deeper tissue layers. Therefore, the slice thickness of 500 μm appears to be sufficient for cell protection within the tissue while ensuring adequate nutrient perfusion through motion-assisted diffusion. Furthermore, CLSM shows preservation of cartilage-specific cell architecture within the tissue even after three weeks of culture. Cartilage is divided into three distinct cellular zones: The superficial zone (densely packed with spindle-shaped cells), the middle zone (pearl cord-like alignment) and the deep zone (columnar chondrocyte alignment). Maintenance of the cellular zones depended on nutrient supply and physiological cartilage infrastructure, suggesting minimal cellular stress from malnutrition and/or hypoxia. However, as Secretan et al., already mentioned in their explant model, the disadvantage of the standard optical live/dead analysis of ex-plants is the exclusive possibility of endpoint analysis and the uncertainty about apoptotic cells that may have been cleared in the meantime [18]. Therefore, the high correlation between cell vitality as determined by CLSM and viability determined by resazurin assay enable the utilization of the inexpensive and easy-to-handle resazurin assay for multi-point analyses in this culture form. This is particularly advantageous for high sample quantities, which can be created by this cutting method. Long-term analysis of cell viability revealed very stable viability values over 21 days with only minor fluctuations from the baseline. Interestingly, this stability was achieved in a regular cell culture medium without serum supplementation. Most explant cultures published to date use serum mixtures between 2–10% during cultivation [18–20]. While the addition of serum is a standard cell culture procedure, it is highly desirable, especially in light of pharmacological testing, if serum were not required as an undefined and potentially interacting, interfering or confounding factor for culture maintenance. This incentive is evident from the immense increase in absolute values and variation in viability values in the short-term culture with FBS addition, where toxicity effects would presumably not be visible due to the increased metabolic activity.

In terms of long-term stability, the slice explants provide similar characteristics to conventional punch explants. Bian et al. were able to demonstrate relative stability regarding the glycosaminoglycan content in serum-free cultivation of 3 mm thick explants over several weeks [21]. While we observed a significant decrease in the histomorphometrically determined Safranin-O staining intensity on day 7, it stabilized again on days 14 and 21. This could be due to an initial outflow of glycosaminoglycans at the cut edges of the cartilage, which account for a larger proportion of the total cartilage volume than in conventional punch explants. Regarding cartilage gene expression, the results are also similar to previously published analyses of explant gene expression. Different studies also described an initial increase of aggrecan followed by a decrease after 14 days and a decrease of the collagen type II expression of >50% after three weeks of cultivation following an initial stable phase [19,22]. *COMP* as a very sensitive marker for cartilage synthesis is the only gene in the analyzed panel to show a constant, almost linear decrease over time [23,24].

Stimulation of osteochondral slices with biological stimuli showed that chondrocytes in slice cultures responded adequately to external stimulation with catabolic molecules. TNF-α is known to be a proinflammatory cytokine in the joint and to induce cartilage matrix degradation both in vivo and in vitro [25,26], but other explant models either took significantly longer for a similarly strong reduction in matrix expression and degradation of proteoglycans or required additional catabolic stimuli such as oncostatin-M or interleukin-1β [11,27,28]. Here, the short perfusion distance between the medium and cells could be an advantage for pharmacological testing, since a shorter diffusion distance results in a higher and faster penetration by the corresponding factors than in thicker explant cultures. In addition to the decrease in anabolic biomarkers such as *COL2A1*, catabolic biomarkers such as *MMP13* also responded to external stimuli. Stimulation of the cultures with TGF-β3 resulted in close to complete suppression of *MMP13* expression more clearly observed in the serum free culture. Meanwhile, stimulation with TNF-α did not significantly increase *MMP13* expression. This suggests that due to the osteoarthritic damage and semi-static nature of the culture, only decreases catabolic marker genes are suitable as indicators of efficacy in pharmacological studies.

In studies aimed at analyzing pathological processes in cartilage or the long-term effects of an external stimulus rather than large-scale screening, it would also be beneficial to examine the distribution of the different collagen subtypes histologically, as these provide the most accurate information on cartilaginous remodeling processes.

Analogous to the viability measurement, it was also shown that when serum was added to the culture, the influences of the stimuli on the chondrocytes were significantly lower. In the serum-containing group, only the decrease of *COL2A1* expression following higher-dose TNF-α stimulation and the TGF-β3-dependent increase of *COMP* on day seven reached statistical significance compared to the control. Furthermore, analysis of the proliferation marker *Ki-67* showed that in the serum-containing group, all stimulated groups including the negative control showed a huge increase, whereas, in the F$^-$ group, only TGF-β3 stimulation resulted in higher expression of *Ki-67*. This is further evidence of nonspecific responses by serum addition masking the specific effects of other stimuli, rendering it neither necessary nor advisable for pharmacological testing.

The method is limited by donor variability, the increased effort in handling, the use of priorly diseased tissue and its static nature. In comparison to conventional explants, which are merely punched out of the tissue specimen, slice cultures require several processing steps until successfully produced. Since the chondrocyte phenotype is strongly related to mechanical stimulation, several approaches are currently aiming to increase the dynamics and longevity of explant cultures by applying mechanical pressure [13,29–31]. This approach is more suitable for thicker, cylindrical explants and would, for the thin sections, be very difficult to implement. Therefore, the native tissue statues is inherently limited to a window of 3 to 4 weeks using this preparation method. This also limits the model in particular to the analysis of toxic-catabolic processes. Anabolic stimuli such as TGF-β3, while showing an increase in matrix protein expression at the transcriptional level, are associated with the simultaneous presence of mechanical stimuli [32]. A prior induction of catabolism would most likely be required to study the effects of an anabolic stimulus as previously described by Schlichting et al. [8,33]. Furthermore, the exact reproduction of slice thickness can be impaired by different qualities of bone density. Stronger bone calcification can make it necessary to cut the slice 100–200 μm thicker as the brittleness causes the bone to crush while being cut, resulting in unusable slices. Due to these slight variations in the cutting process, every donor must be related to itself when performing multipoint analysis. Therefore, the availability of a progredient analysis method like the resazurin assay is necessary to monitor individual slice viability. In accordance with this, a proteoglycan assay from the culture supernatants would also be conceivable for the analysis of the ECM. This could also provide continuous data from a slice culture instead of having to sacrifice the culture for histological endpoint analysis.

4. Materials and Methods

4.1. Sample Acquisition and Slice Production

Whole tibial plateaus (TPs; n = 23; 13 female, 10 male, 61–89 years, ⌀ 72 years) were acquired from patients undergoing knee arthroplasty comprising TP removal. The specimens were transported in serum-free cell culture medium (Dulbecco's Modified Eagle Medium with 1 g/L glucose; 1% Penicillin/Streptomycin; 2% HEPES, Merck, Darmstadt Germany) to the laboratory with a maximum delay of 1 h. TPs were then immediately placed in Petri dishes filled with medium prewarmed to 37 °C under a laminar flow cabinet. After macroscopical inspection for an osteochondral site with a well-preserved cartilage-to-bone ratio (criteria: at least 1 mm high cartilage layer; no sclerosed subchondral bone below the cartilage), an orthopedic tissue punch (OATS®, Arthrex, Naples, FL, USA) press was used to create an osteochondral cylinder punch of 20 × 10 mm (Figure 4a). The cylinder was inserted into a custom 3D-printed microtome insert (see Supplemental Figure S2 for exact insert dimensions) and then cut into eight disc-shaped cuts with a thickness of 500–800 μm using a standard rotary microtome (Cut4060, MicroTec, Brixen, Italy). An 8 mm N35 microtome blade (FEATHER, Osaka, Japan) was used for cutting, which was exchanged after the preparation of 3 osteochondral cylinders. To produce a precise cut, the rotary handle was pulled downward at the point of maximum height in a powerful swing to exert maximum force on the cutting surface and thus prevent the bone from breaking. The cuts were then split into 3 cuboid-shaped slices using a scalpel, resulting in 24–36 individual slices per punch (Figure 4b). The remains of the cylinders were then discarded.

Two slices were immediately conserved either in 5% formaldehyde or in RNAlater® (Thermo Fisher, Waltham, MA, USA), posing as day 0 samples for histological analysis and real-time quantitative polymerase chain reaction (RT-qPCR). Slices in RNAlater were subsequently stored at −80 °C. The remaining 22 slices were placed into hanging inserts (in a standing position with the cartilage facing up and leaning onto the upper rim of the inserts) of 24-well tissue culture plates with an 8 μm pore diameter (Transwell®, Corning, New York, NY, USA) for optimal perfusion. All treatments of the tissue were performed with sterile surgical gloves and instruments. Tissue culture plates were cultured at 37 °C and 5% CO_2 on a horizontal shaker at 10 rpm (Figure 4c).

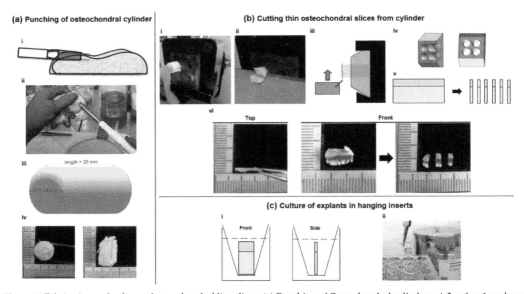

Figure 4. Fabrication and culture of osteochondral live slices. (**a**) Punching of Osteochondral cylinders. A 2 × 1 × 1 cm long osteochondral cylinder is punched out of the macroscopically unaffected area of a recently explanted human tibial plateau under sterile conditions using an orthopedic OATS® Tissue Punch (i,ii). The resulting cylinder is shown schematically in iii, cartilaginous areas are highlighted in yellow. Front and side views of the cylinder are shown in iv. (**b**) Cutting of osteochondral slices from cylinder. The cylinder is inserted into a 3D-printed microtome insert (iv) with no additional fixation (i), and 500–800 μm thick cuts are cut out from the cylinder (ii). Fixation of the cylinder is shown schematically in iii. The resulting disc-shaped cuts (schematic: v) are cut into three parallelepipedal slices using a scalpel (vi). (**c**) Slices are immediately transferred to a hanging insert of a multi-well plate and covered in cell culture medium (i,ii). Plates are then placed on a horizontal shaker for culture at 37 °C and 5% CO_2.

4.2. Maintenance and Stimulation

Slices of donors 1–6 were divided into a serum-free (F$^-$) culture group and a serum-containing group (F$^+$). The F$^+$ group was cultured in the same medium as mentioned above with an additional 10% fetal bovine serum (FBS; Gibco, Thermo Fisher, Waltham, MA, USA). In both groups, four slices each were stimulated with either 0.3 nM (10 ng/mL) TNF-α, 1.2 nM (40 ng/mL) TNF-α or 0.8 nM (20 ng/mL) TGF-β3 (all Peprotech, Rocky Hill, NJ, USA) or no additives. Stimulating factors were pipetted with low-binding tips (Corning, New York, NY, USA) for minimal protein loss. Medium and stimulating factors were exchanged completely every three days. Analyses of slices for viability, gene expression and proteoglycan content were performed on days 0 and 7. Slices of the additional 17 donors were cultured without additional stimulating factors or FBS for 21 days in a large group viability and gene expression analysis (Figure 5). The medium was completely exchanged twice a week.

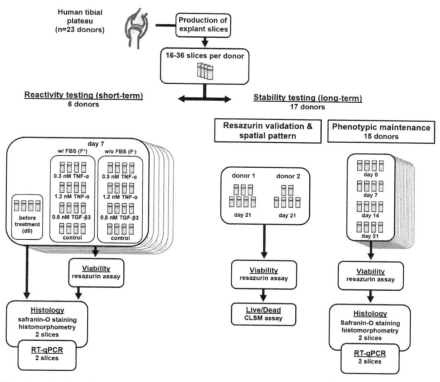

Figure 5. Flowchart depicting donor sample acquisition and distribution. Samples were obtained and then distributed for use in short-term (7 days, donors 1–6) stimulation experiments or long-term (21 days, donors 7–23) viability and gene expression experiments.

4.3. Resazurin Viability Analysis

Resazurin stock solution (AlamarBlue®, Thermo Fisher, Waltham, MA, USA) was diluted 1:10 with serum-free cell culture medium. Slices were taken out of their hanging insert, washed once with phosphate-buffered saline (PBS) and transferred into a well of a 96-well plate filled with 300 µL resazurin solution. Incubation of slices was performed for 2 h at 37 °C and 5% CO_2. After the incubation period, duplicates of 100 µL of the resazurin supernatant of each well were transferred to a fresh 96-well-plate. Fluorescence was determined on a plate reader (Synergy, BioTek, Winooski, VT, USA), applying excitation/emission wavelengths of 540/590 nm. Slices were placed back into their hanging inserts after viability determination.

4.4. Confocal Laser Scanning Microscopy

To validate results from the resazurin assay and to evaluate the spatial distribution of living and dead cells, additional live/dead determination using confocal laser scanning microscopy (CLSM) was performed on 13 slices of two donors (7 and 8) after three weeks of culture. Prior to the resazurin assay, two slices were heated to 60 °C for 30 or 60 min to decrease intra-tissue cell viability to a minimum and obtain a portion of low-viability slices in comparison to the control. Subsequently, a resazurin assay was performed on all slices. Afterward, the slices were analyzed optically via live/dead staining with fluorescein diacetate (FDA) and propidium iodide (PI; both Sigma Aldrich, St. Louis, MO, USA). Slices were taken out of their hanging inserts, washed twice with PBS and incubated in 6 µg/mL FDA in PBS solution (25 min), followed by a 0.1 mg/mL PI in PBS solution (3 min). After a washing step, slices were immediately transferred into the microscopes incubating chamber. Tissue imaging was carried out with a Nikon Scanning Confocal A1Rsi+ (Nikon, Tokyo, Japan) at 37 °C in DMEM without phenol red (Thermo Fisher, Waltham, MA, USA). Excitation/Emission wavelengths were set at 488/590 nm for PI and 485/514 nm for FDA. The scanning area was set at 2.82 mm^2. Pictures were stitched with a 20% overlap and their corresponding volume was determined using Nikon Capture NX-D software (version 1.6.2, Nikon, Tokyo, Japan). Z-stacking was performed with 10 µm spacing. Z-stacks were rendered into a 3D image with living cells depicted in green and dead cells in red. Living cells were counted using ImageJ software (version 1.8.0. [34]). For comparison of both methods, resazurin assay viability data was correlated to the number of living cells per mm^3 sample using linear regression.

4.5. RNA Extraction and Real-Time Quantitative PCR

For RNA isolation, cartilage was carefully dissected from bony tissue, the resulting slices were soaked in RNAlater (Thermo Fisher, Waltham, MA, USA) and then stored at −80 °C overnight. The following day, the frozen tissue was transferred into liquid nitrogen and pulverized using a Biopulverizer (BioSpec, Bartlesville, OK, USA). Pulverized samples were transferred into a 90% TriReagent®, 10% 4-Bromo-2-chlorophenol solution (both Sigma-Aldrich, St. Louis, MO, USA) followed by centrifugation for 45 min at 13,000× *g*. The aqueous phase was collected, and nucleic acids were precipitated by the addition of an equal volume of ice-cold 70% isopropanol. After 30 min of incubation, precipitated nucleic acids were collected and resolved in RNA isolation buffer RLT (Qiagen, Hilden, Germany). Further purification was performed using a PicoPure™ Kit (Thermo Fisher, Waltham, MA, USA) according to the manufacturer's instructions. The integrity and purity of RNA were analyzed using an Agilent Bioanalyzer 2100 (Agilent, Palo Alto, CA, USA); RNA concentration was assessed with a NanoDrop 1000 spectrophotometer (Thermo Fisher, Waltham, MA, USA). RNA was reversely transcribed using a cDNA synthesis kit (iScript™, BioRad, Hercules, CA, USA). RT-qPCR was performed in triplicates in 96-well plates (Becton Dickinson, Franklin Lakes, NJ, USA) on a Mastercycler® ep gradient realplex (Eppendorf, Hamburg, Germany) using expression assays for TaqMan probes and primer sets (Thermo Fisher, Waltham, MA, USA; order no. in parentheses): collagen type II alpha 1 (*COL2A1*, Ss03373344_g1), collagen type I alpha 1 (*COL1A1*, Ss003373341_g1), aggrecan (*ACAN*, SS03373387_S1), Ki-67 (*MKI67*, qHsaCID0011882) and cartilage oligomeric matrix protein (*COMP*, Hs01572837_g1). Expression analysis for matrix metalloproteinase 13 (*MMP13*, Ss033733279_m1) was only performed on short-term cultured slices. Succinate dehydrogenase complex, subunit A (*SDHA*, Hs00188166_m1) was used as reference gene. Marker gene expression is given as fold change compared to *SHDA* or control sample expression applying the efficiency corrected ∆∆-Ct method [35].

4.6. Histological Analysis

Slices of each donor were fixated overnight in 5% formaldehyde solution and subsequently decalcified for 21 days in Osteosoft® solution (Merck, Darmstadt, Germany). Afterward, slices were frozen in liquid nitrogen and subsequently cut into 4 µm thin sections using a CM19000 cryotome (Leica, Wetzlar, Germany). For Safranin-O staining, sections were stained for 30 min with 0.7% Safranin-O in 66% ethanol, counterstaining was performed with 0.2% Fast Green in 0.3% acetic acid (all Thermo Fisher, Waltham, MA, USA) for 1 min. To document ECM formation or loss, sections were mounted on glass slides; stainings were inspected using an AX 10 light microscope (Zeiss, Jena, Germany) and documented with a ProgRes® SpeedXT core 5 microscope-mounted camera system (JENOPTIK, Jena, Germany). The intensity of the Safranin-O staining is directly proportional to the glycosaminoglycan content of the tissue and was therefore analyzed employing a histomorphometrical approach as previously described [8]. Briefly, pictures were taken and all pixels in the areas of interest were valued in the RGB color mode with a tool based on Xcode (Apple, Sunnyvale, CA, USA). When the red value (R) multiplied by 2 was higher than the sum of the green (G) and blue (B) values, the pixel was counted as red. The intensity of each red pixel was calculated as follows: intensity = $2 \times R$-value $- G$-value $- B$-value. Values of the intensity ranged between 1 and 508, and reporting images depicting the intensity distribution were created (see Supplemental Figure S3). The mean intensity (sum of intensities/area of interest) was calculated from each image.

4.7. Statistical Analysis

The significance level of log10-transformed data was determined with the independent two-sample t-test statistics of the Excel 2013 software package (Microsoft, Redmond, WA, USA). Normal distribution was checked applying the Anderson−Darling test, and equal variance of compared sample groups was tested applying the f-test. In all groups, signals were normally distributed. If the equal variance test was passed, student's t-test was used, if not Welch's t-test was applied. p-values < 0.05 were considered significant.

5. Conclusions

Native human osteochondral live slice explants represent a valid culture alternative to conventional punch explants. Its strengths lie in the greatly increased availability of tissue samples, as the thin nature of the slices allows for up to 50–100 pieces to be prepared from a single sample, the ease of fabrication and the simplicity of the culture in hanging inserts. This enables high-throughput screening of three-dimensional tissue processes and reactions in the native state that would otherwise require weeks of preparation in a tissue-based 3D culture or even in an animal model. Our results have shown that despite the stress of sharp dissection, the tissue fully retains its microarchitecture, and the cells retain their tissue-specific phenotype as well as their ability to properly respond to various stimuli. They also suggest that the short perfusion distance between cells and medium could also have a beneficial effect on the response strength of the cells to test stimuli, as the factors reliably reach cells embedded in the tissue. In addition, it was shown that the use of serum for cell expansion/survival is redundant in this culture form, which otherwise could mask adverse effects on tissue in the context of toxicity and degeneration analyses.

In summary, this production method is very well suited to produce native slice explants, which offer an interesting alternative to conventional explant cultures, especially in terms of pharmacological testing.

Supplementary Materials: The following are available online at https://www.mdpi.com/article/10.3390/ijms22126394/s1, Figure S1: *MMP13* gene expression analysis. Figure S2: technical details of custom-made microtome insert. Figure S3: examples of histomorphometrical analysis output.

Author Contributions: Conceptualization, J.S., T.D., L.K.S., U.S., A.A.K., C.R.; methodology, J.S., L.K.S. and T.D.; validation, J.S., L.K.S., A.A.K. and T.D.; formal analysis, T.D., S.H.-S. and C.R.; resources, C.R., U.S., D.K. and M.S.; data curation, J.S. and L.K.S.; writing—original draft preparation, J.S., L.K.S. and T.D.; writing—review and editing, J.S., L.K.S., T.D., C.R., A.A.K., S.H.-S., D.K. and M.S.; supervision, T.D., D.K. and M.S.; project administration, S.H.-S. and M.S. All authors have read and agreed to the published version of the manuscript.

Funding: This research was funded by the Einstein Centre for Regenerative Therapies and Elke-Kröner-Fresenius Stiftung (Grant Number FKZ 2018_T12).

Institutional Review Board Statement: The study was conducted in accordance with the Declaration of Helsinki, and the protocol was approved by the Ethics Committee of Charité-Universitätsmedizin Berlin (EA4/072/18).

Informed Consent Statement: Informed consent was obtained from all subjects involved in the study.

Data Availability Statement: The data presented in this study are available on request from the corresponding author. The data are not publicly available due to the use of patient material and the protection of personal data.

Acknowledgments: We thank our colleagues from Charité Research Workshop for crafting special instruments for slice culture manufacturing. We thank Christoph Müller and Anja Fleischmann for their assistance with tissue culture maintenance. We would also like to show our gratitude to the core unit cell harvest for organizing the logistics of the live tissue transport. Furthermore, we thank Henrik Mei from DRFZ for his excellent advice in the field of immunology of arthritic diseases.

Conflicts of Interest: The authors declare no conflict of interest.

References

1. Puig-Junoy, J.; Ruiz Zamora, A. Socio-economic costs of osteoarthritis: A systematic review of cost-of-illness studies. *Semin. Arthritis Rheum.* **2015**, *44*, 531–541. [CrossRef] [PubMed]
2. Vina, E.R.; Kwoh, C.K. Epidemiology of osteoarthritis: Literature update. *Curr. Opin. Rheumatol.* **2018**, *30*, 160–167. [CrossRef]
3. Knecht, S.; Erggelet, C.; Endres, M.; Sittinger, M.; Kaps, C.; Stüssi, E. Mechanical testing of fixation techniques for scaffold-based tissue-engineered grafts. *J. Biomed. Mater. Res. Part B Appl. Biomater.* **2007**, *83B*, 50–57. [CrossRef] [PubMed]
4. Deng, Z.H.; Li, Y.S.; Gao, X.; Lei, G.H.; Huard, J. Bone morphogenetic proteins for articular cartilage regeneration. *Osteoarthr. Cartil.* **2018**, *26*, 1153–1161. [CrossRef] [PubMed]
5. Foldager, C.B. Advances in autologous chondrocyte implantation and related techniques for cartilage repair. *Dan. Med. J.* **2013**, *60*, B4600. [PubMed]
6. Jimenez, P.A.; Glasson, S.S.; Trubetskoy, O.V.; Haimes, H.B. Spontaneous osteoarthritis in Dunkin Hartley guinea pigs: Histologic, radiologic, and biochemical changes. *Lab. Anim. Sci.* **1997**, *47*, 598–601.
7. Kuyinu, E.L.; Narayanan, G.; Nair, L.S.; Laurencin, C.T. Animal models of osteoarthritis: Classification, update, and measurement of outcomes. *J. Orthop. Surg. Res.* **2016**, *11*, 1–27. [CrossRef]
8. Schlichting, N.; Dehne, T.; Mans, K.; Endres, M.; Stuhlmüller, B.; Sittinger, M.; Kaps, C.; Ringe, J. Suitability of Porcine Chondrocyte Micromass Culture To Model Osteoarthritis In Vitro. *Mol. Pharm.* **2014**, *11*, 2092–2105. [CrossRef]
9. Jorgensen, C.; Simon, M. In Vitro Human Joint Models Combining Advanced 3D Cell Culture and Cutting-Edge 3D Bioprinting Technologies. *Cells* **2021**, *10*, 596. [CrossRef]
10. Rothbauer, M.; Schobesberger, S.; Byrne, R.; Kiener, H.P.; Tögel, S.; Ertl, P. A human joint-on-a-chip as alternative to animal models in osteoarthritis. *Osteoarthr. Cartil.* **2020**, *28*, S89. [CrossRef]
11. Pretzel, D.; Pohlers, D.; Weinert, S.; Kinne, R.W. In vitro model for the analysis of synovial fibroblast-mediated degradation of intact cartilage. *Arthritis Res. Ther.* **2009**, *11*, 1–20. [CrossRef]
12. Haltmayer, E.; Ribitsch, I.; Gabner, S.; Rosser, J.; Gueltekin, S.; Peham, J.; Giese, U.; Dolezal, M.; Egerbacher, M.; Jenner, F. Co-culture of osteochondral explants and synovial membrane as in vitro model for osteoarthritis. *PLoS ONE* **2019**, *14*, e0214709. [CrossRef]
13. Vainieri, M.L.; Wahl, D.; Alini, M.; Van Osch, G.; Grad, S. Mechanically stimulated osteochondral organ culture for evaluation of biomaterials in cartilage repair studies. *Acta Biomater.* **2018**, *81*, 256–266. [CrossRef]
14. Maroudas, A. Transport of solutes through cartilage: Permeability to large molecules. *J. Anat.* **1976**, *122*, 335–347.
15. Schwarz, N.; Uysal, B.; Welzer, M.; Bahr, J.C.; Layer, N.; Löffler, H.; Stanaitis, K.; Pa, H.; Weber, Y.G.; Hedrich, U.; et al. Long-term adult human brain slice cultures as a model system to study human CNS circuitry and disease. *eLife* **2019**, *8*, e48417. [CrossRef] [PubMed]
16. Zwerina, J.; Redlich, K.; Polzer, K.; Joosten, L.; Krönke, G.; Distler, J.; Hess, A.; Pundt, N.; Pap, T.; Hoffmann, O.; et al. TNF-induced structural joint damage is mediated by IL-1. *Proc. Natl. Acad. Sci. USA* **2007**, *104*, 11742–11747. [CrossRef]
17. Finnson, K.W.; Chi, Y.; Bou-Gharios, G.; Leask, A.; Philip, A. TGF-b signaling in cartilage homeostasis and osteoarthritis. *Front. Biosci.* **2012**, *4*, 251–268. [CrossRef]
18. Secretan, C.; Bagnall, K.M.; Jomha, N.M. Effects of introducing cultured human chondrocytes into a human articular cartilage explant model. *Cell Tissue Res.* **2010**, *339*, 421–427. [CrossRef] [PubMed]
19. Gavénis, K.; Andereya, S.; Schmidt-Rohlfing, B.; Mueller-Rath, R.; Silny, J.; Schneider, U. Millicurrent stimulation of human articular chondrocytes cultivated in a collagen type-I gel and of human osteochondral explants. *BMC Complement. Altern Med.* **2010**, *10*, 43. [CrossRef] [PubMed]
20. Lyman, J.R.; Chappell, J.D.; Morales, T.I.; Kelley, S.S.; Lee, G.M. Response of Chondrocytes to Local Mechanical Injury in an Ex Vivo Model. *Cartilage* **2012**, *3*, 58–69. [CrossRef]
21. Bian, L.; Lima, E.; Angione, S.; Ng, K.; Williams, D.; Xu, D.; Stoker, A.; Cook, J.; Ateshian, G.; Hung, C. Mechanical and biochemical characterization of cartilage explants in serum-free culture. *J. Biomech.* **2008**, *41*, 1153–1159. [CrossRef]
22. Ragan, P.M.; Badger, A.M.; Cook, M.; Chin, V.I.; Gowen, M.; Grodzinsky, A.J.; Lark, M.W. Down-regulation of Chondrocyte Aggrecan and Type-II Collagen Gene Expression Correlates with Increases in Static Compression Magnitude and Duration. *J. Bone Jt. Surg.-Am. Vol.* **2000**, *82*, 32. [CrossRef]
23. Zaucke, F.; Dinser, R.; Maurer, P.; Paulsson, M. Cartilage oligomeric matrix protein (COMP) and collagen IX are sensitive markers for the differentiation state of articular primary chondrocytes. *Biochem. J.* **2001**, *358*, 17. [CrossRef] [PubMed]
24. Sharma, A.; Jagga, S.; Lee, S.-S.; Nam, J.-S. Interplay between Cartilage and Subchondral Bone Contributing to Pathogenesis of Osteoarthritis. *Int. J. Mol. Sci.* **2013**, *14*, 19805–19830. [CrossRef] [PubMed]

25. Manicourt, D.-H.; Poilvache, P.; Van Egeren, A.; Devogelaer, J.-P.; Lenz, M.-E.; Thonar, E.J.-M.A. Synovial fluid levels of tumor necrosis factor α and oncostatin M correlate with levels of markers of the degradation of crosslinked collagen and cartilage aggrecan in rheumatoid arthritis but not in osteoarthritis. *Arthritis Rheum.* **2000**, *43*, 281. [CrossRef]

26. Hui, W.; Rowan, A.D.; Richards, C.D.; Cawston, T.E. Oncostatin M in combination with tumor necrosis factor α induces cartilage damage and matrix metalloproteinase expression in vitro and in vivo. *Arthritis Rheum.* **2003**, *48*, 3404–3418. [CrossRef] [PubMed]

27. Thudium, C.S.; Engstrom, A.; Groen, S.S.; Karsdal, M.A.; Bay-Jensen, A.-C. An Ex Vivo Tissue Culture Model of Cartilage Remodeling in Bovine Knee Explants. *J. Vis. Exp.* **2019**, e59467. [CrossRef]

28. Clutterbuck, A.L.; Mobasheri, A.; Shakibaei, M.; Allaway, D.; Harris, P. Interleukin-1β-Induced Extracellular Matrix Degradation and Glycosaminoglycan Release Is Inhibited by Curcumin in an Explant Model of Cartilage Inflammation. *Ann. N. Y. Acad. Sci.* **2009**, *1171*, 428–435. [CrossRef]

29. Theodoropoulos, J.S.; De Croos, A.J.N.; Petrera, M.; Park, S.; Kandel, R.A. Mechanical stimulation enhances integration in an in vitro model of cartilage repair. *Knee Surgery Sport. Traumatol. Arthrosc.* **2016**, *24*, 2055–2064. [CrossRef]

30. Spitters, T.W.; Leijten, J.C.; Deus, F.D.; Costa, I.B.; Van Apeldoorn, A.A.; Van Blitterswijk, C.A.; Karperien, M. A Dual Flow Bioreactor with Controlled Mechanical Stimulation for Cartilage Tissue Engineering. *Tissue Eng. Part C Methods* **2013**, *19*, 774–783. [CrossRef]

31. Qu, P.; Qi, J.; Han, Y.; Zhou, L.; Xie, D.; Song, H.; Geng, C.; Zhang, K.; Wang, G. Effects of Rolling-Sliding Mechanical Stimulation on Cartilage Preserved In Vitro. *Cell Mol. Bioeng.* **2019**, *12*, 301–310. [CrossRef] [PubMed]

32. Elder, B.D.; Athanasiou, K.A. Synergistic and Additive Effects of Hydrostatic Pressure and Growth Factors on Tissue Formation. *PLoS ONE* **2008**, *3*, e2341. [CrossRef] [PubMed]

33. Lüderitz, L.; Dehne, T.; Sittinger, M.; Ringe, J. Dose-Dependent Effect of Mesenchymal Stromal Cell Recruiting Chemokine CCL25 on Porcine Tissue-Engineered Healthy and Osteoarthritic Cartilage. *Int. J. Mol. Sci.* **2018**, *20*, 52. [CrossRef] [PubMed]

34. Schneider, C.A.; Rasband, W.S.; Eliceiri, K.W. NIH Image to ImageJ: 25 years of image analysis. *Nat. Methods* **2012**, *9*, 671–675. [CrossRef] [PubMed]

35. Pfaffl, M.W. A new mathematical model for relative quantification in real-time RT–PCR. *Nucleic Acids Res.* **2001**, *29*, e45. [CrossRef] [PubMed]

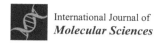

International Journal of
Molecular Sciences

MDPI

Review

Role of Physical Exercise and Nutraceuticals in Modulating Molecular Pathways of Osteoarthritis

Alessandro de Sire [1,*], Nicola Marotta [1], Cinzia Marinaro [1], Claudio Curci [2], Marco Invernizzi [3,4] and Antonio Ammendolia [1]

[1] Department of Medical and Surgical Sciences, University of Catanzaro "Magna Graecia", 88100 Catanzaro, Italy; nicola.marotta@unicz.it (N.M.); cinziamarinaro83@gmail.com (C.M.); ammendolia@unicz.it (A.A.)

[2] Physical Medicine and Rehabilitation Unit, Department of Neurosciences, ASST Carlo Poma, 46100 Mantova, Italy; claudio.curci@asst-mantova.it

[3] Physical Medicine and Rehabilitation, Department of Health Sciences, University of Eastern Piedmont, 28100 Novara, Italy; marco.invernizzi@med.uniupo.it

[4] Translational Medicine, Dipartimento Attività Integrate Ricerca e Innovazione (DAIRI), Azienda Ospedaliera S.S. Antonio e Biagio e Cesare Arrigo, 15121 Alessandria, Italy

* Correspondence: alessandro.desire@unicz.it; Tel.: +39-0961-712819

Abstract: Osteoarthritis (OA) is a painful and disabling disease that affects millions of patients. Its etiology is largely unknown, but it is most likely multifactorial. OA pathogenesis involves the catabolism of the cartilage extracellular matrix and is supported by inflammatory and oxidative signaling pathways and marked epigenetic changes. To delay OA progression, a wide range of exercise programs and naturally derived compounds have been suggested. This literature review aims to analyze the main signaling pathways and the evidence about the synergistic effects of these two interventions to counter OA. The converging nutrigenomic and physiogenomic intervention could slow down and reduce the complex pathological features of OA. This review provides a comprehensive picture of a possible signaling approach for targeting OA molecular pathways, initiation, and progression.

Keywords: exercise; physical activity; nutraceuticals; osteoarthritis; dietary supplements; inflammation; aging; inflammaging

Citation: de Sire, A.; Marotta, N.; Marinaro, C.; Curci, C.; Invernizzi, M.; Ammendolia, A. Role of Physical Exercise and Nutraceuticals in Modulating Molecular Pathways of Osteoarthritis. *Int. J. Mol. Sci.* **2021**, *22*, 5722. https://doi.org/10.3390/ijms22115722

Academic Editor: Magali Cucchiarini

Received: 29 April 2021
Accepted: 26 May 2021
Published: 27 May 2021

Publisher's Note: MDPI stays neutral with regard to jurisdictional claims in published maps and institutional affiliations.

1. Introduction

Osteoarthritis (OA) is one of the most common degenerative musculoskeletal disorders, characterized by a progressive loss of joint cartilage, synovial inflammation, formation of osteophytes, and subchondral bone remodeling [1–3]. This detrimental condition has a complex pathogenesis due to its multifactorial nature [4–6]. More specifically, the aberrant expression of degradative proteases or catabolic mediators might be induced in the chondrocytes, which contribute to cartilage erosion [7,8]. This imbalance between anabolic and catabolic processes might damage the structural integrity of the joint cartilage, resulting in stiffness, pain, and limited range of motion (ROM) in the later stages of OA [9,10]. Thus, subsequent loss of function, increased disability, lower performance in the activities of daily living (ADL), and reduction of health-related quality of life (HRQoL) are common findings in these patients [11].

In this scenario, an early diagnosis supported by the detailed understanding of the molecular pathways underpinning OA could help to develop tailored conservative therapeutic approaches aimed to avoid surgical and joint replacement treatments [12]. To date, several non-surgical treatments have been proposed in the last years for OA patients, including pharmacological treatments (e.g., acetaminophen, nonsteroidal anti-inflammatory drugs (NSAIDs), duloxetine, and opioids) [13], intra-articular injections with hyaluronic acid and glucocorticoids [14], focal muscle vibration [15], intra-articular oxygen-ozone therapy [16], radiofrequency ablation of genicular nerves [17], adipose-derived mesenchymal stem cell therapy [18], and platelet-rich plasma injections [19]. However, physical exercise is recommended by several guidelines as the first-line intervention in OA patients [13,20,21], which plays a crucial role in the prevention and treatment of the disabling sequelae of this severe chronic disease [22,23].

Nowadays, other alternative therapeutic interventions to treat OA have come to the fore, such as nutraceuticals, defined as substances that can be considered as a food or part of a food and provides medical or health benefits, including OA prevention and treatment [24,25]. In vitro and in vivo studies showed that epigenetic changes are triggered by micronutrients commonly present in diets (e.g., vitamins, carotenoids, and flavonoids) that might modulate OA mediator pathways [26–28]. Indeed, myoblasts and chondrocytes seem to share similar pathological targets and pathways and close anatomical location, suggesting the possible existence of a paracrine network [29]. In this context, an adequate prescription of physical exercise and nutritional supplementation might have a positive impact not only in terms of OA molecular pathways modulation, but also in terms of functioning and HRQoL improvement.

Therefore, in the present comprehensive review, we sought to describe the state-of-the-art about the role that physical exercise and nutraceuticals might play in the complex management of OA, in terms of modulation of its molecular pathways.

2. Osteoarthritis Molecular Pathways

The pathogenic involvement in OA pathogenesis of pro-inflammatory cytokines released by chondrocytes and synoviocytes is well known and described in the scientific literature [7]. These cellular mediator patterns develop from cell signaling and gene expression pathways, which amplify the already altered cellular transduction, releasing additional inflammatory compounds and enzymes [30].

2.1. Reactive Oxygen Species

OA etiopathogenesis is influenced by several genetic and environmental factors not already fully explained. Recent studies have shown the involvement of oxidative stress and reactive oxygen species (ROS) in OA onset and progression [31]. ROS are unstable and highly reactive oxygen-containing free radicals combined with molecules to achieve chemical stability. Cells have developed antioxidant systems to scavenge ROS and maintain intracellular redox milieu. However, ROS are also key components of many physiological processes, and, at moderate concentrations, they act as indispensable second messengers. Their activity is based on the alterations of the cellular chemical environment, consisting of oxidative modification of proteins, influencing signal transduction, gene regulation, and cell cycling, in a complex process called redox biology [32]. The ability of cells to discriminate between the opposing effects of ROS is dependent on intensity, duration, and context of signaling and cellular redox status. When the cellular antioxidant capacity is insufficient to detoxify, ROS reacts with DNA, proteins, and lipids, disrupting their normal structure, impairing function, and leading to cytotoxicity in a process called oxidative stress [33].

Articular cartilage exists in relatively hypoxic conditions as a unique tissue thriving in a mechanically active environment. Despite living in a low O_2 environment, chondrocytes are characterized by abundant and active mitochondria that contribute to adenosine triphosphate (ATP) production [34]. Disruption of mitochondrial function, leading to increased levels of intracellular ROS, has been hypothesized to disrupt cartilage homeostasis and is considered as one of the main contributors of OA-related cartilage damage [35].

In physiological conditions, ROS are produced at low concentrations in chondrocytes mitochondria through oxidative phosphorylation and in cytoplasm by nicotinamide adenine dinucleotide phosphate (NADPH) oxidase. The overproduction of ROS observed in OA impairs mitochondrial functions through mtDNA damage, inducing chondrocyte senescence and apoptosis, increasing cartilage degradation, and reducing matrix synthesis along with subchondral bone disfunction and synovial inflammation [36–38]. Evidence for ROS implication in cartilage degradation comes from the presence of lipid peroxidation products, nitrite, and nitrated products in the biological fluids in OA animal models [36]. On the contrary, antioxidant enzyme concentrations are decreased in OA patients, confirming the role that oxidative stress might play in OA pathogenesis [39].

Prolonged oxidative stress induces in the cartilaginous tissue the synthesis of large amounts of proteolytic enzymes, which in turn favors the shift towards catabolic reactions through several kinases such as p38 mitogen-activated protein kinase/nuclear factor kappa-light-chain-enhancer of activated B cells (p38MAPK/NF-κB) and activin receptor-like kinase 1 (ALK1) pathways [30]. In response to the proinflammatory stimuli, the overproduction of nitric oxide (NO) suppresses the cartilage matrix synthesis, enhances matrix metalloproteinases (MMPs) activity and induces chondrocyte apoptosis [40]. Taken together, all these mechanisms increase ROS concentrations leading to the membrane potential alterations that result in the release of cytochrome c and increase in Caspase-3 activity leading to apoptosis [41]. Lastly, oxidative stress-mediated inflammation is also responsible for the increased rate of hyaluronan degradation in synovial fluid [42].

On the other hand, chondrocytes respond to hypoxia and ROS damage, increasing the production of hypoxia-inducible factor-1 (HIF-1). HIF-1α can alleviate hypoxia-induced apoptosis, senescence, and matrix degradation in chondrocytes through mitophagy enhancing BCL2/adenovirus E1B 19-kDa-interacting protein 3 (BNIP3) expression [43].

2.2. Cellular Apoptosis

In the context of cellular autophagy, the phosphatidylinositol 3-kinase/protein kinase B (PI3K/AKT)/mechanistic target of rapamycin (mTOR) survival pathway plays a crucial role in OA pathogenesis. However, the role of Wnt/β-catenin and extracellular signal-regulated kinases (ERKs) pathway in OA pathogenesis is less elucidated [44]. In PI3K/mTOR signaling, AKT phosphorylated by PI3K modulates mTOR through a direct activation or an indirect block of one of its inhibitors. Activation of PI3K/mTOR pathway curbs the pro-apoptotic machinery resulting in enhanced cell survival through Caspase-3 inhibition [44,45]. Indeed, PI3K/mTOR is inactivated in IL-1b mediated chondrocyte apoptosis [46]. Alongside these mechanisms, Wnt proteins stand out through two characteristic pathways: β-catenin-independent pathway and β-catenin-dependent pathway [47]. In the independent process, the β-catenin undergoes phosphorylation, resulting in ubiquitination and consequent proteasomal degradation. On the other hand, in the β-catenin-dependent pathway, after the binding of Wnt ligands to the transmembrane frizzled (Fzd) receptor, the disheveled protein prevents the phosphorylation of β-catenin inducing the translocation into the nucleus where it stimulates the transcription of anti-apoptotic genes including c-Myc and cyclin D1 [48,49]. Lastly, recent studies seem to show that ERKs might be able to increase rather than decrease the levels of anabolic biomarkers in degenerative human chondrocyte [50–52].

2.3. Pro-Inflammatory Signaling

Alongside chondrocyte apoptosis, the scientific literature has recently focused on the mediation of inflammatory gene expression and inflammatory pathways role in OA pathogenesis. NF-κB is a protein complex that controls transcription of DNA and cytokine production [53]. In unstimulated cells, the NF-κB dimers are sequestered in the cytoplasm by a family of inhibitors called inhibitors of κB (IκBs) [54]. High Mobility Group Box 1 (HMGB1) is a non-histone DNA binding protein and is considered a damage-associated molecular pattern protein (DAMP) [55]. The binding of the extracellular ligand HMGB1 to the advanced glycation end product receptor (RAGE) has been described to activate IκB kinase (IKK), resulting in phosphorylation and degradation of IκBα [56].

Subsequently, p65 protein is released and phosphorylated for NF-κB heterodimer formation, and this complex is then translocated from the cytoplasm to the nucleus, inducing the expression of several genes such as cyclooxygenase (COX), Matrix metalloproteinases (MMPs), and pro inflammatory cytokines [10].

This pathway is associated with mitogen-activated protein kinase (MAPK) signaling which constitutes a family of serine/threonine kinases (p38 MAPK; c-Jun amino-terminal kinase (JNK); and ERK1/2) characterized by a multilevel crosstalk and activated by a large array of inflammatory and stressful conditions [57,58]. In addition to the ERKs, the activated p38 MAPK can translocate into the nucleus upregulating kinases and transcription factors promoting cell autophagy in some cells while enhancing survival, growth, and differentiation in other cells [57]. Lastly, the phosphorylation of JNK via specific tyrosine and threonine residues is able to increase pro-inflammatory gene expression [58].

2.4. Anti-Inflammatory Signaling

Nuclear erythroid factor 2 (Nrf2) is a distress mediator involved in oxidative stress reduction [59]. It operates as a transcription factor binding to the antioxidant response elements (AREs) in the promoter region of antioxidant genes. In unstimulated chondrocytes, Nrf2 is kept quiescent through the association with kelch-like ECH-associated protein 1 (Keap1) in the cytosol, hence restricting its translocation into the nucleus to bind the AREs [60]. DJ-1 is a sensitive redox protein that serves as a stabilizer of Nrf2; in DJ-1 knockout animal models, the downregulation of Nrf2 could lead to an increase in oxidative stress. In the same context, heme oxygenase-1 (HO-1) is an Nrf2 downstream effector and both proteins are compensatory mediators that recognize pro-oxidative stressors and induce the production of antioxidant enzymes to neutralize the ROS [61]. Emerging evidence showed that the activation of DJ-1/Nrf2 signaling in chondrocytes is crucial to protecting these cells against oxidative insults, downregulating HMGB1 and NF-κB protein expression, and activating the PI3K/mTOR pathway [62].

In summary, the activation of NF kB, p38MAPK, and JNK is involved in the expression of several inflammatory genes that boost OA pathogenesis and progression. On the other hand, the upregulation of NRf2 could allow the expression of genes leading to a suppression of inflammation and inhibition of the activation of NF-κB. In this scenario, the PI3K/mTOR, Wnt, and ERK pathways appear to block cell apoptosis and promote proliferation.

3. Physical Exercise as a Modulator of Osteoarthritis Molecular Pathways

Physical exercise has been recognized as a safe, effective, and multifaceted therapeutic treatment to reduce pain and disability in OA patients [13,20,22,23,63].

The American College of Sports Medicine guidelines and EULAR recommend physical activity and exercise as positive and effective interventions on physical fitness as well as disease-specific and general outcomes in people with hip and knee OA. Moreover, these guidelines suggest that physical activity and exercise should be considered as integral parts of standard care [64,65].

Recommended exercise programs include land-based therapeutic exercise and water physiotherapy interventions [66,67]. Indeed, a recent systematic review confirmed that Pilates, aerobic, and strengthening exercise programs performed for 8–12 weeks, 3–5 sessions per week, with each session lasting 1 h, could be considered as an effective treatment in OA patients [68].

The exact protective mechanism of action of physical exercise on cartilage is not yet known, albeit several studies performed on animal models highlighted key molecules that could help define the best therapeutic exercise regimen.

Exercise modulates transcription in several metabolic pathways associated with extracellular matrix (ECM) biosynthesis and inflammation/immune responses in normal cartilage of rats undergoing treadmill walking (12 m/min, 45 min/day for 2, 5, or 15 days). More specifically, low-intensity exercises were able to regulate the different pathways involving PI3K-AKT, NF-κB, Ras, Rap, MAPK, cAMP, and Ptgs2. Moreover, exercise was able to suppress the expression of genes involved in ECM degradation, bone formation, and initiation of pro-inflammatory cascades, which are known to be upregulated in OA (Mmp9,

Mmp8, Igf1, Col1a1, Adamts3, Adamts14). Conversely, exercise can upregulate genes involved in ECM synthesis that are commonly downregulated in OA (Chrdl2, Tnfrsf11b, Timp4, Thbs2, Tgfb1, Mmp3, Il1r1, Il1r2, Cilp, and Bmp5) [29]. Taken together, these results suggest a crucial and multifaceted role of physical exercise in several molecular pathways involved in OA pathogenesis and progression.

3.1. Chondroprotective Role of Physical Exercise

OA animal models have been widely used in the research field to investigate the role of physical exercise in modulating molecular pathways involved in OA pathogenesis, highlighting a positive effect on cartilage preservation.

Iijima and colleagues showed that low-speed treadmill walking exercise (12 m/min for 30 min/day, 5 days/week performed for 2–4 weeks) prevented the progression of post-traumatic bone and cartilage lesions and increased BMP-2 and BMP-6 expression in the chondrocytes of the joint superficial zone of 24 male Wistar rats with induced damage to knee joints [69].

Assis et al. studied the effects of aerobic exercise performed with treadmill, training 3 days/week at 16 m/min for 50 min/day for 8 weeks, on an animal experimental model of knee OA. At the end of the treatment protocol, the exercise group had a better pattern of cartilage organization with less fibrillation and irregularities along the articular surface and a lower degenerative process, compared with controls. Moreover, animals in the exercise group had a lower chondrocyte nuclear or nucleolar expression of IL-1β, Caspase-3, and MMP-13, confirming the ability of aerobic exercise to downregulate proinflammatory, proteolytic, and apoptotic pathways [70]. Similarly, treadmill exercise with moderate-intensity (18 m/min, 60 min/day, 5 days/week for 8 weeks) could have a chondroprotective effect in an OA animal model through the inhibition of NF-κB expression, resulting in a potent inhibition of MMP-13 gene expression [71].

Moderate-intensity exercise performed for only 4 weeks can also inhibit nuclear translocation of HDAC3/NF-κB complex, leading to the decreased expression of inflammatory proteins and cartilage protection in a rat model of OA. Similarly, in isolated primary rat chondrocytes mimicking OA-like pathologies, RGFP966, an HDAC3-specific inhibitor, could reduce IL-1β-induced inflammation and ROS production through the inhibition of nuclear translocation of NF-κB. Moreover, the same results were observed in a OA rat model, suggesting a role of RGFP966 in exerting exercise mediated chondroprotective effects [72]. Lastly, Castrogiovanni et al. demonstrated that a moderate-intensity physical activity protocol could lead to a decreased expression of OA-related biomarkers (IL-1, TNFα, MMP-13) and an increased expression of chondroprotective ones (IL-4, IL-10, and lubricin) in the synovium of an OA-induced rat model, highlighting the beneficial effects of exercise on cartilage preservation [73].

3.2. Anti-Inflammatory and Anti-Apoptotic Role of Physical Exercise on Murine Models

The anti-inflammatory effects of physical exercise in OA have been widely investigated on murine models. Here, a short review of the main findings showing the positive effects of physical exercise at different levels in OA damaged joints will be performed.

One hour treadmill activity showed an increase in Maresin-1 content, a strong anti-inflammatory molecule, in intra-articular lavage fluid of MIA-induced rat OA. Maresin-1 was able to decrease MMP13, activate the PI3k/Akt pathway, and suppress the NF-κB p65 pathway in IL-1β-induced rat fibroblast-like synoviocytes in vitro, suggesting a pivotal role of Maresin-1 in exerting the anti-inflammatory activity of exercise [74].

Similarly, four weeks of moderate exercise in a monosodium iodoacetate (MIA)-induced OA model determined IL-1β reduction and IL-4 increase in both serum and intra-articular lavage fluid, resulting in anti-inflammatory effect at cartilage tissue level. Furthermore, immunohistochemical assays showed that exercise markedly promoted the expression of autophagosome proteins LC3B, SQSTM1, and LC3II in the whole cartilage tissue, suggesting a positive role of exercise in autophagosome's reaction to pathological stimuli [75].

Moderate intensity treadmill training in MIA-induced OA determined an increase in 15-hydroxyeicosatetraenoic acid (15-HETE) concentration in knee joint. 15-HETE is a well-known anti-inflammatory molecule and was also able to inhibit IL-1β-induced inflammation in primary chondrocytes and increase p-Akt levels in vitro. Moreover, 15-HETE injection in knee OA alleviated cartilage damage through the inhibition of MMP-13 expression and the concomitant increase in COL2 expression in joint cartilage tissue [76].

Other animal experimental models of OA included anterior cruciate ligament transection. A study performed on this specific animal model revealed that 4 months of moderate exercise determined the reduction of Caspase3 expression and concomitant overexpression of Hsp70, an antiapoptotic factor, in both superficial and deep zones of the knee medial compartment [77]. Similarly, in surgically-induced rat knee OA, low-speed treadmill exercise (12 m/min, 5 days/week for 4 weeks) increased pSmad-5, Id1 and BMP-2, BMP-4, BMP-6, and BMP receptor 2 expression in the superficial zone chondrocytes and suppressed cartilage degeneration [69].

In this scenario, it should be noted that physical exercise could provide beneficial effects in OA according to several factors, including adherence to exercise regimens, frequency of exercise, and actual loading of the symptomatic compartment [76,78]. Nam et al. [78] demonstrated that the extent of cartilage damage could play a key role in achieving the optimal effects of exercise. They conducted a study using a common treadmill exercise protocol (speed of 12 m/min for 45 min/day) after MIA-induction damage at knee level in rats, demonstrating that exercise significantly prevented the OA progression, albeit its efficacy appeared to be inversely related to the extent of cartilage damage. Transcriptome-wide gene expression analysis revealed that gentle treadmill activity started 1 day post–MIA OA induction significantly suppressed inflammation-associated genes through NF-κB network downregulation, with crucial effects on apoptosis and cell cycle (Cdkn1a and Bcl2), matrix breakdown (Mmp12 and Mmp14), and proinflammatory responses (IL15 and IL18) in murine models. On the other hand, a delayed intervention after grade 1 cartilage damage could be less effective in suppressing proinflammatory genes or upregulating matrix synthesis. These effects were mainly related to Sox9 suppression leading to the down-regulation of alkaline phosphatase, Cilp, Cilp2, and Mgp, which are crucial mediators required for correct matrix assembly [78].

3.3. Beneficial Effects of Physical Exercise on Osteoarthritis Patients

Evidence observed on rat and mouse OA models have provided further insights that have been translated to humans since the early disease stages. The beneficial effect of exercise has been already showed in subjects at high risk of developing OA and alterations in articular cartilage composition could be a good marker of early OA pathological modifications [79].

In a randomized trial, patients at a high risk of developing radiographic OA for partial medial meniscus resection were subjected to 4 months weight-bearing exercise protocol. Cartilage quality, comprising GAG, was evaluated through fixed-charge density tissue measurement by gadolinium-enhanced MRI (dGEMRIC). The exercise group showed an improvement in dGEMRIC, compared with controls ($p = 0.036$), suggesting that human cartilage has a potential to adapt to loading changes [80]. This adaptation consequent to exercises varies between different locations within the joint, and the largest beneficial effect is observed in the load-bearing cartilage, such as the lateral posterior cartilage [81].

dGEMRIC index changes were also investigated in the study of Munukka et al. The authors evaluated 87 postmenopausal women with mild knee OA performing leisure-time physical activity (LTPA). After a period of 12 months, a linear relationship between higher LTPA level and increased dGEMRIC index changes in the posterior region of the lateral and medial femoral cartilage, were observed. These results suggested that higher LTPA level is related to regional increases in estimated glycosaminoglycan content of tibiofemoral cartilage [82]. Similarly, a randomized controlled trial conducted on 43 post-menopausal women with mild knee OA performing lower limb aquatic resistance training, showed a significantly reduction of T2-MRI scores in the posterior region of the medial femoral condyle after 4 months of physical activity. A decrease in T2 scores is suggestive of improved integrity and orientation of the collagen fibers and a decrease in hydration of articular cartilage [82].

Another promising technique to assess OA-related cartilage modifications is the microdialysis method. Helmark et al. obtained information about the effect of a single-leg knee-extension protocol on cartilage biomarkers and cytokines, both inside the joint as well as in the synovium, in a group of women affected by knee OA. In this RCT, over a period of three hours, a single bout of mechanical loading resulted in a significant decrease in cartilage oligomeric matrix proteins (COMP) and an increase in the anti-inflammatory mediator IL-10 in both intra-articular and peri-synovium spaces, compared with controls ($p < 0.05$). Significant increases were also registered for IL-6 and IL-8 in both groups, whereas TNF-α increased peri-synovially in the experimental group only [83].

Similarly, a pilot RCT performed by Hunt et al. demonstrated that a 10-week exercise protocol, consisting of hip abductors, quadriceps, and hamstrings muscle strengthening, performed on seventeen subjects with radiographically confirmed medial tibiofemoral OA, could lead to a reduction in serum of the cartilage degradation marker COMP levels, compared with controls (2.11 log U/L vs. 2.36 log U/L; $p < 0.04$). Moreover, a significant relationship emerged between dynamic measure of knee joint load and the ratio between two molecular markers increased in OA patient biological fluids (the urinary C-telopeptide of type II collagen/serum C-propeptide of type II procollagen ratio $\beta = 1.11$, 95% CI = 0.15, 2.07; $p = 0.04$) [84]. Lastly, the combined nutritional and exercise intervention also seem to act on cartilage biomarkers. A recent study demonstrated that an 18-month period aerobic walking and strength training in combination with an intensive diet determined the reduction of serum collagen type I (C1M) and II (C2M) in obese elderly patients affected by tibiofemoral OA [85].

3.4. Physical Exercise as an Antioxidant Intervention

The role of physical activity on oxidative stress and redox biology balance has recently obtained an emerging interest in the scientific literature. It is already known that physical activity might improve antioxidant defenses and lowers lipid peroxidation levels in both adults and aged individuals [86]. At cellular level, the beneficial role of physical exercise in OA comes through the increased expression of chondrogenic transcription factors SOX9 in circulating mesenchymal progenitors associated with autophagy. Autophagy regulates mitochondrial activity in stem cells to provide the best metabolic conditions, thus limiting ROS production and preventing metabolic stress and genome damage [87].

Furthermore, aerobic exercise modulates the chondrocyte response according to the balance between redox milieu and mechano-transduction mechanisms. Chondrocytes subjected to mechanical stimulation activate the NF-κB signaling pathway, which is considered a possible link between loading and chondrocytic responses to proinflammatory cytokines [88].

Nrf2 is a stress response protein in OA chondrocytes with anti-oxidative and anti-apoptotic function and acts via ERK1/2/ELK1-P70S6K-P90RSK signaling axis in vitro [89]. Physical exercise could activate Nrf2 in response to the ROS increase, leading to the expression of antioxidant genes such as phase-II antioxidant enzymes such as glutathione and NADPH through Nrf2/Maf/ARE pathways activation [90].

Although researchers and clinicians have demonstrated a particular attention to the role of physical exercise antioxidant effects on OA, at present, evidence in literature about this issue is scarce. In MIA-induced OA rat model, 8 weeks of endurance exercise training (13 m/min, 50 min/day for 3 days/week) promoted free radicals generation that could stimulate both exercise adaptation and mitochondrial biogenesis. In this scenario, exercise promoted a significant increase in myeloperoxidase and superoxide dismutase activity in the articular capsule [91]. Similarly, a two-group cross-sectional study showed that strengthening exercises could changes antioxidant status of systemic markers in knee OA patients. More specifically, ten obese women affected by knee OA, following an acute bout of isokinetic exercise, showed an immediate post-exercise rise of non-enzymatic antioxidant capacity of serum sustained by scavenging activity of 1,1-diphenyl-2-picrylhydrazyl. This finding suggests that the up-regulation of the body's antioxidant defense could be probably related to the mobilization of antioxidant reserves in plasma [92].

In the complex management of OA, physical exercise turned out to be effective also in synergy with other innovative therapies (i.e., mesenchymal cell implants or injections). In this scenario, autologous chondrocyte implants and bone marrow-derived mesenchymal cell implants or injections are innovative therapeutic interventions in OA focused on articular cartilage and subchondral bone damage treatment [93–95]. Studies in humans showed that exercise might enhance joint recruitment of bone marrow-derived mesenchymal stem cells and upregulates the expression of osteogenic and chondrogenic genes (Runx, MSx1, Sox9, COL2A1, ATG3), osteogenic microRNAs, and osteogenic growth factors (BMP2, BMP6) [87,96,97]. In experimental rodent models, physical exercise enhanced the osteogenic potential of bone marrow-derived mesenchymal stem cells and reduced their adipogenic potential. Moreover, exercise performed after stem cell implantation could enhance stem cell transplant viability [98–102]. Taken together, these results suggest a complex and multifaceted role of physical exercise on different antioxidant pathways corroborating the physiological basis supporting its efficacy in the treatment of OA.

3.5. Challenges and Potential Controversies

Despite its countless scientifically proven beneficial effects, physical exercise in certain conditions could be detrimental to articular cartilage health. Studies on human subjects reported that even moderate exercise, recommended as a treatment for OA, might increase markers of cartilage degradation in OA-affected joints [103,104]. Due to these controversies, the investigation of the imbalances in the molecular pathways involved in OA pathogenesis and progression could help in providing more insights about this controversial issue.

In an exercise-induced OA rat model, two weeks of 16 m/min treadmill activity showed that Ctnnb1, β-catenin, and Wnt-3a participate in the pro-inflammatory OA pathogenesis through an abnormal activation of the Wnt/β-catenin pathway due to excessive mechanical load [105]. Similarly a high-impact exercise protocol comprising flexion, extension, and compression of the limbs for two weeks resulted in IL-1β overexpression and IL-10 down-regulation in an advanced stage of OA induced in a rat model [106]. Siebelt et al. highlighted the impact of a 6-week treadmill intense exercise protocol in rats highlighting the loss of proteoglycan content in the exercised compared with sedentary OA joints induced by papain injection [104]. In surgically-induced rat knee OA, the same treadmill velocity was not able to modulate the effect of BMP pathway on OA pathological modifications, leading to the progression of morphological alterations [69]. Similarly, anterior cruciate ligament transected-animals running at a lower speed (18 m/min for 6 weeks) underwent advanced cartilage degradation, compared with the sedentary animals [107].

In humans affected by OA, Jayabalan et al. observed that 45 min of continuous walking resulted in a cumulative increase in COMP concentration, a marker of cartilage turnover, whereas interval walking was associated with COMP concentrations comparable to baseline. This study shed light about the possibility that incorporating resting periods in walking regimens may impact the potentially deleterious effects of longer continuous walking bouts on the knee joint [108].

In conclusion, the above-mentioned controversies might be due to the performance of high-intensity exercises for a long time. Indeed, they are not commonly recommended by the recent International Guidelines for frail OA patients [64,65].

4. Nutrigenomic: Role of Nutraceuticals on Osteoarthritis

Nutraceuticals are considered as dietary supplements including a concentrated form of a presumed bioactive substance, originally derived from a food, aimed to improve health status particularly in "active aging" [109]. In this scenario, nutraceuticals play a pivotal role on osteoarthritis pathogenesis with specific targets in modulating OA pathways (see Table 1).

Table 1. Characteristics of the studies included with the nutrigenomic targets.

Nutraceutical	OA Pathways Involved	Modulation Action	Main Findings	Journal	Authors	Year
Apigenin	⊣ HIF 2α	↓ ADAMTS-4 ↓ COX-2 ↓ MMP	Apigenin blocks osteoarthritis development as Hif-2α inhibitor.	*Journal of Cellular and Molecular Medicine*	Cho et al. [110]	2019
Berberine	→ PI3K/AKT ⊣ NF-κB	↓ ADAMTS-4 ↓ COX-2 ↓ MMP	Berberine activates PI3K/Akt and NF-κB pathways.	*Phytomedicine*	Wong et al. [111]	2019
Chondroitin Sulfate	⊣ NF-κB	↓ ADAMTS-4 ↓ COX-2 ↓ MMP	Separate administration of chondroitin sulfate raised expression of Comp and reduced TLRs, and NF-κB expressions in cartilage.	*Probiotics and Antimicrobial Proteins*	Korotkyi et al. [112]	2021
Curcumin	→ ERK1/2	↓ Chondrocyte Apoptosis	Curcumin inhibits apoptosis of chondrocytes through activation ERK1/2 signaling pathways induced autophagy.	*Nutrients*	Li et al. [52]	2017
	⊣ NF-κB	↓ ADAMTS-4 ↓ COX-2 ↓ MMP	Curcumin reduces inflammation in knee osteoarthritis through blocking TLR4/MyD88/NF-κB signal pathway.	*Drug Development Research*	Zhang et al. [113]	2018
	→ Nrf2/HO-1	↑ GPX1,3,4 ↑ SOD1 ↑ CAT ↑ GST	Curcumin inhibits chondrocytes inflammation through the Nrf2/ARE signaling pathway, thereby exerting cartilage protective effects.	*Cell Stress and Chaperones*	Jiang et al. [114]	2020
	⊣ TLR4/NF-κB	↓ ADAMTS-4 ↓ COX-2 ↓ MMP	Curcumin improve neuroinflammatory process by reducing microglia/macrophage activation and neuronal apoptosis through a mechanism involving the TLR4/NF-κB signaling pathway in microglia/macrophages.	*International Journal of Molecular Sciences*	Panaro et al. [115]	2020
	⊣ NF-κB	↓ ADAMTS-4 ↓ COX-2 ↓ MMP	Curcumin reduces expression of NF-κB and ROCK1.	*Journal of Cellular and Molecular Medicine*	Qiu et al. [116]	2020

Table 1. *Cont.*

Nutraceutical	OA Pathways Involved	Modulation Action	Main Findings	Journal	Authors	Year
Eupatilin	⊣ NF-κB ⊣ JNK ⊣ p38MAPK	↓ ADAMTS-4 ↓ COX-2 ↓ MMP	Eupatilin suppressed expression of MMPs, ADAMTSs in chondrocytes by reducing JNK phosphorylation and NF-κB and MAPK signaling.	*Pharmaceuticals*	Lee et al. [117]	2021
Genistein	→ Nrf2/HO-1	↑ GPX1,3,4 ↑ SOD1 ↑ CAT ↑ GST	Genistein downregulates MMPs, ADAMTSs via NF-κB signaling pathway by blocking IκB degradation and activating Keap1/Nrf2 pathway.	*Nutrients*	Liu et al. [118]	2019
Genistein	⊣ NF-κB	↓ ADAMTS-4 ↓ COX-2 ↓ MMP	Genistein downregulates MMPs, ADAMTSs via NF-κB signaling pathway by blocking IκB degradation and activating Keap1/Nrf2 pathway.	*BioMed Research International*	Yaun et al. [119]	2019
Genistein				*Molecular Medicine Report*	Zou et al. [120]	2020
Glucosamine	→ mTOR	↓ Chondrocyte Apoptosis	Glucosamine promotes osteoblast proliferation by modulating autophagy via the mTOR pathway.	*Biomedicine & Pharmacotherapy*	Lv et al. [121]	2018
Glucosamine	→ Wnt/β-catenin	↓ Chondrocyte Apoptosis	GlcN increases β-catenin nuclear translocation, thus promoting chondrocyte proliferation.	*International Journal of Molecular Medicine*	Ma et al. [49]	2018
Green tea polyphenol	⊣ NF-κB	↓ ADAMTS-4 ↓ COX-2 ↓ MMP	L-theanine inhibits upregulation of MMPs, as well as inhibiting NF-κB	*Nutrients*	Bai et al. [122]	2020
Green tea polyphenol			Green tea catechins increase NF-κB inhibitors expression	*Antioxidants*	Luk et al. [123]	2020
Green tea polyphenol	→PI3K/AKT	↓ FOX-O1	Epigallocatechin-3-gallate modulating AKT-FoxO1 via upregulating miR-486-5p.	*Archives of Biochemistry and Biophysics*	Chang et al. [124]	2020
Jaceosidin	⊣ NF-κB	↓ ADAMTS-4 ↓ COX-2 ↓ MMP	Jaceosidin attenuates cartilage destruction by suppressing MMPs, ADAMTSs and the NFκB signaling pathway by blocking IκB degradation.	*Journal of Cellular and Molecular Medicine*	Lee et al. [117]	2019
Omega-3 PUFA	⊣ p38MAPK	↓ Chondrocyte Apoptosis	PUFA inactivates of p38MAPK	*International Journal of Molecular Medicine*	Wang et al. [58]	2016
Omega-3 PUFA	→ PI3K/AKT ⊣ NF-κB	↓ MMPs	PUFA metabolite suppresses MMP-13 secretion by activating PI3K/AKT pathway directly, while inhibiting NF-κB pathway.	*Connective Tissue Research*	Lu et al. [74]	2020

Table 1. *Cont.*

Nutraceutical	OA Pathways Involved	Modulation Action	Main Findings	Journal	Authors	Year
OOP	⊣ NF-κB ⊣ p38MAPK	↓ ADAMTS-4 ↓ COX-2 ↓ MMP	OOPs inhibited IL-1β-induced expression of inflammatory mediators through suppressing NF-κB and MAPK activation in chondrocytes.	*Food & Function*	Feng et al. [125]	2017
	→ Nrf2/HO-1 ⊣ NF-κB	↓ ADAMTS-4 ↓ COX-2 ↓ MMP	OOPs can activate Nrf-2 signaling and the blockage of NF-κB nuclear translocation	*Cells*	Serrelli et al. [126]	2020
	⊣ NF-κB	↓ ADAMTS-4 ↓ COX-2 ↓ MMP	OOPs reduce the inflammatory and catabolic factors mediated by NF-κB (IL-1ß, IL-6, COX-2 and MMP-3	*Aging*	Varela-Eirín et al. [127]	2020
	⊣ NF-κB	↓ ADAMTS-4 ↓ COX-2 ↓ MMP	Mechanistically, OOPs exhibited an anti-inflammatory effect by inactivating the PI3K/AKT/NF-κB pathway.	*Journal of Cellular Physiology*	Chen et al. [128]	2021
Quercitin	⊣ NF-κB	↓ ADAMTS-4 ↓ COX-2 ↓ MMP	Quercetin inhibits IL-1b and TNF-a production via TLR-4/NF-κB pathway.	*Journal of International Medical Research*	Zhang et al. [129]	2019
Resveratrol	→Wnt/β-catenin	↓ Chondrocyte Apoptosis	Rev increased osteoblastogenesis and bone formation through stimulation of Wnt signaling pathway.	*Journal of Cell Physiology*	Ashrafizadeh et al. [47]	2020
	→Nrf2/HO-1	↑ GPX1,3,4 ↑ SOD1 ↑ CAT ↑ GST	Res modulates the Nrf2 activation by inhibiting Keap1, Nrf2 gene expression, changing the upstream mediators of Nrf2, and potentiating the nuclear translocation of Nrf2.	*Biomedicine & Pharmacotherapy*	Farkhondeh et al. [130]	2020
	→PI3K/AKT	↓ FOX-O1	Resveratrol may exert anti-OA effect by enhancing the self-limiting mechanism of inflammation through TLR4/Akt/FoxO1 axis.	*Drug Design, Development and Therapy*	Xu et al. [131]	2020
	⊣ NF-κB	↓ ADAMTS-4 ↓ COX-2 ↓ MMP	Resveratrol alleviates the interleukin-1β-induced chondrocytes injury through the NF-κB signaling pathway.	*Journal of Orthopaedic Surgery and Research*	Yi et al. [132]	2020

Table 1. *Cont.*

Nutraceutical	OA Pathways Involved	Modulation Action	Main Findings	Journal	Authors	Year
Sulforaphane	→ Nrf2/HO-1	↑ GPX1,3,4 ↑ SOD1 ↑ CAT ↑ GST	Sulforaphane ameliorates oxidative stress suppressing inflammatory cytokines and activating Keap1/Nrf2 pathway.	*Free Radical Biology and Medicine*	Yang et al. [133]	2020
			Sulforaphane inhibits the production of inflammatory cytokines.	*PLoS ONE*	Moon et al. [134]	2021
	⊣ JNK	↓ ADAMTS-4 ↓ COX-2 ↓ MMP	Sulforaphane inhibits osteoclastogenesis by suppressing autophagy modulating JNK pathway.	*Molecules*	Lou et al. [135]	2021
Wogonin	⊣ NF-κB	↓ ADAMTS-4 ↓ COX-2 ↓ MMP	Wogonin downregulates NF-κB pathway and genes involved in inflammatory-response.	*Nature: Scientific Report*	Khan et al. [136]	2017

Abbreviations: ADAMTS = A disintegrin and metalloproteinase with thrombospondin motifs; AKT = Tyrosine kinase A; CAT = Catalase; COX-2 = Cyclooxygenase-2; ERK = Extracellular signal-regulated kinases; FOX-O1 = Forkhead box protein O1; GPX = glutathione peroxidase; GST = Glutatione S-transferasi; HIF-2α = Hypoxia-inducible factor; HO-1 = Heme oxygenase 1; MAPK = Mitogen-activated protein kinases; MMP = Matrix metalloproteinase; mTOR = mammalian target of rapamycin; NF-κB = Nuclear factor kappa-light-chain-enhancer of activated B cells; Nrf2 = Nuclear factor-erythroid factor-2; OOP = Olive Oil Polyphenols; PI3K = Fosfoinositide 3-chinasi; PUFA = Polyunsaturated Fatty Acids; SOD = Superoxide dismutase; TLR4 = Toll-like receptor; Wnt = Wingless-related integration site.

Long-chain polyunsaturated fatty acids (PUFAs) include alpha-linolenic (ALA), eicosapentaenoic (EPA) and docosahexaenoic (DHA) and are structural components of cell membranes. However, they also exert their action in a high number of intracellular signaling and metabolic pathways [26]. PUFAs and their metabolites act as second messengers when intercalated in the cell membrane, inhibiting the expression of MMP-13 through the inactivation of the p38MAPK and NF-κB p65 pathway, and promoting the activation of the PI3k/Akt signaling [58,74].

In the recent literature, the isolated administration of Chondroitin Sulfate has been shown to increase the transcription of the gene for Cartilage Oligomeric Matrix Protein (COMP) and decrease the expression of Toll-like receptors, thus inhibiting the Nfkb1 pathway in chondrocytes [112].

Glucosamine (GlcN) is an amino monosaccharide component of glycosaminoglycan (GAG) chains, usually in the form of sulfate or hydrochloride salts derived from the chitin of the exoskeleton of crustaceans and from mushrooms [26]. Glucosamine promotes the proliferation of human osteoblasts modulating the mTOR pathway and enhancing β-catenin nuclear translocation with consequent activation of cell proliferation via cyclin D1 expression [49,121,137].

Sulforaphane is an isothiocyanate derived from its glucosinolate precursor glucoraphanin, which is found in edible cruciferous vegetables, especially in broccoli. It can ameliorate ROS-induced oxidative stress and cartilage matrix degradation suppressing pro-inflammatory cytokines such as IL-6, TNF-α, and IL-17, inhibiting the JNK signaling and activating Keap1/Nrf2 pathway [133–135].

Berberine is an isoquinoline alkaloid, produced by many plants, as Coptis japonica Makino, Coptis, Berberis petiolaris and B. vulgaris [138]. It modulates the PI3K/Akt and NF-κB pathways regulating cytoskeletal reorganization and dedifferentiation in chondrocytes, improving the progression of OA [111].

Apigenin is a natural product belonging to the flavone class that is the aglycone of several naturally occurring glycosides. As an isolated compound from Cirsium japonicum var. maackii, it blocks MMP3, MMP13, and COX-2 expression through Hif-2α inhibition via the NF-κB and JNK signaling pathways [110]. Therefore, downstream of the NF-κB and JNK signal expression might block the translation of the pro-inflammatory factor HIF2a.

Eupatilin is an O-methylated flavonoid present in Artemisia asiatica (Asteraceae), which suppresses the expression of pro-inflammatory genes in chondrocytes through the reduction of JNK phosphorylation, NF-κB, and MAPK activation pathway [28].

Other nutraceuticals that could have a role in modulating the OA pathways seem to be the green tea catechins (GTCs), which could protect against cartilage loss and reduce the progression of OA through the modulation of NF-κB inhibitor expression and targeting the PI3K/AKT pathway. Another main component of the green tea is the epigallo-catechin-3 gallate that might inhibit NF-κB nuclear translocation by blocking IkB degradation in human chondrocytes stimulated with IL-1β [122–124].

Genistein, an isoflavone from soy (Glycine max), inhibits the NF-κB pathway and the consequent expression of catabolic factors, while stimulating the expression of Ho-1, associated with the activation of Nrf-2 in human chondrocytes [118–120].

Furthermore, Jaceosidin, an extract of *Artemisia argyi*, showed to reduce the damage to OA cartilage by blocking the degradation of IκB and inhibiting the nuclear translocation of NF-κB [117].

Quercitin is a hydroxyflavonoid widely contained in the flowers, leaves, and fruits of different plants. It improved OA via dose-dependent effects on the Toll-like Receptor-4 (TRL-4)/NF-κB pathway in vivo, inducing a cytosolic down expression of TLR-4 [129].

Moreover, Wogonin is an O-methylated flavone present in *Scutellaria baicalensis* with a positive effect on OA, which may be related to the inhibition of pro-inflammatory genes expression via the NF-κB pathway [136].

Curcumin, the main polyphenol component from the roots of turmeric (*Curcuma longa*), improves the inflammatory pattern through NF-κB signaling inhibition and Nrf2/ARE signaling activation. In addition, curcumin inhibits cell autophagy via ERK1/2 signaling pathway activation [52,113–116].

Olive oil polyphenols (OOPs), as oleocanthal (OC), oleuropein (OP), tyrosol (TY), and hydroxytyrosol (HT), could modulate inflammatory and degenerative OA molecular patterns. OOPs inhibit pro-inflammatory genes expression through the suppression of NF-κB and MAPK activation, while enhancing Nrf-2 signaling [125–128].

Lastly, resveratrol, a phenol extracted from the skin of grapes, wines, mulberries, and peanuts, belongs to the phytoalexins that protect plants from microbial infections. Resveratrol increases cell proliferation via stimulation of Wnt signaling dependent pathway and might exert self-limiting mechanism of inflammation through PI3K/Akt and Nrf2 axis activation and concomitant NF-κB inhibition [47,86,139,140].

Therefore, nutraceuticals and physical exercise are involved in molecular pathways OA with apoptotic, pro-, or anti-inflammatory targets (see Figure 1 for further details).

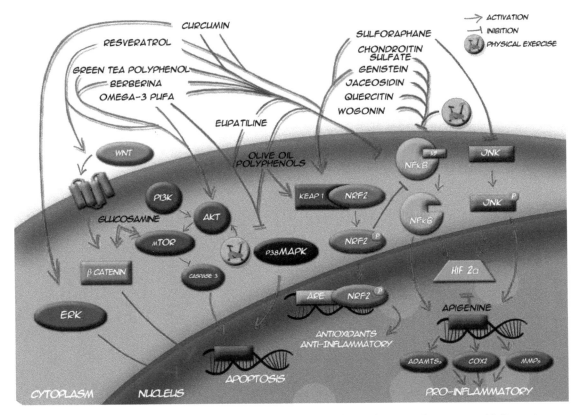

Figure 1. Involvement of nutraceuticals and exercise in molecular pathways for apoptotic, pro-, or anti-inflammatory signaling.

5. Conclusions

In this comprehensive review, we described the main molecular pathways underpinning OA pathogenesis and progression, highlighting the different mechanisms of action and potential targets for innovative therapeutic interventions. Moreover, we described common targets of physical activity and nutraceuticals suggesting a possible therapeutical synergism of these two interventions. The decrease in ROS production upstream of physical exercise can guarantee a beneficial approach regardless of the nutraceutical chosen, whereas the mutual connections on a cellular mediator would suggest the composition of the compounds in an ad hoc logic.

In conclusion, despite the limitations related to the low characterizations of some molecular pathways, the current review provides intriguing insights regarding molecular pathophysiological mechanisms, innovative therapeutical target pathways, and synergistic interventions that could improve the complex framework of OA management.

Author Contributions: Study conceptualization, A.d.S.; methodology, A.d.S.; writing—original draft preparation, A.d.S., N.M., and C.M.; writing—review and editing, M.I. and A.A.; visualization, C.C.; supervision, A.d.S. All authors have read and agreed to the published version of the manuscript.

Funding: Not applicable.

Institutional Review Board Statement: Not applicable.

Informed Consent Statement: Not applicable.

Data Availability Statement: Not applicable.

Conflicts of Interest: The authors declare no conflict of interest.

References

1. Cross, M.; Smith, E.; Hoy, D.; Nolte, S.; Ackerman, I.; Fransen, M.; Bridgett, L.; Williams, S.; Guillemin, F.; Hill, C.L.; et al. The global burden of hip and knee osteoarthritis: Estimates from the Global Burden of Disease 2010 study. *Ann. Rheum. Dis.* **2014**, *73*, 1323–1330. [CrossRef]
2. Agel, J.; Akesson, K.; Amadio, P.C.; Anderson, M.; Badley, E.; Balint, G.; Bellamy, N.; Bigos, S.; Bishop, N.; Bivans, B.; et al. *The Burden of Musculoskeletal Conditions at the Start of the New Millennium*; WHO Technical Report Series; World Health Organization: Geneva, Switzerland, 2003.
3. Martel-Pelletier, J.; Boileau, C.; Pelletier, J.P.; Roughley, P.J. Cartilage in normal and osteoarthritis conditions. *Best Pract. Res. Clin. Rheumatol.* **2008**, *22*, 351–384. [CrossRef]
4. Wang, M.N.; Liu, L.; Zhao, L.P.; Yuan, F.; Fu, Y.B.; Xu, X.B.; Li, B. Research of inflammatory factors and signaling pathways in knee osteoarthritis. *Zhongguo Gu Shang* **2020**, *33*, 388–392. [PubMed]
5. Hong, J.I.; Park, I.Y.; Kim, H.A. Understanding the molecular mechanisms underlying the pathogenesis of arthritis pain using animal models. *Int. J. Mol. Sci.* **2020**, *21*, 533. [CrossRef] [PubMed]
6. Al-Modawi, R.N.; Brinchmann, J.E.; Karlsen, T.A. Multi-pathway Protective Effects of MicroRNAs on Human Chondrocytes in an In Vitro Model of Osteoarthritis. *Mol. Ther. Nucleic Acids* **2019**. [CrossRef]
7. Zheng, L.; Zhang, Z.; Sheng, P.; Mobasheri, A. The role of metabolism in chondrocyte dysfunction and the progression of osteoarthritis. *Ageing Res. Rev.* **2021**, *66*, 101249. [CrossRef]
8. Kraus, V.B.; Karsdal, M.A. Osteoarthritis: Current Molecular Biomarkers and the Way Forward. *Calcif. Tissue Int.* **2020**, 1–10. [CrossRef]
9. Xu, L.; Li, Y. A Molecular Cascade Underlying Articular Cartilage Degeneration. *Curr. Drug Targets* **2020**. [CrossRef]
10. Chow, Y.Y.; Chin, K.Y. The Role of Inflammation in the Pathogenesis of Osteoarthritis. *Mediat. Inflamm.* **2020**, *2020*, 1–19. [CrossRef] [PubMed]
11. McDonough, C.M.; Jette, A.M. The contribution of osteoarthritis to functional limitations and disability. *Clin. Geriatr. Med.* **2010**, *26*, 387–399. [CrossRef]
12. Iolascon, G.; Gimigliano, F.; Moretti, A.; de Sire, A.; Migliore, A.; Brandi, M.L.; Piscitelli, P. Early osteoarthritis: How to define, diagnose, and manage. A systematic review. *Eur. Geriatr. Med.* **2017**. [CrossRef]
13. McAlindon, T.E.; Bannuru, R.R.; Sullivan, M.C.; Arden, N.K.; Berenbaum, F.; Bierma-Zeinstra, S.M.; Hawker, G.A.; Henrotin, Y.; Hunter, D.J.; Kawaguchi, H.; et al. OARSI guidelines for the non-surgical management of knee osteoarthritis. *Osteoarthr. Cartil.* **2014**. [CrossRef]
14. Santilli, V.; Mangone, M.; Paoloni, M.; Agostini, F.; Alviti, F.; Bernetti, A. Comment on "early efficacy of intra-articular HYADD® 4 (Hymovis®) injections for symptomatic knee osteoarthritis". *Joints* **2018**, *5*, 79. [CrossRef]
15. Rabini, A.; De Sire, A.; Marzetti, E.; Gimigliano, R.; Ferriero, G.; Piazzini, D.B.; Iolascon, G.; Gimigliano, F. Effects of focal muscle vibration on physical functioning in patients with knee osteoarthritis: A randomized controlled trial. *Eur. J. Phys. Rehabil. Med.* **2015**, *51*, 513–520.
16. De Sire, A.; Stagno, D.; Minetto, M.A.; Cisari, C.; Baricich, A.; Invernizzi, M. Long-term effects of intra-articular oxygen-ozone therapy versus hyaluronic acid in older people affected by knee osteoarthritis: A randomized single-blind extension study. *J. Back Musculoskelet. Rehabil.* **2020**. [CrossRef]
17. El-Hakeim, E.H.; Elawamy, A.; Kamel, E.Z.; Goma, S.H.; Gamal, R.M.; Ghandour, A.M.; Osman, A.M.; Morsy, K.M. Fluoroscopic guided radiofrequency of genicular nerves for pain alleviation in chronic knee osteoarthritis: A single-blind randomized controlled trial. *Pain Physician* **2018**. [CrossRef]
18. Roato, I.; Ferracini, R. Is the adipose-derived mesenchymal stem cell therapy effective for treatment of knee osteoarthritis? *Ann. Transl. Med.* **2019**. [CrossRef]
19. Southworth, T.M.; Naveen, N.B.; Tauro, T.M.; Leong, N.L.; Cole, B.J. The Use of Platelet-Rich Plasma in Symptomatic Knee Osteoarthritis. *J. Knee Surg.* **2019**. [CrossRef]
20. Kolasinski, S.L.; Neogi, T.; Hochberg, M.C.; Oatis, C.; Guyatt, G.; Block, J.; Callahan, L.; Copenhaver, C.; Dodge, C.; Felson, D.; et al. 2019 American College of Rheumatology/Arthritis Foundation Guideline for the Management of Osteoarthritis of the Hand, Hip, and Knee. *Arthritis Rheumatol.* **2020**. [CrossRef]
21. Meiyappan, K.P.; Cote, M.P.; Bozic, K.J.; Halawi, M.J. Adherence to the American Academy of Orthopaedic Surgeons Clinical Practice Guidelines for Nonoperative Management of Knee Osteoarthritis. *J. Arthroplast.* **2020**. [CrossRef]
22. Mazor, M.; Best, T.M.; Cesaro, A.; Lespessailles, E.; Toumi, H. Osteoarthritis biomarker responses and cartilage adaptation to exercise: A review of animal and human models. *Scand. J. Med. Sci. Sport.* **2019**, *29*, 1072–1082. [CrossRef]
23. de Sire, A.; de Sire, R.; Petito, V.; Masi, L.; Cisari, C.; Gasbarrini, A.; Scaldaferri, F.; Invernizzi, M. Gut–joint axis: The role of physical exercise on gut microbiota modulation in older people with osteoarthritis. *Nutrients* **2020**, *12*, 574. [CrossRef]

24. Pérez-Lozano, M.L.; Cesaro, A.; Mazor, M.; Esteve, E.; Berteina-Raboin, S.; Best, T.M.; Lespessailles, E.; Toumi, H. Emerging natural-product-based treatments for the management of osteoarthritis. *Antioxidants* **2021**, *10*, 265. [CrossRef]
25. Aghamohammadi, D.; Dolatkhah, N.; Bakhtiari, F.; Eslamian, F.; Hashemian, M. Nutraceutical supplements in management of pain and disability in osteoarthritis: A systematic review and meta-analysis of randomized clinical trials. *Sci. Rep.* **2020**, *10*. [CrossRef] [PubMed]
26. D'Adamo, S.; Cetrullo, S.; Panichi, V.; Mariani, E.; Flamigni, F.; Borzì, R.M. Nutraceutical Activity in Osteoarthritis Biology: A Focus on the Nutrigenomic Role. *Cells* **2020**, *9*, 1232. [CrossRef] [PubMed]
27. Deligiannidou, G.E.; Papadopoulos, R.E.; Kontogiorgis, C.; Detsi, A.; Bezirtzoglou, E.; Constantinides, T. Unraveling natural products' role in osteoarthritis management—An overview. *Antioxidants* **2020**, *9*, 348. [CrossRef]
28. Lee, H.; Zhao, X.; Son, Y.O.; Yang, S. Therapeutic single compounds for osteoarthritis treatment. *Pharmaceuticals* **2021**, *14*, 131. [CrossRef]
29. Blazek, A.D.; Nam, J.; Gupta, R.; Pradhan, M.; Perera, P.; Weisleder, N.L.; Hewett, T.E.; Chaudhari, A.M.; Lee, B.S.; Leblebicioglu, B.; et al. Exercise-driven metabolic pathways in healthy cartilage. *Osteoarthr. Cartil.* **2016**. [CrossRef]
30. Hui, W.; Young, D.A.; Rowan, A.D.; Xu, X.; Cawston, T.E.; Proctor, C.J. Oxidative changes and signalling pathways are pivotal in initiating age-related changes in articular cartilage. *Ann. Rheum. Dis.* **2016**. [CrossRef]
31. Li, D.; Xie, G.; Wang, W. Reactive oxygen species: The 2-edged sword of osteoarthritis. *Am. J. Med. Sci.* **2012**, *344*, 486–490. [CrossRef]
32. Schieber, M.; Chandel, N.S. ROS function in redox signaling and oxidative stress. *Curr. Biol.* **2014**, *24*, R453–R462. [CrossRef]
33. Jones, D.P. Radical-free biology of oxidative stress. *Am. J. Physiol. Cell Physiol.* **2008**, *295*, C849–C868. [CrossRef]
34. Blanco, F.J.; Rego, I.; Ruiz-Romero, C. The role of mitochondria in osteoarthritis. *Nat. Rev. Rheumatol.* **2011**, *7*, 161–169. [CrossRef]
35. Mao, X.; Fu, P.; Wang, L.; Xiang, C. Mitochondria: Potential Targets for Osteoarthritis. *Front. Med.* **2020**, *7*, 7. [CrossRef]
36. Lepetsos, P.; Papavassiliou, A.G. ROS/oxidative stress signaling in osteoarthritis. *Biochim. Biophys. Acta Mol. Basis Dis.* **2016**, *1862*, 576–591. [CrossRef]
37. Rahmati, M.; Nalesso, G.; Mobasheri, A.; Mozafari, M. Aging and osteoarthritis: Central role of the extracellular matrix. *Ageing Res. Rev.* **2017**, *40*, 20–30. [CrossRef]
38. Henrotin, Y.E.; Bruckner, P.; Pujol, J.P.L. The role of reactive oxygen species in homeostasis and degradation of cartilage. *Osteoarthr. Cartil.* **2003**, *11*, 747–755. [CrossRef]
39. Regan, E.A.; Bowler, R.P.; Crapo, J.D. Joint fluid antioxidants are decreased in osteoarthritic joints compared to joints with macroscopically intact cartilage and subacute injury. *Osteoarthr. Cartil.* **2008**. [CrossRef]
40. Hwang, H.S.; Kim, H.A. Chondrocyte apoptosis in the pathogenesis of osteoarthritis. *Int. J. Mol. Sci.* **2015**, *16*, 26035–26054. [CrossRef]
41. Zahan, O.M.; Serban, O.; Gherman, C.; Fodor, D. The evaluation of oxidative stress in osteoarthritis. *Med. Pharm. Rep.* **2020**, *93*, 12–22. [CrossRef]
42. Setti, T.; Arab, M.G.L.; Santos, G.S.; Alkass, N.; Andrade, M.A.P.; Lana, J.F.S.D. The protective role of glutathione in osteoarthritis. *J. Clin. Orthop. Trauma* **2021**, *15*, 145–151. [CrossRef]
43. Hu, S.; Zhang, C.; Ni, L.; Huang, C.; Chen, D.; Shi, K.; Jin, H.; Zhang, K.; Li, Y.; Xie, L.; et al. Stabilization of HIF-1α alleviates osteoarthritis via enhancing mitophagy. *Cell Death Dis.* **2020**. [CrossRef]
44. Malemud, C.J. The PI3K/Akt/PTEN/mTOR pathway: A fruitful target for inducing cell death in rheumatoid arthritis? *Future Med. Chem.* **2015**, *7*, 1137–1147. [CrossRef]
45. Li, Z.; Wang, J.; Deng, X.; Huang, D.; Shao, Z.; Ma, K. Compression stress induces nucleus pulposus cell autophagy by inhibition of the PI3K/AKT/mTOR pathway and activation of the JNK pathway. *Connect. Tissue Res.* **2020**. [CrossRef] [PubMed]
46. Rao, Z.; Wang, S.; Wang, J. Peroxiredoxin 4 inhibits IL-1β-induced chondrocyte apoptosis via PI3K/AKT signaling. *Biomed. Pharmacother.* **2017**. [CrossRef]
47. Ashrafizadeh, M.; Ahmadi, Z.; Farkhondeh, T.; Samarghandian, S. Resveratrol targeting the Wnt signaling pathway: A focus on therapeutic activities. *J. Cell. Physiol.* **2020**, *235*, 4135–4145. [CrossRef] [PubMed]
48. Bouaziz, W.; Sigaux, J.; Modrowski, D.; Devignes, C.S.; Funck-Brentano, T.; Richette, P.; Ea, H.K.; Provot, S.; Cohen-Solal, M.; Haÿ, E. Interaction of HIF1α and β-catenin inhibits matrix metalloproteinase 13 expression and prevents cartilage damage in mice. *Proc. Natl. Acad. Sci. USA* **2016**. [CrossRef] [PubMed]
49. Ma, Y.; Zheng, W.; Chen, H.; Shao, X.; Lin, P.; Liu, X.; Li, X.; Ye, H. Glucosamine promotes chondrocyte proliferation via the Wnt/β-catenin signaling pathway. *Int. J. Mol. Med.* **2018**. [CrossRef] [PubMed]
50. Khan, N.M.; Haseeb, A.; Ansari, M.Y.; Devarapalli, P.; Haynie, S.; Haqqi, T.M. Wogonin, a plant derived small molecule, exerts potent anti-inflammatory and chondroprotective effects through the activation of ROS/ERK/Nrf2 signaling pathways in human Osteoarthritis chondrocytes. *Free Radic. Biol. Med.* **2017**. [CrossRef]
51. Zhao, Y.P.; Liu, B.; Tian, Q.Y.; Wei, J.L.; Richbourgh, B.; Liu, C.J. Progranulin protects against osteoarthritis through interacting with TNF-α and β-Catenin signalling. *Ann. Rheum. Dis.* **2015**. [CrossRef]
52. Li, X.; Feng, K.; Li, J.; Yu, D.; Fan, Q.; Tang, T.; Yao, X.; Wang, X. Curcumin inhibits apoptosis of chondrocytes through activation ERK1/2 signaling pathways induced autophagy. *Nutrients* **2017**, *9*, 414. [CrossRef]

53. Imagawa, K.; de Andrés, M.C.; Hashimoto, K.; Pitt, D.; Itoi, E.; Goldring, M.B.; Roach, H.I.; Oreffo, R.O.C. The epigenetic effect of glucosamine and a nuclear factor-kappa B (NF-κB) inhibitor on primary human chondrocytes—Implications for osteoarthritis. *Biochem. Biophys. Res. Commun.* **2011**. [CrossRef]
54. Vincent, T.L. Mechanoflammation in osteoarthritis pathogenesis. *Semin. Arthritis Rheum.* **2019**. [CrossRef]
55. Qin, Y.; Chen, Y.; Wang, W.; Wang, Z.; Tang, G.; Zhang, P.; He, Z.; Liu, Y.; Dai, S.M.; Shen, Q. HMGB1-LPS complex promotes transformation of osteoarthritis synovial fibroblasts to a rheumatoid arthritis synovial fibroblast-like phenotype. *Cell Death Dis.* **2014**. [CrossRef] [PubMed]
56. Millerand, M.; Berenbaum, F.; Jacques, C. Danger signals and inflammaging in osteoarthritis. *Clin. Exp. Rheumatol.* **2019**, *37*, 48–56. [PubMed]
57. Sun, J.; Nan, G. The Mitogen-Activated Protein Kinase (MAPK) Signaling Pathway as a Discovery Target in Stroke. *J. Mol. Neurosci.* **2016**, *59*, 90–98. [CrossRef]
58. Wang, Z.; Guo, A.; Ma, L.; Yu, H.; Zhang, L.; Meng, H.; Cui, Y.; Yu, F.; Yang, B. Docosahexenoic acid treatment ameliorates cartilage degeneration via a p38 MAPK-dependent mechanism. *Int. J. Mol. Med.* **2016**. [CrossRef]
59. Marchev, A.S.; Dimitrova, P.A.; Burns, A.J.; Kostov, R.V.; Dinkova-Kostova, A.T.; Georgiev, M.I. Oxidative stress and chronic inflammation in osteoarthritis: Can NRF2 counteract these partners in crime? *Ann. N. Y. Acad. Sci.* **2017**, *1404*, 114–135. [CrossRef]
60. Sun, Z.; Zhang, S.; Chan, J.Y.; Zhang, D.D. Keap1 Controls Postinduction Repression of the Nrf2-Mediated Antioxidant Response by Escorting Nuclear Export of Nrf2. *Mol. Cell. Biol.* **2007**. [CrossRef]
61. Tonelli, C.; Chio, I.I.C.; Tuveson, D.A. Transcriptional Regulation by Nrf2. *Antioxid. Redox Signal.* **2018**, *29*, 1727–1745. [CrossRef]
62. He, F.; Ru, X.; Wen, T. NRF2, a transcription factor for stress response and beyond. *Int. J. Mol. Sci.* **2020**, *21*, 4777. [CrossRef]
63. Jevsevar, D.S.; Brown, G.A.; Jones, D.L.; Matzkin, E.G.; Manner, P.A.; Mooar, P.; Schousboe, J.T.; Stovitz, S.; Sanders, J.O.; Bozic, K.J.; et al. The American Academy of Orthopaedic Surgeons evidence-based guideline on: Treatment of osteoarthritis of the knee, 2nd edition. *J. Bone Jt. Surg. Am.* **2013**. [CrossRef]
64. Garber, C.E.; Blissmer, B.; Deschenes, M.R.; Franklin, B.A.; Lamonte, M.J.; Lee, I.M.; Nieman, D.C.; Swain, D.P. Quantity and quality of exercise for developing and maintaining cardiorespiratory, musculoskeletal, and neuromotor fitness in apparently healthy adults: Guidance for prescribing exercise. *Med. Sci. Sports Exerc.* **2011**. [CrossRef] [PubMed]
65. Rausch Osthoff, A.K.; Niedermann, K.; Braun, J.; Adams, J.; Brodin, N.; Dagfinrud, H.; Duruoz, T.; Esbensen, B.A.; Günther, K.P.; Hurkmans, E.; et al. 2018 EULAR recommendations for physical activity in people with inflammatory arthritis and osteoarthritis. *Ann. Rheum. Dis.* **2018**, *77*, 1251–1260. [CrossRef]
66. Fransen, M. When is physiotherapy appropriate? *Best Pract. Res. Clin. Rheumatol.* **2004**. [CrossRef]
67. Rahmann, A. Exercise for people with hip or knee osteoarthritis: A comparison of land-based and aquatic interventions. *Open Access J. Sport. Med.* **2010**. [CrossRef]
68. Raposo, F.; Ramos, M.; Lúcia Cruz, A. Effects of exercise on knee osteoarthritis: A systematic review. *Musculoskelet. Care* **2021**. [CrossRef]
69. Iijima, H.; Aoyama, T.; Ito, A.; Tajino, J.; Yamaguchi, S.; Nagai, M.; Kiyan, W.; Zhang, X.; Kuroki, H. Exercise intervention increases expression of bone morphogenetic proteins and prevents the progression of cartilage-subchondral bone lesions in a post-traumatic rat knee model. *Osteoarthr. Cartil.* **2016**. [CrossRef]
70. Assis, L.; Milares, L.P.; Almeida, T.; Tim, C.; Magri, A.; Fernandes, K.R.; Medalha, C.; Muniz Renno, A.C. Aerobic exercise training and low-level laser therapy modulate inflammatory response and degenerative process in an experimental model of knee osteoarthritis in rats. *Osteoarthr. Cartil.* **2016**, *24*, 169–177. [CrossRef]
71. Yang, Y.; Wang, Y.; Kong, Y.; Zhang, X.; Bai, L. The effects of different frequency treadmill exercise on lipoxin A4 and articular cartilage degeneration in an experimental model of monosodium iodoacetate-induced osteoarthritis in rats. *PLoS ONE* **2017**, *12*. [CrossRef]
72. Zhang, H.; Ji, L.; Yang, Y.; Wei, Y.; Zhang, X.; Gang, Y.; Lu, J.; Bai, L. The Therapeutic Effects of Treadmill Exercise on Osteoarthritis in Rats by Inhibiting the HDAC3/NF-KappaB Pathway in vivo and in vitro. *Front. Physiol.* **2019**, *10*. [CrossRef]
73. Castrogiovanni, P.; Di Rosa, M.; Ravalli, S.; Castorina, A.; Guglielmino, C.; Imbesi, R.; Vecchio, M.; Drago, F.; Szychlinska, M.A.; Musumeci, G. Moderate physical activity as a prevention method for knee osteoarthritis and the role of synoviocytes as biological key. *Int. J. Mol. Sci.* **2019**, *20*, 511. [CrossRef]
74. Lu, J.; Feng, X.; Zhang, H.; Wei, Y.; Yang, Y.; Tian, Y.; Bai, L. Maresin-1 suppresses IL-1β-induced MMP-13 secretion by activating the PI3K/AKT pathway and inhibiting the NF-κB pathway in synovioblasts of an osteoarthritis rat model with treadmill exercise. *Connect. Tissue Res.* **2020**. [CrossRef] [PubMed]
75. Zhang, X.; Yang, Y.; Li, X.; Zhang, H.; Gang, Y.; Bai, L. Alterations of autophagy in knee cartilage by treatment with treadmill exercise in a rat osteoarthritis model. *Int. J. Mol. Med.* **2019**, *43*, 336–344. [CrossRef] [PubMed]
76. Tian, Y.; Gou, J.; Zhang, H.; Lu, J.; Jin, Z.; Jia, S.; Bai, L. The anti-inflammatory effects of 15-HETE on osteoarthritis during treadmill exercise. *Life Sci.* **2021**. [CrossRef]
77. Galois, L.; Etienne, S.; Grossin, L.; Watrin-Pinzano, A.; Cournil-Henrionnet, C.; Loeuille, D.; Netter, P.; Mainard, D.; Gillet, P. Dose-response relationship for exercise on severity of experimental osteoarthritis in rats: A pilot study. *Osteoarthr. Cartil.* **2004**. [CrossRef]
78. Nam, J.; Perera, P.; Liu, J.; Wu, L.C.; Rath, B.; Butterfield, T.A.; Agarwal, S. Transcriptome-wide gene regulation by gentle treadmill walking during the progression of monoiodoacetate-induced arthritis. *Arthritis Rheum.* **2011**. [CrossRef]

79. Bricca, A.; Juhl, C.B.; Steultjens, M.; Wirth, W.; Roos, E.M. Impact of exercise on articular cartilage in people at risk of, or with established, knee osteoarthritis: A systematic review of randomised controlled trials. *Br. J. Sports Med.* **2019**. [CrossRef]
80. Roos, E.M.; Dahlberg, L. Positive effects of moderate exercise on glycosaminoglycan content in knee cartilage: A four-month, randomized, controlled trial in patients at risk of osteoarthritis. *Arthritis Rheum.* **2005**. [CrossRef]
81. Hawezi, Z.K.; Lammentausta, E.; Svensson, J.; Roos, E.M.; Dahlberg, L.E.; Tiderius, C.J. Regional dGEMRIC analysis in patients at risk of osteoar thritis provides additional information about activity related changes in car tilage structure. *Acta Radiol.* **2016**. [CrossRef]
82. Munukka, M.; Waller, B.; Häkkinen, A.; Nieminen, M.T.; Lammentausta, E.; Kujala, U.M.; Paloneva, J.; Kautiainen, H.; Kiviranta, I.; Heinonen, A. Physical Activity Is Related with Cartilage Quality in Women with Knee Osteoarthritis. *Med. Sci. Sports Exerc.* **2017**. [CrossRef] [PubMed]
83. Helmark, I.C.; Mikkelsen, U.R.; Børglum, J.; Rothe, A.; Petersen, M.C.H.; Andersen, O.; Langberg, H.; Kjaer, M. Exercise increases interleukin-10 levels both intraarticularly and peri-synovially in patients with knee osteoarthritis: A randomized controlled trial. *Arthritis Res. Ther.* **2010**. [CrossRef] [PubMed]
84. Hunt, M.A.; Pollock, C.L.; Kraus, V.B.; Saxne, T.; Peters, S.; Huebner, J.L.; Sayre, E.C.; Cibere, J. Relationships amongst osteoarthritis biomarkers, dynamic knee joint load, and exercise: Results from a randomized controlled pilot study. *BMC Musculoskelet. Disord.* **2013**. [CrossRef] [PubMed]
85. Messier, S.P.; Mihalko, S.L.; Legault, C.; Miller, G.D.; Nicklas, B.J.; DeVita, P.; Beavers, D.P.; Hunter, D.J.; Lyles, M.F.; Eckstein, F.; et al. Effects of intensive diet and exercise on knee joint loads, inflammation, and clinical outcomes among overweight and obese adults with knee osteoarthritis: The IDEA randomized clinical trial. *JAMA J. Am. Med. Assoc.* **2013**. [CrossRef]
86. Simioni, C.; Zauli, G.; Martelli, A.M.; Vitale, M.; Sacchetti, G.; Gonelli, A.; Neri, L.M. Oxidative stress: Role of physical exercise and antioxidant nutraceuticals in adulthood and aging. *Oncotarget* **2018**, *9*, 17181–17198. [CrossRef] [PubMed]
87. Dalle Carbonare, L.; Mottes, M.; Cheri, S.; Deiana, M.; Zamboni, F.; Gabbiani, D.; Schena, F.; Salvagno, G.L.; Lippi, G.; Valenti, M.T. Increased Gene Expression of RUNX2 and SOX9 in Mesenchymal Circulating Progenitors Is Associated with Autophagy during Physical Activity. *Oxid. Med. Cell. Longev.* **2019**. [CrossRef]
88. Hunter, C.J.; Imler, S.M.; Malaviya, P.; Nerem, R.M.; Levenston, M.E. Mechanical compression alters gene expression and extracellular matrix synthesis by chondrocytes cultured in collagen I gels. *Biomaterials* **2002**. [CrossRef]
89. Khan, N.M.; Ahmad, I.; Haqqi, T.M. Nrf2/ARE pathway attenuates oxidative and apoptotic response in human osteoarthritis chondrocytes by activating ERK1/2/ELK1-P70S6K-P90RSK signaling axis. *Free Radic. Biol. Med.* **2018**, *116*, 159–171. [CrossRef]
90. Vargas-Mendoza, N.; Morales-González, Á.; Madrigal-Santillán, E.O.; Madrigal-Bujaidar, E.; Álvarez-González, I.; García-Melo, L.F.; Anguiano-Robledo, L.; Fregoso-Aguilar, T.; Morales-Gonzalez, J.A. Antioxidant and adaptive response mediated by Nrf2 during physical exercise. *Antioxidants* **2019**, *8*, 196. [CrossRef]
91. Cifuentes, D.J.; Rocha, L.G.; Silva, L.A.; Brito, A.C.; Rueff-Barroso, C.R.; Porto, L.C.; Pinho, R.A. Decrease in oxidative stress and histological changes induced by physical exercise calibrated in rats with osteoarthritis induced by monosodium iodoacetate. *Osteoarthr. Cartil.* **2010**. [CrossRef]
92. Germanou, E.I.; Chatzinikolaou, A.; Malliou, P.; Beneka, A.; Jamurtas, A.Z.; Bikos, C.; Tsoukas, D.; Theodorou, A.; Katrabasas, I.; Margonis, K.; et al. Oxidative stress and inflammatory responses following an acute bout of isokinetic exercise in obese women with knee osteoarthritis. *Knee* **2013**. [CrossRef] [PubMed]
93. Freitag, J.; Bates, D.; Boyd, R.; Shah, K.; Barnard, A.; Huguenin, L.; Tenen, A. Mesenchymal stem cell therapy in the treatment of osteoarthritis: Reparative pathways, safety and efficacy—A review. *BMC Musculoskelet. Disord.* **2016**, *17*, 1–13. [CrossRef]
94. Song, J.S.; Hong, K.T.; Kim, N.M.; Jung, J.Y.; Park, H.S.; Chun, Y.S.; Kim, S.J. Cartilage regeneration in osteoarthritic knees treated with distal femoral osteotomy and intra-lesional implantation of allogenic human umbilical cord blood-derived mesenchymal stem cells: A report of two cases. *Knee* **2019**. [CrossRef]
95. Minas, T.; Ogura, T.; Bryant, T. Autologous chondrocyte implantation. *JBJS Essent. Surg. Tech.* **2016**. [CrossRef]
96. Schmidt, A.; Bierwirth, S.; Weber, S.; Platen, P.; Schinköthe, T.; Bloch, W. Short intensive exercise increases the migratory activity of mesenchymal stem cells. *Br. J. Sports Med.* **2009**. [CrossRef]
97. Valenti, M.T.; Deiana, M.; Cheri, S.; Dotta, M.; Zamboni, F.; Gabbiani, D.; Schena, F.; Dalle Carbonare, L.; Mottes, M. Physical Exercise Modulates miR-21-5p, miR-129-5p, miR-378-5p, and miR-188-5p Expression in Progenitor Cells Promoting Osteogenesis. *Cells* **2019**, *8*, 742. [CrossRef]
98. Smith, J.K. Exercise as an adjuvant to cartilage regeneration therapy. *Int. J. Mol. Sci.* **2020**, *21*, 9471. [CrossRef] [PubMed]
99. Emmons, R.; Niemiro, G.M.; Owolabi, O.; De Lisio, M. Acute exercise mobilizes hematopoietic stem and progenitor cells and alters the mesenchymal stromal cell secretome. *J. Appl. Physiol.* **2016**. [CrossRef]
100. Bourzac, C.; Bensidhoum, M.; Pallu, S.; Portier, H. Use of adult mesenchymal stromal cells in tissue repair: Impact of physical exercise. *Am. J. Physiol. Cell Physiol.* **2019**, *317*, C642–C654. [CrossRef] [PubMed]
101. Ocarino, N.M.; Boeloni, J.N.; Goes, A.M.; Silva, J.F.; Marubayashi, U.; Serakides, R. Osteogenic differentiation of mesenchymal stem cells from osteopenic rats subjected to physical activity with and without nitric oxide synthase inhibition. *Nitric Oxide Biol. Chem.* **2008**. [CrossRef] [PubMed]
102. Hell, R.C.R.; Ocarino, N.M.; Boeloni, J.N.; Silva, J.F.; Goes, A.M.; Santos, R.L.; Serakides, R. Physical activity improves age-related decline in the osteogenic potential of rats' bone marrow-derived mesenchymal stem cells. *Acta Physiol.* **2012**, *205*, 292–301. [CrossRef]

103. Andersson, M.L.E.; Thorstensson, C.A.; Roos, E.M.; Petersson, I.F.; Heinegård, D.; Saxne, T. Serum levels of Cartilage Oligomeric Matrix Protein (COMP) increase temporarily after physical exercise in patients with knee osteoarthritis. *BMC Musculoskelet. Disord.* **2006**, *7*. [CrossRef] [PubMed]

104. Siebelt, M.; Groen, H.C.; Koelewijn, S.J.; de Blois, E.; Sandker, M.; Waarsing, J.H.; Müller, C.; van Osch, G.J.V.M.; de Jong, M.; Weinans, H. Increased physical activity severely induces osteoarthritic changes in knee joints with papain induced sulfate-glycosaminoglycan depleted cartilage. *Arthritis Res. Ther.* **2014**, *16*. [CrossRef]

105. Liu, S.S.; Zhou, P.; Zhang, Y. Abnormal expression of key genes and proteins in the canonical Wnt/β-catenin pathway of articular cartilage in a rat model of exercise-induced osteoarthritis. *Mol. Med. Rep.* **2016**, *13*, 1999–2006. [CrossRef] [PubMed]

106. Rojas-Ortega, M.; Cruz, R.; Vega-López, M.A.; Cabrera-González, M.; Hernández-Hernández, J.M.; Lavalle-Montalvo, C.; Kouri, J.B. Exercise modulates the expression of IL-1β and IL-10 in the articular cartilage of normal and osteoarthritis-induced rats. *Pathol. Res. Pract.* **2015**. [CrossRef]

107. Coyle, C.H.; Henry, S.E.; Haleem, A.M.; O'Malley, M.J.; Chu, C.R. Serum CTXii Correlates with Articular Cartilage Degeneration After Anterior Cruciate Ligament Transection or Arthrotomy Followed by Standardized Exercise. *Sports Health* **2012**. [CrossRef]

108. Jayabalan, P.; Gustafson, J.; Sowa, G.A.; Piva, S.R.; Farrokhi, S. A Stimulus-Response Framework to Investigate the Influence of Continuous Versus Interval Walking Exercise on Select Serum Biomarkers in Knee Osteoarthritis. *Am. J. Phys. Med. Rehabil.* **2019**. [CrossRef] [PubMed]

109. Iolascon, G.; Gimigliano, R.; Bianco, M.; de Sire, A.; Moretti, A.; Giusti, A.; Malavolta, N.; Migliaccio, S.; Migliore, A.; Napoli, N.; et al. Are dietary supplements and nutraceuticals effective for musculoskeletal health and cognitive function? A scoping review. *J. Nutr. Heal. Aging* **2017**. [CrossRef]

110. Cho, C.; Kang, L.J.; Jang, D.; Jeon, J.; Lee, H.; Choi, S.; Han, S.J.; Oh, E.; Nam, J.; Kim, C.S.; et al. Cirsium japonicum var. maackii and apigenin block Hif-2α-induced osteoarthritic cartilage destruction. *J. Cell. Mol. Med.* **2019**. [CrossRef]

111. Wong, S.K.; Chin, K.Y.; Ima-Nirwana, S. Berberine and musculoskeletal disorders: The therapeutic potential and underlying molecular mechanisms. *Phytomedicine* **2020**, *73*, 152892. [CrossRef]

112. Korotkyi, O.; Huet, A.; Dvorshchenko, K.; Kobyliak, N.; Falalyeyeva, T.; Ostapchenko, L. Probiotic Composition and Chondroitin Sulfate Regulate TLR-2/4-Mediated NF-κB Inflammatory Pathway and Cartilage Metabolism in Experimental Osteoarthritis. *Probiotics Antimicrob. Proteins* **2021**. [CrossRef]

113. Zhang, Y.; Zeng, Y. Curcumin reduces inflammation in knee osteoarthritis rats through blocking TLR4 /MyD88/NF-κB signal pathway. *Drug Dev. Res.* **2019**. [CrossRef]

114. Jiang, C.; Luo, P.; Li, X.; Liu, P.; Li, Y.; Xu, J. Nrf2/ARE is a key pathway for curcumin-mediated protection of TMJ chondrocytes from oxidative stress and inflammation. *Cell Stress Chaperones* **2020**. [CrossRef] [PubMed]

115. Panaro, M.A.; Corrado, A.; Benameur, T.; Paolo, C.F.; Cici, D.; Porro, C. The emerging role of curcumin in the modulation of TLR-4 signaling pathway: Focus on neuroprotective and anti-rheumatic properties. *Int. J. Mol. Sci.* **2020**, *21*, 2299. [CrossRef] [PubMed]

116. Qiu, B.; Xu, X.; Yi, P.; Hao, Y. Curcumin reinforces MSC-derived exosomes in attenuating osteoarthritis via modulating the miR-124/NF-κB and miR-143/ROCK1/TLR9 signalling pathways. *J. Cell. Mol. Med.* **2020**. [CrossRef]

117. Lee, H.; Jang, D.; Jeon, J.; Cho, C.; Choi, S.; Han, S.J.; Oh, E.; Nam, J.; Park, C.H.; Shin, Y.S.; et al. Seomae mugwort and jaceosidin attenuate osteoarthritic cartilage damage by blocking IκB degradation in mice. *J. Cell. Mol. Med.* **2020**, *24*, 8126–8137. [CrossRef]

118. Liu, F.C.; Wang, C.C.; Lu, J.W.; Lee, C.H.; Chen, S.C.; Ho, Y.J.; Peng, Y.J. Chondroprotective effects of genistein against osteoarthritis induced joint inflammation. *Nutrients* **2019**, *11*, 1180. [CrossRef] [PubMed]

119. Yuan, J.; Ding, W.; Wu, N.; Jiang, S.; Li, W. Protective Effect of Genistein on Condylar Cartilage through Downregulating NF- B Expression in Experimentally Created Osteoarthritis Rats. *Biomed Res. Int.* **2019**. [CrossRef]

120. Zou, Y.; Liu, Q.; Guo, P.; Huang, Y.; Ye, Z.; Hu, J. Anti-chondrocyte apoptosis effect of genistein in treating inflammation-induced osteoarthritis. *Mol. Med. Rep.* **2020**, *22*, 2032–2042. [CrossRef]

121. Lv, C.; Wang, L.; Zhu, X.; Lin, W.; Chen, X.; Huang, Z.; Huang, L.; Yang, S. Glucosamine promotes osteoblast proliferation by modulating autophagy via the mammalian target of rapamycin pathway. *Biomed. Pharmacother.* **2018**. [CrossRef]

122. Bai, H.; Zhang, Z.; Li, Y.; Song, X.; Ma, T.; Liu, C.; Liu, L.; Yuan, R.; Wang, X.; Gao, L. L-theanine reduced the development of knee osteoarthritis in rats via its anti-inflammation and anti-matrix degradation actions: In vivo and in vitro study. *Nutrients* **2020**, *12*, 1988. [CrossRef] [PubMed]

123. Luk, H.Y.; Appell, C.; Chyu, M.C.; Chen, C.H.; Wang, C.Y.; Yang, R.S.; Shen, C.L. Impacts of green tea on joint and skeletal muscle health: Prospects of translational nutrition. *Antioxidants* **2020**, *9*, 1050. [CrossRef] [PubMed]

124. Chang, Y.C.; Liu, H.W.; Chan, Y.C.; Hu, S.H.; Liu, M.Y.; Chang, S.J. The green tea polyphenol epigallocatechin-3-gallate attenuates age-associated muscle loss via regulation of miR-486-5p and myostatin. *Arch. Biochem. Biophys.* **2020**. [CrossRef]

125. Feng, Z.; Li, X.; Lin, J.; Zheng, W.; Hu, Z.; Xuan, J.; Ni, W.; Pan, X. Oleuropein inhibits the IL-1β-induced expression of inflammatory mediators by suppressing the activation of NF-κB and MAPKs in human osteoarthritis chondrocytes. *Food Funct.* **2017**. [CrossRef] [PubMed]

126. Serreli, G.; Deiana, M. Extra Virgin Olive Oil Polyphenols: Modulation of Cellular Pathways Related to Oxidant Species and Inflammation in Aging. *Cells* **2020**, *9*, 478. [CrossRef]

127. Varela-Eirín, M.; Carpintero-Fernández, P.; Sánchez-Temprano, A.; Varela-Vázquez, A.; Paíno, C.L.; Casado-Díaz, A.; Continente, A.C.; Mato, V.; Fonseca, E.; Kandouz, M.; et al. Senolytic activity of small molecular polyphenols from olive restores chondrocyte redifferentiation and promotes a pro-regenerative environment in osteoarthritis. *Aging* **2020**. [CrossRef]

128. Chen, Y.L.; Yan, D.Y.; Wu, C.Y.; Xuan, J.W.; Jin, C.Q.; Hu, X.L.; Bao, G.D.; Bian, Y.J.; Hu, Z.C.; Shen, Z.H.; et al. Maslinic acid prevents IL-1β-induced inflammatory response in osteoarthritis via PI3K/AKT/NF-κB pathways. *J. Cell. Physiol.* **2021**. [CrossRef]
129. Zhang, J.; Yin, J.; Zhao, D.; Wang, C.; Zhang, Y.; Wang, Y.; Li, T. Therapeutic effect and mechanism of action of quercetin in a rat model of osteoarthritis. *J. Int. Med. Res.* **2019**. [CrossRef]
130. Farkhondeh, T.; Folgado, S.L.; Pourbagher-Shahri, A.M.; Ashrafizadeh, M.; Samarghandian, S. The therapeutic effect of resveratrol: Focusing on the Nrf2 signaling pathway. *Biomed. Pharmacother.* **2020**, *127*, 110234. [CrossRef]
131. Xu, X.; Liu, X.; Yang, Y.; He, J.; Jiang, M.; Huang, Y.; Liu, X.; Liu, L.; Gu, H. Resveratrol exerts anti-osteoarthritic effect by inhibiting TLR4/NF-κB signaling pathway via the TLR4/Akt/FoxO1 axis in IL-1β-stimulated SW1353 cells. *Drug Des. Devel. Ther.* **2020**. [CrossRef] [PubMed]
132. Yi, H.; Zhang, W.; Cui, Z.M.; Cui, S.Y.; Fan, J.B.; Zhu, X.H.; Liu, W. Resveratrol alleviates the interleukin-1β-induced chondrocytes injury through the NF-κB signaling pathway. *J. Orthop. Surg. Res.* **2020**. [CrossRef]
133. Yang, J.; Song, X.; Feng, Y.; Liu, N.; Fu, Z.; Wu, J.; Li, T.; Chen, H.; Chen, J.; Chen, C.; et al. Natural ingredients-derived antioxidants attenuate H2O2-induced oxidative stress and have chondroprotective effects on human osteoarthritic chondrocytes via Keap1/Nrf2 pathway. *Free Radic. Biol. Med.* **2020**. [CrossRef] [PubMed]
134. Moon, S.J.; Jhun, J.; Ryu, J.; Kwon, J.Y.; Kim, S.Y.; Jung, K.A.; Cho, M.L.; Min, J.K. The anti-arthritis effect of sulforaphane, an activator of Nrf2, is associated with inhibition of both B cell differentiation and the production of inflammatory cytokines. *PLoS ONE* **2021**. [CrossRef] [PubMed]
135. Luo, T.; Fu, X.; Liu, Y.; Ji, Y.; Shang, Z. Sulforaphane Inhibits Osteoclastogenesis via Suppression of the Autophagic Pathway. *Molecules* **2021**, *26*, 347. [CrossRef] [PubMed]
136. Khan, N.M.; Haseeb, A.; Ansari, M.Y.; Haqqi, T.M. A wogonin-rich-fraction of Scutellaria baicalensis root extract exerts chondroprotective effects by suppressing IL-1β-induced activation of AP-1 in human OA chondrocytes. *Sci. Rep.* **2017**. [CrossRef]
137. Ammendolia, A.; Marotta, N.; Marinaro, C.; Demeco, A.; Mondardini, P.; Costantino, C. High Power Laser Therapy and Glucosamine sulfate in the treatment of knee osteoarthritis: A single blinded randomized controlled trial. *Acta Biomed. l'Ateneo Parm.* **2021**. [CrossRef]
138. Zhang, C.; Sheng, J.; Li, G.; Zhao, L.; Wang, Y.; Yang, W.; Yao, X.; Sun, L.; Zhang, Z.; Cui, R. Effects of berberine and its derivatives on cancer: A systems pharmacology review. *Front. Pharmacol.* **2020**, *10*, 1461. [CrossRef]
139. Hou, C.Y.; Tain, Y.L.; Yu, H.R.; Huang, L.T. The effects of resveratrol in the treatment of metabolic syndrome. *Int. J. Mol. Sci.* **2019**, *20*, 535. [CrossRef]
140. Hasan, M.M.; Bae, H. An overview of stress-induced resveratrol synthesis in grapes: Perspectives for resveratrol-enriched grape products. *Molecules* **2017**, *22*, 294. [CrossRef]

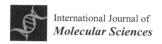

International Journal of
Molecular Sciences

MDPI

Review

Vibrational Spectroscopy in Assessment of Early Osteoarthritis—A Narrative Review

Chen Yu [1,2,†], Bing Zhao [1,2,†], Yan Li [3], Hengchang Zang [1,2,4,5] and Lian Li [1,2,4,*]

1 School of Pharmaceutical Sciences, Cheeloo College of Medicine, Shandong University, Wenhuaxi Road 44, Jinan 250012, China; y17865190891@163.com (C.Y.); zhaobing911@163.com (B.Z.); zanghcw@126.com (H.Z.)
2 NMPA Key Laboratory for Technology Research and Evaluation of Drug Products, Shandong University, Wenhuaxi Road 44, Jinan 250012, China
3 Institute of Materia Medica, Shandong First Medical University and Shandong Academy of Medical Scinces, Jinan 250062, China; liyan091022@126.com
4 Key Laboratory of Chemical Biology (Ministry of Education), Shandong University, Wenhuaxi Road 44, Jinan 250012, China
5 National Glycoengineering Research Center, Shandong University, Wenhuaxi Road 44, Jinan 250012, China
* Correspondence: lilian@sdu.edu.cn; Tel.: +86-531-8838-0268
† These authors contributed equally to this work.

Abstract: Osteoarthritis (OA) is a degenerative disease, and there is currently no effective medicine to cure it. Early prevention and treatment can effectively reduce the pain of OA patients and save costs. Therefore, it is necessary to diagnose OA at an early stage. There are various diagnostic methods for OA, but the methods applied to early diagnosis are limited. Ordinary optical diagnosis is confined to the surface, while laboratory tests, such as rheumatoid factor inspection and physical arthritis checks, are too trivial or time-consuming. Evidently, there is an urgent need to develop a rapid nondestructive detection method for the early diagnosis of OA. Vibrational spectroscopy is a rapid and nondestructive technique that has attracted much attention. In this review, near-infrared (NIR), infrared, (IR) and Raman spectroscopy were introduced to show their potential in early OA diagnosis. The basic principles were discussed first, and then the research progress to date was discussed, as well as its limitations and the direction of development. Finally, all methods were compared, and vibrational spectroscopy was demonstrated that it could be used as a promising tool for early OA diagnosis. This review provides theoretical support for the application and development of vibrational spectroscopy technology in OA diagnosis, providing a new strategy for the nondestructive and rapid diagnosis of arthritis and promoting the development and clinical application of a component-based molecular spectrum detection technology.

Keywords: osteoarthritis; vibrational spectroscopy; near-infrared spectroscopy; infrared spectroscopy; Raman spectroscopy; early diagnosis

Citation: Yu, C.; Zhao, B.; Li, Y.; Zang, H.; Li, L. Vibrational Spectroscopy in Assessment of Early Osteoarthritis—A Narrative Review. *Int. J. Mol. Sci.* **2021**, 22, 5235. https://doi.org/10.3390/ijms22105235

Academic Editor: Walter Herzog

Received: 1 April 2021
Accepted: 13 May 2021
Published: 15 May 2021

1. Introduction

Osteoarthritis (OA) is one of the major diseases affecting public health, and it is caused by both the mechanical and biological degradations of cartilage [1,2]. The 2017 Global Burden of Disease study shows that the annual number of OA patients is increasing, yet there remains no effective medicine to treat it [3]. OA is characterized by joint swelling, pain, and stiffness, causing physical pain to and placing a heavy financial burden on patients [4]. MacDonald et al. reported that the average age of people diagnosed with OA is 47.6, which is 7.7 years later than the onset of symptoms [5]. A Canadian study reported that patients with an OA score greater than or equal to 55 (severe disability) cost 3.5 times more than patients with an OA score of 15 (low severity) [6]. Most patients usually choose to see a doctor after they have obvious symptoms, and the general treatment of OA is often to address the corresponding symptoms, rather than to fundamentally cure the disease [7].

Many physiological and pathological changes may appear in the early stage of OA, which are the starting point for early diagnosis. OA is mainly caused by the inability of chondrocytes to maintain homeostasis between the synthesis and decomposition of intracellular and extracellular components, resulting in the inflammation of the synovium and joint capsule [8]. Moreover, various pathological changes may combine and worsen, leading to cartilage degeneration, subchondral osteosclerosis, angiogenesis, innervation, and other pathological phenomena. The extracellular matrix of chondrocytes is mainly composed of collagen, noncollagen proteins (glycosaminoglycan (GAG), proteoglycan (PG), cartilage oligomer matrix protein (COMP)), hyaluronic acid (HA), fibrin protein, follistatin-like protein 1 (FSTIL-1), glycoproteins, lipids, and water [9]. A number of these proteins are often used as biomarkers for the diagnosis of OA. GAG is the main component of the cartilage matrix. GAG in cartilage is cleaved by proteolytic enzymes, such as matrix metalloproteinases (MMPs) and aggregase, which decrease the expression level of GAG and lead to cartilage destruction. Therefore, GAG is often used as a marker of cartilage destruction in OA [10]. As an important component of synovial fluid (SF), HA can increase joint smoothness, thereby reducing cartilage wear, and it has been shown to be associated with the radiological progression of OA [3]. Subchondral bone can provide mechanical and nutritional support for cartilage. Small molecule diffusion experiments revealed that there is a direct molecular signaling pathway between cartilage and subchondral bone [11], indicating that changes in the microenvironment of subchondral bone may directly or indirectly affect cartilage metabolism. The quality and hardness of bone in patients with OA are decreased, making it more likely for some injuries to occur [12] and eventually leading to the production of osteophytes. In subchondral bone, markers such as the mineral-to-matrix ratio, mineral maturity/crystallinity, relative carbonate content, or relative tissue water content/porosity can provide signs of early OA [13]. The detection of changes in these markers is beneficial for an early diagnosis, which not only improves the treatment effect of OA for patients, but also greatly reduces treatment costs [14]. Considering the importance of an early diagnosis of OA, in this review, we aimed to summarize and analyze the vibrational spectroscopy used in early OA diagnosis to provide theoretical support for its application and development.

The diagnosis of OA primarily involves imaging and laboratory tests. The conventional imaging tests used include magnetic resonance imaging (MRI) [15–18], optical coherence tomography (OCT) [18–21], ultrasonic diagnosis [22–26], and X-ray [27–29]. Their specific applications are shown in Table 1. X-ray is the most accessible tool for assessing OA: it can show damage and other changes related to OA to confirm its severity according to different grading schemes, such as the Kellgren–Lawrence grading scheme [30]. MRI, which does not use radiation, is more expensive than X-ray but can provide better images of cartilage and other structures to detect early abnormalities in OA [16]. OCT is used to generate cross-sectional images of articular cartilage [19], and it can provide quantitative information on the state of articular cartilage, especially for OA caused by changes in collagen structure [31]. In terms of laboratory tests, the main method is joint aspiration, which comprises a needle being inserted into the joint, and fluid is extracted for further analysis to determine the stage of OA, which can help to rule out other forms of arthritis [32].

Table 1. Comparison table of application analysis of traditional imaging methods in relation to osteoarthritis (OA).

Name	Main Inspection Site	Advantages	Disadvantages	Reference
MRI	Structure of cartilage	Observe structural features related to cartilage integrity, no radiation	Expensive, long scan time	[15–18]
OCT	Transverse view of articular cartilage	Good reproducibility and no radiation to living tissue	Depth limitations allow only surface cross-sectional analysis	[18–21]

Table 1. Cont.

Name	Main Inspection Site	Advantages	Disadvantages	Reference
Ultrasonic diagnosis	Periarticular soft tissue	Visible image information, low cost	Poor penetration of bone, inability to observe deeper structures, poor reproducibility	[22–26]
X-ray	Joint appearance	Low cost, high benefit, combined with arthroscopy to assist doctors in diagnosis	Unable to show early symptoms of OA	[27–29]

The methods mentioned above are commonly used in clinical practice but are often time-consuming, expensive, and even destructive. The development of rapid and nondestructive methods is urgent [19,29]. As a promising technique, vibrational spectroscopy has received increasing attention from researchers worldwide. A vibrational spectrum is generated by the vibration of molecules or atomic groups caused by electromagnetic radiation, and vibrational spectroscopy includes a variety of techniques, such as near-infrared (NIR), infrared (IR), and Raman spectroscopy [33]. As shown in Figure 1, NIR/IR/Raman spectra of SF, articular cartilage, and/or subchondral bone were collected to compare the spectral differences between healthy and OA-affected joints. The spectra of SF indicate that the content of protein increased and the content of carotenoid decreased in OA-affected joints [34]. Furthermore, the spectra of articular cartilage characterized changes in the contents of GAG and PG, as well as the orientation of collagen fibers in joints [35]. By analyzing the spectra of subchondral bone, it was concluded that mineralized components increased in OA-affected joints [36]. Extracting and analyzing effective spectral information can help to distinguish OA-affected joints from healthy ones, thereby improving the likelihood of early OA diagnosis. In this review, these new vibrational spectroscopy methods for OA diagnosis are introduced to provide theoretical support for their application and development in relation to the early diagnosis of OA.

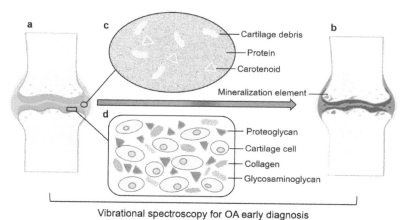

Figure 1. Vibrational spectroscopy is used for early OA diagnosis by detecting changes in the composition and morphology of articular cartilage and changes in synovial fluid (SF) and subchondral bone. The figure depicts (**a**) a healthy joint and (**b**) an OA-affected joint. In an OA-affected joint, the SF composition changes, articular cartilage becomes thinner and its composition changes, and the mineralization element in the subchondral bone increases. The main biomarkers of OA in (**c**) SF and (**d**) articular cartilage are also shown. Vibrational spectroscopy can detect the changes of these components for early OA diagnosis.

2. NIR Spectroscopy

NIR spectroscopy reflects the overtones and/or combination bands of stretching and bending vibrations of C–H, N–H, and O–H bonds ranging from 12,500 to 4000 cm^{-1} [37]. As shown in Figure 2, when a beam of NIR light with continuous wavelength irradiates to the sample, if the vibrational/rotational frequency of some groups in the sample is consistent with that of the NIR light, the molecule will absorb energy for energy-level transition, and the light at that wavelength is absorbed [38]. The sample can then be analyzed according to the transmitted or reflected light. NIR spectroscopy has been widely used in the agriculture [39–42], food [43–46], chemistry [47–49], and pharmaceutical fields [50–53] because it is fast, accurate, nondestructive and labor-saving. However, a limitation of this method is that the spectra are composed of wide overlapping bands [54,55], such that it is difficult to find specific peaks attributed to the complicated component. Chemometrics is a powerful tool for analyzing the NIR spectra and can improve the spectral resolution to help extract useful information from the spectra [56]. With the help of chemometrics, NIR spectroscopy has appeared in OA diagnostic research owing to its fast and nondestructive characteristics [57]. Although most of the work of NIR spectroscopy in OA diagnosis, including SF and tissue analysis, is still restricted to laboratory-scale research [58], it is becoming a useful tool for the diagnosis of OA and has good development prospects.

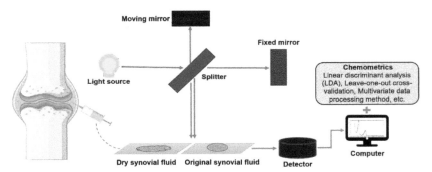

Figure 2. SF is analyzed by NIR spectroscopy. The SF extracted from the joint capsule is dried and either membrane-formed or examined directly. The light source is divided into two beams by the splitter, which are then reflected onto two mirrors—one is a fixed mirror and the other is a moving mirror. After the light is reflected, it is recombined and sent to the sample, and then the change of the light beam after the reflection and absorption of the sample is detected. Finally, the spectral data are analyzed with the help of chemometrics.

2.1. Application of NIR Spectroscopy on OA SF Analysis

Some studies have shown changes in the composition and concentration of SF metabolites in OA [59,60]. Therefore, SF is useful for the investigation of OA based on chemical composition and physical properties. There are two main methods for SF spectra collection: The first is to dry the SF onto a film and then to obtain the reflection spectrum for analysis. This can identify arthritis with a classification rate greater than 95% [61]. The second method is to obtain the SF spectrum through the transmitting module. Shaw et al. [58] collected the NIR spectra of SF and then divided the spectra into three categories by linear discriminant analysis (LDA), which is a kind of subjective measurement and classification based on a series of biochemical or biological diseases, leading to SF physical change. Their results showed that the best classification results were obtained when the spectral range was limited to 2000–2400 nm. This research demonstrated that NIR spectroscopy can determine the type of arthritis and the feasibility of severity ratings by SF analysis, showing that it is a powerful tool for the diagnosis of OA based on SF analysis. However, the application of this technology in SF analysis requires further research, which may help provide new hypotheses to explain the mechanism of OA in the future.

2.2. Application of NIR Spectroscopy on OA Cartilage Analysis

Normal hyaline cartilage contains 70%–80% water, mainly in the form of binding to GAG. In the early stage of OA, cartilage deformities often manifest as complex changes in the matrix, including GAG, moisture, and collagen [62]. Hofmann et al. [63] compared the degree of recognition of OCT, arthroscopy, MRI, and NIR spectroscopy for early OA cartilage change and found that only the result of NIR spectroscopy showed good correlation with the Knee Injury and Osteoarthritis Outcome Score (KOOS). Afara et al. [57] analyzed the NIR spectra of articular cartilage in mice with OA in four stages (1, 2, 4, and 6 weeks), and the spectral data showed that the spectral intensity increased over time, mainly due to changes in the cartilage moisture content; this showed that the method could detect early manifestations of cartilage degeneration. In addition, they applied principal component analysis (PCA) and multiple scattering correction (MSC) to process the two main spectral bands at 8547–$10,361$ cm^{-1} and 6411–6496 cm^{-1} and predict the Mankin score [64,65]. They also designed a genetic algorithm-based model to evaluate GAG content, which further demonstrated the power of NIR spectroscopy in OA diagnosis by detecting tissue integrity and GAG content.

The main feature of OA is cartilage degeneration, and PG and GAG are the key components of cartilage [66], so their effective detection is crucial for early diagnosis of OA. Palukuru et al. [67] identified 20–60 μm thickness of cartilage tissue as most suitable for analysis based on collagen and PG at 1336 and 856 cm^{-1} for linear absorption band intensity changes. They used partial least squares (PLS) modeling in the spectral range of 4000–6000 cm^{-1} to predict the relative content of collagen and PG, as well as the proportion of collagen, from NIR spectroscopy. The error of this method was reduced to 6%, which ultimately improved the accuracy of NIR spectroscopy for cartilage composition quantification.

In addition, a direct manifestation of OA is the reduction and thinning of cartilage [68]. Sarin et al. [69] combined arthroscopy with NIR spectroscopy to evaluate the cartilage thickness in vivo and determine PG content and the collagen orientation angle. Using a one-dimensional neural network, they demonstrated the clinical potential of NIR spectroscopy for evaluating cartilage thickness and composition structure. Afara et al. [70] combined NIR spectroscopy with support vector machines (SVMs), deep neural networks (DNNs), logistic regression (LR), and other methods to distinguish the integrity of cartilage. Their study indicated that the SVM model can distinguish anterior cruciate ligament transection (ACLT) from non-operationally operated control (CNTRL) samples, the DNN model can discriminate between different types of OA, and LR can differentiate between contralateral (CL) and CNTRL samples. NIR spectroscopy, in combination with machine learning techniques, can provide a powerful tool for the classification of cartilage integrity [71], with the potential to accurately distinguish between normal and early osteoarthritic cartilage [72,73].

3. Infrared Spectroscopy

The principle of IR is similar to that of NIR spectroscopy, but the difference lies in the acquisition bands used by the methods. IR spectroscopy technology is used to investigate interactions between molecules in the range of 4000–400 cm^{-1} [74]. It can be used to analyze the characteristic information of absorbed substances by reflecting IR light. Each molecule has a unique IR absorption spectrum, which is determined by its composition and structure, and this can be used for structural analysis and identification [75]. Fourier-transform IR (FTIR) spectroscopy is a simple method used to investigate the composition of macromolecules in biological samples, and it can be analyzed in situ by a probe, so it has advantages in the study of organisms and for early diagnosis of OA [76]. FTIR microspectroscopy (FTIR–MS) comprises an FTIR spectrometer and a traditional optical microscope to achieve chemical imaging, with which the spatial distribution and structure of various biochemical components can be identified [77]. Due to the complexity of the data structure, the required information cannot be revealed without powerful data analysis methods. Therefore, the application of IR spectroscopy in the biomedical field usually requires the combination of advanced multivariate data analysis methods [78]. At present, IR spectroscopy, especially FTIR spectroscopy, has shown great application prospects in the early diagnosis of OA, mainly including SF analysis and tissue analysis.

3.1. Application of IR Spectroscopy to SF Analysis in OA Subsection

The analysis of changes in SF by IR spectroscopy is also an effective method for the early diagnosis of OA. Eysel et al. [79] used LDA and leave-one-out cross-validation to classify 239 SF membrane spectra from 86 patients. Through multivariate analysis, the spectra were successfully divided into four categories, which were consistent with the clinical diagnosis (96.5% correct classification). By collecting the IR spectrum of joint fluid, Hou et al. [80] established an effective diagnostic model, indicating that IR spectrum technology combined with a multivariate data processing method can be used as a simple and effective method for OA diagnosis. In addition, IR spectrum data based on serum and articular fluid were shown to differentiate between samples of healthy dogs and dogs with OA, indicating that IR spectroscopy combined with multivariate data analysis is a simple and accurate diagnostic method for OA.

3.2. Application of FTIR Imaging on Articular Cartilage Analysis in OA

Some manifestations of OA, including dissolution, thinning, compositional changes, mineralization, and subchondral bone thickening [81], can be detected with traditional diagnostic techniques. By using FTIR imaging (FTIRI), both the corresponding spectral image of each pixel and the complete pathological joint image can be obtained, so the diagnostic analysis can be carried out from both the macro and micro perspective. Yin et al. [82] used FTIRI to examine the content of collagen and PG, along with the change of depth in healthy cartilage and OA cartilage. Their results showed that the deep dependence of PG levels was different between healthy and OA-affected subjects. Therefore, the FTIRI technique could be used to detect changes in cartilage composition related to OA for early diagnosis. However, the data analysis of the IR spectrum is complex, and accurate data processing methods are needed to optimize data analysis and gather information. Rieppo et al. [83] carried out optimal variable selection for FTIR spectral analysis of articular cartilage composition, and successfully determined the major components of AC, PG, and collagen using multiple regression.

The IR spectra absorption peaks of PG and collagen often overlap, and a second derivative is normally applied to improve the resolution of the overlapping peaks. Rieppo et al. [84] provided a practical approach for the analysis of articular cartilage composition by a second derivative analysis of collagen protein and polysaccharide. David-Vaudey et al. [85] collected FTIRI spectral images on the surface, middle, and deep layers of samples and then used a reference spectrum to perform Euclidean distance mapping and quantitative PLS on type II collagen and chondroitin sulfate (CS). Their results showed that the FTIRI results were correlated with the Mankin scoring system based on histology, and PLS analysis showed that the relative concentrations of collagen and PG in OA cartilage were relatively low.

Fisher discriminant analysis (FDA) establishes a discriminant function through covariance analysis to classify data sets rapidly. The discriminant principle of FDA is to ensure maximum covariance between different categories and minimum covariance within a category. Mao et al. [86] extracted FTIR images and performed a PCA of IR spectra, and then established a model to identify articular cartilage samples by FDA. Their results showed that all healthy cases in the prediction group were correctly identified, and only a few individual OA cases were misdiagnosed. Similarly, Zhang et al. [87] used FTIRI and PLS–DA methods to identify healthy cartilage and OA cartilage. In the calibration and prediction matrix, the recognition rates of healthy cartilage and injured cartilage were 100% and 90.24%, respectively. Mao et al. [88] predicted that both FTIRI–PLS–DA and FTIRI–PCA–FDA integration technologies would become tools for the microscopic identification of healthy cartilage and OA cartilage specimens and the diagnosis of cartilage lesions.

Oinas et al. [78] used cluster analysis to investigate human articular cartilage samples with different histological levels of OA. Through cluster analysis, the IR spectrum can be used to compare multiple images in order to quantitatively and qualitatively detect changes in the surface and deep layers of articular cartilage at the early stage of OA.

3.3. Application of FTIR in OA In Situ Analysis

One advantage of FTIR is that the IR fiber-optic probe (IFOP) is coupled to the FTIR spectrometer, which provides in situ full-tissue spectral acquisition and has the potential to evaluate OA in vivo. Johansson et al. [89] measured the thickness of articular cartilage based on the principle of broadband diffuse light reflection and conducted an in vitro study on the thickness of articular cartilage in multiple parts of human knee condyles with the specific goal of arthroscopic integration. An exponential model was used to compare the estimated value with the reference cartilage thickness value (obtained after section). A two-dimensional Monte Carlo simulation analysis was used to estimate the thickness of human knee cartilage, and the thickness distribution of cartilage on the joint surface could be visualized. This method provides support for research in the field of arthroscopy. Hanifi et al. [90] applied IFOP to collect spectra from normal and degraded areas of OA and established a multiplex PLS method based on the second derivative to predict the Mankin score of histology with an accuracy of 72%. Similarly, West et al. [91] found that type II collagen degradation was associated with chondrogenic degeneration, which could be used to monitor small changes associated with early cartilage degeneration. This demonstrated that IFOP could be used to perform in situ determination of cartilage integrity during arthroscopy. Yang et al. [92] used FTIR–MS spectroscopy to detect changes in the tibial articular subchondral bone in guinea pigs with increasing age, and their results showed that the ratio of amide III to amide II was consistent at different ages. At the molecular level, this research provides reliable pathological information for subchondral bone histology of OA and technical support for the early diagnosis of OA. However, the novel attenuated total reflectance–mid-IR–hollow optical fiber (ATR–MIR–HOF) probe has more advantages than traditional FTIR and ATR–FTIRI techniques. ATR–HOF–FTIR can obtain reliable ATR–IR spectra without the need for sample pretreatment. Its detection of articular cartilage damage shows that the ATR–MIR–HOF probe can easily detect changes in a small target region in situ and obtain spectral information related to changes in the major components of articular cartilage with good repeatability [93].

4. Raman Spectroscopy

Raman spectroscopy is a vibrational spectroscopy technology based on the Raman scattering principle. Rayleigh scattering and Raman scattering of different wavelengths are generated when a laser shines on a sample [94]. Rayleigh scattering is consistent with the wavelength of the incident light, while Raman scattering is different from the frequency of the incident light and can reflect specific intermolecular vibrations, such as $C-C$, $C=C$, $C-O$, and $C-H$ [95]. Therefore, the characteristic information of the material can be analyzed by collecting Raman spectrum lines. Over recent years, Raman spectroscopy technology has continued to be developed, and researchers have combined Raman spectroscopy technology with a variety of other technologies to make detection technologies more effective, such as confocal Raman microscopy [96], Raman imaging technology [97,98], resonance Raman technology [99], surface-enhanced Raman spectroscopy (SERS) technology [100], and so forth. Raman spectroscopy technology is widely used in the fields of medicine [101], pharmaceuticals [102–104], cosmetics [105,106], carbon materials [107,108], geology [109,110], and life sciences because of its ability to rapidly analyze chemical structures in a nondestructive manner and its powerful imaging functions. Compared with other spectroscopic techniques, Raman spectroscopy has improved analytical performance for samples in aqueous solutions, biological tissues, and cells because the Raman signal of water is very weak. Increased research attention is being paid to the use of Raman spectroscopy for the diagnosis of OA through the analysis of changes in SF, subchondral bone, and articular cartilage, among others.

4.1. Application of Raman Spectroscopy on OA SF Analysis

The early occurrence of OA is accompanied by the degeneration, dissolution, and fragmentation of articular cartilage. Raman spectroscopy can be used to detect changes of SF in joints for the early diagnosis of OA. Esmonde-White et al. [111] conducted a study on the correlation between NIR–Raman spectroscopy of SF and radiological scores of knee joint injury in patients with OA. Changes in the SF composition of patients were studied by NIR–Raman spectroscopy, and data were analyzed by *K*-cluster analysis. The results showed that the spectral signals of SF in patients with different grades of OA differed. HA, a main component of SF, is an important biomarker in the diagnosis of OA [112,113]. With the development of OA, the amounts of amide III (1250 cm^{-1}) and C–C, C–O bonds (1155 cm^{-1}) in HA increased [114], which showed the potential of Raman spectroscopy in relation to the diagnosis of OA by SF analysis.

Researchers have been searching for biomarkers in SF that can be used to diagnose OA earlier and with greater reliability. However, the composition of SF is complex, and it is difficult to effectively study its single components, so it requires the development of signal enhancement techniques [115]. As an important component of SF, HA has attracted the attention of researchers. Mandair et al. [116] found that SERS could greatly enhance the signal intensity of HA, such that the minimum detectable concentration could be as low as 0.5 mg/mL. At the same time, effective protein removal techniques, including the trichloroacetic acid precipitation method, centrifugal method, and droplet deposition method, can effectively remove the influence of protein on Raman spectrum to observe HA more clearly. Bocsa et al. [34] studied SF using resonance Raman technology combined with SERS. They found low carotenoid levels in advanced OA patients, and using a PCA–LDA analysis method to classify OA patients, they achieved an accuracy of 100%. With the development of various Raman enhancement techniques, Raman spectroscopy analysis of biomarkers in SF has become a good prospect for the early diagnosis of OA.

4.2. Application of Raman Spectroscopy in Subchondral Bone Analysis in OA

As one of the main manifestations of OA is the proliferation of subchondral bone, OA can be diagnosed by analyzing changes in it [117,118]. Researchers compared the internal and external Raman spectroscopies of knee subchondral bone in OA patients and healthy people. Using multivariate analysis, they found that both the internal and external components of subchondral bone in OA patients were altered, and there were significant spectral differences between OA and healthy people ($p < 0.001$). Differences primarily manifested in the phosphate band (954 and 966 cm^{-1}), amide I (1668 and 1685 cm^{-1}), and shoulder (941 cm^{-1}), and the proportion of type I collagen chain in OA was significantly higher [119–121].

The development of OA can be distinguished by observing changes in subchondral bone composition [122]. Das Gupta [123] investigated subchondral bone and changes of calcified cartilage-specific biochemical composition in OA with NIR–Raman spectroscopy technology. *K*-means clustering analysis and hierarchical cluster analysis (HCA) showed that calcified knees (CCs) were more mineralized than the subchondral bone plate (SBP), and that the mineral had a higher crystallinity. The degree of mineralization of the two tissues began to change from the early stage of OA. In the late stage of OA, the mineral crystals were rich in carbonate, but the overall mineralization had decreased. The Raman spectra of subchondral bone collected during in situ analysis are often doped with cartilage or even cancellous bone signals. Esmonde-White et al. [124] used Raman arthroscopy to conduct an in situ analysis of OA and compared the Raman spectra of the articular surface with the standard spectra of isolated articular cartilage and subchondral bone in order to study the influence of cartilage thickness on the Raman spectra of articular cartilage. The in situ spectrum reflected the mixed signal of articular cartilage and subchondral bone that as the cartilage becomes thicker, the spectral expression of subchondral bone and cancellous bone decreases. This study provides theoretical support for the further study of the Raman probe in relation to diagnosis of OA.

4.3. Raman Spectroscopy Analysis of Articular Cartilage in OA

OA is mainly manifested by the degeneration of articular cartilage and reduced elasticity, thinning, or even dissolution and fragmentation of articular cartilage, leading to the decrease of joint lubricity [122]. As shown in Figure 3, OA can be diagnosed and analyzed by observing changes in the articular cartilage with Raman spectroscopy. The main components of articular cartilage are GAG and collagen [123], and changes in them can be used as indicators for the early diagnosis of OA. Mason et al. [125] used Raman multivariate curve resolution (MCR) to analyze the cartilage surface, and their results showed that Raman MCR could accurately quantify the cartilage subcomponent distribution on the entire surface, with a depth of up to 0.5 mm. Jensen et al. [126] collected Raman spectra from the cartilage tissue model and found that there were slight differences in the spectra of different tissue regions, which represented the orientation of collagen fibers, proving that polarized Raman spectroscopy can distinguish between collagen fiber orientations in the cartilage explant model system. In another study, Lim et al. [127] examined real pig cartilage, and their spectral results showed that the amide III spectral band had a red shift from 1264 to 1274 cm^{-1}, reflecting the compression possibility of CN vibration in collagen fiber. Furthermore, a decrease of 1042 cm^{-1} in the GAG-related pyran saccharide band indicated a decrease in GAG content in OA patients. Kumar et al. [128] classified cartilage according to the definition provided by the International Cartilage Maintenance Society (ICRS) of OA, and then collected Raman spectra and analyzed them using PCA. Their results showed that, in the early stage of OA, the content of helical collagen is significantly increased, while only in the late stage of OA could an obvious difference in GAG be shown. De Souza et al. [129] used Raman spectroscopy to detect molecular changes related to OA induced chemically and by treadmill exercise. Their results showed that both OA experimental models significantly increased the Raman ratio of tissue remodeling associated with mineralization. Compared with the chemical induction model, the content of phenylalanine in the treadmill exercise induction model was significantly lower and the crystallinity was higher. Their study showed that Raman spectroscopy can not only diagnose and detect cartilage damage at the molecular level, but also monitor and analyze subchondral bone and cancellous bone in the pathogenesis of OA.

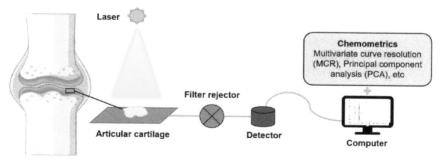

Figure 3. Articular cartilage is detected by Raman spectroscopy. The laser light source irradiates the articular cartilage, and the scattering light is generated through the scattering of the sample. Raman scattering light is obtained by the filter, and the Raman spectrum is presented after its detection and processing by a detector. Spectral data are analyzed with the help of chemometrics.

Raman spectroscopy can be analyzed at the cellular level for early diagnosis of OA. Kumar et al. [130] showed that Raman spectroscopy can distinguish between stages of OA. According to their analysis, the contents of amide I (1612–1696 cm^{-1}) and protein decrease with increasing severity of OA, and the intensity of the spectral band at 1302–1307 cm^{-1} with the peak value at 1304 cm^{-1} increases, which may indicate a change of lipids. Similarly, Takahashi et al. [36] studied the changes of OA cartilage by NIR–Raman spectroscopy and found that changes in the amide III bands are different in patients with different stages of OA. The changes in the amide III were derived from structural and direction changes in collagen fiber bundles, and the amide III band ratio (1241/1269 cm^{-1}) can be considered to be a sensitive indicator of a disordered knee cartilage collagen secondary structure, which has significance for the early detection of OA. Oshima et al. [131] divided mice into control and model groups and collected Raman spectra from them, examining the amide I, CH$_2$ deformation, amide III, phenylalanine, and hydroxyproline peaks. Their results showed that the phosphate and collagen bands in the OA group were significantly different from those in the control group, and a PCA method could successfully distinguish between the two experimental groups.

Fiber-optic Raman technology, Raman probe [132–134], Raman arthroscopy, and other related technologies are constantly developing, and their applications in OA are attracting more attention from researchers. Bergholt et al. [135] used fiber-optic Raman technology to quantify the extracellular matrix (ECM) of living-tissue constructs online. In addition, the similarity between natural cartilage and tissue cartilage constructed from living cells was quantitatively evaluated, and the growth ability of living tissues in different cycles was monitored by this technique, which provided theoretical support for the development of engineered cartilage. Esmonde-White et al. [132] carried out Raman signal collection in cartilage, subchondral bone, and cancellous bone and used a human tissue model to determine the influence of cartilage thickness on Raman signal collection, providing support for further study of the Raman probe. Oshima et al. [136] studied the PG content and collagenous fiber arrangement in a cartilage matrix, which may be related to degenerative changes caused by OA. Moreover, they designed an original Raman device for remote sensing in arthroscopic surgery, and a grading system for cartilage defects was defined based on the results of Raman spectroscopy. Furthermore, the Raman detection system for early cartilage degenerative injury was evaluated, which proves that it may be a useful new tool for the diagnosis of OA.

5. Summary and Prospect

As a degenerative disease with no specific medical treatment, OA is affecting the health of an increasing number of people worldwide. Early diagnosis can effectively prevent the deterioration in OA, reducing the pain experienced by patients and the cost of treatment. However, there are limitations associated with using complex and expensive imaging methods such as MRI, OCT, and X-ray for early diagnosis. They are commonly used in clinical practice but are often time-consuming, expensive, or even destructive. Vibrational spectroscopy techniques, including NIR, IR, and Raman spectroscopy, have attracted the attention of OA researchers because of their advantages of being fast, nondestructive, and low cost. The characteristics of these three vibrational spectroscopy techniques are summarized in Table 2. Research on the diagnosis of OA by vibrational spectroscopy at the laboratory stage is currently ongoing.

Table 2. Comparison table of application analysis of vibrational spectroscopy.

Vibrational Spectroscopy	Working Principle	Advantages	Disadvantages	Application in OA
NIR spectroscopy	Reflects the overtones and/or combination bands of stretching and bending vibrations of C–H, N–H, and O–H bonds ranging from 12,500 to 4000 cm^{-1}	Fast, accurate, nondestructive, labor-saving	Wide band, high spectral overlap, difficult to distinguish characteristic peak	Has a high penetration depth but can only provide a full spectral signal of the cartilage
IR spectroscopy	Studies the structural changes in the range (4000–400 cm^{-1}) caused by the transition of vibrational and rotational energy levels of molecules	Fast, accurate, and nondestructive; reflects information of most organic matter	Low sensitivity, complex band, sample limitations	Detects a variety of components in the cartilage and can achieve high-speed imaging
Raman spectroscopy	Reflects the vibrational information between molecules based on the principle of Raman scattering	Weak water signal, fast, simple, reflects biological signal	Raman scattering area can be affected by the optical system, fluorescence interference	Reflects physiological changes of OA at tissue, cell, and molecular levels

NIR spectroscopy has strong sensitivity and can be used as an effective method for the early diagnosis of OA through the identification of biomarkers. Therefore, qualitative and quantitative analyses of biomarkers are important research topics for the development of NIR spectroscopy in terms of the early diagnosis of OA. Although it is difficult to determine specific cartilage regions under diffuse reflection, NIR spectroscopy can display full spectral signals and can be used for arthroscopic evaluation of articular cartilage status. Further development of the sample collection methodology, in combination with chemometrics and the exploration of more spectral processing methods, will be conducive to its future development [137,138]. Meanwhile, IR spectroscopy based on the strongest fundamental frequency vibration in molecules, especially FTIR spectroscopy technology, is becoming increasingly advanced for the early diagnosis of OA [139]. Some major research technologies, such as IR probe spectral acquisition technology and FTIR–MS imaging technology, are important means of IR spectroscopy in the early diagnosis of OA. Compared with Raman imaging and NIR spectroscopy, FTIRI has the advantage of speed and is most suitable for large-area chemical imaging in unstained tissue sections. Moreover, since the thickness of the tissue section and the infrared light penetration distance are known, it is feasible to use FTIRI for quantitative analysis. Raman spectroscopy has the advantage of being used to perform molecular analysis, but there are technical limitations of this method, such as tissue autofluorescence, low signal intensity, or phototoxic effects, that may occur after prolonged exposure to laser light [140,141]. Solutions to these limitations currently being explored include using low-energy NIR lasers to optimize parameters and establishing standardized protocols for mathematical and computational modeling involving spectral data processing and analysis. In addition, NIR–Raman spectroscopy is one of the best spectroscopic techniques with high specificity of biomolecules. NIR excitation light can selectively resonate with valuable signal molecules to enhance the Raman signals and effectively avoid fluorescence background interference [35]. This method has been used to detect the vibration of biomolecules and reveal highly specific biochemical structures and conformations of tissues and cells. The application of vibrational spectroscopy in the early diagnosis of OA has attracted increased research focus. Although there are still some limitations, it is being actively developed to achieve more accurate, rapid, and nondestructive diagnostic tools.

Author Contributions: Conceptualization, L.L.; writing—original draft preparation, B.Z. and C.Y.; writing—review and editing, Y.L. and H.Z. All authors have read and agreed to the published version of the manuscript.

Funding: This research was funded by the National Natural Science Foundation of China (NSFC) (81703403), China-Australia Centre for Health Sciences Research (CACHSR) (2019GJ03), General Financial Grant from China Postdoctoral Science Foundation (2017M622224), Shandong Province Postdoctoral Innovation Project (201701009), Fundamental Research Funds of Shandong University (2019GN092), and Future Scholar Program of Shandong University.

Conflicts of Interest: The authors declare no conflict of interest.

References

1. Wang, Q.; Rozelle, A.L.; Lepus, C.M.; Scanzello, C.R.; Song, J.J.; Larsen, D.M.; Crish, J.F.; Bebek, G.; Ritter, S.Y.; Lindstrom, T.M.; et al. Identification of a central role for complement in osteoarthritis. *Nat. Med.* **2011**, *17*, 1674–1679. [CrossRef] [PubMed]
2. Nguyen, L.T.; Sharma, A.R.; Chakraborty, C.; Saibaba, B.; Ahn, M.E.; Lee, S.S. Review of Prospects of Biological Fluid Biomarkers in Osteoarthritis. *Int. J. Mol. Sci.* **2017**, *18*, 601. [CrossRef] [PubMed]
3. Safiri, S.; Kolahi, A.A.; Smith, E.; Hill, C.; Bettampadi, D.; Mansournia, M.A.; Hoy, D.; Ashrafi-Asgarabad, A.; Sepidarkish, M.; Almasi-Hashiani, A.; et al. Global, regional and national burden of osteoarthritis 1990–2017: A systematic analysis of the Global Burden of Disease Study 2017. *Ann. Rheum. Dis.* **2020**, *79*, 819–828. [CrossRef]
4. Collins, J.E.; Losina, E.; Nevitt, M.C.; Roemer, F.W.; Guermazi, A.; Lynch, J.A.; Katz, J.N.; Kent Kwoh, C.; Kraus, V.B.; Hunter, D.J. Semiquantitative Imaging Biomarkers of Knee Osteoarthritis Progression: Data From the Foundation for the National Institutes of Health Osteoarthritis Biomarkers Consortium. *Arthritis Rheumatol.* **2016**, *68*, 2422–2431. [CrossRef] [PubMed]
5. MacDonald, K.V.; Sanmartin, C.; Langlois, K.; Marshall, D.A. Symptom onset, diagnosis and management of osteoarthritis. *Health Rep.* **2014**, *25*, 10–17. [PubMed]
6. Bitton, R. The economic burden of osteoarthritis. *Am. J. Manag. Care* **2009**, *15*, S230–S235.
7. Gamble, R.; Wyeth-Ayerst, J.; Johnson, E.L. Recommendations for the medical management of osteoarthritis of the hip and knee: 2000 update. American College of Rheumatology Subcommittee on Osteoarthritis Guidelines. *Arthritis Rheum.* **2000**, *43*, 1905–1915. [CrossRef]
8. Bobinac, D.; Spanjol, J.; Zoricic, S.; Maric, I. Changes in articular cartilage and subchondral bone histomorphometry in osteoarthritic knee joints in humans. *Bone* **2003**, *32*, 284–290. [CrossRef]
9. Garvican, E.R.; Vaughan-Thomas, A.; Clegg, P.D.; Innes, J.F. Biomarkers of cartilage turnover. Part 2: Non-collagenous markers. *Vet. J.* **2010**, *185*, 43–49. [CrossRef]
10. Neame, P.J.; Tapp, H.; Azizan, A. Noncollagenous, nonproteoglycan macromolecules of cartilage. *Cell Mol. Life Sci.* **1999**, *55*, 1327–1340. [CrossRef]
11. Chen, Y.; Jiang, W.; Yong, H.; He, M.; Yang, Y.; Deng, Z.; Li, Y. Macrophages in osteoarthritis: Pathophysiology and therapeutics. *Am. J. Transl. Res.* **2020**, *12*, 261–268.
12. Dall'Ara, E.; Ohman, C.; Baleani, M.; Viceconti, M. Reduced tissue hardness of trabecular bone is associated with severe osteoarthritis. *J. Biomech.* **2011**, *44*, 1593–1598. [CrossRef]
13. Yang, Y.T.; Li, P.R.; Zhu, S.S.; Bi, R.Y. Comparison of early-stage changes of osteoarthritis in cartilage and subchondral bone between two different rat models. *Peerj* **2020**, *8*. [CrossRef]
14. Le, T.K.; Montejano, L.B.; Cao, Z.; Zhao, Y.; Ang, D. Healthcare costs associated with osteoarthritis in US patients. *Pain Pract.* **2012**, *12*, 633–640. [CrossRef]
15. Zhao, J.; Link, T.M. MRI in degenerative arthritides: Structural and clinical aspects. *Ann. N. Y. Acad. Sci.* **2009**, *1154*, 115–135. [CrossRef]
16. Chaudhari, A.S.; Kogan, F.; Pedoia, V.; Majumdar, S.; Gold, G.E.; Hargreaves, B.A. Rapid Knee MRI Acquisition and Analysis Techniques for Imaging Osteoarthritis. *J. Magn. Reson. Imaging* **2020**, *52*, 1321–1339. [CrossRef]
17. Zhang, X.M.; Tong, H.Y.; Zhang, J.; Xu, J.Y.; Xia, S.Y. Diagnostic Value of 3.0T MRI in Cartilage Injury Grading of Knee Osteoarthritis. *J. Med. Imaging Health Inform.* **2020**, *10*, 2979–2984. [CrossRef]
18. Pishgar, F.; Guermazi, A.; Roemer, F.W.; Link, T.M.; Demehri, S. Conventional MRI-based subchondral trabecular biomarkers as predictors of knee osteoarthritis progression: Data from the Osteoarthritis Initiative. *Eur. Radiol.* **2020**. [CrossRef] [PubMed]
19. Herz, P.; Bourquin, S.; Hsiung, P.L.; Ko, T.; Schneider, K.; Fujimoto, J.; Adams, S.; Roberts, M.; Patel, N.; Brezinski, M. Imaging of cartilage degeneration in vivo using ultrahigh resolution OCT. *Opt. Coherence Tomogr. Coherence Tech.* **2003**, *5140*, 152–154. [CrossRef]
20. Kushida, Y.; Ozeki, N.; Mizuno, M.; Katano, H.; Otabe, K.; Tsuji, K.; Koga, H.; Kishima, K.; Soma, Y.; Sekiya, I. Two- and three-dimensional optical coherence tomography to differentiate degenerative changes in a rat meniscectomy model. *J. Orthop. Res.* **2020**, *38*, 2592–2600. [CrossRef] [PubMed]
21. Zhou, X.; Eltit, F.; Yang, X.; Maloufi, S.; Alousaimi, H.; Liu, Q.H.; Huang, L.; Wang, R.Z.; Tang, S. Detecting human articular cartilage degeneration in its early stage with polarization-sensitive optical coherence tomography. *Biomed. Opt. Express* **2020**, *11*, 2745–2760. [CrossRef] [PubMed]
22. Radunovic, G.L.; Pilipovic, N.; Stanisic, M.; Damjanov, N.S. Assessment of knee osteoarthritis: X-ray or ultrasonography? *Ann. Rheum. Dis.* **2003**, *62*, 262.
23. Novakofski, K.D.; Pownder, S.L.; Koff, M.F.; Williams, R.M.; Potter, H.G.; Fortier, L.A. High-Resolution Methods for Diagnosing Cartilage Damage In Vivo. *Cartilage* **2016**, *7*, 39–51. [CrossRef]

24. Rocha, B.D.; Torres, R.C.S. Ultrasonic and radiographic study of laxity in hip joints of young dogs. *Arq. Bras. Med. Vet. Zoo.* **2007**, *59*, 90–96. [CrossRef]
25. Saarakkala, S.; Toyras, J.; Hirvonen, J.; Laasanen, M.S.; Lappalainen, R.; Jurvelin, J.S. Ultrasonic quantitation of superficial degradation of articular cartilage. *Ultrasound Med. Biol.* **2004**, *30*, 783–792. [CrossRef] [PubMed]
26. Viren, T.; Timonen, M.; Tyrvainen, H.; Tiitu, V.; Jurvelin, J.S.; Toyras, J. Ultrasonic evaluation of acute impact injury of articular cartilage in vitro. *Osteoarthr. Cartil.* **2012**, *20*, 719–726. [CrossRef]
27. Shamir, L.; Ling, S.M.; Scott, W.W.; Bos, A.; Orlov, N.; Macura, T.J.; Eckley, D.M.; Ferrucci, L.; Goldberg, I.G. Knee X-Ray Image Analysis Method for Automated Detection of Osteoarthritis. *IEEE Trans. Bio-Med. Eng.* **2009**, *56*, 407–415. [CrossRef] [PubMed]
28. Saleem, M.; Farid, M.S.; Saleem, S.; Khan, M.H. X-ray image analysis for automated knee osteoarthritis detection. *Signal. Image Video Process.* **2020**, *14*, 1079–1087. [CrossRef]
29. Chen, S.B.; Lin, S.B.; Li, Y.Q.; Liu, Y.T. Characteristics of musculoskeletal ultrasound versus X-ray in their differential diagnosis of knee osteoarthritis. *Int. J. Clin. Exp. Med.* **2020**, *13*, 8734–8739.
30. Yong, C.W.; Teo, K.; Murphy, B.P.; Hum, Y.C.; Tee, Y.K.; Xia, K.J.; Lai, K.W. Knee osteoarthritis severity classification with ordinal regression module. *Multimed. Tools Appl.* **2021**. [CrossRef]
31. Chu, C.R.; Williams, A.; Tolliver, D.; Kwoh, C.K.; Bruno, S.; Irrgang, J.J. Clinical Optical Coherence Tomography of Early Articular Cartilage Degeneration in Patients With Degenerative Meniscal Tears. *Arthritis Rheum.* **2010**, *62*, 1412–1420. [CrossRef]
32. Adarmes, H.; Croxatto, A.; Galleguillos, M.; Gonzalez, E. Concentration of glycosaminoglycan, aldehydes and protein in synovial fluid from normal and damaged equine metacarpophalangeal joints. *Arch. Med. Vet.* **2006**, *38*, 47–52. [CrossRef]
33. dos Santos, C.A.T.; Pascoa, R.N.M.J.; Lopes, J.A. A review on the application of vibrational spectroscopy in the wine industry: From soil to bottle. *Trac-Trend Anal. Chem.* **2017**, *88*, 100–118. [CrossRef]
34. Bocsa, C.D.; Moisoiu, V.; Stefancu, A.; Leopold, L.F.; Leopold, N.; Fodor, D. Knee osteoarthritis grading by resonant Raman and surface-enhanced Raman scattering (SERS) analysis of synovial fluid. *Nanomed. Nanotechnol.* **2019**, *20*. [CrossRef] [PubMed]
35. Ma, D.Y.; Zhao, Y.; Shang, L.W.; Zhu, Y.K.; Fu, J.J.; Lu, Y.F.; Yin, J.H. Research Progress of Raman Spectroscopy Application for Articular Cartilage and Osteoarthritis. *Spectrosc. Spect. Anal.* **2020**, *40*, 2029–2034. [CrossRef]
36. Takahashi, Y.; Sugano, N.; Takao, M.; Sakai, T.; Nishii, T.; Pezzotti, G. Raman spectroscopy investigation of load-assisted microstructural alterations in human knee cartilage: Preliminary study into diagnostic potential for osteoarthritis. *J. Mech. Behav. Biomed. Mater.* **2014**, *31*, 77–85. [CrossRef]
37. Li, L.; Zang, H.; Li, J.; Chen, D.; Li, T.; Wang, F. Identification of anisodamine tablets by Raman and near-infrared spectroscopy with chemometrics. *Spectrochim. Acta Part A Mol. Biomol. Spectrosc.* **2014**, *127*, 91–97. [CrossRef] [PubMed]
38. Zhang, H.; Song, Y.; Leng, J.; Jiang, Z.D. Near Infrared Spectroscopy Analysis Technology. *Chin. J. Spectrosc. Lab.* **2007**, *24*, 388–395.
39. Badaro, A.T.; Garcia-Martin, J.F.; Lopez-Barrera, M.D.C.; Barbin, D.F.; Alvarez-Mateos, P. Determination of pectin content in orange peels by near infrared hyperspectral imaging. *Food Chem.* **2020**, *323*, 126861. [CrossRef]
40. Schopf, M.; Wehrli, M.C.; Becker, T.; Jekle, M.; Scherf, K.A. Fundamental characterization of wheat gluten. *Eur. Food Res. Technol.* **2021**, *247*, 985–997. [CrossRef]
41. Thomson, A.L.; Karunaratne, S.B.; Copland, A.; Stayches, D.; McNabb, E.M.; Jacobs, J. Use of traditional, modern, and hybrid modelling approaches for in situ prediction of dry matter yield and nutritive characteristics of pasture using hyperspectral datasets. *Anim. Feed. Sci. Tech.* **2020**, *269*. [CrossRef]
42. Xia, J.A.; Zhang, W.Y.; Zhang, W.X.; Yang, Y.W.; Hu, G.Y.; Ge, D.K.; Liu, H.; Cao, H.X. A cloud computing-based approach using the visible near-infrared spectrum to classify greenhouse tomato plants under water stress. *Comput. Electron. Agr.* **2021**, *181*. [CrossRef]
43. Arndt, M.; Rurik, M.; Drees, A.; Ahlers, C.; Feldmann, S.; Kohlbacher, O.; Fischer, M. Food authentication: Determination of the geographical origin of almonds (Prunus dulcis MILL.) via near-infrared spectroscopy. *Microchem. J.* **2021**, *160*. [CrossRef]
44. Chang, Y.T.; Hsueh, M.C.; Hung, S.P.; Lu, J.M.; Peng, J.H.; Chen, S.F. Prediction of specialty coffee flavors based on near-infrared spectra using machine- and deep-learning methods. *J. Sci. Food Agr.* **2021**. [CrossRef]
45. Gao, B.; Xu, X.D.; Han, L.J.; Liu, X. A novel near infrared spectroscopy analytical strategy for meat and bone meal species discrimination based on the insight of fraction composition complexity. *Food Chem.* **2021**, *344*. [CrossRef] [PubMed]
46. Nakajima, S.; Genkawa, T.; Miyamoto, A.; Ikehata, A. Useful tissues in cabbage head for freshness evaluation with visible and near infrared spectroscopy. *Food Chem.* **2021**, *339*, 128058. [CrossRef] [PubMed]
47. Ishikawa, H.T.; Aoki, W.; Kotani, T.; Kuzuhara, M.; Omiya, M.; Reiners, A.; Zechmeister, M. Elemental abundances of M dwarfs based on high-resolution near-infrared spectra: Verification by binary systems. *Publ. Astron. Soc. Jpn.* **2020**, *72*. [CrossRef]
48. Rubini, M.; Feuillerat, L.; Cabaret, T.; Leroyer, L.; Leneveu, L.; Charrier, B. Comparison of the performances of handheld and benchtop near infrared spectrometers: Application on the quantification of chemical components in maritime pine (Pinus Pinaster) resin. *Talanta* **2021**, *221*. [CrossRef] [PubMed]
49. Yamazaki, Y.; Umemura, K. Sensing of epigallocatechin gallate and tannic acid based on near infrared optical spectroscopy of DNA-wrapped single-walled carbon nanotube hybrids. *J. Near Infrared Spec.* **2020**. [CrossRef]
50. Chen, X.Y.; Sun, X.F.; Hua, H.M.; Yi, Y.; Li, H.L.; Chen, C. Quality evaluation of decoction pieces of Rhizoma Atractylodis Macrocephalae by near infrared spectroscopy coupled with chemometrics. *Spectrochim. Acta A* **2019**, *221*. [CrossRef] [PubMed]

51. Li, L.Q.; Pan, X.P.; Chen, W.L.; Wei, M.M.; Feng, Y.C.; Yin, L.H.; Hu, C.Q.; Yang, H.H. Multi-manufacturer drug identification based on near infrared spectroscopy and deep transfer learning. *J. Innov. Opt. Health Sci.* **2020**, *13*. [CrossRef]

52. Mishra, P.; Nordon, A.; Roger, J.M. Improved prediction of tablet properties with near-infrared spectroscopy by a fusion of scatter correction techniques. *J. Pharm. Biomed.* **2021**, *192*. [CrossRef]

53. Sun, F.; Zhao, W.J.; Wang, K.Y.; Wang, S.M.; Liang, S.W. Near-infrared spectroscopy to assess typhaneoside and isorhamnetin-3-O-glucoside in different processed products of pollen typhae. *Spectrosc. Lett.* **2019**, *52*, 423–430. [CrossRef]

54. Moros, J.; Garrigues, S.; de la Guardia, M. Vibrational spectroscopy provides a green tool for multi-component analysis. *Trac-Trend Anal. Chem.* **2010**, *29*, 578–591. [CrossRef]

55. Bec, K.B.; Grabska, J.; Huck, C.W. Near-Infrared Spectroscopy in Bio-Applications. *Molecules* **2020**, *25*, 2948. [CrossRef]

56. Biancolillo, A.; Marini, F.; Ruckebusch, C.; Vitale, R. Chemometric Strategies for Spectroscopy-Based Food Authentication. *Appl. Sci.* **2020**, *10*, 6544. [CrossRef]

57. Afara, I.O.; Prasadam, I.; Arabshahi, Z.; Xiao, Y.; Oloyede, A. Monitoring osteoarthritis progression using near infrared (NIR) spectroscopy. *Sci. Rep.* **2017**, *7*. [CrossRef] [PubMed]

58. Shaw, R.A.; Kotowich, S.; Eysel, H.H.; Jackson, M.; Thomson, G.T.D.; Mantsch, H.H. Arthritis diagnosis based upon the near infrared spectrum of synovial fluid. *Rheumatol. Int.* **1995**, *15*, 159–165. [CrossRef]

59. Mickiewicz, B.; Kelly, J.J.; Ludwig, T.E.; Weljie, A.M.; Wiley, J.P.; Schmidt, T.A.; Vogel, H.J. Metabolic analysis of knee synovial fluid as a potential diagnostic approach for osteoarthritis. *J. Orthop. Res.* **2015**, *33*, 1631–1638. [CrossRef]

60. Mickiewicz, B.; Heard, B.J.; Chau, J.K.; Chung, M.; Hart, D.A.; Shrive, N.G.; Frank, C.B.; Vogel, H.J. Metabolic Profiling of Synovial Fluid in a Unilateral Ovine Model of Anterior Cruciate Ligament Reconstruction of the Knee Suggests Biomarkers for Early Osteoarthritis. *J. Orthop. Res.* **2015**, *33*, 71–77. [CrossRef] [PubMed]

61. Esmonde-White, K.A.; Mandair, G.S.; Raaii, F.; Jacobson, J.A.; Miller, B.S.; Urquhart, A.G.; Roessler, B.J.; Morris, M.D. Raman spectroscopy of synovial fluid as a tool for diagnosing osteoarthritis. *J. Biomed. Opt.* **2009**, *14*. [CrossRef] [PubMed]

62. Chhol, K.Z.; Bykov, V.A.; Nikolaeva, S.S.; Rebrova, G.A.; Roshina, A.A.; Rumjantseva, N.V.; Yakovleva, L.B.; Korolyova, O.A.; Rebrov, L.B. The changes of biochemical characteristics of collagen and nature of water in human osteoarthrotic cartilage. *Vopr. Med. Khimii* **2001**, *47*, 498–505.

63. Hofmann, G.O.; Marticke, J.; Grosstuck, R.; Hoffmann, M.; Lange, M.; Plettenberg, H.K.; Braunschweig, R.; Schilling, O.; Kaden, I.; Spahn, G. Detection and evaluation of initial cartilage pathology in man: A comparison between MRT, arthroscopy and near-infrared spectroscopy (NIR) in their relation to initial knee pain. *Pathophysiology* **2010**, *17*, 1–8. [CrossRef]

64. Murat, N.; Karadam, B.; Ozkal, S.; Karatosun, V.; Gidener, S. Quantification of papain-induced rat osteoarthritis in relation to time with the Mankin score. *Acta Orthop. Traumatol. Turc.* **2007**, *41*, 233–237.

65. van der Sluijs, J.A.; Geesink, R.G.; van der Linden, A.J.; Bulstra, S.K.; Kuyer, R.; Drukker, J. The reliability of the Mankin score for osteoarthritis. *J. Orthop. Res.* **1992**, *10*, 58–61. [CrossRef] [PubMed]

66. Watanabe, H.; Watanabe, H.; Kimata, K. The roles of proteoglycans for cartilage. *Clin. Calcium* **2006**, *16*, 1029–1033.

67. Palukuru, U.P.; Hanifi, A.; McGoverin, C.M.; Devlin, S.; Lelkes, P.I.; Pleshko, N. Near infrared spectroscopic imaging assessment of cartilage composition: Validation with mid infrared imaging spectroscopy. *Anal. Chim. Acta* **2016**, *926*, 79–87. [CrossRef] [PubMed]

68. Buck, R.J.; Wirth, W.; Dreher, D.; Nevitt, M.; Eckstein, F. Frequency and spatial distribution of cartilage thickness change in knee osteoarthritis and its relation to clinical and radiographic covariates—Data from the osteoarthritis initiative. *Osteoarthr. Cartil.* **2013**, *21*, 102–109. [CrossRef]

69. Sarin, J.K.; Te Moller, N.C.R.; Mancini, I.A.D.; Brommer, H.; Visser, J.; Malda, J.; van Weeren, P.R.; Afara, I.O.; Toyras, J. Arthroscopic near infrared spectroscopy enables simultaneous quantitative evaluation of articular cartilage and subchondral bone in vivo. *Sci. Rep.* **2018**, *8*, 13409. [CrossRef]

70. Afara, I.O.; Sarin, J.K.; Ojanen, S.; Finnila, M.A.J.; Herzog, W.; Saarakkala, S.; Korhonen, R.K.; Toyras, J. Machine Learning Classification of Articular Cartilage Integrity Using Near Infrared Spectroscopy. *Cell. Mol. Bioeng.* **2020**, *13*, 219–228. [CrossRef] [PubMed]

71. Sarin, J.K.; Torniainen, J.; Prakash, M.; Rieppo, L.; Afara, I.O.; Toyras, J. Dataset on equine cartilage near infrared spectra, composition, and functional properties. *Sci. Data* **2019**, *6*, 164. [CrossRef]

72. Chen, Y.; Li, C.; Wang, X.; Chu, Q.; Long, Z. Detection of knee osteoarthritis with near infrared spectroscopy in vivo. *J. Optoelectron. Laser* **2014**, *25*, 1023–1026.

73. Kafian-Attari, I.; Semenov, D.; Nippolainen, E.; Hauta-Kasari, M.; Toyras, J.; Afara, I.O. Optical properties of articular cartilage in the near-infrared spectral range are related to its proteoglycan content. *Tissue Opt. Photonics* **2020**, *11363*. [CrossRef]

74. Maddams, W.F.; Willis, H.A. The principles and applications of mathematical peak finding procedures in vibrational spectra IR spectroscopy. *Proc. SPIE Int. Soc. Opt. Eng.* **1988**, *917*, 35–46.

75. Ichimura, K.T.T.; Suzuki, Y. Fourier transform technique and infrared analysis. *J. Jpn. Soc. Infrared Sci. Technol.* **1995**, *5*, 36–48.

76. Tiernan, H.; Byrne, B.; Kazarian, S.G. ATR-FTIR spectroscopy and spectroscopic imaging for the analysis of biopharmaceuticals. *Spectrochim. Acta A* **2020**, *241*. [CrossRef]

77. Bunaciu, A.A.; Hoang, V.D.; Aboul-Enein, H.Y. Vibrational Micro-Spectroscopy of Human Tissues Analysis: Review. *Crit. Rev. Anal. Chem.* **2017**, *47*, 194–203. [CrossRef] [PubMed]

78. Oinas, J.; Rieppo, L.; Finnila, M.A.J.; Valkealahti, M.; Lehenkari, P.; Saarakkala, S. Imaging of Osteoarthritic Human Articular Cartilage using Fourier Transform Infrared Microspectroscopy Combined with Multivariate and Univariate Analysis. *Sci. Rep.* **2016**, *6*. [CrossRef]

79. Eysel, H.H.; Jackson, M.; Nikulin, A.; Somorjai, R.L.; Thomson, G.T.D.; Mantsch, H.H. A novel diagnostic test for arthritis: Multivariate analysis of infrared spectra of synovial fluid. *Biospectroscopy* **1997**, *3*, 161–167. [CrossRef]

80. Hou, S.Y. Development of diagnostic models for canine osteoarthritis based on serum and joint fluid mid-infrared spectral data using five different discrimination and classification methods. *J. Chemom.* **2016**, *30*, 663–681. [CrossRef]

81. Ren, P.L.; Niu, H.J.; Cen, H.P.; Jia, S.W.; Gong, H.; Fan, Y.B. Biochemical and Morphological Abnormalities of Subchondral Bone and Their Association with Cartilage Degeneration in Spontaneous Osteoarthritis. *Calcif. Tissue Int.* **2021**. [CrossRef]

82. Yin, J.H.; Xia, Y.; Xiao, Z.Y. Comparison of Macromolecular Component Distributions in Osteoarthritic and Healthy Cartilages by Fourier Transform Infrared Imaging. *J. Innov. Opt. Health Sci.* **2013**, *6*. [CrossRef]

83. Rieppo, L.; Saarakkala, S.; Jurvelin, J.S.; Rieppo, J. Optimal variable selection for Fourier transform infrared spectroscopic analysis of articular cartilage composition. *J. Biomed. Opt.* **2014**, *19*. [CrossRef] [PubMed]

84. Rieppo, L.; Saarakkala, S.; Narhi, T.; Helminen, H.J.; Jurvelin, J.S.; Rieppo, J. Application of second derivative spectroscopy for increasing molecular specificity of fourier transform infrared spectroscopic imaging of articular cartilage. *Osteoarthr. Cartil.* **2012**, *20*, 451–459. [CrossRef] [PubMed]

85. David-Vaudey, E.; Burghardt, A.; Keshari, K.; Brouchet, A.; Ries, M.; Majumdar, S. Fourier Transform Infrared Imaging of focal lesions in human osteoarthritic cartilage. *Eur. Cell Mater.* **2005**, *10*, 51–60. [CrossRef]

86. Mao, Z.H.; Zhang, X.X.; Wu, Y.C.; Yin, J.H.; Xia, Y. Fourier Transform Infrared Microscopic Imaging and Fisher Discriminant Analysis for Identification of Healthy and Degenerated Articular Cartilage. *Chin. J. Anal. Chem.* **2015**, *43*, 518–522. [CrossRef]

87. Zhang, X.X.; Yin, J.H.; Mao, Z.H.; Xia, Y. Discrimination of healthy and osteoarthritic articular cartilages by Fourier transform infrared imaging and partial least squares-discriminant analysis. *J. Biomed. Opt.* **2015**, *20*. [CrossRef]

88. Mao, Z.H.; Wu, Y.C.; Zhang, X.X.; Gao, H.; Yin, J.H. Comparative study on identification of healthy and osteoarthritic articular cartilages by fourier transform infrared imaging and chemometrics methods. *J. Innov. Opt. Health Sci.* **2017**, *10*. [CrossRef]

89. Johansson, A.; Sundqvist, T.; Kuiper, J.H.; Oberg, P.A. A spectroscopic approach to imaging and quantification of cartilage lesions in human knee joints. *Phys. Med. Biol.* **2011**, *56*, 1865–1878. [CrossRef]

90. Hanifi, A.; Bi, X.H.; Yang, X.; Kavukcuoglu, B.; Lin, P.C.; DiCarlo, E.; Spencer, R.G.; Bostrom, M.P.G.; Pleshko, N. Infrared Fiber Optic Probe Evaluation of Degenerative Cartilage Correlates to Histological Grading. *Am. J. Sport Med.* **2012**, *40*, 2853–2861. [CrossRef]

91. West, P.A.; Torzilli, P.A.; Chen, C.; Lin, P.; Camacho, N.P. Fourier transform infrared imaging spectroscopy analysis of collagenase-induced cartilage degradation. *J. Biomed. Opt.* **2005**, *10*. [CrossRef]

92. Yang, L.P.; Liu, J.L.; Song, Q.H.; Zhu, J.; Zhang, W.Q.; Kong, H.Y.; Zhao, T.J. FTIR Microspectroscopic Investigation of the Age-Related Changes of Subchondral Bone of the Knee in Guinea Pig. *Spectrosc. Spect. Anal.* **2013**, *33*, 2369–2373. [CrossRef]

93. Zhao, Y.; Lu, Y.F.; Zhu, Y.K.; Wu, Y.C.; Zhai, M.Y.; Wang, X.; Yin, J.H. Submillimetric FTIR detection of articular cartilage by home-made ATR-MIR-Hollow optical fiber probe. *Infrared Phys. Tech.* **2019**, *98*, 236–239. [CrossRef]

94. Akhmanov, S.A.; Koroteyev, N.I. Spectroscopy of Light-Scattering and Nonlinear Optics, Nonlinear Optical Methods in Active Spectroscopy of Raman and Rayleigh-Scattering. *Sov. Phys. Uspekhi* **1977**, *123*, 405–471. [CrossRef]

95. Cialla-May, D.; Schmitt, M.; Popp, J. Theoretical principles of Raman spectroscopy. *Phys. Sci. Rev.* **2019**, *4*. [CrossRef]

96. Brenan, C.J.; Hunter, I.W. Chemical imaging with a confocal scanning Fourier-transform-Raman microscope. *Appl. Opt.* **1994**, *33*, 7520–7528. [CrossRef]

97. Lu, J.; Zhu, S.S.; Cui, X.Y.; Chen, S.; Yao, Y.D. Raman Spectroscopic Imaging Technology and Its Biomedical Applications. *Chin. J. Lasers* **2018**, *45*. [CrossRef]

98. Chernenko, T.; Sawant, R.R.; Miljkovic, M.; Quintero, L.; Diem, M.; Torchilin, V. Raman microscopy for noninvasive imaging of pharmaceutical nanocarriers: Intracellular distribution of cationic liposomes of different composition. *Mol. Pharm.* **2012**, *9*, 930–936. [CrossRef] [PubMed]

99. Chen, C.L.; Heglund, D.L.; Ray, M.D.; Harder, D.; Dobert, R.; Leung, K.P.; Wu, M.T.; Sedlacek, A.J. Application of resonance Raman lidar for chemical species identification. *Proc. SPIE Int. Soc. Opt. Eng.* **1997**, *3065*, 279–285.

100. Fikiet, M.A.; Khandasammy, S.R.; Mistek, E.; Ahmed, Y.; Halamkova, L.; Bueno, J.; Lednev, I.K. Surface enhanced Raman spectroscopy: A review of recent applications in forensic science. *Spectrochim. Acta A Mol. Biomol. Spectrosc.* **2018**, *197*, 255–260. [CrossRef]

101. Alvarez-Figueroa, M.J.; Narvaez-Araya, D.; Armijo-Escalona, N.; Carrasco-Flores, E.A.; Gonzalez-Aramundiz, J.V. Design of Chitosan Nanocapsules with Compritol 888 ATO (R) for Imiquimod Transdermal Administration. Evaluation of Their Skin Absorption by Raman Microscopy. *Pharm. Res. Dordr.* **2020**, *37*. [CrossRef]

102. Dadou, S.M.; Tian, Y.W.; Li, S.; Jones, D.S.; Andrews, G.P. The optimization of process analytical technology for the inline quantification of multiple drugs in fixed dose combinations during continuous processing. *Int. J. Pharm.* **2021**, *592*. [CrossRef]

103. Starciuc, T.; Guinet, Y.; Hedoux, A.; Shalaev, E. Water content thresholds in glycerol/water system: Low- and high-wavenumber Raman spectroscopy study. *J. Mol. Liq.* **2021**, *321*. [CrossRef]

104. Dohrn, S.; Luebbert, C.; Lehmkemper, K.; Kyeremateng, S.O.; Degenhardt, M.; Sadowski, G. Solvent influence on the phase behavior and glass transition of Amorphous Solid Dispersions. *Eur. J. Pharm. Biopharm.* **2021**, *158*, 132–142. [CrossRef]

105. Franzen, L.; Anderski, J.; Windbergs, M. Quantitative detection of caffeine in human skin by confocal Raman spectroscopy—A systematic in vitro validation study. *Eur. J. Pharm. Biopharm.* **2015**, *95*, 110–116. [CrossRef] [PubMed]

106. Stella, A.; Bonnier, F.; Tfayli, A.; Yvergnaux, F.; Byrne, H.J.; Chourpa, I.; Munnier, E.; Tauber, C. Raman mapping coupled to self-modelling MCR-ALS analysis to estimate active cosmetic ingredient penetration profile in skin. *J. Biophotonics* **2020**, *13*, e202000136. [CrossRef]

107. Kim, J.H.; Lee, J.H.; Kang, Y.S.; Jang, K.T.; Im, J.; Seong, M.J. Evolution of amorphous carbon films into nano-crystalline graphite with increasing growth temperature in plasma-enhanced chemical vapor deposition. *Curr. Appl Phys.* **2021**, *23*, 52–56. [CrossRef]

108. Lee, J.; Kim, H.S.; Osawa, E.; Hoang, G.C.; Lee, K.H. Predicting the Number of Graphene-Like Layers on Surface for Commercial Fumed Nanodiamonds with Raman Spectra and Model Calculations. *J. Nanosci. Nanotechnol.* **2021**, *21*, 1815–1819. [CrossRef]

109. Gibbons, E.; Leveille, R.; Berlo, K. Data fusion of laser-induced breakdown and Raman spectroscopies: Enhancing clay mineral identification. *Spectrochim. Acta B* **2020**, *170*. [CrossRef]

110. Yao, C.; Song, H.; Li, Q.; Li, N.; Zhang, G.Y. Micro Raman Spectral Characteristics and Implication of Pyrite in the Jiaojia Gold Deposit, Jiaodong Area, Shandong Province, China. *Spectrosc. Spect. Anal.* **2020**, *40*, 2479–2483. [CrossRef]

111. Esmonde-White, K.A.; Mandair, G.S.; Esmonde-White, F.W.L.; Raaii, F.; Roessler, B.J.; Morris, M.D. Osteoarthritis Screening using Raman Spectroscopy of Dried Human Synovial Fluid Drops. *Opt. Bone Biol. Diagn.* **2009**, *7166*. [CrossRef]

112. Matisioudis, N.; Rizos, E.; Tyrnenopoulou, P.; Papazoglou, L.; Diakakis, N.; Aggeli, A. Comparative Studies of Hyaluronic Acid Concentration in Normal and Osteoarthritic Equine Joints. *Fluids* **2019**, *4*, 193. [CrossRef]

113. Sun, Z.P.; Wu, S.P.; Liang, C.D.; Zhao, C.X.; Sun, B.Y. The synovial fluid neuropeptide PACAP may act as a protective factor during disease progression of primary knee osteoarthritis and is increased following hyaluronic acid injection. *Innate Immun.* **2019**, *25*, 255–264. [CrossRef] [PubMed]

114. Timchenko, E.; Timchenko, P.; Volova, L.; Dolgushkin, D.; Markova, M.; Yagofarova, E. The synovial fluid analysis by using Raman Scattering spectroscopy in order to educe the synovial joint pathology. *Int. Conf. Phys.* **2018**, *1038*. [CrossRef]

115. Chaudhari, A.; Dhonde, S.B. A Review on Speech Enhancement Techniques. In Proceedings of the 2015 International Conference on Pervasive Computing (ICPC), Pune, India, 8–10 January 2015.

116. Mandair, G.S.; Dehring, K.A.; Roessler, B.J.; Morris, M.D. Detection of potential osteoarthritis biomarkers using surface-enhanced Raman spectroscopy in the near-infrared. *Biomed. Vib. Spectrosc. Adv. Res. Ind.* **2006**, *6093*. [CrossRef]

117. Galli, M.M.; Protzman, N.M.; Bleazey, S.T.; Brigido, S.A. Role of Demineralized Allograft Subchondral Bone in the Treatment of Shoulder Lesions of the Talus: Clinical Results With Two-Year Follow-Up. *J. Foot Ankle Surg.* **2015**, *54*, 717–722. [CrossRef] [PubMed]

118. Zhou, F.; Chu, L.Y.; Liu, X.Q.; He, Z.H.; Han, X.Q.; Yan, M.N.; Qu, X.H.; Li, X.F.; Yu, Z.F. Subchondral Trabecular Microstructure and Articular Cartilage Damage Variations Between Osteoarthritis and Osteoporotic Osteoarthritis: A Cross-sectional Cohort Study. *Front. Med.* **2021**, *8*. [CrossRef]

119. Kerns, J.G.; Buckley, K.; Gikas, P.D.; Birch, H.L.; McCarthy, I.D.; Keen, R.; Parker, A.W.; Matousek, P.; Goodship, A.E. Raman spectroscopy reveals evidence for early bone changes in osteoarthritis. *Int. J. Exp. Pathol.* **2015**, *96*, A3.

120. Dehring, K.A.; Roessle, B.J.; Morris, M.D. Correlating chemical changes in subchondral bone mineral due to aging or defective type II collagen by Raman spectroscopy. *Adv. Biomed. Clin. Diagn. Syst. V* **2007**, *6430*. [CrossRef]

121. Dehring, K.A.; Crane, N.J.; Smukler, A.R.; McHugh, J.B.; Roessler, B.J.; Morris, M.D. Identifying chemical changes in subchondral bone taken from murine knee joints using Raman spectroscopy. *Appl. Spectrosc.* **2006**, *60*, 1134–1141. [CrossRef] [PubMed]

122. Stack, J.; McCarthy, G.M. Cartilage calcification and osteoarthritis: A pathological association? *Osteoarthr. Cartil.* **2020**, *28*, 1301–1302. [CrossRef] [PubMed]

123. Das Gupta, S.; Finnila, M.A.J.; Karhula, S.S.; Kauppinen, S.; Joukainen, A.; Kroger, H.; Korhonen, R.K.; Thambyah, A.; Rieppo, L.; Saarakkala, S. Raman microspectroscopic analysis of the tissue-specific composition of the human osteochondral junction in osteoarthritis: A pilot study. *Acta Biomater.* **2020**, *106*, 145–155. [CrossRef] [PubMed]

124. Esmonde-White, K.A.; Esmonde-White, F.W.; Morris, M.D.; Roessler, B.J. Fiber-optic Raman spectroscopy of joint tissues. *Analyst* **2011**, *136*, 1675–1685. [CrossRef]

125. Mason, D.; Murugkar, S.; Speirs, A.D. Measurement of cartilage sub-component distributions through the surface by Raman spectroscopy-based multivariate analysis. *J. Biophotonics* **2021**, *14*. [CrossRef]

126. Jensen, M.; Horgan, C.C.; Vercauteren, T.; Albro, M.B.; Bergholt, M.S. Multiplexed polarized hypodermic Raman needle probe for biostructural analysis of articular cartilage. *Opt. Lett.* **2020**, *45*, 2890–2893. [CrossRef]

127. Lim, N.S.J.; Hamed, Z.; Yeow, C.H.; Chan, C.; Huang, Z.W. Early detection of biomolecular changes in disrupted porcine cartilage using polarized Raman spectroscopy. *J. Biomed. Opt.* **2011**, *16*. [CrossRef]

128. Kumar, R.; Gronhaug, K.M.; Afseth, N.K.; Isaksen, V.; Davies, C.D.; Drogset, J.O.; Lilledahl, M.B. Optical investigation of osteoarthritic human cartilage (ICRS grade) by confocal Raman spectroscopy: A pilot study. *Anal. Bioanal. Chem.* **2015**, *407*, 8067–8077. [CrossRef]

129. de Souza, R.A.; Xavier, M.; Mangueira, N.M.; Santos, A.P.; Pinheiro, A.L.B.; Villaverde, A.B.; Silveira, L. Raman spectroscopy detection of molecular changes associated with two experimental models of osteoarthritis in rats. *Laser Med. Sci.* **2014**, *29*, 797–804. [CrossRef]

130. Kumar, R.; Singh, G.P.; Gronhaug, K.M.; Afseth, N.K.; Davies, C.D.; Drogset, J.O.; Lilledahl, M.B. Single Cell Confocal Raman Spectroscopy of Human Osteoarthritic Chondrocytes: A Preliminary Study. *Int. J. Mol. Sci.* **2015**, *16*, 9341–9353. [CrossRef] [PubMed]

131. Oshima, Y.; Akehi, M.; Kiyomatsu, H.; Miura, H. Label-free characterization of degenerative changes in articular cartilage by Raman spectroscopy. *Biomed. Imaging Sens. Conf.* **2017**, *10251*. [CrossRef]

132. Sirleto, L.; Ferrara, M.A. Fiber Amplifiers and Fiber Lasers Based on Stimulated Raman Scattering: A Review. *Micromachines* **2020**, *11*, 247. [CrossRef] [PubMed]

133. Sun, Z.H.; Song, B.; Li, X.; Zou, Y.; Wang, Y.; Yu, Z.G.; Huang, M.Z. A smart optical fiber probe for Raman spectrometry and its application. *J. Opt.* **2017**, *46*, 62–67. [CrossRef]

134. Xu, H.; Zhu, Y.K.; Lu, Y.F.; Yin, J.H. Development and Biomedical Application of Raman Probe. *Laser Optoelectron. Prog.* **2019**, *56*. [CrossRef]

135. Bergholt, M.S.; Albro, M.B.; Stevens, M.M. Online quantitative monitoring of live cell engineered cartilage growth using diffuse fiber-optic Raman spectroscopy. *Biomaterials* **2017**, *140*, 128–137. [CrossRef] [PubMed]

136. Oshima, Y.; Ishimaru, Y.; Kiyomatsu, H.; Hino, K.; Miura, H. Evaluation of degenerative changes in articular cartilage of osteoarthritis by Raman spectroscopy. *Imaging Manip. Anal. Biomol. Cells Tissues Xvi* **2018**, *10497*. [CrossRef]

137. Pester, J.K.; Stumpfe, S.T.; Steinert, S.; Marintschev, I.; Plettenberg, H.K.; Aurich, M.; Hofmann, G.O. Histological, Biochemical and Spectroscopic Changes of Articular Cartilage in Osteoarthritis: Is There a Chance for Spectroscopic Evaluation? *Z. Orthop. Unf.* **2014**, *152*, 469–479. [CrossRef]

138. Slooter, M.D.; Bierau, K.; Chan, A.B.; Lowik, C.W. Near infrared fluorescence imaging for early detection, monitoring and improved intervention of diseases involving the joint. *Connect. Tissue Res.* **2015**, *56*, 153–160. [CrossRef] [PubMed]

139. Paraskevaidi, M.; Hook, P.D.; Morais, C.L.M.; Anderson, J.R.; White, R.; Martin-Hirsch, P.L.; Peffers, M.J.; Martin, F.L. Attenuated total reflection Fourier-transform infrared (ATR-FTIR) spectroscopy to diagnose osteoarthritis in equine serum. *Equine Vet. J.* **2020**, *52*, 46–51. [CrossRef] [PubMed]

140. Bartick, E. Forensic analysis by Raman spectroscopy: An emerging technology. *Meet. Int. Assoc. Forensic Sci.* **2002**, 45–50.

141. Downes, A.; Elfick, A. Raman Spectroscopy and Related Techniques in Biomedicine. *Sensors* **2010**, *10*, 1871–1889. [CrossRef]

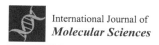

International Journal of
Molecular Sciences

Article

Exploring the Crosstalk between Hydrostatic Pressure and Adipokines: An In Vitro Study on Human Osteoarthritic Chondrocytes

Sara Cheleschi [1,*], Sara Tenti [1], Marcella Barbarino [2,3], Stefano Giannotti [4], Francesca Bellisai [1], Elena Frati [1] and Antonella Fioravanti [1]

1 Rheumatology Unit, Department of Medicine, Surgery and Neuroscience, Azienda Ospedaliera Universitaria Senese, Policlinico Le Scotte, 53100 Siena, Italy; sara_tenti@hotmail.it (S.T.); f.bellisai@ao-siena.toscana.it (F.B.); fratielena@unisi.it (E.F.); fioravanti7@virgilio.it (A.F.)
2 Department of Medical Biotechnologies, University of Siena, 53100 Siena, Italy; marcella.barbarino@unisi.it
3 Center for Biotechnology, Sbarro Institute for Cancer Research and Molecular Medicine, College of Science and Technology, Temple University, Philadelphia, PA 19122, USA
4 Department of Medicine, Surgery and Neurosciences, Section of Orthopedics and Traumatology, University of Siena, Policlinico Le Scotte, 53100 Siena, Italy; stefano.giannotti@unisi.it
* Correspondence: saracheleschi@hotmail.com; Tel.: +39-0577-233471

Abstract: Obesity is a risk factor for osteoarthritis (OA) development and progression due to an altered biomechanical stress on cartilage and an increased release of inflammatory adipokines from adipose tissue. Evidence suggests an interplay between loading and adipokines in chondrocytes metabolism modulation. We investigated the role of loading, as hydrostatic pressure (HP), in regulating visfatin-induced effects in human OA chondrocytes. Chondrocytes were stimulated with visfatin (24 h) and exposed to high continuous HP (24 MPa, 3 h) in the presence of visfatin inhibitor (FK866, 4 h pre-incubation). Apoptosis and oxidative stress were detected by cytometry, B-cell lymphoma (*BCL*)2, metalloproteinases (*MMPs*), type II collagen (*Col2a1*), antioxidant enzymes, miRNA, *cyclin D1* expressions by real-time PCR, and β-catenin protein by western blot. HP exposure or visfatin stimulus significantly induced apoptosis, superoxide anion production, and *MMP-3*, -13, antioxidant enzymes, and miRNA gene expression, while reducing *Col2a1* and *BCL2* mRNA. Both stimuli significantly reduced β-catenin protein and increased *cyclin D1* gene expression. HP exposure exacerbated visfatin-induced effects, which were counteracted by FK866 pre-treatment. Our data underline the complex interplay between loading and visfatin in controlling chondrocytes' metabolism, contributing to explaining the role of obesity in OA etiopathogenesis, and confirming the importance of controlling body weight for disease treatment.

Keywords: hydrostatic pressure; adipokines; visfatin; Wnt/β-catenin; mechanical loading; osteoarthritis; obesity; chondrocytes; microRNA; oxidative stress

Citation: Cheleschi, S.; Tenti, S.; Barbarino, M.; Giannotti, S.; Bellisai, F.; Frati, E.; Fioravanti, A. Exploring the Crosstalk between Hydrostatic Pressure and Adipokines: An In Vitro Study on Human Osteoarthritic Chondrocytes. *Int. J. Mol. Sci.* **2021**, 22, 2745. https://doi.org/10.3390/ijms22052745

Academic Editor: Nicola Veronese

Received: 13 February 2021
Accepted: 2 March 2021
Published: 9 March 2021

Publisher's Note: MDPI stays neutral with regard to jurisdictional claims in published maps and institutional affiliations.

1. Introduction

Obesity represents one of the most influential risk factors for osteoarthritis (OA) incidence, progression, and disability [1]. Its effect on the joint has been traditionally attributed to altered mechanical loading on the articular cartilage of weight-bearing joints [2–5]; indeed, different mechanical forces in the form of compression, shear stress, and hydrostatic pressure (HP) can affect cartilage homeostasis, leading to irreversible and deleterious effects [5].

Several in vitro studies demonstrated that the application of injurious static HP induced chondrocyte catabolic processes, including degradation of extracellular matrix (ECM) components, production of inflammatory cytokines, oxidative stress, and dysregulation of miRNA expression [6–14].

Obesity also increases the risk in developing OA in non-weight-bearing joints, ascribing a prominent role of metabolic factors in the OA pathogenesis [2,15,16]. Interestingly, obesity induces a low-grade chronic inflammatory state mainly through the production of inflammatory mediators, such as adipokines, cytokines, chemokines, and complement factors by white adipose tissue [17]. Adipokines, including adiponectin, leptin, resistin, chemerin, and visfatin, are metabolically active proteins that emerged as crucial regulators of immune system response and chronic inflammation [18,19]. Their critical role in the pathogenesis of immune-mediated rheumatic diseases and degenerative OA has been amply demonstrated [20–23]. Among them, visfatin is a functionally multi-faceted and ubiquitously protein with insulin-mimetic properties and pro-inflammatory and immunomodulating functions [23–25]. Circulating visfatin levels were found higher in patients with OA than those in healthy controls [20,26]; furthermore, pro-inflammatory, catabolic, and pro-degradative effects of visfatin in OA chondrocytes and synovial fibroblasts were revealed [27–30].

Interestingly, some in vitro studies demonstrated the effect of shear stress or mechanical overloading on adipokine-induced OA damage, exacerbating the loss of chondrocyte homeostasis and accelerating the formation of OA phenotype [31–33]. However, the results are still limited and inconclusive, and further investigations to address the characteristics of the interplay between loading and adipokines in the regulation of chondrocytes metabolism and function are needed.

Therefore, the purpose of the present study was to investigate the in vitro role of 3 h of a high continuous HP (24 MPa) in regulating visfatin-induced effects in human OA chondrocyte cultures. In particular, we evaluated the cell viability, the apoptosis ratio, the transcriptional levels of the anti-apoptotic marker B-cell lymphoma *(BCL)2* and of the main extracellular matrix-degrading enzymes, metalloproteinase *(MMP)-3, MMP-13*, and of collagen type II alpha 1 chain *(Col2a1)*. The production of mitochondrial superoxide anion and the gene expression of antioxidant enzymes (superoxide dismutase *(SOD)-2*, catalase *(CAT)*, glutathione peroxidase *(GPx)4*, of nuclear factor erythroid 2 like 2 *(NRF2)*), and of a pattern of miRNA *(mir-27a, miR-34a, mir-140, miR-146a, miR-155, miR-181a*, and *miR-let7e)* involved in OA pathogenesis were also assessed.

Furthermore, based on our previous results, we analyzed the regulation of the Wnt/β-catenin signaling pathway following HP exposure. To confirm the role of visfatin effects on underlying mechanisms of chondrocytes, cells were pre-treated for 4 h with the visfatin inhibitor FK866.

2. Results

2.1. HP Regulates Cellular Apoptosis and Cartilage Turnover

Figure 1 summarizes the effects of 3 h-application of high continuous HP of 24 MPa on viability, apoptosis ratio, and the regulation of matrix-degrading enzymes, MMP-3, -13, and of Col2a1. The exposure of the cells to HP significantly reduced the percentage of survival and the transcriptional levels of the anti-apoptotic marker *BCL2*, while it raised apoptosis and induced an up-regulation of *MMP-3, MMP-13* gene expression, and a decrease of *Col2a1*, in comparison to the basal condition ($p < 0.01$, Figure 1A–F).

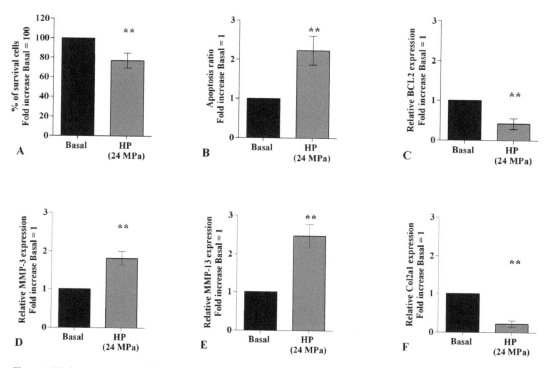

Figure 1. Hydrostatic pressure (HP) exposure regulates chondrocyte metabolism. Human osteoarthritic (OA) chondrocytes were examined at basal condition and after 3 h of high continuous HP (24 MPa). (**A**) Evaluation of cell viability by MTT assay. (**B**) Apoptosis detection performed by flow cytometry analysis and measured with Annexin Alexa fluor 488 assay. Data were expressed as the percentage of positive cells for Annexin-V and propidium iodide (PI) staining. (**C–F**) Expression levels of B-cell lymphoma (*BCL2*), metalloproteinase (*MMP*)-3, -13, type II collagen (*Col2a1*), analyzed by quantitative real-time PCR. The percentage of survival cells, the ratio of apoptosis, and the gene expression were referenced to the ratio of the value of interest and the value of basal condition, reported equal to 100 or 1. Data were expressed as mean ± standard deviation (SD) of triplicate values. ** $p < 0.01$ versus basal condition.

2.2. HP Influences Oxidative Stress Balance and miRNA Expression Profile

High HP significantly promoted the production of mitochondrial superoxide anion ($p < 0.01$) and the gene expression of the antioxidant enzymes, *SOD-2* ($p < 0.001$), *CAT* ($p < 0.05$), and of the transcriptional factor *NRF2* ($p < 0.01$), with respect to baseline (Figure 2A–C,E). On the contrary, no detectable changes have been observed in *GPx4* mRNA levels (Figure 2D).

Figure 3 shows the effect of continuous HP of 24 MPa in regulating the gene expression of a pattern of miRNA known to be implicated in OA pathogenesis. The transcriptional levels of *miR-27a* and *miR-140* resulted significantly reduced ($p < 0.01$) in cells exposed to HP in comparison to those at the basal condition (Figure 3A,C). On the other hand, the studied pressurization upregulated, in a significant manner, the gene levels of *miR-34a* ($p < 0.01$), *miR-146a* ($p < 0.01$), *miR-155* ($p < 0.001$), *miR-181a* ($p < 0.01$), and *miR-let7e* ($p < 0.01$) (Figure 3B,D–G).

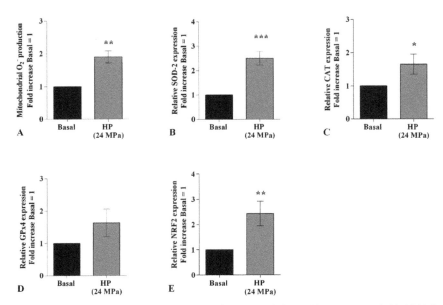

Figure 2. Hydrostatic pressure (HP) exposure regulates oxidative stress balance. Human osteoarthritic (OA) chondrocytes were examined at the basal condition and after 3 h of high continuous HP (24 MPa). (**A**) Mitochondrial superoxide anion production evaluated by MitoSox Red staining at flow cytometry. (**B–E**) Expression levels of superoxide dismutase (*SOD*)-2, catalase (*CAT*), glutathione peroxidase (*GPx*)4, nuclear factor erythroid 2 like 2 (*NRF2*) analyzed by quantitative real-time PCR. The production of superoxide anion and gene expression were referenced to the ratio of the value of interest and the value of basal condition, reported equal to 1. Data were expressed as mean ± standard deviation (SD) of triplicate values. * $p < 0.05$, ** $p < 0.01$, *** $p < 0.001$ versus basal condition.

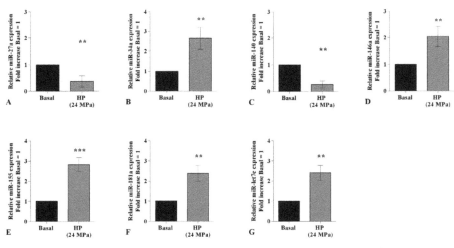

Figure 3. Hydrostatic pressure (HP) exposure modulates miRNA expression. Human osteoarthritic (OA) chondrocytes were examined at the basal condition and after 3 h of high continuous HP (24 MPa). (**A–G**) Expression levels of *miR-27a*, *miR-34a*, *miR-140*, *miR-146a*, *miR-155*, *miR-181a*, and *miR-let7e* analyzed by quantitative real-time PCR. The gene expression was referenced to the ratio of the value of interest and the value of basal condition, reported equal to 1. Data were expressed as mean ± standard deviation (SD) of triplicate values. ** $p < 0.01$, *** $p < 0.001$ versus basal condition.

2.3. Visfatin Induces Cellular Apoptosis and Regulates Cartilage Turnover

To confirm the direct effect of visfatin in the modulation of the apoptosis process and cartilage metabolism, OA chondrocytes were incubated for 4 h with 10 µM of visfatin inhibitor (FK866) prior to 24 h of treatment with visfatin (10 µg/mL) (Figure 4). The stimulus of chondrocytes with visfatin significantly reduced the percentage of cell viability ($p < 0.01$) and the expression levels of *BCL2* ($p < 0.05$), while increasing the amount of apoptotic cells ($p < 0.05$), in comparison to baseline (Figure 4A–C). Furthermore, visfatin induced the over-expression of *MMP-3* and *MMP-13* genes ($p < 0.05$) and the downregulation of *Col2a1* ($p < 0.05$) (Figure 4D–F). The incubation of the cells with the FK866 inhibitor significantly counteracted visfatin-induced effects (Figure 4A–F).

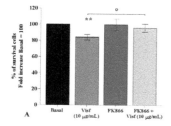
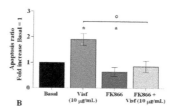
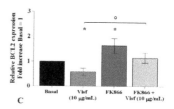
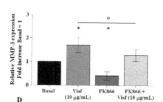
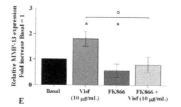
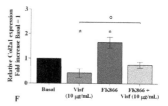

Figure 4. Visfatin regulates chondrocyte metabolism. Human osteoarthritic (OA) chondrocytes were examined at basal condition, after 4 h of pre-incubation with Nicotinamide Phosphoribosyltransferase Inhibitor (FK866, 10 µM), and after 24 h of incubation with visfatin (10 µg/mL). (**A**) Evaluation of cell viability by MTT assay. (**B**) Apoptosis detection performed by flow cytometry analysis and measured with Annexin Alexa fluor 488 assay. Data were expressed as the percentage of positive cells for Annexin-V and propidium iodide (PI) staining. (**C–F**) Expression levels of B-cell lymphoma (*BCL2*), metalloproteinase (*MMP*)-3, -13, type II collagen (*Col2a1*), analyzed by quantitative real-time PCR. The percentage of survival cells, the ratio of apoptosis, and the gene expression were referenced to the ratio of the value of interest and the value of basal condition, reported equal to 100 or 1. Data were expressed as mean ± standard deviation (SD) of triplicate values. * $p < 0.05$, ** $p < 0.01$ versus basal condition. ° $p < 0.05$ versus visfatin.

2.4. Visfatin Modulates Oxidant/Antioxidant System and miRNA Expression Profile

The potential role of visfatin in the regulation of oxidant/antioxidant balance was assessed in visfatin-stimulated chondrocytes pre-treated with a visfatin inhibitor (FK866) (Figure 5).

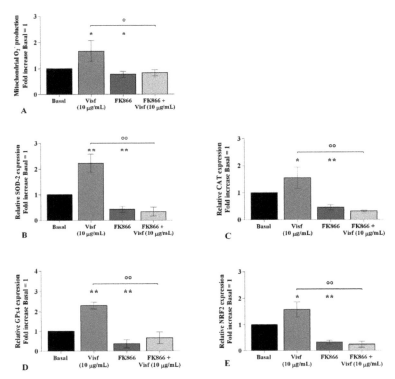

Figure 5. Visfatin regulates oxidative stress balance. Human osteoarthritic (OA) chondrocytes were examined at the basal condition, after 4 h of pre-incubation with nicotinamide phosphoribosyltransferase inhibitor (FK866, 10 μM), and after 24 h of incubation with visfatin (10 μg/mL). (**A**) Mitochondrial superoxide anion production evaluated by MitoSox Red staining at flow cytometry. (**B–E**) Expression levels of superoxide dismutase (SOD)-2, catalase (CAT), glutathione peroxidase (GPx)4, and nuclear factor erythroid 2 like 2 (NRF2) analyzed by quantitative real-time PCR. The production of superoxide anion and the gene expression were referenced to the ratio of the value of interest and the value of basal condition, reported equal to 1. Data were expressed as mean ± standard deviation (SD) of triplicate values. * $p < 0.05$, ** $p < 0.01$ versus basal condition. ° $p < 0.05$, °° $p < 0.01$ versus visfatin.

Flow cytometry and PCR analysis demonstrated a significant increase of mitochondrial superoxide anion production ($p < 0.05$) and of *SOD-2* ($p < 0.01$), *CAT* ($p < 0.05$), *GPx4* ($p < 0.01$), and *NRF2* ($p < 0.05$) transcriptional levels in cells stimulated with visfatin compared to baseline (Figure 5A–E). Conversely, the incubation of the cells with FK866 significantly reduced the ROS production ($p < 0.05$) and antioxidant enzymes' gene expression ($p < 0.05$, $p < 0.01$) (Figure 5A–E).

Furthermore, pre-treatment of chondrocytes with the inhibitor decreased the ROS release ($p < 0.05$) and the expression of *SOD-2*, *CAT*, *GPx4*, and *NRF2* ($p < 0.01$) induced by visfatin, in comparison to the cells incubated with the adipokine alone (Figure 5A–E).

The evaluation of the miRNA expression profile showed a significant down-regulation of *miR-27a* and *miR-140* ($p < 0.05$) gene levels, and an over-expression of *miR-34a* ($p < 0.05$), *miR-146a* ($p < 0.05$), *miR-155* ($p < 0.01$), *miR-181a* ($p < 0.05$), and *miR-let7e* ($p < 0.01$) in visfatin-stimulated cells in comparison to the control cultures (Figure 6A–G). As expected, opposite regulation on the miRNA expression profile was obtained in OA cells incubated with visfatin inhibitor (Figure 6A–G).

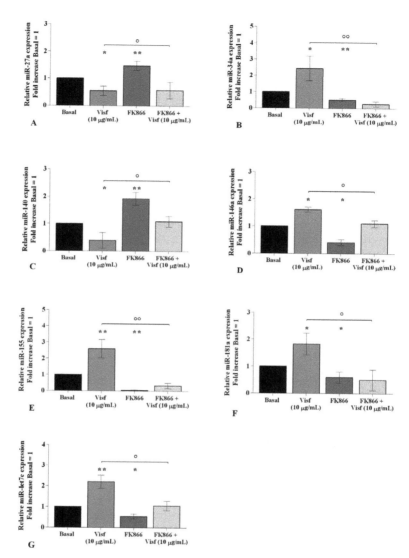

Figure 6. Visfatin modulates miRNA expression. Human osteoarthritic (OA) chondrocytes were examined at the basal condition, after 4 h of pre-incubation with the nicotinamide phosphoribosyltransferase inhibitor (FK866, 10 µM), and after 24 h of incubation with visfatin (10 µg/mL). (**A–G**) Expression levels of *miR-27a*, *miR-34a*, *miR-140*, *miR-146a*, *miR-155*, *miR-181a*, and *miR-let7e* analyzed by quantitative real-time PCR. The gene expression was referenced to the ratio of the value of interest and the value of the basal condition, reported equal to 1. Data were expressed as mean ± standard deviation (SD) of triplicate values. * $p < 0.05$, ** $p < 0.01$ versus basal condition. ° $p < 0.05$, °° $p < 0.01$ versus visfatin.

2.5. HP Increases Cellular Apoptosis and Cartilage Damage Caused by Visfatin

Figure 7 shows the implication of HP in regulating visfatin-induced effects on cartilage metabolism; human OA chondrocytes were treated for 24 h with visfatin 10 µg/mL (4 h pre-incubation with 10 µM of visfatin inhibitor, FK866) and, then exposed to 3 h of continuous HP (24 MPa). The concomitant exposure of the cells to visfatin and a cycle of HP significantly exacerbated the regulation on chondrocyte survival, apoptosis, and cartilage turnover caused by the only stimulus with visfatin or HP (Figure 7A–F). In addition, the pre-treatment of chondrocytes with FK866 significantly limited the effects of HP in comparison to what is observed after the pressurization alone (Figure 7A–F).

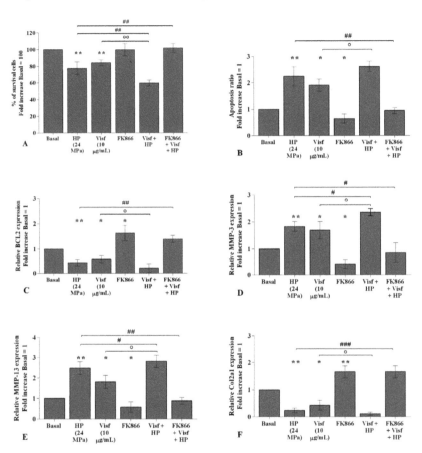

Figure 7. Hydrostatic pressure (HP) exposure exacerbates the effect of visfatin on chondrocyte metabolism. Human osteoarthritic (OA) chondrocytes were examined at the basal condition, after 24 h of incubation with visfatin (10 μg/mL) (4 h of pre-incubation with nicotinamide phosphoribosyl-transferase inhibitor (FK866, 10 μM)), and after 3 h of high continuous HP (24 MPa). (**A**) Evaluation of cell viability by MTT assay. (**B**) Apoptosis detection performed by flow cytometry analysis and measured with Annexin Alexa fluor 488 assay. Data were expressed as the percentage of positive cells for Annexin-V and propidium iodide (PI) staining. (**C–F**) Expression levels of B-cell lymphoma (*BCL2*), metalloproteinase (*MMP*)-3, -13, type II collagen (*Col2a1*), analyzed by quantitative real-time PCR. The percentage of survival cells, the ratio of apoptosis, and the gene expression were referenced to the ratio of the value of interest and the value of basal condition, reported equal to 100 or 1. Data were expressed as mean ± standard deviation (SD) of triplicate values. * $p < 0.05$, ** $p < 0.01$ versus basal condition. ° $p < 0.05$, °° $p < 0.01$ versus visfatin. # $p < 0.05$, ## $p < 0.01$, ### $p < 0.001$ versus HP.

2.6. HP Exacerbates Oxidative Stress Balance Caused by Visfatin

The effects of visfatin in the regulation of oxidative stress balance were significantly increased ($p < 0.05$) when chondrocytes were also subjected to a high HP of 24 MPa, in comparison to only visfatin stimulus or HP exposure (Figure 8A–E). Furthermore, the activation of oxidant/antioxidant factors was significantly reduced in pressurized cells pre-incubated with FK866 with respect to the only HP exposure (Figure 8A–E).

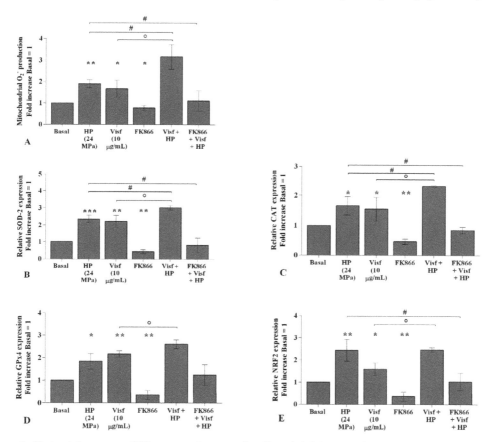

Figure 8. Hydrostatic pressure (HP) exposure increases the effect of visfatin on oxidative stress balance. Human osteoarthritic (OA) chondrocytes were examined at the basal condition, after 24 h of incubation with visfatin (10 μg/mL) (4 h of pre-incubation with nicotinamide phosphoribosyltransferase inhibitor (FK866, 10 μM)), and after 3 h of high continuous HP (24 MPa). (**A**) Mitochondrial superoxide anion production evaluated by MitoSox Red staining at flow cytometry. (**B–E**) Expression levels of superoxide dismutase (*SOD*)-2, catalase (*CAT*), glutathione peroxidase (*GPx*)4, nuclear factor erythroid 2 like 2 (*NRF2*) analyzed by quantitative real-time PCR. The production of superoxide anion and gene expression were referenced to the ratio of the value of interest and the value of basal condition, reported equal to 1. Data were expressed as mean ± standard deviation (SD) of triplicate values. * $p < 0.05$, ** $p < 0.01$, *** $p < 0.001$ versus basal condition. ° $p < 0.05$ versus visfatin. # $p < 0.05$ versus HP.

2.7. HP Enhances Visfatin Effect on miRNA Gene Expression Profile

The effect of visfatin on miRNA expression became significantly more intensive ($p < 0.05$) when OA chondrocytes were also exposed to a cycle of HP with respect to HP or visfatin stimulus alone (Figure 9A–G). In addition, the pre-treatment of the cells with FK866 limited, in a significant manner, the simultaneous effect of visfatin and HP on miRNA regulation in comparison to only visfatin or HP treatments (Figure 9A–G).

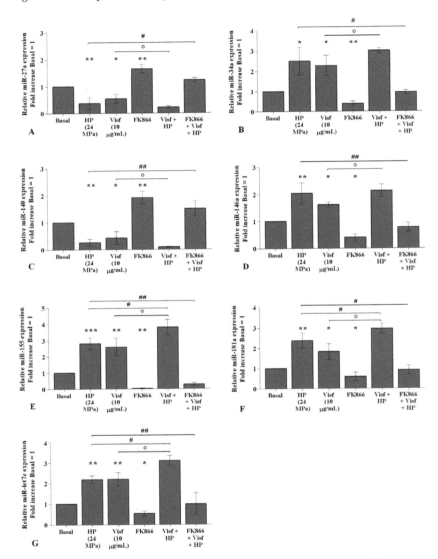

Figure 9. Hydrostatic pressure (HP) exposure increases the effect of visfatin on miRNA expression. Human osteoarthritic (OA) chondrocytes were examined at the basal condition, after 24 h of incubation with visfatin (10 μg/mL) (4 h of pre-incubation with nicotinamide phosphoribosyltransferase inhibitor (FK866, 10 μM)), and after 3 h of high continuous HP (24 MPa). (**A–G**) Expression levels of *miR-27a*, *miR-34a*, *miR-140*, *miR-146a*, *miR-155*, *miR-181a*, and *miR-let7e* analyzed by quantitative real-time PCR. The gene expression was referenced to the ratio of the value of interest and the value of the basal condition, reported equal to 1. Data were expressed as mean ± standard deviation (SD) of triplicate values. * $p < 0.05$, ** $p < 0.01$, *** $p < 0.001$ versus basal condition. ° $p < 0.05$ versus visfatin. # $p < 0.05$, ## $p < 0.01$ versus HP.

2.8. HP Influences the Regulation of the Wnt/β-Catenin Pathway Induced by Visfatin

Figure 10 describes the regulation of HP on the Wnt/β-catenin pathway activated by visfatin. For the detection of β-catenin protein levels, OA chondrocytes were treated for 4 h with visfatin 10 μg/mL (4 h pre-incubation with 10 μM of visfatin inhibitor, FK866), and then exposed to 3 h of high continuous HP of 24 MPa. Western blot analysis of cell lysates showed the β-catenin band at approximately 92 KDa. The densitometric quantification of the bands revealed that β-catenin protein levels were significantly reduced in OA cells subjected to HP ($p < 0.05$) or following 4 h of visfatin stimulus ($p < 0.05$) in comparison to baseline, while no changes upon the incubation with FK866 inhibitor were observed (Figure 10A,B). A significant increase of β-catenin protein expression ($p < 0.05$) was found in visfatin-treated chondrocytes pre-incubated with FK866 compared to visfatin stimulus alone. Furthermore, FK866 pre-treatment of OA cells simultaneously stimulated with visfatin and HP induced a significant increase of β-catenin expression ($p < 0.05$) with respect to visfatin or HP stimuli alone (Figure 10A,B).

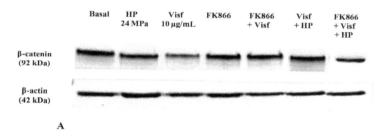

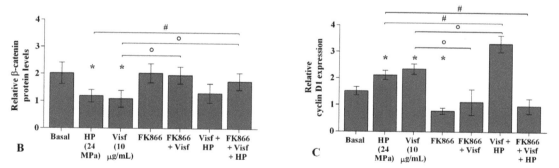

Figure 10. Hydrostatic pressure HP exposure regulates the effect of visfatin on Wnt/β-catenin pathway. Human osteoarthritic (OA) chondrocytes were examined at basal condition, after 4 h of incubation with visfatin (10 μg/mL) (4 h of pre-incubation with nicotinamide phosphoribosyltransferase inhibitor (FK866, 10 μM)), and after 3 h of high continuous (24 MPa) hydrostatic pressure (HP). (**A,B**) Representative immunoblotting image and densitometric analysis of β-catenin protein levels by western blot. (**C**) Expression levels of *cyclin D1* analyzed by quantitative real-time PCR. The protein levels and the gene expression were referenced to the ratio of the value of interest and the value of the basal condition, reported equal to 1. Data were expressed as mean ± standard deviation (SD) of triplicate values. * $p < 0.05$ versus basal condition. ° $p < 0.05$ versus visfatin. # $p < 0.05$ versus HP.

The stimulus of the cells with visfatin or their exposure to HP significantly up-regulated the gene levels of *cyclin D1* ($p < 0.05$) in comparison to those at basal condition, whereas a significant reduction after FK866 incubation was observed ($p < 0.05$) (Figure 10C). FK866 pre-incubation of visfatin-treated chondrocytes significantly reduced the expression of *cyclin D1* ($p < 0.05$) compared to visfatin stimulus alone (Figure 10C). A significant increase of *cyclin D1* expression levels ($p < 0.05$) was observed in OA cells simultaneously exposed to visfatin and HP compared to only visfatin or HP stimulus; the increase of *cyclin D1* was counteracted by the pre-incubation with FK866 inhibitor ($p < 0.05$) (Figure 10C).

3. Discussion

Accumulating evidence reported the complex interplay between mechanical loading and adipokines in the development and the progression of OA [3,13,20,34], even if the exact mechanisms underlying this relationship has not completely elucidated and additional studies are required.

The present research aimed to evaluate the potential role of HP in regulating visfatin-induced effects on cartilage turnover, apoptosis, and oxidative stress, and on the modulation of a pattern of miRNA, in human OA chondrocytes. Our experiments were performed using a prototype of the HP system, developed for in vitro cell cultures. In particular, we tested a high continuous HP of 24 MPa, exceeding the range of physiological loading measured in vivo [35]; this pressurization, applied for a period of 3 consecutive hours, approximately reproduced the conditions that occur in the human joints [6,36,37]. Furthermore, to inhibit the enzymatic activity of visfatin, our cultures were pre-treated with FK866, in agreement with other authors [38]. FK866 is a pharmacologic competitive inhibitor that binds the catalytic pocket of nicotinamide and reduces the intracellular NAD content in a time- and concentration-dependent manner [38].

Our results showed the up-regulation of the gene expression of matrix-degrading enzymes, *MMP-3* and *MMP-13*, and the reduction of *Col2a1* in OA chondrocytes exposed to HP or stimulated with visfatin, in agreement with previous studies [6,8,9,13,27,29,39–43].

Furthermore, we first demonstrated that the effect of visfatin on MMPs and Col2a1 was increased when OA chondrocytes were simultaneously subjected to high continuous HP, while the use of visfatin inhibitor limited both visfatin- and HP-induced effects. Evidence from Su et al. [32] partially confirmed our data even if the studies are not comparable. The authors showed a higher increase of cyclooxygenase (COX)-2 gene expression in OA chondrocytes treated for 4 h with resistin and meanwhile exposed to fluid shear stress than the resistin stimulus alone.

The continuous HP of 24 MPa applied to our OA chondrocytes raised the percentage of apoptotic cells, with a concomitant reduction of the gene expression of the anti-apoptotic marker *BCL2*, in agreement with previous studies. Indeed, an increase of apoptosis rate has been reported in human cartilage explants exposed to a single static pressure of 14 MPa for 500 ms under radially unconfined compression [44], and in human or bovine OA chondrocytes subjected to 10 or 20 MPa of loading for a maximum timing of 3 h [13,45,46].

The activation of apoptosis signaling and the reduced expression of the anti-apoptotic marker was also observed when our cell cultures were stimulated for 24 h with visfatin; according to our results, other authors previously revealed the pro-apoptotic effect of this adipokine in endothelial progenitor cells and human OA chondrocytes [13,27,47]. To the best of our knowledge, we found, for the first time, a significant increase of apoptosis exposing OA chondrocytes to visfatin and high continuous HP compared to stimulus with visfatin or HP alone. These results were significantly counteracted upon the pre-incubation with the visfatin inhibitor FK866.

Oxidative stress has been increasingly recognized to be involved in joint damage that occurs in OA. The failure of oxidant/antioxidant balance in chondrocytes determines an altered redox status in favor of catabolic processes, contributing to OA pathogenesis [8,48]. The results of the present study showed an increased production of mitochondrial superoxide anion and an upregulation of the transcriptional levels of the main antioxidant enzymes, *SOD*, *CAT*, *GPx4*, and *NRF2*, after the exposure of OA chondrocytes to HP or visfatin. Similarly, it has been previously reported an excessive ROS production upon the application of 24 h of static compression ranged from 40 to 120 psi or 3 h of static continuous HP of 10 MPa, in porcine and human OA chondrocytes [13,49]. Furthermore, an increase of mitochondrial ROS release and antioxidant enzymes expression was shown in human OA chondrocytes and synoviocytes stimulated with visfatin [29,30]. To our knowledge, this is the first paper showing that the concomitant treatment of OA cultures with visfatin and a cycle of high pressurization significantly exacerbated ROS release and antioxidant enzymes expression; these effects were significantly counterbalanced by FK866 pre-incubation.

An altered expression of some miRNA was associated with the regulation of chondrocyte metabolism, inflammatory response, and oxidative stress during OA damage [29,50–53]. In this experience, we confirmed the up-regulation of *miR-34a*, *miR-146a*, and *miR-181a* gene expression in OA chondrocytes stimulated with HP, in line with the growing body of evidence [8,13,46,50,53–55]. Besides, we first demonstrated the dysregulation of *miR-27a*, *miR-140*, *miR-155*, and *miR-let7e* after the application of this pressurization schedule. Previous studies showed an up-regulation of *miR-27a*, *miR-140*, *miR-146a*, and a decrease of *miR-155* and *miR-181a* gene levels in OA chondrocytes subjected to 3 h of cyclic low HP (1–5 MPa) [8,10].

Moreover, in the present study, the evaluation of visfatin effects on miRNA regulation showed a reduction of *miR-27a* and *miR-140* gene levels, and an increase of *miR-34a*, *miR-146a*, *miR-155*, *miR-181a*, and *miR-let7e* in OA chondrocytes, according to our previous findings in human OA chondrocytes and synoviocytes [27,30].

Finally, we reported a significantly altered expression of the studied miRNA when OA chondrocytes were simultaneously treated with visfatin and exposed to high continuous HP. This combined effect was counteracted by the pre-incubation of the cells with FK866 inhibitor.

The pivotal role of the canonical Wnt/β-catenin signaling pathway in articular cartilage homeostasis and joint disease has been extensively reported [56,57].

Based on our previous findings, in this study we evaluated the regulation of Wnt/β-catenin signaling after a cycle of mechanical loading and/or adipokines stimulus. The exposure of our OA chondrocytes to HP or visfatin stimulus showed a reduction of total β-catenin protein expression. This expression resulted intensified when the cells were simultaneously treated with visfatin and high HP, while it was partially counteracted by the pre-treatment with FK866.

Previous studies found increased protein levels of Wnt-3a and β-catenin in articular cartilage of an injured exercise-induced OA rat model and in OA rat chondrocytes cultures subjected to cyclic mechanical strain with a 0.5 Hz sinusoidal curve at 10% elongation for 8 h/day [58,59]. Recently, Cheleschi et al. showed a reduction of β-catenin protein expression in OA chondrocytes exposed to 3 h of low cyclic sinusoidal HP (1–5 MPa) [8], while its increase was found upon the application of a static continuous HP of 10 MPa [13].

Furthermore, increased protein levels of Wnt-3a and β-catenin were reported after the incubation of human chondrocyte cell lines (C-28/I2 and T/C-28a2) and human OA primary osteoblasts for 24 h with leptin and resistin, respectively [60,61].

Our results seem to be in contrast with the current literature since the apparent non-activation of the signaling pathway following the negative stimuli applied to our cultures. However, this discrepancy could be related to the use, in our experiments, of a non-specific antibody for the assessment of β-catenin expression; indeed, our antibody seemed to be useful in detecting the total β-catenin protein levels, while not able to discriminate between the active non-phosphorylated form and the inactivate phospho-β-catenin labeled for ubiquitination and proteasomal degradation [8,62,63]. In this regard, to confirm the activation of the studied pathway, we also investigated the transcriptional levels of *cyclin D1*, a downstream target gene of Wnt/β-catenin signaling cascade and a central player in cell cycle regulation, cell proliferation, and apoptosis during OA [64]. In this experience, we observed the up-regulation of *cyclin D1* gene expression when OA chondrocytes were exposed to HP and/or to visfatin stimulus. Similar results were found after the exposure of osteoblastic cell lines to 5 h of 3400 microstrains of mechanical loading (2 Hz, 7200 cycles/h) or upon the application of 12 h of 12% cyclical tensile stress at human osteosarcoma cell lines [65,66]. Furthermore, the stimulus of endometrial carcinoma cell lines with visfatin for 24 h induced the expression of *cyclin D1*, which was reduced following FK866 [67].

Finally, we first observed the strong increase of *cyclin D1* gene levels after the combined treatment of chondrocytes with visfatin and HP; the HP effect was reduced by the pre-incubation of the cells with FK866 inhibitor.

4. Materials and Methods

4.1. Isolation and Culture of Human OA Chondrocytes

Human OA articular cartilage was obtained from femoral heads of five non-obese (body mass index ranging from 20 to 24 kg/m^2) and non-diabetic patients (two men and three women, age ranging from 63 to 76) with coxarthrosis according to American College of Rheumatology criteria [68], undergoing to hip replacement surgery. OA grades ranged from moderate to severe, and cartilage showed typical OA changes, with the presence of chondrocyte clusters, fibrillation, and loss of metachromasia (Mankin degree 3–7) [69]. The femoral heads were supplied by the Orthopaedic Surgery, University of Siena, Italy. The use of human articular samples was permitted after the authorization of the Ethic Committee of Azienda Ospedaliera Universitaria Senese/Siena University Hospital (decision no. 13931/18), and the informed consent of the donor.

After surgery, cartilage fragments were aseptically dissected from each donor and processed by an enzymatic digestion as previously described [29]. For growth and expansion, cells were cultured in Dulbecco's modified eagle medium (DMEM) (Euroclone, Milan, Italy) with phenol red and 4 mM L-glutamine (Euroclone, Milan, Italy), supplemented with 10% fetal bovine serum (FBS) (Euroclone, Milan, Italy), 200 U/mL penicillin, and 200 µg/mL streptomycin (P/S) (Sigma–Aldrich, Milan, Italy). The medium was changed every 2–3 days and the cell morphology was examined daily with an inverted microscope (Olympus IMT-2, Tokyo, Japan) [70]. For each single experiment, a cell culture from a unique donor was used.

4.2. OA Chondrocytes Exposure to HP

The HP was generated by a unique prototype of pressurization system described in detail by Nerucci et al. [35]; the system has been validated in a number of in vitro studies [6,8,13,71].

In the present study, OA chondrocytes were seeded in Petri dishes (35 × 10 mm^2) (Euroclone, Milan, Italy) at a starting density of 1 × 10^5 cells, until they became 85% confluent, in DMEM supplemented with 10% FBS for 24 h. Then, the medium was removed, and substituted with DMEM with 0.5% FBS for the treatment procedure. Petri dishes were completely filled with the culture medium and sealed with a special membrane (Surlyn 1801 Bynel CXA 3048 bilayer membrane, Du Pont, Biesterfeld polychem s.r.l, Milan, Italy), excluding air to avoid implosions due to the presence of air between the membrane and the medium, suitable for preserving a stable environment. The dishes were arranged inside the pressure chamber filled with distilled water at a temperature of 37 °C. Then, the cells were subjected to a high continuous pressure of 24 MPa, for a period of 3 h. Some dishes, used as controls, were maintained in the same culture conditions without receiving any pressurization. Chondrocytes at basal condition and immediately after receiving pressure were collected to perform flow cytometry, quantitative real-time PCR, and western blot analysis.

4.3. OA Chondrocytes Treatment

Human OA chondrocytes were plated in 6-well dishes at a starting density of 1×10^5 cells/well until 85% confluence. Human recombinant visfatin (Sigma–Aldrich, Milan, Italy) was dissolved in phosphate buffered saline (PBS) (Euroclone, Milan, Italy), in accordance with the manufacturer's instructions, and then directly diluted in the culture medium for the treatment in order to obtain the final concentration required.

The cells were cultured in DMEM enriched with 0.5% FBS and 2% P/S, and stimulated for 24 h with visfatin at concentration of 10 μg/mL, according to previous studies [27,29,47]. Some dishes were pre-incubated for 4 h with 10 μM of nicotinamide phosphoribosyltransferase inhibitor, FK866 (Sigma–Aldrich, Milan, Italy) [63].

After the treatment, the cells were recovered and immediately processed to carry out flow cytometry, quantitative real-time PCR, and western blot analysis.

4.4. Cell Viability

The viability of the cells was evaluated by MTT (3-[4,4-dimethylthiazol-2-yl]-2,5-diphenyl-tetrazoliumbromide) (Sigma–Aldrich, Milan, Italy) for each experimental condition. The experimental procedure was performed as previously described [30]. The percentage of survival cells was evaluated as (absorbance of considered sample)/(absorbance of control) $\times$ 100. Data were reported as OD units per 10^4 adherent cells.

4.5. Apoptosis Detection

Apoptotic cells were measured by using an Annexin V-FITC and propidium iodide (PI) kit (ThermoFisher Scientific, Milan, Italy). OA chondrocytes were seeded in 12-well plates (8×10^4 cells/well) for 24 h in DMEM with 10% FBS, before replacement with 0.5% FBS used for the treatment. The procedure was performed as previously described [13]. A total of 10,000 events (1×10^4 cells per assay) were measured by the instrument. The results were examined with Cell Quest software (Version 4.0, Becton Dickinson, San Jose, CA, USA).

The instrument permitted to discriminate intact cells (annexin-V and PI-negative), early apoptosis (annexin-V-positive and PI-negative), and late apoptosis (annexin-V and PI positives). Cells simultaneously stained with Alexa Fluor 488 annexin-V and PI were considered for the evaluation of apoptosis [72]. The results were expressed as the percentage of positive cells to each dye (total apoptosis).

4.6. Mitochondrial Superoxide Anion ($\cdot O2-$) Assessment

OA chondrocyte were seeded in 12 well-plates (8×10^4 cells/well) for 24 h in DMEM with 10% FCS, before replacement with 0.5% FBS used for the treatment procedure. The procedure has been performed as previously described [13]. A density of 1×10^4 cells per assay (a total of 10,000 events) were measured by flow cytometry and data were analyzed with CellQuest software (Version 4.0, Becton Dickinson, San Jose, CA, USA). Results were collected as the median of fluorescence (AU) and represented the mean of three independent experiments.

4.7. RNA Isolation and Quantitative Real-Time PCR

OA chondrocyte were grown and maintained in 6-well dishes at a starting density of 1×10^5 cells/well until they became 85% confluent in DMEM supplemented with 10% FBS, before replacement with 0.5% FBS used for the treatment. After treatment, cells were collected and total RNA, including miRNA, was extracted using TriPure Isolation Reagent (Euroclone, Milan, Italy) according to the manufacturer's instructions. The concentration, purity, and integrity of RNA were evaluated by measuring the OD at 260 nm and the 260/280 and 260/230 ratios by Nanodrop-1000 (Celbio, Milan, Italy).

Five hundred nanograms of RNA of target genes and miRNA were reverse transcribed by using the QuantiTect Reverse Transcription (Qiagen, Hilden, German) and the cDNA miScript PCR Reverse Transcription (Qiagen, Hilden, German) kits, respectively, according to the manufacturer's instructions.

Target genes and miRNA were assessed by real-time PCR using QuantiFast SYBR Green PCR (Qiagen, Hilden, German) and miScript SYBR Green (Qiagen, Hilden, German) kits, respectively. Primers used for PCR reactions are listed in Table S1.

All qPCR reactions were achieved in glass capillaries by a LightCycler 1.0 (Roche Molecular Biochemicals, Mannheim, Germany) with LightCycler Software Version 3.5. The reaction procedure for miRNA and target genes has described in detail by our previous studies [13,29].

For the data analysis, the Ct values of each sample and the efficiency of the primer set were calculated through LinReg Software [73] and then converted into relative quantities and normalized according to Pfaffl model [74]. The normalization was performed considering actin beta (*ACTB*) for target genes and small nucleolar RNA, C/D Box 25 (*SNORD-25*) for miRNA, as the housekeeping genes [75].

4.8. Western Blot

OA chondrocytes at first passage were seeded in Petri dishes (35×10 mm^2) at a starting density of 1×10^5 cells/chamber in DMEM supplemented with 10% FBS for 24 h. After this period, the medium was removed and the cells were cultured in DMEM with 0.5% FBS for the experiment. After treatment, cells were collected and total lysates were obtained with M-PER™ Mammalian Protein Extraction Reagent (Thermo Fisher Scientific, Rockford, IL, USA) containing a protease inhibitor cocktail (Sigma–Aldrich, Milan, Italy). For each experimental condition, ten micrograms were loaded into 10% sodium dodecyl sulphate-polyacrylamide electrophoresis gels and separated by molecular size. Proteins were then transferred to a nitrocellulose membrane and, after blocking step, incubated at 4 °C overnight with mouse monoclonal anti-total β-catenin primary antibody (sc-59737, Santa Cruz Biotechnology, Milan, Italy) (dilution 1:250), and then with secondary goat anti-mouse IgG (H + L)-HRP conjugate antibody (1:5000) (Bio-Rad Laboratories S.r.l., Milan, Italy). The reaction was assessed by chemiluminescence (Bio-Rad Laboratories S.r.l., Milan, Italy). The blots were re-probed with HRP-conjugated β-actin (Sigma-Aldrich, Milan, Italy) used as the loading control. Images of the bands were digitized and the densitometric quantification was performed by Image-J software (LOCI, University of Wisconsin-Madison, Madison, WI, USA). Results were normalized with the relative loading control.

4.9. Statistical Analysis

Three independent experiments were carried out and the results were expressed as the mean ± standard deviation (SD) of triplicate values for each experiment. Data normal distribution was evaluated by Shapiro–Wilk, D'Agostino and Pearson, and Kolmogorov–Smirnov tests. Flow cytometry and western blot results were analyzed by ANOVA with a Bonferroni post-hoc test. Quantitative real-time PCR data were evaluated by one-way ANOVA with a Tukey's post-hoc test using $2^{-\Delta\Delta CT}$ values for each sample. All analyses were performed through the SAS System (SAS Institute Inc., Cary, NC, USA) and GraphPad Prism 6.1. A p-value < 0.05 was defined as statistically significant.

5. Conclusions

The results of the present study contribute to increasing knowledge about the complex interplay between HP and visfatin in regulating metabolism in human OA chondrocyte cultures, via the Wnt/β-catenin signaling pathway.

We showed that a cycle of high continuous HP of 24 MPa (3 h), exceeding the physiological loading range measured in in vivo joint, caused cartilage degradation, activated apoptosis signaling, increased oxidative stress, and regulated the expression profile of a miRNA pattern and β-catenin expression and cyclin D1 proteins. Similar and detrimental effects were obtained after 24 h of treatment with visfatin.

Further, the simultaneous exposure of OA cells to visfatin stimulus and high continuous HP seemed to be more effective overall than each single treatment.

Finally, the pre-incubation of the cells with a specific visfatin inhibitor, FK866, reversed both visfatin and HP-induced effects on the analyzed cellular processes.

Taken together, our data support the dual role of obesity in the OA pathogenesis, ascribing a prominent function both to mechanical overloading and the adipose tissue-induced low-grade of chronic inflammation, confirming the importance of controlling body weight in treating the disease.

However, this study reported preliminary results and additional experiments are required to confirm our hypothesis. The implementation of the same analysis on healthy primary chondrocytes could be useful to better understand the involvement of HP and visfatin on chondrocyte homeostasis and, in particular, their relevance in the OA pathogenesis. Furthermore, a deeper analysis of the upstream molecular mechanism responsible for the visfatin-induced effects may contribute to finding out the exact role of mechanical loading in this process. Finally, the use of a specific Wnt/β-catenin inhibitor points out the involvement of the pathway in this complex mechanism.

Supplementary Materials: Supplementary materials are available online at https://www.mdpi.com/1422-0067/22/5/2745/s1.

Author Contributions: Conceptualization, S.C., S.T., and A.F.; data curation, S.C. and M.B.; funding acquisition, S.G. and E.F.; investigation, S.C. and M.B.; methodology, S.C. and M.B.; resources, E.F. and A.F.; validation, M.B.; visualization, S.C.; writing—original draft, S.C. and A.F.; writing—review and editing, S.C., S.T., S.G., F.B., E.F., and A.F. All authors have read and agreed to the published version of the manuscript.

Funding: This work was partially supported by a grant (funds for the research) from the University of Siena, PAR-2021.

Informed Consent Statement: Informed consent was obtained from all subjects involved in the study.

Conflicts of Interest: The authors declare no conflict of interest. The funders had no role in the design of the study; in the collection, analyses, or interpretation of data; in the writing of the manuscript, or in the decision to publish the results.

References

1. Hunter, D.J.; Bierma-Zeinstra, S. Osteoarthritis. *Lancet* **2019**, *393*, 1745–1759. [CrossRef]
2. Issa, R.I.; Griffin, T.M. Pathobiology of Obesity and Osteoarthritis: Integrating Biomechanics and Inflammation. *Pathobiol. Aging Age Relat. Dis.* **2012**, *2*. [CrossRef]
3. Francisco, V.; Pérez, T.; Pino, J.; López, V.; Franco, E.; Alonso, A.; Gonzalez-Gay, M.A.; Mera, A.; Lago, F.; Gómez, R.; et al. Biomechanics, Obesity, and Osteoarthritis. The role of Adipokines: When the Levee Breaks. *J. Orthop. Res.* **2018**, *36*, 594–604. [CrossRef] [PubMed]
4. Herger, S.; Vach, W.; Liphardt, A.M.; Egloff, C.; Nüesch, C.; Mündermann, A. Dose-response Relationship Between Ambulatory Load Magnitude and Load-induced Changes in COMP in Young Healthy Adults. *Osteoarthr. Cartil.* **2019**, *27*, 106–113. [CrossRef] [PubMed]
5. Hunt, M.A.; Charlton, J.M.; Esculier, J.F. Osteoarthritis Year in Review 2019: Mechanics. *Osteoarthr. Cartil.* **2020**, *28*, 267–274. [CrossRef] [PubMed]
6. Fioravanti, A.; Collodel, G.; Petraglia, A.; Nerucci, F.; Moretti, E.; Galeazzi, M. Effect of Hydrostatic Pressure of Various Magnitudes on Osteoarthritic Chondrocytes Exposed to IL-1beta. *Indian J. Med. Res.* **2010**, *132*, 209–217. [PubMed]
7. Pascarelli, N.A.; Collodel, G.; Moretti, E.; Cheleschi, S.; Fioravanti, A. Changes in Ultrastructure and Cytoskeletal Aspects of Human Normal and Osteoarthritic Chondrocytes Exposed to Interleukin-1β and Cyclical Hydrostatic Pressure. *Int. J. Mol. Sci.* **2015**, *16*, 26019–26034. [CrossRef] [PubMed]

8. Cheleschi, S.; De Palma, A.; Pecorelli, A.; Pascarelli, N.A.; Valacchi, G.; Belmonte, G.; Carta, S.; Galeazzi, M.; Fioravanti, A. Hydrostatic Pressure Regulates MicroRNA Expression Levels in Osteoarthritic Chondrocyte Cultures via the Wnt/β-Catenin Pathway. *Int. J. Mol. Sci.* **2017**, *18*, 133. [CrossRef] [PubMed]

9. Montagne, K.; Onuma, Y.; Ito, Y.; Aiki, Y.; Furukawa, K.S.; Ushida, T. High Hydrostatic Pressure Induces Pro-osteoarthritic Changes in Cartilage Precursor Cells: A Transcriptome Analysis. *PLoS ONE* **2017**, *12*, e0183226. [CrossRef]

10. De Palma, A.; Cheleschi, S.; Pascarelli, N.A.; Giannotti, S.; Galeazzi, M.; Fioravanti, A. Hydrostatic Pressure as Epigenetic Modulator in Chondrocyte Cultures: A Study on miRNA-155, miRNA-181a and miRNA-223 Expression Levels. *J. Biomech.* **2018**, *66*, 165–169. [CrossRef]

11. Rieder, B.; Weihs, A.M.; Weidinger, A.; Szwarc, D.; Nürnberger, S.; Redl, H.; Rünzler, D.; Huber-Gries, C.; Teuschl, A.H. Hydrostatic Pressure-generated Reactive Oxygen Species Induce Osteoarthritic Conditions in Cartilage Pellet Cultures. *Sci. Rep.* **2018**, *8*, 17010. [CrossRef] [PubMed]

12. Tworkoski, E.; Glucksberg, M.R.; Johnson, M. The Effect of the Rate of Hydrostatic Pressure Depressurization on Cells in Culture. *PLoS ONE* **2018**, *13*, e0189890. [CrossRef] [PubMed]

13. Cheleschi, S.; Barbarino, M.; Gallo, I.; Tenti, S.; Bottaro, M.; Frati, E.; Giannotti, S.; Fioravanti, A. Hydrostatic Pressure Regulates Oxidative Stress through microRNA in Human Osteoarthritic Chondrocytes. *Int. J. Mol. Sci.* **2020**, *21*, 3653. [CrossRef] [PubMed]

14. Dai, H.; Chen, R.; Gui, C.; Tao, T.; Ge, Y.; Zhao, X.; Qin, R.; Yao, W.; Gu, S.; Jiang, Y.; et al. Eliminating Senescent Chondrogenic Progenitor Cells Enhances Chondrogenesis under Intermittent Hydrostatic Pressure for the Treatment of OA. *Stem Cell Res. Ther.* **2020**, *11*, 199. [CrossRef] [PubMed]

15. Zeddou, M. Osteoarthritis Is a Low-Grade Inflammatory Disease: Obesity's Involvement and Herbal Treatment. *Evid. Based Complement. Alternat. Med.* **2019**, *2019*, 2037484. [CrossRef]

16. Silvestre, M.P.; Rodrigues, A.M.; Canhão, H.; Marques, C.; Teixeira, D.; Calhau, C.; Branco, J. Cross-Talk between Diet-Associated Dysbiosis and Hand Osteoarthritis. *Nutrients* **2020**, *12*, 3469. [CrossRef] [PubMed]

17. Xie, C.; Chen, Q. Adipokines: New Therapeutic Target for Osteoarthritis? *Curr. Rheumatol. Rep.* **2019**, *21*, 71. [CrossRef] [PubMed]

18. Recinella, L.; Orlando, G.; Ferrante, C.; Chiavaroli, A.; Brunetti, L.; Leone, S. Adipokines: New Potential Therapeutic Target for Obesity and Metabolic, Rheumatic, and Cardiovascular Diseases. *Front. Physiol.* **2020**, *11*, 578966. [CrossRef] [PubMed]

19. Neumann, E.; Hasseli, R.; Ohl, S.; Lange, U.; Frommer, K.W.; Müller-Ladner, U. Adipokines and Autoimmunity in Inflammatory Arthritis. *Cells* **2021**, *10*, 216. [CrossRef] [PubMed]

20. Fioravanti, A.; Cheleschi, S.; De Palma, A.; Addimanda, O.; Mancarella, L.; Pignotti, E.; Pulsatelli, L.; Galeazzi, M.; Meliconi, R. Can Adipokines Serum Levels be Used as Biomarkers of Hand Osteoarthritis? *Biomarkers* **2018**, *23*, 265–270. [CrossRef] [PubMed]

21. Fioravanti, A.; Tenti, S.; Bacarelli, M.R.; Damiani, A.; Li Gobbi, F.; Bandinelli, F.; Cheleschi, S.; Galeazzi, M.; Benucci, M. Tocilizumab Modulates Serum Levels of Adiponectin and Chemerin in Patients with Rheumatoid Arthritis: Potential Cardiovascular Protective Role of IL-6 Inhibition. *Clin. Exp. Rheumatol.* **2019**, *37*, 293–300. [PubMed]

22. Carrión, M.; Frommer, K.W.; Pérez-García, S.; Müller-Ladner, U.; Gomariz, R.P.; Neumann, E. The Adipokine Network in Rheumatic Joint Diseases. *Int. J. Mol. Sci.* **2019**, *20*, 4091. [CrossRef]

23. MacDonald, I.J.; Liu, S.C.; Huang, C.C.; Kuo, S.J.; Tsai, C.H.; Tang, C.H. Associations between Adipokines in Arthritic Disease and Implications for Obesity. *Int. J. Mol. Sci.* **2019**, *20*, 1505. [CrossRef]

24. Francisco, V.; Ruiz-Fernández, C.; Pino, J.; Mera, A.; González-Gay, M.A.; Gómez, R.; Lago, F.; Mobasheri, A.; Gualillo, O. Adipokines: Linking Metabolic Syndrome, the Immune System, and Arthritic Diseases. *Biochem. Pharmacol.* **2019**, *165*, 196–206. [CrossRef] [PubMed]

25. Han, D.F.; Li, Y.; Xu, H.Y.; Li, R.H.; Zhao, D. An Update on the Emerging Role of Visfatin in the Pathogenesis of Osteoarthritis and Pharmacological Intervention. *Evid. Based Complement. Alternat. Med.* **2020**, *2020*, 8303570. [CrossRef] [PubMed]

26. Fioravanti, A.; Giannitti, C.; Cheleschi, S.; Simpatico, A.; Pascarelli, N.A.; Galeazzi, M. Circulating Levels of Adiponectin, Resistin, and Visfatin after Mud-bath Therapy in Patients with Bilateral Knee Osteoarthritis. *Int. J. Biometeorol.* **2015**, *59*, 1691–1700. [CrossRef] [PubMed]

27. Cheleschi, S.; Giordano, N.; Volpi, N.; Tenti, S.; Gallo, I.; Di Meglio, M.; Giannotti, S.; Fioravanti, A. A Complex Relationship between Visfatin and Resistin and microRNA: An In Vitro Study on Human Chondrocyte Cultures. *Int. J. Mol. Sci.* **2018**, *19*, 3909. [CrossRef] [PubMed]

28. Wu, M.H.; Tsai, C.H.; Huang, Y.L.; Fong, Y.C.; Tang, C.H. Visfatin Promotes IL-6 and TNF-α Production in Human Synovial Fibroblasts by Repressing miR-199a-5p through ERK, p38 and JNK Signaling Pathways. *Int. J. Mol. Sci.* **2018**, *19*, 190. [CrossRef] [PubMed]

29. Cheleschi, S.; Tenti, S.; Mondanelli, N.; Corallo, C.; Barbarino, M.; Giannotti, S.; Gallo, I.; Giordano, A.; Fioravanti, A. MicroRNA-34a and MicroRNA-181a Mediate Visfatin-Induced Apoptosis and Oxidative Stress via NF-κB Pathway in Human Osteoarthritic Chondrocytes. *Cells* **2019**, *8*, 874. [CrossRef] [PubMed]

30. Cheleschi, S.; Gallo, I.; Barbarino, M.; Giannotti, S.; Mondanelli, N.; Giordano, A.; Tenti, S.; Fioravanti, A. MicroRNA Mediate Visfatin and Resistin Induction of Oxidative Stress in Human Osteoarthritic Synovial Fibroblasts Via NF-κB Pathway. *Int. J. Mol. Sci.* **2019**, *20*, 5200. [CrossRef] [PubMed]

31. Adyshev, D.M.; Elangovan, V.R.; Moldobaeva, N.; Mapes, B.; Sun, X.; Garcia, J.G. Mechanical Stress Induces Pre-B-cell Colony-enhancing Factor/NAMPT Expression via Epigenetic Regulation by miR-374a and miR-568 in Human Lung Endothelium. *Am. J. Respir. Cell Mol. Biol.* **2014**, *50*, 409–418. [CrossRef] [PubMed]

32. Su, Y.P.; Chen, C.N.; Chang, H.I.; Huang, K.C.; Cheng, C.C.; Chiu, F.Y.; Lee, K.C.; Lo, C.M.; Chang, S.F. Low Shear Stress Attenuates COX-2 Expression Induced by Resistin in Human Osteoarthritic Chondrocytes. *J. Cell Physiol.* **2017**, *232*, 1448–1457. [CrossRef] [PubMed]
33. Liu, L.; He, Z.; Xu, L.; Lu, L.; Feng, H.; Leong, D.J.; Kim, S.J.; Hirsh, D.M.; Majeska, R.J.; Goldring, M.B.; et al. CITED2 Mediates the Mechanical Loading-induced Suppression of Adipokines in the Infrapatellar Fat Pad. *Ann. N. Y. Acad. Sci.* **2019**, *1442*, 153–164. [CrossRef] [PubMed]
34. Fang, T.; Zhou, X.; Jin, M.; Nie, J.; Li, X. Molecular Mechanisms of Mechanical Load-induced Osteoarthritis. *Int. Orthop.* **2021**. [CrossRef]
35. Nerucci, F.; Fioravanti, A.; Cicero, M.R.; Marcolongo, R.; Spinelli, G. Preparation of a Pressurization System to Study the Effect of Hydrostatic Pressure on Chondrocyte Cultures. *In Vitro Cell. Dev. Biol. Anim.* **1998**, *34*, 9–10. [CrossRef] [PubMed]
36. Buckwalter, J.A.; Anderson, D.D.; Brown, T.D.; Tochigi, Y.; Martin, J.A. The Roles of Mechanical Stresses in the Pathogenesis of Osteoarthritis: Implications for Treatment of Joint Injuries. *Cartilage* **2013**, *4*, 286–294. [CrossRef] [PubMed]
37. Nordberg, R.C.; Mellor, L.F.; Krause, A.R.; Donahue, H.J.; Loboa, E.G. LRP Receptors in Chondrocytes are Modulated by Simulated Microgravity and Cyclic Hydrostatic Pressure. *PLoS ONE* **2019**, *14*, e0223245. [CrossRef] [PubMed]
38. Laiguillon, M.C.; Houard, X.; Bougault, C.; Gosset, M.; Nourissat, G.; Sautet, A.; Jacques, C.; Berenbaum, F.; Sellam, J. Expression and Function of Visfatin (Nampt), an Adipokine-enzyme Involved in Inflammatory Pathways of Osteoarthritis. *Arthritis Res. Ther.* **2014**, *16*, R38. [CrossRef] [PubMed]
39. Zhang, Z.; Xing, X.; Hensley, G.; Chang, L.W.; Liao, W.; Abu-Amer, Y.; Sandell, L.J. Resistin Induces Expression of Proinflammatory Cytokines and Chemokines in Human Articular Chondrocytes via Transcription and Messenger RNA Stabilization. *Arthritis Rheum.* **2010**, *62*, 1993–2003. [CrossRef] [PubMed]
40. Correia, C.; Pereira, A.L.; Duarte, A.R.; Frias, A.M.; Pedro, A.J.; Oliveira, J.T.; Sousa, R.A.; Reis, R.L. Dynamic Culturing of Cartilage Tissue: The Significance of Hydrostatic Pressure. *Tissue Eng. Part A* **2012**, *18*, 1979–1991. [CrossRef] [PubMed]
41. Pérez-García, S.; Gutiérrez-Cañas, I.; Seoane, I.V.; Fernández, J.; Mellado, M.; Leceta, J.; Tío, L.; Villanueva-Romero, R.; Juarranz, Y.; Gomariz, R.P. Healthy and Osteoarthritic Synovial Fibroblasts Produce a Disintegrin and Metalloproteinase with Thrombospondin Motifs 4, 5, 7, and 12: Induction by IL-1β and Fibronectin and Contribution to Cartilage Damage. *Am. J. Pathol.* **2016**, *186*, 2449–2461. [CrossRef] [PubMed]
42. Nazempour, A.; Quisenberry, C.R.; Abu-Lail, N.I.; Van Wie, B.J. Combined Effects of Oscillating Hydrostatic Pressure, Perfusion and Encapsulation in a Novel Bioreactor for Enhancing Extracellular Matrix Synthesis by Bovine Chondrocytes. *Cell Tissue Res.* **2017**, *370*, 179–193. [CrossRef] [PubMed]
43. Machado, C.R.L.; Resende, G.G.; Macedo, R.B.V.; do Nascimento, V.C.; Branco, A.S.; Kakehasi, A.M.; Andrade, M.V. Fibroblast-like Synoviocytes from Fluid and Synovial Membrane from Primary Osteoarthritis Demonstrate Similar Production of Interleukin 6, and Metalloproteinases 1 and 3. *Clin. Exp. Rheumatol.* **2019**, *37*, 306–309. [PubMed]
44. D'Lima, D.D.; Hashimoto, S.; Chen, P.C.; Colwell, C.W., Jr.; Lotz, M.K. Human Chondrocyte Apoptosis in Response to Mechanical Injury. *Osteoarthr. Cartil.* **2001**, *9*, 712–719. [CrossRef] [PubMed]
45. Loening, A.M.; James, I.E.; Levenston, M.E.; Badger, A.M.; Frank, E.H.; Kurz, B.; Nuttall, M.E.; Hung, H.H.; Blake, S.M.; Grodzinsky, A.J.; et al. Injurious Mechanical Compression of Bovine Articular Cartilage Induces Chondrocyte Apoptosis. *Arch. Biochem. Biophys.* **2000**, *381*, 205–212. [CrossRef] [PubMed]
46. Jin, L.; Zhao, J.; Jing, W.; Yan, S.; Wang, X.; Xiao, C.; Ma, B. Role of miR-146a in Human Chondrocyte Apoptosis in Response to Mechanical Pressure Injury in Vitro. *Int. J. Mol. Med.* **2014**, *34*, 451–463. [CrossRef]
47. Gosset, M.; Berenbaum, F.; Salvat, C.; Sautet, A.; Pigenet, A.; Tahiri, K.; Jacques, C. Crucial Role of Visfatin/Pre-B cell Colony-enhancing Factor in Matrix Degradation and Prostaglandin E2 Synthesis in Chondrocytes: Possible Influence on Osteoarthritis. *Arthritis Rheum.* **2008**, *58*, 1399–1409. [CrossRef] [PubMed]
48. Zahan, O.M.; Serban, O.; Gherman, C.; Fodor, D. The Evaluation of Oxidative Stress in Osteoarthritis. *Med. Pharm. Rep.* **2020**, *93*, 12–22. [CrossRef] [PubMed]
49. Young, I.C.; Chuang, S.T.; Gefen, A.; Kuo, W.T.; Yang, C.T.; Hsu, C.H.; Lin, F.H. A Novel Compressive Stress-based Osteoarthritis-like Chondrocyte System. *Exp. Biol. Med.* **2017**, *242*, 1062–1071. [CrossRef]
50. De Palma, A.; Cheleschi, S.; Pascarelli, N.A.; Tenti, S.; Galeazzi, M.; Fioravanti, A. Do MicroRNAs Have a Key Epigenetic Role in Osteoarthritis and in Mechanotransduction? *Clin. Exp. Rheumatol.* **2017**, *35*, 518–526.
51. Lu, T.X.; Rothenberg, M.E. MicroRNA. *J. Allergy. Clin. Immunol.* **2018**, *141*, 1202–1207. [CrossRef] [PubMed]
52. Xie, F.; Liu, Y.L.; Chen, X.Y.; Li, Q.; Zhong, J.; Dai, B.Y.; Shao, X.F.; Wu, G.B. Role of MicroRNA, LncRNA, and Exosomes in the Progression of Osteoarthritis: A Review of Recent Literature. *Orthop. Surg.* **2020**, *12*, 708–716. [CrossRef] [PubMed]
53. Yang, X.; Guan, Y.; Tian, S.; Wang, Y.; Sun, K.; Chen, Q. Mechanical and IL-1β Responsive miR-365 Contributes to Osteoarthritis Development by Targeting Histone Deacetylase 4. *Int. J. Mol. Sci.* **2016**, *17*, 436. [CrossRef] [PubMed]
54. Feng, C.; Liu, M.; Fan, X.; Yang, M.; Liu, H.; Zhou, Y. Intermittent Cyclic Mechanical Tension Altered the microRNA Expression Profile of Human Cartilage Endplate Chondrocytes. *Mol. Med. Rep.* **2018**, *17*, 5238–5246. [CrossRef] [PubMed]
55. Stadnik, P.S.; Gilbert, S.J.; Tarn, J.; Charlton, S.; Skelton, A.J.; Barter, M.J.; Duance, V.C.; Young, D.A.; Blain, E.J. Regulation of microRNA-221, -222, -21 and -27 in Articular Cartilage Subjected to Abnormal Compressive Forces. *J. Physiol.* **2021**, *599*, 143–155. [CrossRef] [PubMed]

56. Lories, R.J.; Monteagudo, S. Review Article: Is Wnt Signaling an Attractive Target for the Treatment of Osteoarthritis? *Rheumatol. Ther.* **2020**, *7*, 259–270. [CrossRef]

57. Zhou, X.; Cao, H.; Yuan, Y.; Wu, W. Biochemical Signals Mediate the Crosstalk between Cartilage and Bone in Osteoarthritis. *Biomed. Res. Int.* **2020**, *2020*, 5720360. [CrossRef]

58. Niu, Q.; Li, F.; Zhang, L.; Xu, X.; Liu, Y.; Gao, J.; Feng, X. Role of the Wnt/β-catenin Signaling Pathway in the Response of Chondrocytes to Mechanical Loading. *Int. J. Mol. Med.* **2016**, *37*, 755–762. [CrossRef] [PubMed]

59. Xu, H.G.; Zheng, Q.; Song, J.X.; Li, J.; Wang, H.; Liu, P.; Wang, J.; Wang, C.D.; Zhang, X.L. Intermittent Cyclic Mechanical Tension Promotes Endplate Cartilage Degeneration via Canonical Wnt Signaling Pathway and E-cadherin/β-catenin Complex Cross-talk. *Osteoarthr. Cartil.* **2016**, *24*, 158–168. [CrossRef] [PubMed]

60. Ohba, S.; Lanigan, T.M.; Roessler, B.J. Leptin Receptor JAK2/STAT3 Signaling Modulates Expression of Frizzled Receptors in Articular Chondrocytes. *Osteoarthr. Cartil.* **2010**, *18*, 1620–1629. [CrossRef] [PubMed]

61. Philp, A.M.; Collier, R.L.; Grover, L.M.; Davis, E.T.; Jones, S.W. Resistin Promotes the Abnormal Type I Collagen Phenotype of Subchondral Bone in Obese Patients with End Stage Hip Osteoarthritis. *Sci. Rep.* **2017**, *7*, 4042. [CrossRef] [PubMed]

62. Denysenko, T.; Annovazzi, L.; Cassoni, P.; Melcarne, A.; Mellai, M.; Schiffer, D. WNT/β-catenin Signaling Pathway and Downstream Modulators in Low- and High-grade Glioma. *Cancer Genom. Proteom.* **2016**, *13*, 31–45.

63. Sun, Y.; Wang, F.; Sun, X.; Wang, X.; Zhang, L.; Li, Y. CX3CR1 Regulates Osteoarthrosis Chondrocyte Proliferation and Apoptosis via Wnt/β-catenin Signaling. *Biomed. Pharmacother.* **2017**, *96*, 1317–1323. [CrossRef] [PubMed]

64. Bougault, C.; Priam, S.; Houard, X.; Pigenet, A.; Sudre, L.; Lories, R.J.; Jacques, C.; Berenbaum, F. Protective Role of Frizzled-related Protein B on Matrix Metalloproteinase Induction in Mouse Chondrocytes. *Arthritis Res. Ther.* **2014**, *16*, R137. [CrossRef]

65. Robinson, J.A.; Chatterjee-Kishore, M.; Yaworsky, P.J.; Cullen, D.M.; Zhao, W.; Li, C.; Kharode, Y.; Sauter, L.; Babij, P.; Brown, E.L.; et al. Wnt/beta-catenin Signaling is a Normal Physiological Response to Mechanical Loading in Bone. *J. Biol. Chem.* **2006**, *281*, 31720–31728. [CrossRef]

66. Li, F.F.; Zhang, B.; Cui, J.H.; Chen, F.L.; Ding, Y.; Feng, X. Alterations in β-catenin/E-cadherin Complex Formation During the Mechanotransduction of Saos-2 Osteoblastic Cells. *Mol. Med. Rep.* **2018**, *18*, 1495–1503. [CrossRef] [PubMed]

67. Wang, Y.; Gao, C.; Zhang, Y.; Gao, J.; Teng, F.; Tian, W.; Yang, W.; Yan, Y.; Xue, F. Visfatin Stimulates Endometrial cancer cell proliferation via activation of PI3K/Akt and MAPK/ERK1/2 signalling pathways. *Gynecol. Oncol.* **2016**, *143*, 168–178. [CrossRef] [PubMed]

68. Altman, R.; Alarcón, G.; Appelrouth, D.; Bloch, D.; Borenstein, D.; Brandt, K.; Brown, C.; Cooke, T.D.; Daniel, W.; Feldman, D.; et al. The American College of Rheumatology Criteria for the Classification and Reporting of Osteoarthritis of the Hip. *Arthritis Rheum.* **1991**, *34*, 505–514. [CrossRef]

69. Mankin, H.J.; Dorfman, H.; Lippiello, L.; Zarins, A. Biochemical and Metabolic Abnormalities in Articular Cartilage from Osteo-arthritic Human Hips. II. Correlation of Morphology with Biochemical and Metabolic Data. *J. Bone Joint Surg. Am.* **1971**, *53*, 523–537. [CrossRef] [PubMed]

70. Francin, P.J.; Guillaume, C.; Humbert, A.C.; Pottie, P.; Netter, P.; Mainard, D.; Presle, N. Association between the Chondrocyte Phenotype and the Expression of Adipokines and Their Receptors: Evidence for a Role of Leptin but not Adiponectin in the Expression of Cartilage-specific Markers. *J. Cell. Physiol.* **2011**, *226*, 2790–2797. [CrossRef]

71. Fioravanti, A.; Cantarini, L.; Chellini, F.; Manca, D.; Paccagnini, E.; Marcolongo, R.; Collodel, G. Effect of Hyaluronic Acid (MW 500-730 kDa) on Proteoglycan and Nitric Oxide Production in Human Osteoarthritic Chondrocyte Cultures Exposed to Hydrostatic Pressure. *Osteoarthr. Cartil.* **2005**, *13*, 688–696. [CrossRef] [PubMed]

72. Cheleschi, S.; Calamia, V.; Fernandez-Moreno, M.; Biava, M.; Giordani, A.; Fioravanti, A.; Anzini, M.; Blanco, F. In Vitro Comprehensive Analysis of VA692 a New Chemical Entity for the Treatment of Osteoarthritis. *Int. Immunopharmacol.* **2018**, *64*, 86–100. [CrossRef] [PubMed]

73. Ramakers, C.; Ruijter, J.M.; Deprez, R.H.; Moorman, A.F. Assumption-free Analysis of Quantitative Real-time Polymerase Chain Reaction (PCR) Data. *Neurosci. Lett.* **2003**, *339*, 62–66. [CrossRef]

74. Pfaffl, M.W. A new Mathematical Model for Relative Quantification in Real-time RT-PCR. *Nucleic Acids Res.* **2001**, *29*, e45. [CrossRef] [PubMed]

75. Vandesompele, J.; De Preter, K.; Pattyn, F.; Poppe, B.; Van Roy, N.; De Paepe, A.; Speleman, F. Accurate Normalization of Real-time Quantitative RT-PCR Data by Geometric Averaging of Multiple Internal Control Genes. *Genome Biol.* **2002**, *3*, RESEARCH0034. [CrossRef] [PubMed]

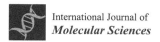

International Journal of
Molecular Sciences

MDPI

Review

Control of the Autophagy Pathway in Osteoarthritis: Key Regulators, Therapeutic Targets and Therapeutic Strategies

Maria Teresa Valenti [1], Luca Dalle Carbonare [1,*], Donato Zipeto [2] and Monica Mottes [2]

1 Department of Medicine, Section of Internal Medicine, University of Verona, 37134 Verona, Italy;
mariateresa.valenti@univr.it
2 Department of Neurosciences, Biomedicine and Movement Sciences, Section of Biology and Genetics,
University of Verona, 37134 Verona, Italy; donato.zipeto@univr.it (D.Z.); monica.mottes@univr.it (M.M.)
* Correspondence: luca.dallecarbonare@univr.it; Tel.: +39-045-8126062

Abstract: Autophagy is involved in different degenerative diseases and it may control epigenetic modifications, metabolic processes, stem cells differentiation as well as apoptosis. Autophagy plays a key role in maintaining the homeostasis of cartilage, the tissue produced by chondrocytes; its impairment has been associated to cartilage dysfunctions such as osteoarthritis (OA). Due to their location in a reduced oxygen context, both differentiating and mature chondrocytes are at risk of premature apoptosis, which can be prevented by autophagy. AutophagomiRNAs, which regulate the autophagic process, have been found differentially expressed in OA. AutophagomiRNAs, as well as other regulatory molecules, may also be useful as therapeutic targets. In this review, we describe and discuss the role of autophagy in OA, focusing mainly on the control of autophagomiRNAs in OA pathogenesis and their potential therapeutic applications.

Keywords: mesenchymal stem cells; chondrocytic commitment; autophagy; osteoarthritis; miRNAs

Citation: Valenti, M.T.; Dalle Carbonare, L.; Zipeto, D.; Mottes, M. Control of the Autophagy Pathway in Osteoarthritis: Key Regulators, Therapeutic Targets and Therapeutic Strategies. *Int. J. Mol. Sci.* **2021**, *22*, 2700. https://doi.org/10.3390/ijms22052700

Academic Editor: Nicola Veronese

Received: 16 February 2021
Accepted: 4 March 2021
Published: 7 March 2021

Publisher's Note: MDPI stays neutral with regard to jurisdictional claims in published maps and institutional affiliations.

1. Background

Chondrogenesis, the process by which cartilage is formed, occurs as a result of mesenchymal cell condensation and chondroprogenitor cell differentiation. SOX9 is the master transcription factor for MSCs differentiation into chondrocytes [1]. During development, chondrogenesis is subject to complex regulation by several interplaying factors such as fibroblast growth factor (FGF), transforming growth factor β (TGFβ), bone morphogenetic proteins (BMPs) and Wnt signaling pathways. Among regulatory factors, TGFβ plays a key role in development. TGFβ receptors are present in many cells, and an integrin-applied force is required to release TGF-β from its prodomain. Force application has been shown to occurs through the prodomain of TGF-β and through the β subunit of the integrin [2]. In the process termed endochondral ossification, chondrocytes undergo proliferation and terminal differentiation to hypertrophy and apoptosis, whereby hypertrophic cartilage is replaced by bone tissue. In mature articular cartilage, instead, chondrocytes are responsible for the production and homeostatic maintenance of the extracellular matrix (ECM) components.

Structural ECM components are: collagens (mainly type II collagen), proteoglycans, (including aggrecan, decorin, biglycan and fibromodulin) and noncollagenous proteins, such as cartilage oligomeric protein (COMP), cartilage matrix protein (CMP) and fibronectin. The primary matrix degrading enzymes involved in cartilage turnover are metalloproteinases (MMPs) and cathepsins (CTS). In healthy articular cartilage, balanced degradation and synthesis by chondrocytes ensure tissue homeostasis.

Autophagy plays a key role in the preservation of cartilage integrity [3]. Besides playing a crucial role in adaptive response to different stimuli, it is also required for intracellular quality control and is involved in removing and recycling misfolded proteins, damaged organelles or dysfunctional cell components [4].

Authophagy may be distinguished into (i) macroautophagy; (ii) microautophagy; (iii) chaperone mediated autophagy. Macroautophagy represents the prevalent form of autophagy in different cell types. It starts with a membrane formation, the phagophore, which expands to engulf the cellular cargo, generating the autophagosome. This latter structure matures through fusion with lysosomes. mTOR is a major player in autophagy and acts as a signaling control point downstream of growth factor receptor signaling, hypoxia, ATP levels and insulin signaling. It is activated downstream of Akt kinase, PI3-kinase and growth factor receptor and acts to inhibit autophagy by modulating the Ulk1 (Atg1) complex. In response to the autophagy cascade activation, the IIIPI3K complex produces PI3P and induces other Atg proteins, such as the Atg12-Atg5-Atg-16 and LC3 (Atg8)-phosphatidylethanolamine complexes. After translation, proLC3 is proteolytically cleaved generating LC3-I. Upon induction of autophagy, LC3-I is conjugated by the Atg7, Atg3 and Atg12-Atg5-Atg16L complexes to the highly lipophilic phosphatidylethanolamine (PE) moiety to generate LC3-II. Finally, PE promotes integration of LC3-II into lipid membranes allowing autophagosomes formation. Due to its crucial role as a natural defense mechanism against inflammatory, infectious and degenerative disorders, the autophagic process must be tightly regulated. Several molecular mechanisms of autophagy regulation have been investigated: microRNAs (miRNAs) stand out, among others [5]. These small non-coding RNAs act as negative regulators of specific target mRNAs expression. One single miRNA can act as a post-transcriptional repressor by binding to partially complementary sequences in the 3′UTR sites of various mRNAs. miRNAs which regulate the autophagic process, predominantly targeting the pathway early stages, are called autophagomiRNAs. In several pathological conditions, e.g., degenerative disorders, autophagomiRNAs have been found to be differentially expressed [6].

Increasing evidence suggests that autophagy dysregulation is closely related to the pathogenesis of osteoarthritis (OA) [7] (Figure 1).

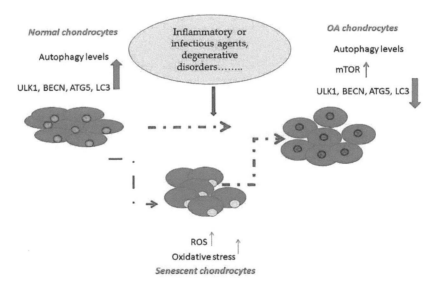

Figure 1. Schematic representation showing changes occurring in the autophagic process in normal versus osteoarthritic chondrocytes.

OA, a chronic, age-related degenerative disease of articular cartilage, is associated with dramatic changes in cartilage homeostasis, due to an imbalance between degradation and synthesis by chondrocytes. Age-related changes that occur in joints are thought to represent a major risk factor for OA development. OA may develop in any joint, but most commonly, it affects the knee, hip, hand, spine and foot.

Incidence is higher in women than in men, especially beyond age 50. Worldwide estimates indicate that 10% of men and 18% of women $\geq$ 60 years have symptomatic OA. Disease progression is usually slow but can ultimately lead to joint failure with pain and disability, with considerable socio-economic impact [8].

2. Role of the Autophagic Process in Chondrogenic Differentiation

Autophagy is involved in different cellular processes such as the control of epigenetic modifications, metabolic processes, cellular senescence and apoptosis, as well as stem cells differentiation steps [9]. Recent studies have demonstrated that the autophagic process is crucial for stem cell functioning [10,11]. Mesenchymal stem cells have trilineage potency (adipocyte, osteoblast and chondrocyte); they are essential for homeostasis maintenance and tissues repair. Chondrogenesis is a dynamic process associated with morphological changes and metabolic stress [12]. Healthy chondrocytes are essential for a functional cartilage, but their regenerative potential is very limited; hence, both chondrocytic homeostasis and cartilage extracellular matrix integrity are required [11]. Endochondral ossification, a process where chondrocytes differentiate to form the growth plate, is essential in mammalian bone formation. As the growth plate is poorly vascularized, chondrocytes grow in an hypoxic environment [13]. In such a context, autophagy is induced, preventing premature apoptosis of differentiating and mature chondrocytes. In fact, the chondrocytic maturation phase is regulated by mTOR and AMP kinase (AMPK) activity [14]. AMPK, a molecule involved in the regulation of cellular metabolism, acts by inducing autophagy, whereas mTOR, a regulator of cell growth, inhibits autophagy [15]. AMPK and mTORC (complex1 of mTOR) provide an integrated signal by phosphorylating ULK 1 protein kinase in a coordinated way so that the cells are able to respond appropriately to external factors [15]. During endochondral ossification, chondrocytes produce extracellular matrix components: the endoplasmic reticulum (ER), involved in the secretory process, is in a stressful condition. Consequently, ER stress induces autophagy in order to maintain its homeostasis [16]. Recently, it has been demonstrated that a faulty autophagic process induces ER stress and affects chondrogenesis [8]. Under mechanical stimuli, such as compression, autophagy preserves intervertebral disc degeneration. However, a persistent compression stimulus can induce excessive autophagy leading to cellular apoptosis [17]. Ma et al. demonstrated that autophagy is mediated by ROS (reactive oxygen species) in nucleus pulposus cells of rats exposed to compressive stimuli [18]. The levels of reactive oxygen and nitrogen species (RONS) induced by IL-1 can be influenced by oxygen tension. Indeed, environmental oxygen tension in articular chondrocytes has been shown to play an important role in determining their ability to counteract RONS exposure in OA [19]. In addition, we have demonstrated increased expression during physical activity of chondrogenic transcription factors SOX9 in circulating mesenchymal progenitors associated with autophagy [20]. This finding suggests the beneficial role of physical exercise in preserving chondrogenesis. Autophagy adjusts mitochondrial activity in stem cells in order to provide the best metabolic conditions, thus limiting ROS production, preventing metabolic stress and genome damage. Mitochondria, as cellular energy producers, are involved in many vital processes [21]. Mitochondria dysfunctions cause cellular damages in many aging-related diseases such as osteoarthritis [22]. Maintenance of a correct mitochondrial functionality appears therefore very important. Mitophagy, the autophagy process involving damaged mitochondria, contributes to a correct mitochondrial activity [23]. Different mitophagy mechanisms as well as different mitophagy inducers have been investigated. Generally, mitophagy can be PRKN (parkin RBR E3 ubiquitin protein ligase)-dependent or PRKN-independent [24]. In animal models, it has been demonstrated that the chondrogenic commitment involves LC3-Dependent Mitophagy [25] and that mitophagy improves the chondrogenic differentiation potential of Adipose Stem Cells [26]. Additionally, mitophagy regulators such as PINK1, PRKN, BNIP3 and MFN2 were shown to be involved in OA pathogenesis [24]. In particular, the PINK1-PRKN pathway plays an important role in the induction of mitophagy in chondrocytes [24]. Therefore, mitophagy appears as an effective contrast tool against OA development.

3. MicroRNAs Involvement in the Autophagy Process

Autophagy dysfunctions are involved in cartilage deterioration, whereas induction of autophagy can counteract cartilage degeneration. ULK1, LC3 and beclin, autophagy-related proteins, are expressed in cartilage. However, their expression is reduced in OA disorder [27]. In addition, the expression of LC3, ULK-1, P62 and Beclin-1 in chondrocytes is downregulated by miR-411 [28]. Recently, it has been demonstrated that miR-375 worsens knee osteoarthritis by targeting the autophagy related protein ATG2B [29]. Reduced circulating miR let-7e levels are associated to increased apoptosis and reduced autophagy in knee OA cartilage [30]. Undoubtedly, miRNAs play a crucial role in cartilage homeostasis as well as in the autophagic process. In particular, level changes in miRNAs targeting the autophagic pathway (autophagomiRNAs) may influence the development of OA [31].

MiRNAs may be recovered from biological samples such as plasma, serum, cartilage and synovial fluid, as they are secreted from cells in exosomes or encapsulated within microvesicles. Quantification and analysis of several autophagomiRNAs reveal differential expression levels in samples from OA patients, compared with healthy controls [4]. Panels of cartilage miRNAs, which appear deregulated in OA, have been proposed as diagnostic/prognostic markers. A sample of those cited in this review is shown in Figure 2.

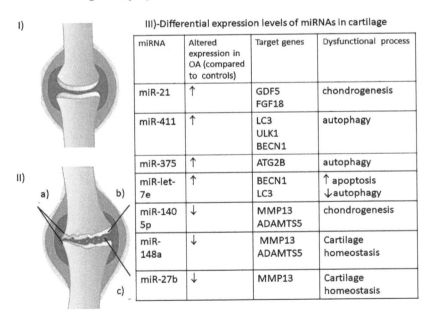

III)-Differential expression levels of miRNAs in cartilage

miRNA	Altered expression in OA (compared to controls)	Target genes	Dysfunctional process
miR-21	↑	GDF5 FGF18	chondrogenesis
miR-411	↑	LC3 ULK1 BECN1	autophagy
miR-375	↑	ATG2B	autophagy
miR-let-7e	↑	BECN1 LC3	↑ apoptosis ↓autophagy
miR-140 5p	↓	MMP13 ADAMTS5	chondrogenesis
miR-148a	↓	MMP13 ADAMTS5	Cartilage homeostasis
miR-27b	↓	MMP13	Cartilage homeostasis

Figure 2. Schematic representation of changes that occur in a healthy knee joint (**I**) upon OA degenerative process (**II**): (a) osteophytes production; (b) cartilage thinning; (c) cartilage fragmentation. (**III**) The table reports a few miRNAs cited within the text, which are differentially expressed in OA cartilage, compared to healthy cartilage. ↑ = enhanced expression; ↓ = lowered expression.

4. Transcription Factors in OA

Transcription factors are DNA-binding proteins which play a central role in regulating gene expression [32] and, consequently, are involved in cell signaling as well as in cellular proliferation and differentiation [33].

Some transcription factors, defined Master regulators, commit progenitor cells differentiation by inducing the expression of lineage-specific genes [34]. Generally, transcription factors recognize highly conserved sequences (6 to 12 bp long) upstream target genes [35]. Notably, the same transcription factors can differently modulate gene expression on the basis of specific interactions [36]. Furthermore, posttranslational modifications, such as phosphorylation/dephosphorylation, may regulate transcription factors efficiency [37]. Transcription factor SOX9 is the master regulator of chondrogenic differentiation. It acts by inducing mesenchymal cells condensation and proliferation and inhibits chondrocyte senescence [38]. Cartilage is absent in Sox9-knockout murine embryonic stem cells; human SOX9 haploinsufficiency induces lethal skeletal malformations [39].

The expression of SOX9 is reduced in chondrocytes of OA patients [40]. In cartilage, it has been shown that SOX9 regulates miR-140 levels in zebrafish and mammalian cells [41], while miR-1247 as well as MiR-30a and miR-145 target SOX9 [42–44].

By performing an enrichment analysis, it has been observed that transcription factors, such as activator protein 1 (AP-1), CCAAT-enhancer-binding protein (C/EBP) and the activator of transcription 3 (STAT3), may be involved in the regulation of genes whose expression is altered in OA [45]. A transcriptome study showed altered expression of transcription factors such as JUN, EGR1, JUND, FOSL2, MYC, KLF4, RelA and FOXO in the cartilage of OA human knee [46].

The transcription factors AP-1, runt-related transcription factor 2 (RUNX2), NFkB, HIF2 α and T-cell factor/lymphoid enhancer factor (TCF/LEF) regulate the cartilage ECM-degrading molecules MMP3 and MMP13 (collagenases), whereas ADAMTS4 and ADAMTS5 (aggrecanases) are regulated by the transcription factors NFAT, RUNX2, SOX4, SOX11 and NFkB [47,48]. Interestingly, during chondrogenesis in human adipose-derived stem cells (hADSCs), it has been demonstrated that miR-193b, miR-199a-3p/has-miR-199b-3p, miR-455-3p, miR-210, miR-381 and miR-92a target RUNX2 [49].

The upregulation of SOX4 and SOX11 in mouse cartilage is associated to impaired cartilage and increased expression of ADAMTS5 and MMP13 [48]; chondrocyte proteins ACAN and COL2A1 are regulated by the transcription factors SOX5, SOX6 and SOX9 [50]. During cartilage formation, miR-193b targets SOX4 and miR-455-3p targets SOX-4, SOX5, SOX6 and SOX9 [49].

Transcription factor EB (TFEB) and the zinc-finger protein with KRAB and SCAN domains 3 (ZKSCAN3) are important master regulators of autophagy. TFEB, known to induce autophagy in HeLa cells [51], is reduced in a OA mouse model and in OA human knee cartilage [52]. On the contrary, ZKSCAN3 inhibits autophagy by blocking the expression of ULK1 and LC3 genes [53]. ZKSCAN3 expression has not been evaluated in chondrocytes; however, it has been demonstrated that ZKSCAN3 knockout induces premature aging in Mesenchymal Stem Cells [54]. SIRT1, whose levels are increased in early chondrocytes but are reduced in severe OA, promotes autophagy by acting on FOXO family transcription factors [55]. FOXO1 and FOXO3 induce autophagy [56]. In fact, ATG genes expression is reduced in chondrocytes under oxidative stress conditions due to FOXO1 or FOXO1/FOXO3 knockdown [57], while a constitutively expressed mutant FOXO1 increased the expression of LC3 and Beclin in normal chondrocytes [58]. Interestingly, in osteoarthritis samples, transcription factors FOXO are reduced [46] and the activated serine/threonine kinase AKT, which phosphorylates the FOXO transcription factors, is higher in OA cartilage compared to normal cartilage [59]. By performing in silico analysis and also in vitro and in vivo experiments, it has been demonstrated that during skeletogenesis FOXO1 is targeted by miR-182 [60]; bioinformatic analysis has shown that miR182 plays a critical role in OA [61].

5. In Vitro and In Vivo Models for OA Studies

Different models have been employed to investigate OA pathogenesis. In vitro systems have been established by using human or murine primary cultures and cell lines. Usually, a mechanical load or inflammatory cytokines are applied to cells in order to mimic OA conditions. In particular, OA mimic conditions are applied to cells growing in a monolayer, in a scaffold or in a co-culture system [62]. The use of 3D cell models may represent a good alternative to 2D cultures. 3D models for the in vitro analysis of subchondral bone and articular cartilage currently exist in a variety of forms, including explants and scaffold-based or scaffold-free systems, each of which has its own advantages and disadvantages. 3D systems make it possible to observe the various cellular interactions and to evaluate any changes due to the addition of therapeutic molecules [63]. However, investigations of explanted tissues allow assessment of the extracellular matrix and cellular interactions to recapitulate in vivo alterations [64].

In vivo models provide the possibility to evaluate pain, cartilage degeneration and the bone remodeling process. OA in animal models can be induced or spontaneous. In particular, OA can be induced surgically or chemically; induced models can also be generated genetically [65]. Animal models with naturally occurring OA, such as aged animals, can also be used.

Usual animal models for OA are: mouse, rat, Syrian hamster, rabbit, horse and also cat and dog [65]. Zebrafish has also been employed for the study of OA. The zebrafish model, due to its ease of being genetically manipulated and its rapid development, appears to be very useful. For example, a COL10A1 knockout zebrafish model has been generated for the study of OA [66].

In fact, the craniofacial cartilage of zebrafish larvae is as mechanically sensitive as the human one [67]. Different models for the zebrafish jaw development are available, including wild-type fish [68] and mutants [68]. In addition, zebrafish larvae in different gravitational fields have been used [68]. The zebrafish model is also suitable for studying miR-mediated joint degeneration. In particular, zebrafish dicer1 mutant shows impaired craniofacial development and overexpression of SOX10 [69]. SOX9 controls miR140 and miR-29; miR92a regulates BMP signaling in zebrafish cartilage [41,70].

The introduction of the CRISPR/Cas9 technology in recent years has further expanded the possibilities of originating cellular and animal models to study the role of different genes and regulatory factors involved in degeneration, regeneration and inflammatory processes associated with OA. The CRISPR/Cas9 system in fact not only allows to knock out specific genes and functions, but by using modified versions of the Cas9 enzyme, it becomes possible to originate recombinant proteins that can act as transcriptional activators and repressors, as well as epigenetic modulators [71], to study in a more precise way the regulation of specific genes [72]. The possibility to originate new cellular and animal models [73,74] will be very helpful to overcome the limited availability of animal models of the disease. In addition, the availability of different models will make drug screening aimed at identifying new therapies much more efficient, as will the possibility of studying new therapeutic approaches based on gene therapy [75].

Various treatments have been developed to counteract or, at least delay, OA clinical progression. Anti-inflammatory drugs are employed, as well as non-pharmacological treatments, such as electromagnetic stimulation, shock wave therapy and biomechanical intervention [76]. Surgical treatment (e.g., total joint replacement) is chosen for advanced OA.

6. Therapeutic Targets in OA

6.1. Autophagy

Considering its prominent role in cell pathophysiology, autophagy can be therapeutically targeted and modulated at various points of its pathways in human diseases [77]. Preventing autophagy inhibition and decreasing ROS production are strategies with therapeutic potential against OA. mTOR, a signaling molecule in the autophagy pathway, has been chosen as a target in experimental studies. Rapamycin, an mTOR inhibitor, has been proven to delay cartilage degeneration upon intra-articular injection in a murine OA model [78]. Isoimperatorin and glucosamine can ameliorate osteoarthritis by activating autophagy and inhibiting mTOR pathway [79]. Resveratrol (RSV) can activate Sirtuin 1 (SIRT1), an autophagy promoter, thus inhibiting OA progression [80].

6.2. Inflammation

The existence of an important inflammatory component in OA is well known. Damage-associated molecular patterns (DAMPs) and various sources of oxidative stress contribute to inflammation [81]. An in vitro screening for DMOADs (disease-modifying osteoarthritis drugs) revealed the strong chondrogenic/chondroprotective effects of BNTA (*N*-[2 bromo-4-phenylsulfonyl-3-thienyl]-2-chlorobenzamide) [82]. BNTA beneficial effects may be ascribed to its induction of SOD3 expression and superoxide anions elimination. Resveratrol (RSV), already cited, is a powerful antioxidant as well.

The condroprotective role of Resveratrol (RSV) may also be associated to its ability to inhibit inflammation and the NF-κB signaling pathway. The activation of transcription factor NF-kB, an essential mediator of inflammatory responses, depends on the inducible degradation of its inhibitor, IkBα [83]. In an in vitro model (IL-β1 treated human chondrocytes), the inflammatory response was significantly inhibited by RSV administration [84]. Molecular evidence demonstrated that RSV relieved the inflammatory response by inhibiting IkBα degradation. It is worth recalling that baseline NF-kB activity plays a positive role in healthy cartilage, ensuring chondrocytes differentiation and survival. Environmental and inflammatory cues exacerbate NF-κB response, which leads to the expression of matrix metalloproteinases (MMPs), cyclooxygenases (COX) and inflammatory cytokines (e.g., IL-1, IL-6, IL-8 and TNF). The MMPs family includes several members, which are secreted as inactive pro-forms. Once the pro-domain is cleaved, the active enzymes proceed to ECM proteins degradation. They are involved in physiological processes, such as embryonic development and tissue remodeling and are overexpressed in degenerative processes such as OA. MMP13, also called collagenase 3, is a major enzyme targeting cartilage for degradation. It targets type II collagen, but it also degrades proteoglycans, type IV and type IX collagen, osteonectin and perlecan. MMP13 overexpression is typically observed in OA patients [85,86]. The ADAMTS (a disintegrin and metalloproteinase with thrombospondin motifs) family of aggrecanases also contributes to proteoglycan/aggrecan depletion. ADAMTS 4 and 5 have been identified as the main aggrecanases involved in OA development [87]. The above-mentioned catabolic enzymes play an important role in OA progression, and therefore, represent interesting therapeutic targets for articular cartilage degradation slowdown [88–91].

6.3. Cell Senescence

Cell senescence is a stress-activated molecular program that prevents damaged cells from further proliferation. Autophagy and cellular senescence share several stimuli (e.g., damaged organelles or macromolecules, oxidative stress). Although autophagy is generally considered to suppress cellular senescence, various studies have suggested that it may also promote it [92,93]. Senescent cells (SC) accumulate in chronic age-associated diseases, such as OA. Their inflammatory senescence-associated secretory phenotype (SASP) severely damages neighboring cells. SC appear to be resistant to apoptosis due to the upregulation of pro-survival pathways related to P13K/AKT, p53-p21 and antiapoptotic BCL family members, among others (Figure 3).

Table 1. Examples of Senolytics with Their Respective Targets.

Senolytic Drug	Targeted Molecules/Pathway
FISETIN	⊥ P13/AKT/mTOR ⊥ Bcl2-xL
QUERCETIN	⊥ P13/AKT/mTOR ⊥ Bcl2-w
NAVITOCLAX	⊥ Bcl2, Bcl-xL, Bcl-w
FOXO4-DRI	⊗ FOXO4-p53 interaction, no p53 in the nucleus
USP7 inhibitor	MDM2 ubiquitination
UBX0101	MDM2, p32

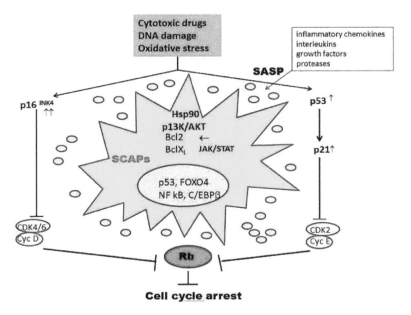

Figure 3. Cellular senescence (i.e., permanent cessation of cell division) is triggered by a variety of stresses. The tumor suppressor p16 ^{INK4}, as well as the p53 and p21 proteins, function as cyclin-dependent kinase inhibitors, preventing phosphorylation of the Rb protein and consequently arresting the cell cycle. They release SASP factors which severely damage neighboring cells. Senescent cells can escape apoptosis by upregulation of pro-survival pathways (SCAPs = senescent cell antiapoptotic pathways). Senolytic therapies primarily target SCAPs, as exemplified in Table 1.

On the basis of the above observations, recently, researchers have started testing molecules known to target pro-survival pathways [94]. Molecules meeting these requirements are called senolytics, as they selectively induce SC apoptosis [95]. Table 1 reports a few examples of senolytics and their targets. Targeting is achieved by nanoparticle-based delivery of senolytics [96].

To our knowledge, there are two current clinical trials in the US involving knee OA patients treated with senolytic regimens:

- UBX0101(NCT04129944).
- Fisetin (NCT04210986).

6.4. microRNAs

Other molecular targets for therapeutic options may be specific miRNAs, whose dysregulation plays an important role in OA. AntagomiRNAs and/or miRNA mimics may be synthesized and delivered into experimental models in order to remodel microRNAs levels. In detail, antagomiRNAs are synthetic oligonucleotides which can inhibit specific endogenous miRNAs by base-pairing, hence hindering miRNA-target mRNAs matching. MiRNA mimics instead act in the opposite way: they can be introduced by transient transfection to enhance the regulatory action of endogenous identical miRNAs. Their therapeutic effectiveness depends on the actual possibility to deliver them to the cartilaginous tissue.

OA animal models (mice and rats) have been employed in promising studies so far. Upregulation of miR21, for example, is associated with OA in humans (Figure 1III) and it has also been observed in experimental OA murine models [97]. Intra-articular injection of miR-21 mimics caused a significant worsening of cartilage degradation, whereas antagomiR-21 injection had the opposite effect. Another experiment on similar OA rat models [98] demonstrated the therapeutic efficacy of miR-140-5p, an autophagy regulator (Figure 1III). Rats were treated with intra-articular injection of human umbilical cord stem cells (hUC-MSCs) ± miR-140-5p mimic. The authors demonstrated that hUC-MSCs+ miR-140-5p mimic differentiated to chondrocytes and induced rat's cartilage repair much more efficiently than hUC-MSCs.

7. Novel Therapeutic Strategies

In addition to the above clinical trials with senolytic molecules, other experimental treatments are based on the use of miRNAs. An efficient way to deliver therapeutic miRNAs involves MSC-derived extracellular vesicles (ECVs) [99] ECVs (100–1000 nm diameter) while exosomes (30–100 nm diameter) are released by several cell types; they are delimited by phospholipid bilayer membranes and carry various cellular components, including miRNAs, which—in this way—are protected from degradation. Surface CD markers allow tracking ECVs' origin while adhesion molecules facilitate internalization by recipient cells. Studies conducted on animal models or in in vitro human models (e.g., Il-1β treated synovial fibroblasts) demonstrated that hMSCs derived exosomes may promote chondrocytes proliferation and cartilage repair [100,101].

Exosomes may also be exploited as therapeutic agents because of their targeting capacity and loading ability. By simple incubation, they can be loaded with hydrophobic molecules, such as curcumin and other antioxidants, ensuring considerable stability and bioavailability [102]. Tissue engineering strategies are under development in order to ensure EVs maintenance within the damaged cartilage [103]. Various scaffold types have been tested. Among others, hyaluronic acid (HA) and collagen hydrogels seemed eligible biomaterials for cartilage regeneration. Liu et al. [104] successfully incorporated EVs obtained from iPSC-MSC into a hydrogel glue, which was then implanted into a rabbit articular defect model. The evolution of 3D printing technology offers new chances to exosome-based tissue engineering strategies. Chen et al. tested a 3D printed cartilage ECM/gelatin methacrylate (GeMA)/exosome scaffold, which restored chondrocyte mitochondrial dysfunction and enhanced chondrocyte migration, facilitating cartilage regeneration in an OA rabbit model. Interestingly, the 3D-printed scaffold could retain exosomes for 14 days in vitro and for ≥7 days in vivo [105].

Innovative therapeutic approaches based on genome editing using the CRISPR/Cas9 technique are also being evaluated. The technique has a high potential in regenerative medicine and cell-based applications for cartilage repair [106].

A first therapeutic approach is based on exogenous-cell-based therapy, by delivering chondrocytes or MSCs previously engineered in vitro. Using this approach, Seidl et al. reported that by targeting the MMP13 gene, increased accumulation of cartilage matrix protein type II collagen was achieved using edited cells [107], while the in vitro knockout of IL1-R1 in chondrocytes before injection reduced inflammation, improving cell-therapy results [108]. Other potential therapeutic target genes which have been investigated are osteocalcin [109] and hyaluronan synthase 2 (HAS2) [110].

An alternative approach relies on intra-articular injection of adeno-associated viral vectors expressing CRISPR/Cas9 components to target MMP13, IL-1β and NGF; Zhao et al. [89] reported that the inactivation of these genes may be useful for both pain management and joint maintenance. Moreover, the Cas9 enzyme may be suitably engineered to originate fusion products with factors such as activators and epigenetic modifiers: activation or repression of genes involved in inflammation could have an important therapeutic potential in OA. Epigenetic editing may also allow programming genes networks to target stem cell differentiation for their clinical employment for regenerative therapy [111].

Delivery systems involving non-viral vectors may be preferable in order to avoid inflammatory responses in joints, which can cause adverse side effects [112]. Studies aimed at evaluating different viral and non-viral vectors for the efficient delivery of the CRISPR/Cas9 system at the joint level are needed before this new technology can be proficiently translated into the clinic.

8. Conclusions and Perspectives

As the human lifespan is progressively expanding, the incidence of degenerative disorders associated with ageing, such as OA, is increasing. Traditional treatment options for OA aim at relieving symptoms (pain, inflammation) and at delaying severe disability in patients. Cell-based therapies focusing on the restoration of damaged articular cartilage have been tested on experimental animal models mimicking the OA phenotype (Figure 4).

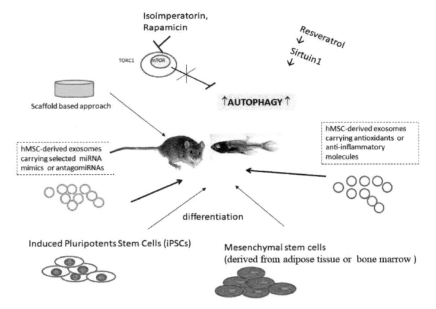

Figure 4. Therapeutic strategies successfully tested in animal OA models (see text).

MicroRNAs involved in the regulation of articular cartilage homeostasis, autophagy and apoptosis show differential expression in OA, i.e., they are either upregulated or downregulated in patients compared to healthy controls. MicroRNAs, which can be recovered from cartilage, blood and synovial fluid, may, therefore, represent diagnostic/prognostic biomarkers. A special attention has been paid to extracellular vesicles-associated miRNAs: they represent the most reliable biomarkers, as they are protected from degradation. Most ECV/exosomes recovered from the OA microenvironment are disease detectors, while

ECVs/exosomes released by MSCs (cartilage progenitor cells) have been shown to exert therapeutic effects on cartilage tissue in experimental models. Bioscaffolds loaded with therapeutic exosomes might be safer and more effective (due to the gradual release) than repeated intra-articular injections. In the future, 3D printed scaffolds might also allow the design of personalized and precision treatments [113]. Cellular senescence, which burdens the OA phenotype, also represents an emerging opportunity for novel therapeutic approaches through the exploitation of senolytics.

Author Contributions: Conceptualization, M.T.V., L.D.C., D.Z. and M.M. All authors have read and agreed to the published version of the manuscript.

Funding: This paper was supported by the FUR-Dep of Medicine, University of Verona (L.D.C.).

Institutional Review Board Statement: Not applicable.

Informed Consent Statement: Not applicable.

Data Availability Statement: Not applicable.

Conflicts of Interest: The authors declare no conflict of interest.

References

1. Lefebvre, V.; Angelozzi, M.; Haseeb, A. SOX9 in cartilage development and disease. *Curr. Opin. Cell Biol.* **2019**, *61*, 39–47. [CrossRef] [PubMed]
2. Dong, X.; Zhao, B.; Iacob, R.E.; Zhu, J.; Koksal, A.C.; Lu, C.; Engen, J.R.; Springer, T.A. Force interacts with macromolecular structure in activation of TGF-β. *Nature* **2017**, *542*, 55–59. [CrossRef] [PubMed]
3. Hügle, T.; Geurts, J.; Nüesch, C.; Müller-Gerbl, M.; Valderrabano, V. Aging and osteoarthritis: An inevitable encounter? *J. Aging Res.* **2012**, *2012*, 950192. [CrossRef] [PubMed]
4. D'Adamo, S.; Cetrullo, S.; Minguzzi, M.; Silvestri, Y.; Borzì, R.M.; Flamigni, F. MicroRNAs and autophagy: Fine players in the control of chondrocyte homeostatic activities in osteoarthritis. *Oxidative Med. Cell. Longev.* **2017**, *2017*, 3720128. [CrossRef]
5. Valenti, M.T.; Carbonare, L.D.; Mottes, M. Role of microRNAs in progenitor cell commitment and osteogenic differentiation in health and disease. *Int. J. Mol. Med.* **2018**, *41*, 2441–2449. [CrossRef] [PubMed]
6. Cheng, N.-T.; Guo, A.; Meng, H. The protective role of autophagy in experimental osteoarthritis, and the therapeutic effects of Torin 1 on osteoarthritis by activating autophagy. *BMC Musculoskelet. Disord.* **2016**, *17*, 1–8. [CrossRef] [PubMed]
7. O'Brien, M.; Philpott, H.T.; McDougall, J.J. Understanding osteoarthritis pain through animal models. *Clin. Exp. Rheumatol.* **2017**, *35* (Suppl. 5), 47–52.
8. Kang, X.; Yang, W.; Feng, D.; Jin, X.; Ma, Z.; Qian, Z.; Xie, T.; Li, H.; Liu, J.; Wang, R. Cartilage-specific autophagy deficiency promotes ER stress and impairs chondrogenesis in PERK-ATF4-CHOP–dependent manner. *J. Bone Miner. Res.* **2017**, *32*, 2128–2141. [CrossRef]
9. Chang, N.C. Autophagy and stem cells: Self-eating for self-renewal. *Front. Cell Dev. Biol.* **2020**, *8*, 138. [CrossRef] [PubMed]
10. Horigome, Y.; Ida-Yonemochi, H.; Waguri, S.; Shibata, S.; Endo, N.; Komatsu, M. Loss of autophagy in chondrocytes causes severe growth retardation. *Autophagy* **2020**, *16*, 501–511. [CrossRef] [PubMed]
11. Luo, P.; Gao, F.; Niu, D.; Sun, X.; Song, Q.; Guo, C.; Liang, Y.; Sun, W. The role of autophagy in chondrocyte metabolism and osteoarthritis: A comprehensive research review. *BioMed Res. Int.* **2019**, *2019*, 5171602. [CrossRef] [PubMed]
12. Kronenberg, H.M. Developmental regulation of the growth plate. *Nature* **2003**, *423*, 332–336. [CrossRef] [PubMed]
13. Settembre, C.; Arteaga-Solis, E.; McKee, M.D.; de Pablo, R.; Al Awqati, Q.; Ballabio, A.; Karsenty, G. Proteoglycan desulfation determines the efficiency of chondrocyte autophagy and the extent of FGF signaling during endochondral ossification. *Genes Dev.* **2008**, *22*, 2645–2650. [CrossRef]
14. Srinivas, V.; Bohensky, J.; Shapiro, I.M. Autophagy: A new phase in the maturation of growth plate chondrocytes is regulated by HIF, mTOR and AMP kinase. *Cells Tissues Organs* **2009**, *189*, 88–92. [CrossRef] [PubMed]
15. Kim, J.; Kundu, M.; Viollet, B.; Guan, K.-L. AMPK and mTOR regulate autophagy through direct phosphorylation of Ulk1. *Nat. Cell Biol.* **2011**, *13*, 132–141. [CrossRef]
16. Houck, S.A.; Ren, H.Y.; Madden, V.J.; Bonner, J.N.; Conlin, M.P.; Janovick, J.A.; Conn, P.M.; Cyr, D.M. Quality control autophagy degrades soluble ERAD-resistant conformers of the misfolded membrane protein GnRHR. *Mol. Cell* **2014**, *54*, 166–179. [CrossRef] [PubMed]
17. Cecconi, F.; Levine, B. The role of autophagy in mammalian development: Cell makeover rather than cell death. *Dev. Cell* **2008**, *15*, 344–357. [CrossRef] [PubMed]
18. Ma, K.-G.; Shao, Z.-W.; Yang, S.-H.; Wang, J.; Wang, B.-C.; Xiong, L.-M.; Wu, Q.; Chen, S.-F. Autophagy is activated in compression-induced cell degeneration and is mediated by reactive oxygen species in nucleus pulposus cells exposed to compression. *Osteoarthr. Cartil.* **2013**, *21*, 2030–2038. [CrossRef]

19. Fermor, B.; Gurumurthy, A.; Diekman, B.O. Hypoxia, RONS and energy metabolism in articular cartilage. *Osteoarthr. Cartil.* **2010**, *18*, 1167–1173. [CrossRef] [PubMed]
20. Dalle Carbonare, L.; Mottes, M.; Cheri, S.; Deiana, M.; Zamboni, F.; Gabbiani, D.; Schena, F.; Salvagno, G.; Lippi, G. Valenti M Increased gene expression of RUNX2 and SOX9 in mesenchymal circulating progenitors is associated with autophagy during physical activity. *Oxidative Med. Cell. Longev.* **2019**, *2019*, 8426259. [CrossRef]
21. Wallace, D.C. A mitochondrial bioenergetic etiology of disease. *J. Clin. Investig.* **2013**, *123*, 1405–1412. [CrossRef] [PubMed]
22. Giorgi, C.; Marchi, S.; Simoes, I.C.; Ren, Z.; Morciano, G.; Perrone, M.; Patalas-Krawczyk, P.; Borchard, S.; Jędrak, P. Pierzynowska K Mitochondria and reactive oxygen species in aging and age-related diseases. *Int. Rev. Cell Mol. Biol.* **2018**, *340*, 209–344.
23. Palikaras, K.; Lionaki, E.; Tavernarakis, N. Mechanisms of mitophagy in cellular homeostasis, physiology and pathology. *Nat. Cell Biol.* **2018**, *20*, 1013–1022. [CrossRef]
24. Sun, K.; Jing, X.; Guo, J.; Yao, X.; Guo, F. Mitophagy in degenerative joint diseases. *Autophagy* **2020**, 1–11. [CrossRef] [PubMed]
25. Forni, M.F.; Peloggia, J.; Trudeau, K.; Shirihai, O.; Kowaltowski, A.J. Murine mesenchymal stem cell commitment to differentiation is regulated by mitochondrial dynamics. *Stem Cells* **2016**, *34*, 743–755. [CrossRef] [PubMed]
26. Marycz, K.; Kornicka, K.; Grzesiak, J.; Śmieszek, A.; Szłapka, J. Macroautophagy and selective mitophagy ameliorate chondrogenic differentiation potential in adipose stem cells of equine metabolic syndrome: New findings in the field of progenitor cells differentiation. *Oxidative Med. Cell. Longev.* **2016**, *2016*, 3718468. [CrossRef]
27. Caramés, B.; Taniguchi, N.; Otsuki, S.; Blanco, F.J.; Lotz, M. Autophagy is a protective mechanism in normal cartilage, and its aging-related loss is linked with cell death and osteoarthritis. *Arthritis Rheum.* **2010**, *62*, 791–801. [CrossRef]
28. Yang, F.; Huang, R.; Ma, H.; Zhao, X.; Wang, G. miRNA-411 Regulates chondrocyte autophagy in osteoarthritis by targeting hypoxia-inducible factor 1 alpha (HIF-1α). *Med. Sci. Monit. Int. Med. J. Exp. Clin. Res.* **2020**, *26*, e921155-1. [CrossRef]
29. Li, H.; Li, Z.; Pi, Y.; Chen, Y.; Mei, L.; Luo, Y.; Xie, J.; Mao, X. MicroRNA-375 exacerbates knee osteoarthritis through repressing chondrocyte autophagy by targeting ATG2B. *Aging* **2020**, *12*, 7248. [CrossRef] [PubMed]
30. Feng, L.; Feng, C.; Wang, C.X.; Xu, D.Y.; Chen, J.J.; Huang, J.F.; Tan, P.L.; Shen, J.M. Circulating microRNA let-7e is decreased in knee osteoarthritis, accompanied by elevated apoptosis and reduced autophagy. *Int. J. Mol. Med.* **2020**, *45*, 1464–1476. [CrossRef]
31. Yu, Y.; Zhao, J. Modulated autophagy by microRNAs in osteoarthritis chondrocytes. *BioMed Res. Int.* **2019**, *2019*, 1484152. [CrossRef] [PubMed]
32. Lambert, S.A.; Jolma, A.; Campitelli, L.F.; Das, P.K.; Yin, Y.; Albu, M.; Chen, X.; Taipale, J.; Hughes, T.R.; Weirauch, M.T. The human transcription factors. *Cell* **2018**, *172*, 650–665. [CrossRef] [PubMed]
33. Accili, D.; Arden, K.C. FoxOs at the crossroads of cellular metabolism, differentiation, and transformation. *Cell* **2004**, *117*, 421–426. [CrossRef]
34. Roeder, R.G. The role of general initiation factors in transcription by RNA polymerase II. *Trends Biochem. Sci.* **1996**, *21*, 327–335. [CrossRef]
35. Maston, G.A.; Evans, S.K.; Green, M.R. Transcriptional regulatory elements in the human genome. *Annu. Rev. Genom. Hum. Genet.* **2006**, *7*, 29–59. [CrossRef]
36. Mullen, A.C.; Orlando, D.A.; Newman, J.J.; Lovén, J.; Kumar, R.M.; Bilodeau, S.; Reddy, J.; Guenther, M.G.; DeKoter, R.P.; Young, R.A. Master transcription factors determine cell-type-specific responses to TGF-β signaling. *Cell* **2011**, *147*, 565–576. [CrossRef] [PubMed]
37. Chen, L.-F.; Williams, S.A.; Mu, Y.; Nakano, H.; Duerr, J.M.; Buckbinder, L.; Greene, W.C. NF-κB RelA phosphorylation regulates RelA acetylation. *Mol. Cell. Biol.* **2005**, *25*, 7966–7975. [CrossRef] [PubMed]
38. Lefebvre, V.; Dvir-Ginzberg, M. SOX9 and the many facets of its regulation in the chondrocyte lineage. *Connect. Tissue Res.* **2017**, *58*, 2–14. [CrossRef]
39. Csukasi, F.; Duran, I.; Zhang, W.; Martin, J.H.; Barad, M.; Bamshad, M.; Weis, M.A.; Eyre, D.; Krakow, D.; Cohn, D.H. Dominant-negative SOX9 mutations in campomelic dysplasia. *Hum. Mutat.* **2019**, *40*, 2344–2352. [CrossRef] [PubMed]
40. Zhong, L.; Huang, X.; Karperien, M.; Post, J.N. Correlation between gene expression and osteoarthritis progression in human. *Int. J. Mol. Sci.* **2016**, *17*, 1126. [CrossRef] [PubMed]
41. Nakamura, Y.; He, X.; Kato, H.; Wakitani, S.; Kobayashi, T.; Watanabe, S.; Iida, A.; Tahara, H.; Warman, M.L.; Watanapokasin, R. Sox9 is upstream of microRNA-140 in cartilage. *Appl. Biochem. Biotechnol.* **2012**, *166*, 64–71. [CrossRef] [PubMed]
42. Martinez-Sanchez, A.; Murphy, C.L. miR-1247 functions by targeting cartilage transcription factor SOX9. *J. Biol. Chem.* **2013**, *288*, 30802–30814. [CrossRef] [PubMed]
43. Zhang, H.; Wang, Y.; Yang, G.; Yu, H.; Zhou, Z.; Tang, M. MicroRNA-30a regulates chondrogenic differentiation of human bone marrow-derived mesenchymal stem cells through targeting Sox9. *Exp. Ther. Med.* **2019**, *18*, 4689–4697. [CrossRef]
44. Yu, X.-M.; Meng, H.-Y.; Yuan, X.-L.; Wang, Y.; Guo, Q.-Y.; Peng, J.; Wang, A.-Y.; Lu, S.-B. MicroRNAs' involvement in osteoarthritis and the prospects for treatments. *Evid. Based Complementary Altern. Med.* **2015**, *2015*, 236179. [CrossRef]
45. Neefjes, M.; van Caam, A.P.; van der Kraan, P.M. Transcription Factors in Cartilage Homeostasis and Osteoarthritis. *Biology* **2020**, *9*, 290. [CrossRef] [PubMed]
46. Fisch, K.M.; Gamini, R.; Alvarez-Garcia, O.; Akagi, R.; Saito, M.; Muramatsu, Y.; Sasho, T.; Koziol, J.A.; Su, A.I.; Lotz, M.K. Identification of transcription factors responsible for dysregulated networks in human osteoarthritis cartilage by global gene expression analysis. *Osteoarthr. Cartil.* **2018**, *26*, 1531–1538. [CrossRef] [PubMed]

47. Kobayashi, H.; Hirata, M.; Saito, T.; Itoh, S.; Chung, U.-I.; Kawaguchi, H. Transcriptional induction of ADAMTS5 protein by nuclear factor-κB (NF-κB) family member RelA/p65 in chondrocytes during osteoarthritis development. *J. Biol. Chem.* **2013**, *288*, 28620–28629. [CrossRef] [PubMed]

48. Takahata, Y.; Nakamura, E.; Hata, K.; Wakabayashi, M.; Murakami, T.; Wakamori, K.; Yoshikawa, H.; Matsuda, A.; Fukui, N.; Nishimura, R. Sox4 is involved in osteoarthritic cartilage deterioration through induction of ADAMTS4 and ADAMTS5. *FASEB J.* **2019**, *33*, 619–630. [CrossRef] [PubMed]

49. Zhang, Z.; Kang, Y.; Zhang, H.; Duan, X.; Liu, J.; Li, X..; Liao, W. Expression of microRNAs during chondrogenesis of human adipose-derived stem cells. *Osteoarthr. Cartil.* **2012**, *20*, 1638–1646. [CrossRef] [PubMed]

50. Hu, G.; Codina, M.; Fisher, S. Multiple enhancers associated with ACAN suggest highly redundant transcriptional regulation in cartilage. *Matrix Biol.* **2012**, *31*, 328–337. [CrossRef]

51. Settembre, C.; Di Malta, C.; Polito, V.A.; Arencibia, M.G.; Vetrini, F.; Erdin, S.; Erdin, S.U.; Huynh, T.; Medina, D.; Colella, P. TFEB links autophagy to lysosomal biogenesis. *Science* **2011**, *332*, 1429–1433. [CrossRef] [PubMed]

52. Zheng, G.; Zhan, Y.; Li, X.; Pan, Z.; Zheng, F.; Zhang, Z.; Zhou, Y.; Wu, Y.; Wang, X.; Gao, W. TFEB, a potential therapeutic target for osteoarthritis via autophagy regulation. *Cell Death Dis.* **2018**, *9*, 1–15. [CrossRef]

53. Chauhan, S.; Goodwin, J.G.; Chauhan, S.; Manyam, G.; Wang, J.; Kamat, A.M.; Boyd, D.D. ZKSCAN3 is a master transcriptional repressor of autophagy. *Mol. Cell* **2013**, *50*, 16–28. [CrossRef]

54. Hu, H.; Ji, Q.; Song, M.; Ren, J.; Liu, Z.; Wang, Z.; Liu, X.; Yan, K.; Hu, J.; Jing, Y. ZKSCAN3 counteracts cellular senescence by stabilizing heterochromatin. *Nucleic Acids Res.* **2020**, *48*, 6001–6018. [CrossRef] [PubMed]

55. Brunet, A.; Sweeney, L.B.; Sturgill, J.F.; Chua, K.F.; Greer, P.L.; Lin, Y.; Tran, H.; Ross, S.E.; Mostoslavsky, R.; Cohen, H.Y. Stress-dependent regulation of FOXO transcription factors by the SIRT1 deacetylase. *Science* **2004**, *303*, 2011–2015. [CrossRef] [PubMed]

56. Pietrocola, F.; Izzo, V.; Niso-Santano, M.; Vacchelli, E.; Galluzzi, L.; Maiuri, M.C.; Kroemer, G. Regulation of autophagy by stress-responsive transcription factors. In *Seminars in Cancer Biology*; Elsevier: Amsterdam, The Netherlands, 2013.

57. Akasaki, Y.; Alvarez-Garcia, O.; Saito, M.; Caramés, B.; Iwamoto, Y.; Lotz, M.K. FoxO transcription factors support oxidative stress resistance in human chondrocytes. *Arthritis Rheumatol.* **2014**, *66*, 3349–3358. [CrossRef] [PubMed]

58. Matsuzaki, T.; Alvarez-Garcia, O.; Mokuda, S.; Nagira, K.; Olmer, M.; Gamini, R.; Miyata, K.; Akasaki, Y.; Su, A.I.; Asahara, H.; et al. FoxO transcription factors modulate autophagy and proteoglycan 4 in cartilage homeostasis and osteoarthritis. *Sci. Transl. Med.* **2018**, *10*, eaan0746. [CrossRef] [PubMed]

59. Xie, J.; Lin, J.; Wei, M.; Teng, Y.; He, Q.; Yang, G.; Yang, X. Sustained Akt signaling in articular chondrocytes causes osteoarthritis via oxidative stress-induced senescence in mice. *Bone Res.* **2019**, *7*, 1–9. [CrossRef] [PubMed]

60. Kim, K.M.; Park, S.J.; Jung, S.H.; Kim, E.J.; Jogeswar, G.; Ajita, J.; Rhee, Y.; Kim, C.H.; Lim, S.K. miR-182 is a negative regulator of osteoblast proliferation, differentiation, and skeletogenesis through targeting FoxO1. *J. Bone Miner. Res.* **2012**, *27*, 1669–1679. [CrossRef]

61. Huang, P.-Y.; Wu, J.-G.; Gu, J.; Zhang, T.-Q.; Li, L.-F.; Wang, S.-Q.; Wang, M. Bioinformatics analysis of miRNA and mRNA expression profiles to reveal the key miRNAs and genes in osteoarthritis. *J. Orthop. Surg. Res.* **2021**, *16*, 1–9. [CrossRef]

62. Duan, R.; Xie, H.; Liu, Z.-Z. The Role of Autophagy in Osteoarthritis. *Front. Cell Dev. Biol.* **2020**, *8*, 1437. [CrossRef] [PubMed]

63. McCorry, M.C.; Puetzer, J.L.; Bonassar, L.J. Characterization of mesenchymal stem cells and fibrochondrocytes in three-dimensional co-culture: Analysis of cell shape, matrix production, and mechanical performance. *Stem Cell Res. Ther.* **2016**, *7*, 1–10. [CrossRef]

64. Samvelyan, H.J.; Hughes, D.; Stevens, C.; Staines, K.A. Models of osteoarthritis: Relevance and new insights. *Calcif. Tissue Int.* **2020**, 1–14. [CrossRef]

65. Guilak, F.; Alexopoulos, L.G.; Upton, M.L.; Youn, I.; Choi, J.B.; Cao, L.; Setton, L.A.; Haider, M.A. The pericellular matrix as a transducer of biomechanical and biochemical signals in articular cartilage. *Ann. N. Y. Acad. Sci.* **2006**, *1068*, 498–512. [CrossRef]

66. Cope, P.; Ourradi, K.; Li, Y.; Sharif, M. Models of osteoarthritis: The good, the bad and the promising. *Osteoarthr. Cartil.* **2019**, *27*, 230–239. [CrossRef]

67. van der Kraan, P. Relevance of zebrafish as an OA research model. *Osteoarthr. Cartil.* **2013**, *21*, 261–262. [CrossRef] [PubMed]

68. Brunt, L.H.; Roddy, K.A.; Rayfield, E.J.; Hammond, C.L. Building finite element models to investigate zebrafish jaw biomechanics. *J. Vis. Exp.* **2016**, *2016*, e54811. [CrossRef] [PubMed]

69. Lawrence, E.A.; Aggleton, J.A.; van Loon, J.J.; Godivier, J.; Harniman, R.L.; Pei, J.; Nowlan, N.; Hammond, C.L. Exposure to hypergravity during zebrafish development alters cartilage material properties and strain distribution. *Bone Jt. Res.* **2021**, *10*, 137–148. [CrossRef] [PubMed]

70. Weiner, A.M.; Scampoli, N.L.; Steeman, T.J.; Dooley, C.M.; Busch-Nentwich, E.M.; Kelsh, R.N.; Calcaterra, N.B. Dicer1 is required for pigment cell and craniofacial development in zebrafish. *Biochim. Biophys. Acta (BBA)-Gene Regul. Mech.* **2019**, *1862*, 472–485. [CrossRef] [PubMed]

71. Sorial, A.K.; Hofer, I.M.; Tselepi, M.; Cheung, K.; Parker, E.; Deehan, D.J.; Rice, S.J.; Loughlin, J. Multi-tissue epigenetic analysis of the osteoarthritis susceptibility locus mapping to the plectin gene PLEC. *Osteoarthr. Cartil.* **2020**, *28*, 1448–1458. [CrossRef]

72. Almarza, D.; Cucchiarini, M.; Loughlin, J. Genome editing for human osteoarthritis–a perspective. *Osteoarthr. Cartil.* **2017**, *25*, 1195–1198. [CrossRef] [PubMed]

73. Moss, J.J.; Hammond, C.L.; Lane, J.D. Zebrafish as a model to study autophagy and its role in skeletal development and disease. *Histochem. Cell Biol.* **2020**, 1–16. [CrossRef] [PubMed]

74. Butterfield, N.C.; Curry, K.F.; Steinberg, J.; Dewhurst, H.; Komla-Ebri, D.; Mannan, N.S.; Adoum, A.-T.; Leitch, V.D.; Logan, J.G.; Waung, J.A. Accelerating functional gene discovery in osteoarthritis. *Nat. Commun.* **2021**, *12*, 1–18. [CrossRef]

75. Brunt, L.; Kague, E.; Hammond, C. Developmental Insights into Osteoarthritis Increase the Applicability of New Animal Models. *J. Musculoskelet. Disord. Treat.* **2016**, *2*, 17.

76. Le, L.T.; Swingler, T.E.; Crowe, N.; Vincent, T.L.; Barter, M.J.; Donell, S.T.; Delany, A.M.; Dalmay, T.; Young, D.A.; Clark, I.M. The microRNA-29 family in cartilage homeostasis and osteoarthritis. *J. Mol. Med.* **2016**, *94*, 583–596. [CrossRef] [PubMed]

77. Cheng, Y.; Ren, X.; Hait, W.N.; Yang, J.-M. Therapeutic targeting of autophagy in disease: Biology and pharmacology. *Pharmacol. Rev.* **2013**, *65*, 1162–1197. [CrossRef] [PubMed]

78. Cooper, C.; Chapurlat, R.; Al-Daghri, N.; Herrero-Beaumont, G.; Bruyère, O.; Rannou, F.; Roth, R.; Uebelhart, D.; Reginster, J.-Y. Safety of oral non-selective non-steroidal anti-inflammatory drugs in osteoarthritis: What does the literature say? *Drugs Aging* **2019**, *36*, 15–24. [CrossRef] [PubMed]

79. Takayama, K.; Kawakami, Y.; Kobayashi, M.; Greco, N.; Cummins, J.H.; Matsushita, T.; Kuroda, R.; Kurosaka, M.; Fu, F.H.; Huard, J. Local intra-articular injection of rapamycin delays articular cartilage degeneration in a murine model of osteoarthritis. *Arthritis Res. Ther.* **2014**, *16*, 1–10. [CrossRef] [PubMed]

80. Ouyang, J.; Jiang, H.; Fang, H.; Cui, W.; Cai, D. Isoimperatorin ameliorates osteoarthritis by downregulating the mammalian target of rapamycin C1 signaling pathway. *Mol. Med. Rep.* **2017**, *16*, 9636–9644. [CrossRef] [PubMed]

81. Sun, M.M.-G.; Beier, F.; Pest, M.A. Recent developments in emerging therapeutic targets of osteoarthritis. *Curr. Opin. Rheumatol.* **2017**, *29*, 96. [CrossRef] [PubMed]

82. Shi, Y.; Hu, X.; Cheng, J.; Zhang, X.; Zhao, F.; Shi, W.; Ren, B.; Yu, H.; Yang, P.; Li, Z. A small molecule promotes cartilage extracellular matrix generation and inhibits osteoarthritis development. *Nat. Commun.* **2019**, *10*, 1–14. [CrossRef] [PubMed]

83. Liu, T.; Zhang, L.; Joo, D.; Sun, S.-C. NF-κB signaling in inflammation. *Signal Transduct. Target. Ther.* **2017**, *2*, 1–9. [CrossRef] [PubMed]

84. Yi, H.; Zhang, W.; Cui, Z.-M.; Cui, S.-Y.; Fan, J.-B.; Zhu, X.-H.; Liu, W. Resveratrol alleviates the interleukin-1β-induced chondrocytes injury through the NF-κB signaling pathway. *J. Orthop. Surg. Res.* **2020**, *15*, 1–9. [CrossRef]

85. Ruan, G.; Xu, J.; Wang, K.; Wu, J.; Zhu, Q.; Ren, J.; Bian, F.; Chang, B.; Bai, X.; Han, W. Associations between knee structural measures, circulating inflammatory factors and MMP13 in patients with knee osteoarthritis. *Osteoarthr. Cartil.* **2018**, *26*, 1063–1069. [CrossRef]

86. Mehana, E.-S.E.; Khafaga, A.F.; El-Blehi, S.S. The role of matrix metalloproteinases in osteoarthritis pathogenesis: An updated review. *Life Sci.* **2019**, *234*, 116786. [CrossRef] [PubMed]

87. Yang, C.-Y.; Chanalaris, A.; Troeberg, L. ADAMTS and ADAM metalloproteinases in osteoarthritis–looking beyond the 'usual suspects'. *Osteoarthr. Cartil.* **2017**, *25*, 1000–1009. [CrossRef]

88. Wang, M.; Sampson, E.R.; Jin, H.; Li, J.; Ke, Q.H.; Im, H.-J.; Chen, D. MMP13 is a critical target gene during the progression of osteoarthritis. *Arthritis Res. Ther.* **2013**, *15*, 1–11. [CrossRef] [PubMed]

89. Zhao, L.; Huang, J.; Fan, Y.; Li, J.; You, T.; He, S.; Xiao, G.; Chen, D. Exploration of CRISPR/Cas9-based gene editing as therapy for osteoarthritis. *Ann. Rheum. Dis.* **2019**, *78*, 676–682. [CrossRef] [PubMed]

90. Fields, G.B. The rebirth of matrix metalloproteinase inhibitors: Moving beyond the dogma. *Cells* **2019**, *8*, 984. [CrossRef]

91. Santamaria, S. ADAMTS-5: A difficult teenager turning 20. *Int. J. Exp. Pathol.* **2020**, *101*, 4–20. [CrossRef] [PubMed]

92. Kang, C.; Elledge, S.J. How autophagy both activates and inhibits cellular senescence. *Autophagy* **2016**, *12*, 898–899. [CrossRef]

93. Di Micco, R.; Krizhanovsky, V.; Baker, D.; d'Adda di Fagagna, F. Cellular senescence in ageing: From mechanisms to therapeutic opportunities. *Nat. Rev. Mol. Cell Biol.* **2020**, *22*, 75–95. [CrossRef]

94. Zhu, Y.; Doornebal, E.J.; Pirtskhalava, T.; Giorgadze, N.; Wentworth, M.; Fuhrmann-Stroissnigg, H.; Niedernhofer, L.J.; Robbins, P.D.; Tchkonia, T.; Kirkland, J.L. New agents that target senescent cells: The flavone, fisetin, and the BCL-XL inhibitors, A1331852 and A1155463. *Aging* **2017**, *9*, 955. [CrossRef] [PubMed]

95. Kirkland, J.L.; Tchkonia, T.; Zhu, Y.; Niedernhofer, L.J.; Robbins, P.D. The clinical potential of senolytic drugs. *J. Am. Geriatr. Soc.* **2017**, *65*, 2297–2301. [CrossRef] [PubMed]

96. Lewinska, A.; Adamczyk-Grochala, J.; Bloniarz, D.; Olszowka, J.; Kulpa-Greszta, M.; Litwinienko, G.; Tomaszewska, A.; Wnuk, M.; Pazik, R. AMPK-mediated senolytic and senostatic activity of quercetin surface functionalized Fe_3O_4 nanoparticles during oxidant-induced senescence in human fibroblasts. *Redox Biol.* **2020**, *28*, 101337. [CrossRef] [PubMed]

97. Deng, Z.; Li, Y.; Liu, H.; Xiao, S.; Li, L.; Tian, J.; Cheng, C.; Zhang, G.; Zhang, F. The role of sirtuin 1 and its activator, resveratrol in osteoarthritis. *Biosci. Rep.* **2019**, *39*, BSR20190189. [CrossRef]

98. Wang, X.-B.; Zhao, F.-C.; Yi, L.-H.; Tang, J.-L.; Zhu, Z.-Y.; Pang, Y.; Chen, Y.-S.; Li, D.-Y.; Guo, K.-J.; Zheng, X. MicroRNA-21-5p as a novel therapeutic target for osteoarthritis. *Rheumatology* **2019**, *58*, 1485–1497. [CrossRef]

99. Geng, Y.; Chen, J.; Alahdal, M.; Chang, C.; Duan, L.; Zhu, W.; Mou, L.; Xiong, J.; Wang, M.; Wang, D. Intra-articular injection of hUC-MSCs expressing miR-140-5p induces cartilage self-repairing in the rat osteoarthritis. *J. Bone Miner. Metab.* **2020**, *38*, 277–288. [CrossRef] [PubMed]

100. Liu, X.; Shortt, C.; Zhang, F.; Bater, M.Q.; Cowman, M.K.; Kirsch, T. Extracellular Vesicles Released From Articular Chondrocytes Play a Major Role in Cell–Cell Communication. *J. Orthop. Res.®* **2020**, *38*, 731–739. [CrossRef] [PubMed]

101. Tao, S.-C.; Yuan, T.; Zhang, Y.-L.; Yin, W.-J.; Guo, S.-C.; Zhang, C.-Q. Exosomes derived from miR-140-5p-overexpressing human synovial mesenchymal stem cells enhance cartilage tissue regeneration and prevent osteoarthritis of the knee in a rat model. *Theranostics* **2017**, *7*, 180. [CrossRef] [PubMed]

102. Mao, G.; Zhang, Z.; Hu, S.; Zhang, Z.; Chang, Z.; Huang, Z.; Liao, W.; Kang, Y. Exosomes derived from miR-92a-3p-overexpressing human mesenchymal stem cells enhance chondrogenesis and suppress cartilage degradation via targeting WNT5A. *Stem Cell Res. Ther.* **2018**, *9*, 1–13. [CrossRef] [PubMed]

103. Qiu, B.; Xu, X.; Yi, P.; Hao, Y. Curcumin reinforces MSC-derived exosomes in attenuating osteoarthritis via modulating the miR-124/NF-kB and miR-143/ROCK1/TLR9 signalling pathways. *J. Cell. Mol. Med.* **2020**, *24*, 10855–10865. [CrossRef]

104. Liu, X.; Yang, Y.; Li, Y.; Niu, X.; Zhao, B.; Wang, Y.; Bao, C.; Xie, Z.; Lin, Q.; Zhu, L. Integration of stem cell-derived exosomes with in situ hydrogel glue as a promising tissue patch for articular cartilage regeneration. *Nanoscale* **2017**, *9*, 4430–4438. [CrossRef]

105. Chen, P.; Zheng, L.; Wang, Y.; Tao, M.; Xie, Z.; Xia, C.; Gu, C.; Chen, J.; Qiu, P.; Mei, S. Desktop-stereolithography 3D printing of a radially oriented extracellular matrix/mesenchymal stem cell exosome bioink for osteochondral defect regeneration. *Theranostics* **2019**, *9*, 2439. [CrossRef]

106. Tanikella, A.S.; Hardy, M.J.; Frahs, S.M.; Cormier, A.G.; Gibbons, K.D.; Fitzpatrick, C.K.; Oxford, J.T. Emerging gene-editing modalities for osteoarthritis. *Int. J. Mol. Sci.* **2020**, *21*, 6046. [CrossRef]

107. Seidl, C.; Fulga, T.; Murphy, C. CRISPR-Cas9 targeting of MMP13 in human chondrocytes leads to significantly reduced levels of the metalloproteinase and enhanced type II collagen accumulation. *Osteoarthr. Cartil.* **2019**, *27*, 140–147. [CrossRef] [PubMed]

108. Karlsen, T.A.; Pernas, P.F.; Staerk, J.; Caglayan, S.; Brinchmann, J. Generation of IL1β-resistant chondrocytes using CRISPR-CAS genome editing. *Osteoarthr. Cartil.* **2016**, *24*, S325. [CrossRef]

109. Lambert, L.J.; Challa, A.K.; Niu, A.; Zhou, L.; Tucholski, J.; Johnson, M.S.; Nagy, T.R.; Eberhardt, A.W.; Estep, P.N.; Kesterson, R.A. Increased trabecular bone and improved biomechanics in an osteocalcin-null rat model created by CRISPR/Cas9 technology. *Dis. Models Mech.* **2016**, *9*, 1169–1179. [CrossRef] [PubMed]

110. Huang, Y.; Askew, E.B.; Knudson, C.B.; Knudson, W. CRISPR/Cas9 knockout of HAS2 in rat chondrosarcoma chondrocytes demonstrates the requirement of hyaluronan for aggrecan retention. *Matrix Biol.* **2016**, *56*, 74–94. [CrossRef] [PubMed]

111. Adkar, S.S.; Brunger, J.M.; Willard, V.P.; Wu, C.-L.; Gersbach, C.A.; Guilak, F. Genome engineering for personalized arthritis therapeutics. *Trends in molecular medicine* **2017**, *23*, 917–931. [CrossRef] [PubMed]

112. Uzieliene, I.; Kalvaityte, U.; Bernotiene, E.; Mobasheri, A. Non-viral Gene Therapy for Osteoarthritis. *Front. Bioeng. Biotechnol.* **2020**, *8*, 8. [CrossRef]

113. Mancuso, P.; Raman, S.; Glynn, A.; Barry, F.; Murphy, J.M. Mesenchymal stem cell therapy for osteoarthritis: The critical role of the cell secretome. *Front. Bioeng. Biotechnol.* **2019**, *7*, 9. [CrossRef] [PubMed]

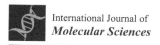

International Journal of
Molecular Sciences

MDPI

Article

Inhibition of Inducible Nitric Oxide Synthase Prevents IL-1β-Induced Mitochondrial Dysfunction in Human Chondrocytes

Annett Eitner [1,*], Sylvia Müller [2], Christian König [3], Arne Wilharm [1], Rebecca Raab [1,4], Gunther O. Hofmann [1], Thomas Kamradt [2] and Hans-Georg Schaible [3]

[1] Department of Trauma, Hand and Reconstructive Surgery, Experimental Trauma Surgery, Jena University Hospital, Friedrich-Schiller-University Jena, 07747 Jena, Germany; Arne.Wilharm@med.uni-jena.de (A.W.); Rebecca@raab-online.de (R.R.); Gunther.Hofmann@med.uni-jena.de (G.O.H.)
[2] Institute of Immunology, Jena University Hospital, Friedrich-Schiller-University Jena, 07743 Jena, Germany; Sylvia.Mueller@med.uni-jena.de (S.M.); Thomas.Kamradt@med.uni-jena.de (T.K.)
[3] Institute of Physiology 1/Neurophysiology, Jena University Hospital, Friedrich-Schiller-University Jena, 07743 Jena, Germany; Christian.Koenig@med.uni-jena.de (C.K.); Hans-Georg.Schaible@med.uni-jena.de (H.-G.S.)
[4] Clinic of Trauma, Orthopedic and Septic Surgery, Hospital St. Georg gGmbH, 04129 Leipzig, Germany
* Correspondence: Annett.Eitner@med.uni-jena.de; Tel.: +49-3641-9397618

Abstract: Interleukin (IL)-1β is an important pro-inflammatory cytokine in the progression of osteoarthritis (OA), which impairs mitochondrial function and induces the production of nitric oxide (NO) in chondrocytes. The aim was to investigate if blockade of NO production prevents IL-1β-induced mitochondrial dysfunction in chondrocytes and whether cAMP and AMP-activated protein kinase (AMPK) affects NO production and mitochondrial function. Isolated human OA chondrocytes were stimulated with IL-1β in combination with/without forskolin, L-NIL, AMPK activator or inhibitor. The release of NO, IL-6, PGE$_2$, MMP3, and the expression of iNOS were measured by ELISA or Western blot. Parameters of mitochondrial respiration were measured using a seahorse analyzer. IL-1β significantly induced NO release and mitochondrial dysfunction. Inhibition of iNOS by L-NIL prevented IL-1β-induced NO release and mitochondrial dysfunction but not IL-1β-induced release of IL-6, PGE$_2$, and MMP3. Enhancement of cAMP by forskolin reduced IL-1β-induced NO release and prevented IL-1β-induced mitochondrial impairment. Activation of AMPK increased IL-1β-induced NO production and the negative impact of IL-1β on mitochondrial respiration, whereas inhibition of AMPK had the opposite effects. NO is critically involved in the IL-1β-induced impairment of mitochondrial respiration in human OA chondrocytes. Increased intracellular cAMP or inhibition of AMPK prevented both IL-1β-induced NO release and mitochondrial dysfunction.

Keywords: osteoarthritis; NO synthase; Interleukin-1β; chondrocytes; mitochondrial dysfunction

Citation: Eitner, A.; Müller, S.; König, C.; Wilharm, A.; Raab, R.; Hofmann, G.O.; Kamradt, T.; Schaible, H.-G. Inhibition of Inducible Nitric Oxide Synthase Prevents IL-1β-Induced Mitochondrial Dysfunction in Human Chondrocytes. *Int. J. Mol. Sci.* **2021**, 22, 2477. https://doi.org/10.3390/ijms22052477

Academic Editor: Nicola Veronese

Received: 20 January 2021
Accepted: 25 February 2021
Published: 1 March 2021

1. Introduction

Pro-inflammatory cytokines contribute significantly to the initiation and progression of osteoarthritis (OA) via up-regulation of catabolic processes [1,2]. In addition, the impairment of the mitochondrial function of chondrocytes is thought to be an important factor in the pathophysiology of OA [3–5]. Experiments showed that Interleukin-1β (IL-1β) can impair the activity of mitochondrial respiratory chain enzyme complexes [6]. However, the mechanism by which IL-1β modulates mitochondrial respiration remains unclear. IL-1β induces upregulation of inducible NO synthase (iNOS) and the production of nitric oxide (NO). This mediator regulates numerous putative pathogenic processes in the cartilage (see below), and may also alter mitochondrial respiration and ATP production in chondrocytes [3]. However, whether IL-1β-induced NO production is causally responsible for mitochondrial impairment and whether inhibition of iNOS can prevent IL-1β-induced mitochondrial dysfunction has not yet been reported.

An increased iNOS expression was found in OA cartilage and synovial tissue [7]. Although NO produced by constitutive NO synthase at low concentration can reduce OA pain probably through the promotion of blood flow, thus improving oxygen supply and reducing ischemic pain [8], NO produced by the cytoplasmic iNOS at high concentration is a pro-inflammatory factor and contributes to OA pathogenesis [9], and can induce cell damage. In chondrocytes, NO increases the release of pro-inflammatory mediators and inhibits the synthesis of cartilage matrix components and increases the activity of matrix-degrading enzymes such as matrix metalloproteinases (MMP) [10]. Exogenous cytokines can increase iNOS expression and NO release of OA cartilage and cultured chondrocytes [11,12]. In addition, NO at high concentration affects cytochrome c oxidase in mitochondria, induces caspase 3, and is presumably responsible for the initiation of apoptosis [13]. It has been reported that mitochondrial dysfunction also increases the responsiveness of chondrocytes for cytokines [14]. An interesting question is, therefore, whether NO-induced mitochondrial dysfunction also increases the IL-1β-induced release of pro-inflammatory mediators.

The expression and activity of iNOS are regulated by various signaling pathways such as cyclic adenosine monophosphate (cAMP)- or AMP-activated protein kinase (AMPK)-pathway, and the effect of activation or inhibition of these pathways differs between cell types. It has been reported that the signaling molecule cAMP can increase iNOS expression in adipocytes, smooth muscle cells, and skeletal muscle cells, whereas in hepatocytes and astrocytes cAMP suppressed iNOS expression [15,16]. Tissue-specific gene expression and an alteration of cell signaling pathways are thought to be responsible for these opposite effects of cAMP [16]. Another regulator of iNOS expression is the AMPK, which is an important regulator of cellular energy metabolism. A high AMP/ATP ratio activates AMPK, which inhibits ATP-consuming pathways and increases ATP production [17]. In many cell types, AMPK exerts anti-inflammatory effects and reduces iNOS expression [18]. In contrast, in hepatocytes, activation of AMPK upregulates the cytokine-induced expression of iNOS and NO production [19]. Presumably, the signaling molecule cAMP and the regulator AMPK are part of two independent pathways for the regulation of iNOS expression. Whether cAMP and AMPK modulate IL-1β-induced NO release and mitochondrial function in chondrocytes is unclear.

The current study aimed to evaluate whether increased NO production is responsible for IL-1β-induced mitochondrial dysfunction in human OA chondrocytes obtained from knee joints during arthroplasty. Of particular interest is to evaluate whether blockade of iNOS activity prevents the negative effects of IL-1β on chondrocytes. Additionally, we analyzed the role of cAMP and AMPK in the regulation of NO production and release from these cells and in IL-1β-induced mitochondrial dysfunction. To understand the regulation of iNOS activity in chondrocytes is important to move forward with the development of OA therapies based on iNOS as a target for OA treatment.

2. Results

2.1. IL-1β-Induced NO Release

After stimulation with IL-1β for 48 h, cultured chondrocytes showed a concentration-dependent NO release (Figure 1a, repeated measures ANOVA: $p < 0.001$). The IL-1β concentration 0.1 ng/mL evoked a high release of NO, which only slightly increased at higher IL-β concentrations (Figure 1a). Therefore, all further experiments were performed with an IL-1β concentration of 0.1 ng/mL.

Co-application of 0.1 ng/mL IL-1β and 10 μM L-NIL, an inhibitor of iNOS, resulted in a significant reduction of IL-1β-induced NO release (Figure 1b, $p = 0.006$), showing that L-NIL is a useful compound to investigate NO-related effects.

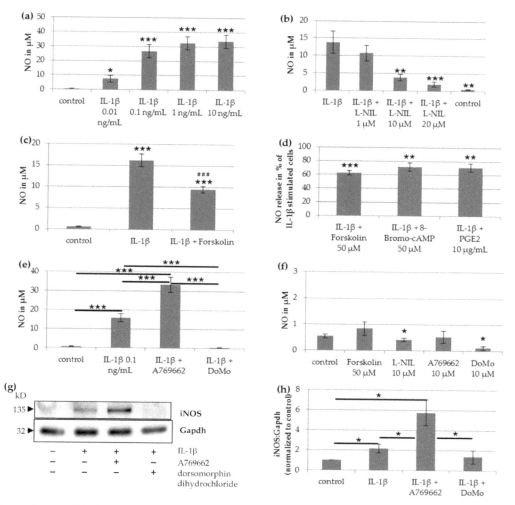

Figure 1. Impact of IL-1β on nitric oxide (NO) release and NO synthase (iNOS) expression of human chondrocytes. (**a**) NO release after stimulation with Interleukin (IL)-1β at different concentrations. Statistical differences vs. unstimulated cells, repeated-measures ANOVA ($n = 7$). (**b**) NO release after stimulation with IL-1β (0.1 ng/mL) and L-NIL at different concentrations. Statistical differences vs. IL-1β-stimulated cells, repeated-measures ANOVA ($n = 7$). (**c**) NO release after stimulation with 0.1 ng/mL IL-1β and 50 μM forskolin. Statistical differences *** vs. unstimulated cells or ### vs. IL-1β-stimulated cells, Wilcoxon signed-rank test and Bonferroni adjustment ($n = 22$). (**d**) NO release after simultaneous stimulation of 0.1 ng/mL IL-1β with 50 μM forskolin ($n = 22$), 50 μM 8-Bromo-cAMP ($n = 10$), or 10 μg/mL PGE$_2$ ($n = 9$) normalized to IL-1β-stimulated cells. Statistical differences vs. IL-1β-stimulated cells, Wilcoxon signed-rank test. (**e**) Impact of activation or inhibition of AMPK on IL-1β-induced NO release. Statistic: Repeated-measures ANOVA with Post Hoc test and Bonferroni adjustment ($n = 9$). (**f**) NO release after stimulation with 50 μM forskolin, 10 μM L-NIL, 10 μM A769662, or 10 μM dorsomorphin dihydrochloride (DoMo). Statistical differences vs. unstimulated cells, Wilcoxon signed-rank test ($n = 5$). (**g**) Representative Western blot of iNOS expression after stimulation with/without 0.1 ng/mL IL-1β, 50 μM forskolin, 10 μM A769662 and 10 μM dorsomorphin dihydrochloride. (**h**) Densitometric quantification of iNOS/Gapdh expression after stimulation with 0.1 ng/mL IL-1β, 10 μM A769662 or 10 μM dorsomorphin dihydrochloride normalized to unstimulated cells ($n = 6$). Statistic: Wilcoxon signed-rank test. Values are reported as mean or percentage ± SD. *** $p < 0.005$, ** $p < 0.01$ and * $p < 0.05$. DoMo: Dorsomorphin dihydrochloride.

Application of forskolin (50 µM), a cell-permeable activator of adenylyl cyclase increasing the intracellular level of cAMP, caused a significant decrease of IL-1β-induced NO production (Figure 1c, $p < 0.001$, Wilcoxon signed-rank test). The reduction of IL-1β-induced NO release by forskolin was on average to 62.7% (Figure 1d). Application of 8-Bromo-cAMP or PGE$_2$, which also induced an increase of intracellular cAMP, reduced the IL-1β-induced NO release on average to 71.9% or 71.0%, respectively (Figure 1d).

To test if the AMPK was involved in the regulation of IL-1β-induced NO release, co-applications of IL-1β with 10 µM A769662, an activator of AMPK, or of IL-1β with 10 µM dorsomorphin dihydrochloride, an inhibitor of AMPK, were performed. Activation of AMPK with A769662 resulted in a significant increase of IL-1β-induced NO release ($p < 0.001$, Wilcoxon signed-rank test with Bonferroni adjustment, Figure 1e). Vice versa, the AMPK-inhibitor dorsomorphin dihydrochloride completely prevented the IL-1β induced NO release to the level of the unstimulated control (Figure 1e).

We found a small basal release of NO. Forskolin or A769662 alone did not influence NO release (Figure 1f). L-NIL or dorsomorphin dihydrochloride alone slightly reduced the basal release of NO compared with the unstimulated control (Figure 1f, $p = 0.028$, Wilcoxon signed-rank test).

2.2. Impact on iNOS Protein Expression

Stimulation with 0.1 ng/mL IL-1β caused a significant upregulation of iNOS protein expression (Figure 1g–h, $p = 0.028$). Co-stimulation of IL-1β with the AMPK activator A769662 resulted in a strong increase of IL-1β-induced iNOS expression compared to IL-1β alone (Figure 1g–h, $p = 0.028$). Co-stimulation of IL-1β with the AMPK inhibitor dorsomorphin dihydrochloride resulted in a low basal iNOS expression comparable to the level of unstimulated cells (Figure 1g–h).

2.3. Impact of IL-1β on Mitochondrial Function

An application of 0.1 ng/mL IL-1β for 24 h resulted in a strong reduction of mitochondrial basal and maximal respiration as well as ATP production (Figure 2a, Wilcoxon signed-rank test with Bonferroni adjustment: All $p < 0.001$), and a significant increase of non-mitochondrial respiration ($p = 0.014$, Wilcoxon signed-rank test with Bonferroni adjustment, Figure 2a). After IL-1β stimulation, the basal mitochondrial respiration decreased to 61.2%, the maximal mitochondrial respiration to 53.4%, and the ATP production to 50.8% of the unstimulated control. However, the non-mitochondrial respiration increased to 128% of the unstimulated control.

Co-application of 0.1 ng/mL IL-1β and 10 µM L-NIL resulted in a complete recovery of mitochondrial function (Figure 2a). The mitochondrial basal respiration, maximal respiration, and ATP production of chondrocytes stimulated with IL-1β and L-NIL simultaneously significantly increased compared with the IL-1β-stimulated cells ($p < 0.001$, Wilcoxon signed-rank test with Bonferroni adjustment) and did not differ significantly from unstimulated cells.

Forskolin also prevented the IL-1β-induced impairment of mitochondrial function (Figure 2a). The values of the mitochondrial basal respiration, maximal respiration, and ATP production were not significantly different after simultaneous application of IL-1β and forskolin compared with unstimulated chondrocytes (Figure 2a). Only the IL-1β-induced increase of non-mitochondrial respiration remained elevated ($p < 0.001$, Wilcoxon signed-rank test with Bonferroni adjustment).

Forskolin alone did not show any influence on the mitochondrial or the non-mitochondrial respiration (Figure 2b). An application of L-NIL alone resulted in a slight but significant reduction of basal respiration (93.6% of unstimulated control, $p = 0.024$, Wilcoxon signed-rank test with Bonferroni adjustment) and maximal respiration (95.8% of unstimulated control, $p = 0.004$, Wilcoxon signed-rank test with Bonferroni adjustment). The ATP production and non-mitochondrial respiration were comparable to unstimulated cells.

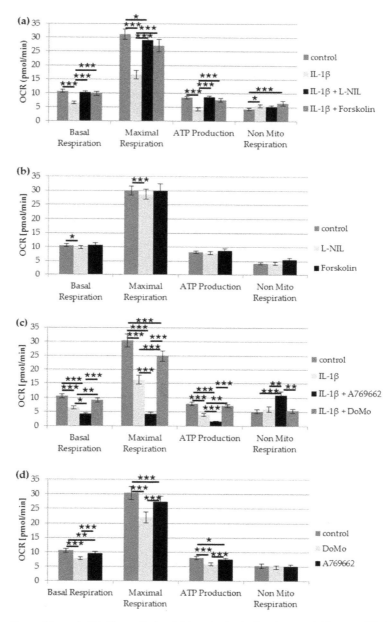

Figure 2. Impact of IL-1β on mitochondrial respiration in chondrocytes. (**a**) Impact of 50 μM forskolin and 10 μM L-NIL (iNOS inhibition) on IL-1β (0.1 ng/mL)-induced mitochondrial dysfunction; $n = 14$. (**b**) Control experiments on the impact of 50 μM forskolin ($n = 11$) and 10 μM L-NIL ($n = 13$) on mitochondrial function. (**c**) Impact of activation or inhibition of AMPK on IL-1β-induced mitochondrial dysfunction ($n = 12$). (**d**) Control experiments on the impact of 10 μM A769662 and 10 μM dorsomorphin dihydrochloride on mitochondrial function ($n = 12$). Statistic: Wilcoxon signed-rang test and Bonferroni adjustment. Values are reported as mean ± SD. *** $p < 0.005$, ** $p < 0.01$ and * $p < 0.05$. OCR: Oxygen consumption rate, DoMo: Dorsomorphin dihydrochloride.

Activation of AMPK with A769662 aggravated IL-1β-induced mitochondrial dysfunction (Figure 2c). Co-application of IL-1β and A769662 resulted in an additional reduction of basal mitochondrial respiration to 66.4% ($p = 0.015$), of maximal mitochondrial respiration to 26.0% ($p < 0.001$), and of ATP production to 39.6% ($p = 0.003$) of IL-1β stimulation alone (all Wilcoxon signed-rank test with Bonferroni adjustment, Figure 2c). The non-mitochondrial respiration increased to 181% of IL-1β-stimulated cells after co-stimulation with IL-1β and A769662 ($p < 0.001$, Wilcoxon signed-rank test with Bonferroni adjustment, Figure 2c). Compared to the unstimulated control, co-application of IL-1β and A769662 reduced the basal mitochondrial respiration to 41.3%, whereas A769662 alone only reduced the basal mitochondrial respiration to 90.6% of the unstimulated control (Figure 2c,d).

Co-application of IL-1β and the AMPK-inhibitor dorsomorphin dihydrochloride resulted in a significant improvement of IL-1β induced mitochondrial dysfunction (Figure 2c). The basal mitochondrial respiration increased to 139% ($p = 0.0059$), the maximal mitochondrial respiration to 153% ($p < 0.001$), and the ATP production to 178% ($p = 0.0059$) of IL-1β stimulation alone (all Wilcoxon signed-rank test with Bonferroni adjustment, Figure 2c). Compared to the unstimulated control, basal mitochondrial respiration, ATP production, and non-mitochondrial respiration were not significantly different after co-application of IL-1β and dorsomorphin dihydrochloride (Figure 2c), even though dorsomorphin dihydrochloride alone caused a significant reduction of basal (73.8%) and maximal mitochondrial respiration (72.4%) as well as ATP production (72.6%) (Figure 2d).

2.4. Effect of iNOS Inhibition by L-NIL on Other Mediators

To test whether the iNOS inhibitor L-NIL also affects IL-1β-induced production of other mediators, the release of IL-6, PGE$_2$, and MMP-3 was measured after co-stimulation of IL-1β and 10 µM L-NIL. Upon IL-1β stimulation, L-NIL had only minor effects on the release of IL-6, PGE$_2$, and MMP-3 (Figure 3a–c). In addition, the production and release of the cartilage matrix protein glycosaminoglycan were not affected by 10 µM L-NIL (Figure 3d). These data suggest that the effect of IL-1β on the release of IL-6, PGE$_2$, MMP3, and GAG did not involve NO.

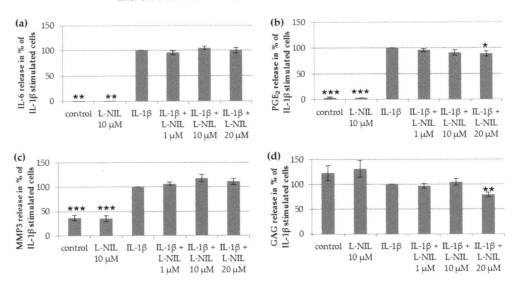

Figure 3. Impact of L-NIL on the IL-1β-induced release of (**a**) IL-6 ($n = 6$), (**b**) PGE$_2$ ($n = 5$), (**c**) MMP3 ($n = 7$), and (**d**) the production of GAG ($n = 6$). Values are reported as percentage ± SD normalized to IL-1β-stimulated cells. Statistical differences vs. IL-1β-stimulated cells, repeated-measures ANOVA with Post Hoc test; *** $p < 0.005$, ** $p < 0.01$ and * $p < 0.05$.

2.5. Impact of Mediators on Vitality of Chondrocytes

To control whether the observed effects were based on cytotoxic effects of the mediators used, an assay was performed to determine the percentage of living and dead chondrocytes after stimulation with different mediators. The percentage of dead cells did not change significantly after stimulation with IL-1β, forskolin, L-NIL, A769662, or dorsomorphin dihydrochloride (Figure 4). After stimulation with IL-1β and forskolin, the viability of chondrocytes was similar to the unstimulated control. L-NIL, A769662, and dorsomorphin dihydrochloride reduced the percentage of living cells slightly, but the observed effect of these mediators on NO release and mitochondrial function cannot be explained by these small effects on the viability. The cytotoxic dimethyl sulfoxide (DMSO) control (1:10) proved the validity of the test, while DMSO 1:200 had no effect.

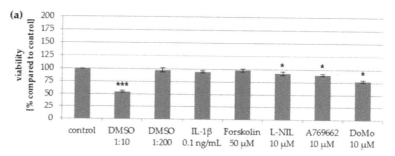

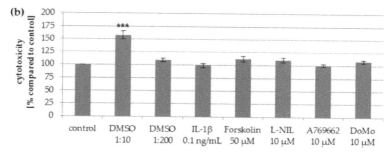

Figure 4. Impact of mediators used on (**a**) viability and (**b**) cytotoxicity of chondrocytes as measured by the LIVE/DEAD viability/cytotoxicity kit, which determines the percentage of living and dead cells. Viability and cytotoxicity values of treated cells are reported as percentage ± SD of control (unstimulated cells), set as 100%. Statistical differences vs. unstimulated cells, Wilcoxon signed-rank test, *** $p < 0.005$ and * $p < 0.05$. DoMo: Dorsomorphin dihydrochloride.

3. Discussion

The results of the current study provide evidence that increased NO production in human chondrocytes is responsible for IL-1β-induced mitochondrial impairment. Inhibition of iNOS by L-NIL prevented the IL-1β-induced reduction of mitochondrial respiration and ATP production. The application or induction of cAMP reduced the IL-1β-induced NO release and impairment of mitochondrial function. Furthermore, the results show that AMPK is an important regulator for the IL-1β-induced NO production in chondrocytes. The activation of AMPK increased the IL-β-induced NO release and, therefore, increased the negative impact of IL-1β on mitochondrial function. The inhibition of AMPK resulted in a strong reduction of NO release and prevented IL-1β-induced impairment of mitochondrial respiration.

Previous studies showed that both IL-1β and NO impaired the activity of respiratory chain enzyme complexes and thus affect mitochondrial function in normal human chondrocytes [6,20]. Therefore, it was supposed that IL-1β-induced NO production may be responsible for the IL-1β-induced mitochondrial dysfunction. Our data now reveal that the effects of IL-1β and NO on mitochondrial function are causally linked. First, the effects of IL-1β on NO release, mitochondrial respiration, and ATP production were prevented by the iNOS inhibitor L-NIL. Second, IL-1β enhanced iNOS expression and NO release in chondrocytes. Third, downregulation of IL-1β-induced NO release by cAMP or the AMPK inhibitor dorsomorphin dihydrochloride was accompanied by a significant improvement of IL-1β-induced mitochondrial impairment.

NO production and iNOS expression were shown to be modulated by cAMP, which activates protein kinases and regulates gene transcription via transcription factors such as CREB. Interestingly, it seems to depend on the cell type whether cAMP increases or decreases iNOS expression and NO production. In our experiment, the stimulation of cAMP synthesis in chondrocytes decreased IL-1β-induced NO production, similar as in hepatocytes and astrocytes, but in cardiac myocytes, macrophages, and vascular smooth muscle cells, NO production was enhanced by cAMP elevation [15,21]. The decrease of NO production by cAMP in hepatocytes and astrocytes was explained by decreasing iNOS mRNA expression, iNOS protein expression, and alteration of iNOS promoter activity. Here, we show for the first time that stimulation of cAMP production by forskolin prevents mitochondrial dysfunction induced by IL-1β, similar to iNOS inhibition, suggesting that the increase of cAMP protects against the negative effect of IL-1β on mitochondrial function by iNOS inhibition or reduced iNOS expression. Since cAMP elevation may also be caused by inflammatory mediators such as PGE_2, this mechanism may limit the mitochondrial impairment of IL-1β in the inflammatory setting.

Activation of AMPK can also influence iNOS activity. AMPK is an important energy-sensing molecule that can switch off ATP-consuming pathways and switch on pathways for ATP production. AMPK is activated by a high AMP/ATP ratio. The effect of AMPK on iNOS activation also depends on the cell type. In myocytes, adipocytes, and macrophages, pharmacological activation of AMPK significantly inhibited iNOS under pro-inflammatory conditions, primarily resulting from post-transcriptional regulation of the iNOS protein [22]. In hepatocytes, however, AMPK activation increased cytokine-induced iNOS expression and NO production [19]. In human chondrocytes, we found a significant increase of IL-1β-induced NO production and iNOS expression after AMPK activation by A769662, and a marked reduction of IL-1β-induced NO production and iNOS expression after AMPK inhibition by dorsomorphin dihydrochloride, thus resembling the effects in hepatocytes. Additionally, our data show that A769662 aggravates IL-1β-induced mitochondrial impairment, whereas dorsomorphin dihydrochloride prevents IL-1β-induced mitochondrial effects. Since the effect of A769662 on NO production and mitochondrial function in chondrocytes was only observed in combination with IL-1β, the mechanism by which AMPK regulates iNOS should be related to the IL-1β pathways. In primary hepatocytes, AMPK affected cytokine-induced NO production and iNOS expression through Akt, c-Jun N-terminal kinase, and NF-kB signaling pathways [19]. Given that the effects of AMPK in hepatocytes and chondrocytes seem to be similar, we assumed analogous regulatory pathways in chondrocytes. IL-1β reduces mitochondrial ATP production through NO production, therefore, it should activate the cytosolic AMPK. As activation of AMPK increased the IL-1β-mediated NO release in chondrocytes, a vicious circle may be produced if AMPK is not inhibited by other mechanisms. Such a mechanism could be the inhibition of phosphodiesterase (PDE), which hydrolyzes cAMP to AMP. Inhibition of AMP production by PDE inhibitors leads to reduced AMPK activity. In human OA chondrocytes, Tenor et al. found that inhibition of PDE4 decreased IL-1β-induced NO production by reducing iNOS protein expression [23], thus resembling the effect of AMPK inhibition observed in the present study. Importantly, our data show that the modulation of NO synthesis by AMPK signaling also affects IL-1β-induced mitochondrial impairment.

In addition to mitochondrial respiration, AMPK regulates glucose uptake and ROS production, protein synthesis, promotor activity, or receptor activity. Thus the AMPK mechanisms in chondrocytes should be further investigated to evaluate the impact on OA mechanisms.

Since chondrocytes mainly utilize glycolysis for ATP production, which does not involve mitochondrial activity, the relative importance of oxidative phosphorylation for ATP supply in chondrocytes has been discussed. However, several studies reported that mitochondrial dysfunction is involved in pathophysiological processes, which include oxidative stress, apoptosis, production of inflammatory mediators, matrix catabolism, and calcification of cartilage matrix [24]. Inhibition of mitochondrial respiratory complexes increased the expression of cyclooxygenase 2 and the level of PGE_2 in normal human chondrocytes [25] as well as the inflammatory responsiveness to cytokines [14]. Furthermore, mitochondrial dysfunction induced apoptosis by inducing ROS and mtDNA damage [24]. Thus, intact mitochondrial respiration is thought to be crucial for the homeostasis and survival of chondrocytes. Since NO induces mitochondrial dysfunction, the regulation of NO production and iNOS expression is of particular interest in this context.

While we identified significant negative NO effects on mitochondrial function, our data did not provide evidence that NO is critically involved in the IL-1β-induced production and release of IL-6, PGE_2, and MMP3. Besides the fact that PGE_2, IL-6, and MMP3 are important molecules in OA processes, several studies found that mitochondrial dysfunction affects the production of these mediators [14,24–26]. In human chondrocytes, mitochondrial dysfunction induced by inhibitors of mitochondrial complexes increased the production of PGE_2 and MMP3 [25,26] and the inflammatory response to IL-1β [14]. According to these studies, we expected a reduced release of IL-6, PGE_2, and MMP3 after incubation with L-NIL and prevention of NO-induced mitochondrial impairment. However, we found that the mediators PGE_2, IL-6, and MMP3 were significantly more released upon stimulation with IL-1β, but the IL-1β-induced release was not affected by L-NIL at concentrations that inhibited the effects of IL-1β on NO production, mitochondrial respiration, and ATP production. Thus, while IL-1β alone reduced mitochondrial function in a NO-dependent manner, this effect was not crucial for the IL-1β-induced release of IL-6, PGE_2, and MMP3 in our experiments. In the study of Vaamonde-Garcia et al., mitochondrial impairment induced by oligomycin alone already enhanced the basal release of pro-inflammatory mediators, oligomycin combined with IL-1β led to an additional increase of these mediators [14]. Thus the mitochondrial dysfunction was directly initiated by inhibitors additionally to the IL-1β-induced mitochondrial impairment. It seems that mitochondrial dysfunction induced by inhibitors of mitochondrial respiration chain complexes results in a slightly different reaction compared to the inhibitory effect of NO on mitochondrial respiration. In addition, anti-inflammatory effects of NO in chondrocytes were described in the literature. In one study, inhibition of NO synthesis enhanced the IL-1β-induced IL-6 and PGE_2 production [27]. Concerning the different mentioned effects of NO and inhibitors, several pathways might converge on mitochondrial respiration and result in different responsiveness to cytokines.

Some limitations of this study should be noted. We did not observe the negative effects of IL-1β on the vitality of chondrocytes upon exposure to IL-1β for two days. Thus mitochondrial dysfunction by IL-1β may not cause rapid cell death. Our study showed putative mechanisms that may protect against IL-1β-induced mitochondrial malfunction. Induction of apoptosis and cytotoxic effects may be observed after a longer stimulation period or higher IL-1β concentrations. Concerning modulation of mitochondrial function by cAMP and AMPK, most experiments were performed with a single concentration of the used mediators according to preliminary experiments and literature. The described effects of cAMP and AMPK could be stronger or weaker with other concentrations or incubation times. In general, in-vitro models presumably do not reflect exactly the in-vivo situation in OA cartilage, but chondrocytes cultured in the monolayer are the most widely used in-vitro model to study the effect of cytokines on molecular pathways of chondrocytes [28].

In summary, our data demonstrate the importance of NO for the IL-1β-induced negative effects on the mitochondrial function in chondrocytes. It supports the concept that inhibition of iNOS could be a beneficial treatment of OA. Treatment with iNOS inhibitors showed chondroprotective effects in animal and human studies [10] and significantly reduced OA progression in an experimental animal model [29]. The chondroprotective effects of iNOS inhibition may result at least in part from the reduction of mitochondrial dysfunction induced by IL-1β.

4. Materials and Methods

4.1. Reagents/Solutions

Human IL-1β was purchased from PeproTech (Rocky Hill, NJ, USA). N^6-(1-iminoethyl)-L-lysine hydrochloride (L-NIL), forskolin, 8-Bromoadenosine-3′,5′-cyclic monophosphate sodium salt (8-Bromo-cAMP), dorsomorphin dihydrochloride, and A769662 were all purchased from Tocris Bioscience (Bristol, UK). Forskolin and A769662 were dissolved in DMSO/water (final DMSO dilution 1:200 and 1:5000, respectively), all other substances were dissolved in water. PGE_2 was from Cayman Chemical (Ann Arbor, MI, USA) and was dissolved in DMSO/water (final DMSO dilution 1:5000). Pronase E was obtained from Merck KGaA (Darmstadt, Germany), and collagenase P from Roche Diagnostics GmbH (Mannheim, Germany). The chondrocytes culture medium contains Chondrocyte Basal Medium + 10% Chondrocyte Growth Medium SupplementMix (both from PromoCell GmbH, Heidelberg, Germany) + 1% Penicillin/Streptomycin Solution (Life Technologies Europe BV, NN Bleiswijk, Netherlands).

4.2. Isolation of Human Chondrocytes

Human chondrocytes were obtained from 37 patients (16 female/21 male) with end-stage knee OA who underwent knee replacement surgery. Patients were on average 63.6 years old (±10.1 years, standard deviation). Patients were informed about the purpose of tissue sampling and gave written consent after the nature of all examinations was fully explained. The study was approved by the Ethical Committee for Clinical Trials of the Friedrich-Schiller-University of Jena (ethic approval code: 3966-12/13; date of approval: 23 January 2014) and performed in accordance with the Declaration of Helsinki.

Directly after surgical removal of the condyles, cartilage was removed from the condyles and was cut into small pieces. Cartilage was treated with 0.01 mg/mL pronase E in Dulbecco's modified Eagles's medium (DMEM) for 30 min at 37 °C following collagenase P (1.3 mg/mL in chondrocyte culture medium) for 16 h at 37 °C. The cells were filtrated, washed, and seeded in cell culture plates.

4.3. Experiments on Release of Mediators

For release experiments, the chondrocytes were plated on 24-well culture plates at a density of 4×10^5 cells/cm^2 and cultured in the chondrocyte culture medium. After 3 days of incubation, the medium was renewed. After an additional 2 days, the cells were stimulated with IL-1β (10–0.01 ng/mL) and the iNOS inhibitor L-NIL (1, 10, and 20 μM) at different concentrations for 48 h to determine the lowest efficient concentration. After preliminary experiments with different concentrations of all mediators in combination with IL-1β, we stimulated the chondrocytes in the final experiments with 50 μM forskolin, 10 μg/mL PGE_2, 50 μM 8-Bromo-cAMP, 10 μM L-NIL, 10 μM A769662 (an activator of AMPK), and 10 μM dorsomorphin dihydrochloride (an inhibitor of AMPK) alone or in combination with IL-1β for 48 h. The supernatant of all experiments was collected and stored at −80 °C until use. The cells were plated in duplicate for each condition. Experiments were performed with a minimum of 5 biological replicates (donors) to ensure reproducibility.

Griess assay: Concentration of nitrite in the supernatant was measured using the Griess Reagent Kit (#G7921, Invitrogen, Thermo Fisher Scientific Inc., Darmstadt, Germany,) according to manufacturer's instruction and used as an indicator for NO synthesis of the cultured chondrocytes.

Measurements of IL-6, PGE_2, and MMP-3: Concentrations of IL-6, PGE_2, and MMP-3 in the supernatant were measured by ELISA using IL-6 human uncoated ELISA Kit (#88-7066-22,

Invitrogen), Prostaglandin E_2 ELISA (DRG Instruments, Marburg, Germany, #EIA-5811), and RayBio human MMP-3 ELISA Kit (RayBiotech Inc., Norcross, GA, USA, #ELH-MMP3-5).

Measurement of GAG: The amount of glycosaminoglycan (GAG) was measured spectrophotometrically using 1,9-dimethylmethylene blue (DMB, Sigma-Aldrich, Taufkirchen, Germany). A standard curve of bovine chondroitin sulfate (Sigma-Aldrich) was generated to calculate the GAG concentration.

4.4. Vitality of Chondrocytes

Chondrocytes were plated on 96-well culture plates at a density of 4×10^5 cells/cm^2. The cells were cultured and stimulated as described above. For testing the impact of mediators used on the viability of chondrocytes, the LIVE/DEAD Viability/Cytotoxicity Kit from Invitrogen (#L3224) was performed according to the manufacturer's instruction. The assay determined the percentage of living and dead cells after stimulation with different mediators.

4.5. Measurement of Mitochondrial Function

Functional parameters of mitochondrial respiration were measured with the Seahorse XF Cell Mito Stress Test Kit using the Seahorse XF Analyzer (Agilent, Santa Clara, CA, USA). The assay included modulators of mitochondrial respiration to measure basal respiration, ATP-linked respiration, maximal respiration, and non-mitochondrial respiration. These functional parameters were calculated by measuring the oxygen consumption rate (OCR) of the cultured chondrocytes using the data analysis tool Seahorse XF Report Generator (Agilent). Oligomycin, carbonyl cyanide-4 (trifluoromethoxy) phenylhydrazone (FCCP), and antimycin A/rotenone were sequentially injected to modulate the mitochondrial respiration.

For this purpose, chondrocytes were plated on Seahorse cell culture plates at a density of 3×10^4 cells/well and cultured in chondrocytes culture medium for 6 days at 37 °C. Thereafter, cells were stimulated with 0.1 ng/mL IL-1β, 50 μM forskolin, 10 μM L-NIL, 10 μM A769662, and 10 μM dorsomorphin dihydrochloride for 24 h. The cells were plated with 8 repetitions for each combination of stimulation. Experiments were performed with a minimum of 5 biological replicates (donors) to ensure reproducibility.

4.6. Western Blot

Isolated chondrocytes were plated on 12-well culture plates at a density of 4×10^5 cells/cm^2. The cells were cultured and stimulated as described above. Chondrocytes were lysed on ice using RIPA lysis buffer (catalog #9806, Cell Signaling, Danvers; MA, USA) freshly supplemented with protease inhibitor cocktail tables (Roche, Mannheim, Germany), transferred in Eppendorf tubes, and frozen at −80 °C. After a freeze-thaw cycle, cell lysates were centrifuged at $15,000 \times g$ for 10 min to remove cellular debris. Protein extracts were mixed with Laemmli-buffer and separated on 10% polyacrylamide gels at 125 V and transferred to a polyvinylidene difluoride membrane (Millipore, Billerica, MA, USA).

Immunoblotting was performed with antibodies against iNOS (Invitrogen, catalog #PA1-036) and Gapdh (Sigma Aldrich, catalog #G8795) at 4 °C overnight following incubation with HRP-linked secondary antibodies (KPL, Gaithersburg, MD, USA). Protein signals were visualized with a chemiluminescence reaction reagent (catalog #34075, Thermo Scientific, Waltham, MA, USA) according to the manufacturer's instruction using a CCD camera system (Synoptics, Cambridge, UK). Densitometry of Western blot images was performed using NIH Image J software (available under: https://imagej.nih.gov/ij/, accessed on 1 January 2021).

4.7. Statistical Analysis

For statistical analyses, the software SPSS statistics 21 (SPSS, Inc, Chicago, IL, USA) was used. Results were expressed as means ± SEM or percent of control. For multiple sample comparison repeated-measures one-way analysis of variance or Friedman test were performed followed by a paired Student's test or Wilcoxon signed-rank test, when appropriate. When required, Bonferroni adjustment was performed for multiple comparisons. Significance was accepted at $p < 0.05$.

5. Conclusions

The results of the current study show that NO is critically involved in the IL-1β-induced mitochondrial dysfunction in human OA chondrocytes. Inhibition of NO production by iNOS inhibitor, cAMP elevation, or AMPK inhibition prevented the IL-1β-induced negative effects on the mitochondrial function. Thus our study supports the idea that treatment with iNOS inhibitors may be chondroprotective by acting against pathogenic IL-1β-effects on mitochondrial function.

Author Contributions: Conceptualization, A.E. and H.-G.S.; methodology, A.E., A.W., C.K. and S.M.; resources, A.W., R.R., S.M., T.K., G.O.H., H.-G.S.; analysis, A.E., C.K, S.M., T.K.; writing—original draft preparation, A.E., H.-G.S., C.K.; writing—review and editing, A.E., G.O.H., T.K., H.-G.S.; supervision, G.O.H., H.-G.S.; project administration, G.O.H., H.-G.S.; funding acquisition, A.E., G.O.H., H.-G.S. All authors have read and agreed to the published version of the manuscript.

Funding: Christian König was supported by the Deutsche Forschungsgemeinschaft (grant numbers: SCHA 404/18-1, EI 1172/2-1). We acknowledge support by the German Research Foundation and the Open Access Publication Fund of the Thueringer Universitaet-und Landesbibliothek Jena Projekt Nr. 433052568.

Institutional Review Board Statement: The study was conducted according to the guidelines of the Declaration of Helsinki, and approved by the Ethics Committee for Clinical Trials of the Friedrich-Schiller-University of Jena (ethic approval code: 3966-12/13; date of approval: 23 January 2014).

Informed Consent Statement: Informed consent was obtained from all patients involved in the study.

Acknowledgments: The authors thank Birgit Lemser for excellent technical support, Thomas Lehmann from the Institute of Medical Statistics, Computer Sciences, and Documentation (Jena University Hospital) for excellent advice in biostatistics and Britt Wildemann for careful review of the final manuscript.

Conflicts of Interest: The authors declare no conflict of interest.

References

1. Goldring, M.B.; Otero, M. Inflammation in osteoarthritis. *Curr. Opin. Rheumatol.* **2011**, *23*, 471–478. [CrossRef] [PubMed]
2. Jenei-Lanzl, Z.; Meurer, A.; Zaucke, F. Interleukin-1β signaling in osteoarthritis–chondrocytes in focus. *Cell. Signal.* **2019**, *53*, 212–223. [CrossRef]
3. Blanco, F.J.; Lopez-Armada, M.J.; Maneiro, E. Mitochondrial dysfunction in osteoarthritis. *Mitochondrion* **2004**, *4*, 715–728. [CrossRef]
4. Maneiro, E.; Martin, M.A.; de Andres, M.C.; Lopez-Armada, M.J.; Fernandez-Sueiro, J.L.; del Hoyo, P.; Galdo, F.; Arenas, J.; Blanco, F.J. Mitochondrial respiratory activity is altered in osteoarthritic human articular chondrocytes. *Arthritis Rheum.* **2003**, *48*, 700–708. [CrossRef] [PubMed]
5. Wu, L.; Liu, H.; Li, L.; Cheng, Q.; Li, H.; Huang, H. Mitochondrial pathology in osteoarthritic chondrocytes. *Curr. Drug Targets* **2014**, *15*, 710–719. [CrossRef] [PubMed]
6. López-Armada, M.J.; Caramés, B.; Martín, M.A.; Cillero-Pastor, B.; Lires-Dean, M.; Fuentes-Boquete, I.; Arenas, J.; Blanco, F.J. Mitochondrial activity is modulated by TNFα and IL-1β in normal human chondrocyte cells. *Osteoarthr. Cartil.* **2006**, *14*, 1011–1022. [CrossRef]
7. Grabowski, P.S.; Wright, P.K.; Van't Hof, R.J.; Helfrich, M.H.; Ohshima, H.; Ralston, S.H. Immunolocalization of inducible nitric oxide synthase in synovium and cartilage in rheumatoid arthritis and osteoarthritis. *Br. J. Rheumatol.* **1997**, *36*, 651–655. [CrossRef] [PubMed]
8. Hancock, C.M.; Riegger-Krugh, C. Modulation of pain in osteoarthritis: The role of nitric oxide. *Clin. J. Pain* **2008**, *24*, 353–365. [CrossRef]
9. Abramson, S.B. Nitric oxide in inflammation and pain associated with osteoarthritis. *Arthritis Res. Ther.* **2008**, *10*, S2. [CrossRef] [PubMed]
10. Leonidou, A.; Lepetsos, P.; Mintzas, M.; Kenanidis, E.; Macheras, G.; Tzetis, M.; Potoupnis, M.; Tsiridis, E. Inducible nitric oxide synthase as a target for osteoarthritis treatment. *Expert Opin. Ther. Targets* **2018**, *22*, 299–318. [CrossRef]
11. Vuolteenaho, K.; Moilanen, T.; Al-Saffar, N.; Knowles, R.G.; Moilanen, E. Regulation of the nitric oxide production resulting from the glucocorticoid-insensitive expression of iNOS in human osteoarthritic cartilage. *Osteoarthr. Cartil.* **2001**, *9*, 597–605. [CrossRef]

12. Vuolteenaho, K.; Moilanen, T.; Jalonen, U.; Lahti, A.; Nieminen, R.; van Beuningen, H.M.; van der Kraan, P.M.; Moilanen, E. TGFbeta inhibits IL-1 -induced iNOS expression and NO production in immortalized chondrocytes. *Inflamm. Res.* **2005**, *54*, 420–427. [CrossRef]

13. Moncada, S.; Erusalimsky, J.D. Does nitric oxide modulate mitochondrial energy generation and apoptosis? *Nat. Rev. Mol. Cell Biol.* **2002**, *3*, 214–220. [CrossRef]

14. Vaamonde-Garcia, C.; Riveiro-Naveira, R.R.; Valcarcel-Ares, M.N.; Hermida-Carballo, L.; Blanco, F.J.; Lopez-Armada, M.J. Mitochondrial dysfunction increases inflammatory responsiveness to cytokines in normal human chondrocytes. *Arthritis Rheum.* **2012**, *64*, 2927–2936. [CrossRef]

15. Pahan, K.; Namboodiri, A.M.; Sheikh, F.G.; Smith, B.T.; Singh, I. Increasing cAMP attenuates induction of inducible nitric-oxide synthase in rat primary astrocytes. *J. Biol. Chem.* **1997**, *272*, 7786–7791. [CrossRef] [PubMed]

16. Zhang, B.; Perpetua, M.; Fulmer, M.; Harbrecht, B.G. JNK signaling involved in the effects of cyclic AMP on IL-1beta plus IFNgamma-induced inducible nitric oxide synthase expression in hepatocytes. *Cell. Signal.* **2004**, *16*, 837–846. [CrossRef] [PubMed]

17. Grahame Hardie, D. AMP-activated protein kinase: A key regulator of energy balance with many roles in human disease. *J. Intern. Med.* **2014**, *276*, 543–559. [CrossRef] [PubMed]

18. Mancini, S.J.; White, A.D.; Bijland, S.; Rutherford, C.; Graham, D.; Richter, E.A.; Viollet, B.; Touyz, R.M.; Palmer, T.M.; Salt, I.P. Activation of AMP-activated protein kinase rapidly suppresses multiple pro-inflammatory pathways in adipocytes including IL-1 receptor-associated kinase-4 phosphorylation. *Mol. Cell. Endocrinol.* **2017**, *440*, 44–56. [CrossRef]

19. Zhang, B.; Lakshmanan, J.; Du, Y.; Smith, J.W.; Harbrecht, B.G. Cell-specific regulation of iNOS by AMP-activated protein kinase in primary rat hepatocytes. *J. Surg. Res.* **2018**, *221*, 104–112. [CrossRef]

20. Maneiro, E.; Lopez-Armada, M.J.; de Andres, M.C.; Carames, B.; Martin, M.A.; Bonilla, A.; Del Hoyo, P.; Galdo, F.; Arenas, J.; Blanco, F.J. Effect of nitric oxide on mitochondrial respiratory activity of human articular chondrocytes. *Ann. Rheum. Dis.* **2005**, *64*, 388–395. [CrossRef] [PubMed]

21. Harbrecht, B.G.; Taylor, B.S.; Xu, Z.; Ramalakshmi, S.; Ganster, R.W.; Geller, D.A. cAMP inhibits inducible nitric oxide synthase expression and NF-kappaB-binding activity in cultured rat hepatocytes. *J. Surg. Res.* **2001**, *99*, 258–264. [CrossRef] [PubMed]

22. Pilon, G.; Dallaire, P.; Marette, A. Inhibition of inducible nitric-oxide synthase by activators of AMP-activated protein kinase: A new mechanism of action of insulin-sensitizing drugs. *J. Biol. Chem.* **2004**, *279*, 20767–20774. [CrossRef]

23. Tenor, H.; Hedbom, E.; Hauselmann, H.J.; Schudt, C.; Hatzelmann, A. Phosphodiesterase isoenzyme families in human osteoarthritis chondrocytes–functional importance of phosphodiesterase 4. *Br. J. Pharmacol.* **2002**, *135*, 609–618. [CrossRef]

24. Blanco, F.J.; Rego, I.; Ruiz-Romero, C. The role of mitochondria in osteoarthritis. *Nat. Rev. Rheumatol.* **2011**, *7*, 161–169. [CrossRef] [PubMed]

25. Cillero-Pastor, B.; Caramés, B.; Lires-Deán, M.; Vaamonde-García, C.; Blanco, F.J.; López-Armada, M.J. Mitochondrial dysfunction activates cyclooxygenase 2 expression in cultured normal human chondrocytes. *Arthritis Rheum.* **2008**, *58*, 2409–2419. [CrossRef]

26. Cillero-Pastor, B.; Rego-Pérez, I.; Oreiro, N.; Fernandez-Lopez, C.; Blanco, F.J. Mitochondrial respiratory chain dysfunction modulates metalloproteases -1, -3 and -13 in human normal chondrocytes in culture. *BMC Musculoskelet. Disord.* **2013**, *14*, 235. [CrossRef]

27. Henrotin, Y.E.; Zheng, S.X.; Deby, G.P.; Labasse, A.H.; Crielaard, J.M.; Reginster, J.Y. Nitric oxide downregulates interleukin 1beta (IL-1beta) stimulated IL-6, IL-8, and prostaglandin E2 production by human chondrocytes. *J. Rheumatol.* **1998**, *25*, 1595–1601.

28. Johnson, C.I.; Argyle, D.J.; Clements, D.N. In vitro models for the study of osteoarthritis. *Vet. J.* **2016**, *209*, 40–49. [CrossRef] [PubMed]

29. Pelletier, J.P.; Jovanovic, D.V.; Lascau-Coman, V.; Fernandes, J.C.; Manning, P.T.; Connor, J.R.; Currie, M.G.; Martel-Pelletier, J. Selective inhibition of inducible nitric oxide synthase reduces progression of experimental osteoarthritis in vivo: Possible link with the reduction in chondrocyte apoptosis and caspase 3 level. *Arthritis Rheum.* **2000**, *43*, 1290–1299. [CrossRef]

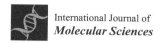

International Journal of
Molecular Sciences

MDPI

Review

Overview of MMP-13 as a Promising Target for the Treatment of Osteoarthritis

Qichan Hu and Melanie Ecker *

Department of Biomedical Engineering, University of North Texas, Denton, TX 76203, USA;
QichanHu@my.unt.edu
* Correspondence: melanie.ecker@unt.edu

Abstract: Osteoarthritis (OA) is a common degenerative disease characterized by the destruction of articular cartilage and chronic inflammation of surrounding tissues. Matrix metalloproteinase-13 (MMP-13) is the primary MMP involved in cartilage degradation through its particular ability to cleave type II collagen. Hence, it is an attractive target for the treatment of OA. However, the detailed molecular mechanisms of OA initiation and progression remain elusive, and, currently, there are no interventions available to restore degraded cartilage. This review fully illustrates the involvement of MMP-13 in the initiation and progression of OA through the regulation of MMP-13 activity at the molecular and epigenetic levels, as well as the strategies that have been employed against MMP-13. The aim of this review is to identify MMP-13 as an attractive target for inhibitor development in the treatment of OA.

Keywords: osteoarthritis; cartilage; type II collagen; matrix metalloproteinases; MMP-13; regulation; inhibitor

Citation: Hu, Q.; Ecker, M. Overview of MMP-13 as a Promising Target for the Treatment of Osteoarthritis. *Int. J. Mol. Sci.* **2021**, *22*, 1742. https://doi.org/10.3390/ijms22041742

Academic Editor: Nicola Veronese
Received: 8 January 2021
Accepted: 4 February 2021
Published: 9 February 2021

Publisher's Note: MDPI stays neutral with regard to jurisdictional claims in published maps and institutional affiliations.

1. Introduction

Osteoarthritis (OA) is one of the most common degenerative joint diseases primarily among the elderly who exhibit typical clinical symptoms such as joint pain, swelling, stiffness, and restricted movement. This may lead to decreased productivity and quality of life among the patients, in addition to an increased socioeconomic burden to the patients and the society as a whole [1,2]. According to the statistics from 2017, over 303 million people worldwide suffer from OA, which makes this disease a non-negligible subject [3].

The specific cause of OA remains elusive. Still, multiple risk factors contribute to the development of OA, including traumatic knee injury, obesity, genetic predisposition, abnormal mechanical stress, and other inflammation caused by infection or surgery, in addition to aging (Figure 1) [4–6]. Recent research has indicated that OA affects the joints' entire structures, including articular cartilage, subchondral bone, synovial membrane, intra-articular fat pads and intraarticular supporting fibrocartilaginous structures (e.g., menisci), particularly those in the knees, hands, and hips [7–10]. The common structural characteristics of OA are chronic inflammation, progressive destruction of articular cartilage, and subchondral bone sclerosis, especially, the irreversible degradation of articular cartilage is central in the pathological process of OA [11].

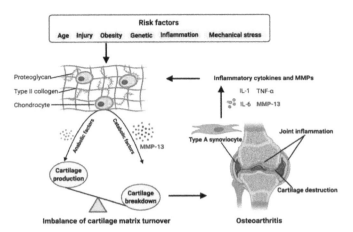

Figure 1. Role of matrix metalloproteinase-13 (MMP-13) in osteoarthritis (OA) pathogenesis. When some OA risk factors lead to increased expression of chondrocytes' catabolic factors, like MMP-13, the balance tips toward a net loss of cartilage. MMP-13 is the primary catabolic factor involved in cartilage degradation through its particular ability to cleave type II collagen. The breakdown products of cartilage stimulate the type A synoviocytes to release inflammatory cytokines and MMPs, like tumor necrosis factor alpha (TNF-α), interleukin (IL)-1, IL-6, and MMP-13, which, in turn, enhance a more comparable catabolic effect on chondrocyte metabolism, accelerating the progression of OA. Created with BioRender.com.

Articular cartilage is a thin layer of connective tissue composed of chondrocytes and extracellular matrix (ECM) without blood vessels. It has a four-layered structure, including the superficial, middle, deep, and calcified cartilage zones, with a sparse distribution of chondrocytes in the ECM of various zones [12]. The ECM is primarily composed of proteoglycans and collagens, and other less-abundant components, such as elastin, gelatin, and matrix glycoproteins [13]. Type II collagen is the major structural protein of cartilage, forming a network structure of ECM with aggrecan and other proteoglycans tangled within it [14]. The regular turnover of these matrix components is very slow and mediated by the chondrocytes, which synthesize these components and the proteolytic enzymes responsible for their breakdown [15]. The balance between anabolism and catabolism in articular cartilage is regulated by a complex network of factors, but it is mainly maintained by MMPs and its endogenous tissue inhibitors of metalloproteinases (TIMPs) [16]. MMP-13 (collagenase 3) is the key enzyme in the cleavage of type II collagen and plays a pivotal role in the breakdown of cartilage in osteoarthritic joints [17].

As shown in Figure 1, risk factors may cause an increased expression of both, anabolic and catabolic factors. However, the catabolic factors increase much more than anabolic factors, causing a disbalance. For example, the chondrocytes secret more MMP-13, resulting in enhanced degradation of ECM, leading to the balance tips toward a net loss of cartilage [18]. The breakdown products of cartilage are released into the synovial fluid and phagocytized by resident macrophages, such as type A synoviocytes containing vacuoles related to phagocytic function [17,19,20]. When the production of these decomposing particles exceeds the system's ability to eliminate them, they become mediators of inflammation. The exposition of digested material through the major histocompatibility complex class I and class II make the type A synoviocytes dialogue with the lymphocytes through their T cell receptors. The invading T cells in the synovial cavity stimulate type A synoviocytes into an inflammatory state, producing various inflammatory cytokines and MMPs, like TNF-α, IL-1, IL-6, and MMP-13, which, in turn, enhance a more comparable catabolic effect on chondrocyte metabolism, accelerating the progression of OA [20]. Several signaling pathways are involved in regulating catabolic events in OA, including nuclear factor kappa-light-chain-enhancer of activated B cells (NF-κB), phosphoinositide 3-kinase/protein kinase B (PI3K/AKT), mitogen-activated protein kinase (MAPK), and others, which modulate the expression of cytokines, chemokines, and matrix-degrading enzymes [21].

Currently, there is no effective treatment to reverse the destructive process of articular cartilage. Thus, the treatment is limited to symptom-relieving approaches involving medications, physical and occupational therapy, and surgical procedures [22]. These treatments aim to relieve pain, maintain joint flexibility, improve joint function and quality of life, and to slow down the disease's progression. However, there are many side effects associated with these conventional approaches. For example, the damage to liver, kidney, and cardiovascular system with long-term use of acetaminophen and non-steroidal anti-inflammatory drugs (NSAIDs) [23], and the risk of reoperation for infectious complications after arthroplasty [24]. Other novel treatments have also been extensively studied, like low-dose radiation [25] and intra-articular injection, including agonist for the transient receptor potential cation channel subfamily V member 1 (e.g., Capsaicin) [26], IL-1α/β dual variable domain immunoglobulin (e.g., Lutikizumab) [27], a humanized monoclonal antibody (e.g., Galcanezumab) [28], and regenerative medicine (e.g., platelet-rich plasma or mesenchymal stem cell) [29,30]. However, these treatments are limited to clinical trials with no or inadequate efficacy.

To overcome current limitations and improve patient outcome, there is an urgent requirement to develop effective therapies that have fewer side effects for OA. A large body of studies revolved around generating and evaluating chemical inhibitors of MMPs, which have shown to inhibit the destruction of cartilage in some animal models of OA [31]. However, owing to the high degree of structural similarity across their active sites, many MMP inhibitors have failed in clinical trials due to low selectivity and side effects [32]. Given this, pharmaceutical research has mainly focused on discovering potent inhibitors of MMP-13 displaying a high degree of selectivity over other MMPs [33].

In this review, the databases used were PubMed and Google Scholar with appropriate keywords (osteoarthritis, pathogenesis, cartilage degradation, MMP-13, epigenetic regulation, and synthetic inhibitor). Overall, approximately 2000 references were initially identified from 2000 until 2020. After the initial screening of titles and abstracts, the articles without mentioning MMP-13 were excluded. We analyzed the included literature to get a comprehensive overview of OA pathogenesis and possible biomarkers and target molecules for OA treatment. Subsequently, determine the topic and component issues. Additional information retrieval was also made when it comes to specific problems.

2. Basic Aspects of MMP-13

2.1. Structure

MMPs are a family of zinc-dependent proteolytic enzymes responsible for the cleavage of a variety of ECM proteins [34]. They are mainly classified into collagenases (MMP-1, -8, -13, and -18), gelatinases (MMP-2 and -9), membrane-type MMPs (MMP-14, -15, -16, -17, -24, and -25) and others (MMP-7, -12, -19, -20, -23, -26, and -28) [35]. MMPs are multi-domain proteins with a highly conserved signal peptide, a propeptide domain, and a catalytic domain. Except for MMP-7, -23, and -26, all MMPs also contain a proline-rich hinge region and a C-terminal hemopexin-like domain [36]. As shown in Figure 2, the spherical catalytic domains share the same structural organization: three α-helixes, five β-sheets, connected by eight loops. Additionally, they contain a catalytic zinc ion coordinated by three histidine residues, a structural zinc ion, and three structural calcium ions required for enzyme stability [37]. The specificity of the MMP-substrate interaction depends on specific subsites or pockets (S) within the MMP molecule that interacts with corresponding substituents (P) in the substrate. The pockets localized on both sides of the catalytic zinc ion (Left: S1, S2, S3, ... Sn; Right: S1', S2', S3', ... Sn') confer binding specificity to the substrate P1, P2, P3, ... Pn and primed P1', P2', P3', ... Pn' substituents, respectively [38]. Of these pockets, the S1' is the most variable in both the amino acid makeup and depth of the pocket [39]. The S1' pocket may be shallow (e.g., MMP-1 and MMP-7), intermediate (e.g., MMP-2, MMP-8 and MMP-9), or deep (e.g., MMP-3, MMP-11, MMP-12, MMP-13 and MMP-14) [40,41]. The large hydrophobic S1′ pocket of MMP-13 has a highly flexible "S1′ specificity loop (Ω-loop)" consisting of residues 245–253, which has been suggested to be a determining factor for the selective binding of inhibitors of MMP-13 [42].

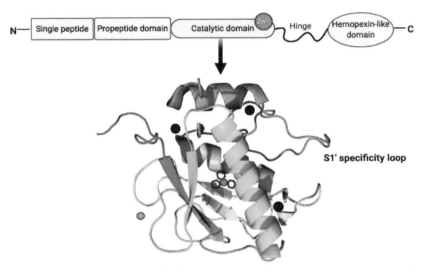

Figure 2. Structure of MMP-13. MMP-13 typically consists of a highly conserved signal peptide, a propeptide domain, a catalytic domain, a proline-rich hinge region, and a C-terminal hemopexin-like domain. The catalytic domain of MMP-13 is represented by the crystal structure. The structural zinc ion is in green, the catalytic zinc ion is in magenta, and three calcium ions are in dark grey. Three histidine residues in black sticks coordinate the catalytic zinc ion. The highly flexible S1′ specificity loop as part of hydrophobic S1′ pocket is a determining factor for the selective inhibitors of MMP-13. Created with BioRender.com.

2.2. Zymogen Activation

MMPs are produced by various tissues and cells [43]. They are synthesized as inactive zymogens (pro-MMPs), and this inactive form is maintained by a "cysteine switch" motif PRCGXPD in which the cysteine residue coordinates with the Zn^{2+} in the catalytic domain [44]. Proteolytical activation of all pro-MMPs often takes place extracellularly through cleavage of their pro-domains by other MMPs and protease [45]. MMP-13 is produced as a 60 kDa precursor form (proMMP-13), which can be activated by MT1-MMP on the cell surface, more efficient in the presence of active MMP-2 [46]. Additionally, plasmin has been shown to activate proMMP-13 with the involvement of the urokinase-type plasminogen activator-plasmin cascade [47].

2.3. Role in OA

Most MMPs, including MMP-1, MMP-2, MMP-3, MMP-8, MMP-9, MMP-10, MMP-13, and MMP-14, are involved in the turnover of ECM and the associated destruction of articular cartilage in OA [48]. Still, the soluble collagenases, MMP-1, MMP-8, and MMP-13, are crucial for this destruction to occur, especially MMP-13 predominates [48]. The preferred substrate for MMP-13 is type II collagen, which is cleaved five times faster than collagen I, six times faster than collagen III, and more readily than by other collagenases [49]. Again, the importance of MMP-13 in type II collagen cleavage is supported by the destabilization of the medial meniscus (DMM) model of OA when performed in MMP-13$^{-/-}$ mice. In this model, MMP-13$^{-/-}$ mice showed less tibial cartilage erosion than wild-type mice at 8 weeks post-surgery [50]. Conversely, cartilage-restricted expression of a constitutively active MMP-13 in mice resulted in joint pathology of the kind observed in OA [51]. Thus, MMP-13 is particularly related to the degradation of articular cartilage in OA by aggressively breakdown of type II collagen. Though, as is mentioned, it is involved principally in the degradation of type II collagen, MMP-13 also targets other matrix molecules such as type I, III, IV, IX, X collagen, perlecan, osteonectin, and proteoglycan [52], and it is likely involved in matrix turnover in healthy cartilage.

3. Molecular Regulation of MMP-13

MMP-13 is a well-known key player in the pathology of early OA due to its capacity to directly or indirectly initiate the degradation of a wide range of downstream matrix and collagen components via its regulatory factors through specific signaling pathways [53]. These factors include endogenous inhibitors, transcriptional factors, promoters, growth factors, receptors, proteases, hormones, and others (Figure 3). They work together in the integrated network to regulate the activity of MMP-13 by triggering specific pathways.

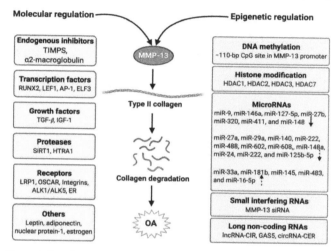

Figure 3. Regulation of MMP-13 in OA with the molecular and epigenetic mechanism. Molecular regulation involves endogenous inhibitors, transcription factors, growth factors, proteases, receptors, and other mediators. Epigenetic regulation contains DNA methylation, histone modification, and non-coding RNAs, which include microRNAs, small interfering RNAs, and long non-coding RNAs. The arrows in the microRNAs frame mean the miRNAs have different types of regulation (solid down-arrow: direct downregulation, dotted down-arrow: indirect downregulation, dotted up-arrow: indirect upregulation). Created with BioRender.com.

3.1. Endogenous Inhibitors

In normal physiology, MMPs are required for various processes such as tissue remodeling, embryonic development, angiogenesis, cell adhesion, and wound healing. Alterations in specific MMPs could lead to various pathological disorders. Therefore, MMP activity is constitutively regulated by endogenous inhibitors, such as tissue inhibitors of metalloproteinases (TIMPs) and α2-macroglobulin [54].

TIMPs (TIMP-1, TIMP-2, TIMP-3, and TIMP-4) are specific inhibitors that bind MMPs in a 1:1 stoichiometry. The overall shape of TIMP molecule is like a wedge, which slots into the active-site cleft of an MMP like that of the substrate. TIMPs inhibit all MMPs tested so far, except that TIMP-1 fails to inhibit MT1-MMP, MT2-MMP, MT3-MMP, and MT5-MMP [55]. They can hinder both activated MMPs and the conversion of pro-MMPs to activated MMPs, as well as regulate a variety of other cellular functions which may or may not directly involve MMPs [56]. TIMP-3, in particular, has been ascribed a chondroprotec-

Int. J. Mol. Sci. **2021**, 22, 1742

tive role in cartilage, which was demonstrated by TIMP-3$^{-/-}$ mice exhibiting increased cartilage collagen destruction [57]. The addition of exogenous TIMP-3 by intraarticular injection blocks cartilage breakdown in a rat meniscal tear model of OA mainly due to the potency against MMP-13 [58]. Although TIMP-3 is elevated in the cartilage of OA patients compared with normal cartilage, MMP-13 is increased more significantly than TIMP-3 [59]. Therefore, TIMP-3 is insufficient to regulate MMP-13 activity, resulting in the progression of OA.

In addition to endogenous TIMPs, α2-macroglobulin is another endogenous MMP inhibitor found in blood and tissue fluids. MMP activity is partly regulated by α2-macroglobulin and related proteins. Human α2-macroglobulin is a glycoprotein consisting of four identical subunits. α2-macroglobulin is a wide-spectrum proteinase inhibitor that inhibits most endopeptidases, including MMPs, by entrapping them within the macroglobulin. The complex is then rapidly internalized and cleared by endocytosis via low-density lipoprotein receptor-related protein-1 [60].

3.2. Transcription Factors

Runt-related transcription factor 2 (Runx2) is a crucial transcription factor associated with OA development [61]. Hirata et al. elucidated its molecular mechanism underlying the endochondral ossification during OA development with the compound knockout of C/EBPb (CCAAT/enhancer-binding protein-b) and Runx2 in mice, showing C/EBPb and RUNX2, with MMP-13 as the target and HIF-2α as the inducer, control cartilage degradation [62]. Lymphoid enhancer-binding factor 1 (LEF1) is a transcription factor primarily involved in the canonical Wnt/β-catenin signaling pathway to regulate MMP-13 expression in chondrocytes induced by IL-1 β [63]. It is accomplished by transactivating MMP-13 promoter activity through LEF1/β-catenin binding to the LEF1 binding site in the 3' region of the MMP-13 genomic locus. Moreover, the same group in another study showed that IL-1β stimulation increases physical interactions between the 3' region-bound LEF1 and promoter-bound transcription factors AP-1 or NF-kB, leading to synergistic upregulation of MMP-13 gene expression [64]. The E-74 like factor 3 (ELF3) is a transcription factor induced by proinflammatory factors in various cell types, including OA cartilage and synovium [65]. ELF3 directly controls MMP-13 promoter activity by targeting an E26 transformation-specific binding site enhanced by IL-1β stimulation in chondrocytes. Consistently, the IL-1β-induced MMP-13 expression is inhibited in primary human chondrocytes by siRNA-ELF3 knockdown and in chondrocytes from ELF3$^{-/-}$ mice, indicating that ELF3 as a procatabolic factor contributes to cartilage remodeling and degradation by regulating MMP-13 gene transcription [66]. Hairy and enhancer of split-1 (Hes1) is a transcription factor that is activated by Notch signaling. Sugita et al. reported that Hes1 is involved in the upregulation of expression of MMP-13 [67]. Hes1-knockout mice exhibited the suppression of cartilage destruction and decreased MMP-13 expression in a surgically induced OA model, suggesting that Hes1 acts through Notch-Hes1 signaling [67].

3.3. Growth Factors

Transforming growth factor-β (TGF-β) plays a critical role in the development, homeostasis, and repair of the cartilage. TGF-β sub-pathway have a protective function in articular cartilage, but the expected role is altered in human OA cartilage because the expression levels of TGF-β isoforms are negatively correlated with the expressions of main proteins in human cartilage, i.e., type II collagen and aggrecan [68]. The results are consistent with a strong correlation between expressions of TGFβ1 and MMP-13 in OA-affected cartilage that TGF-β can upregulate the levels of MMP13 primarily through the SMAD independent pathway, suggesting TGF-β switches from a protective role observed from in vitro studies to a negative factor in OA-affected cartilage [69]. Insulin-like growth factor-1 (IGF-1) is another biomarker associated with the production of cartilage matrix proteins and cell proliferation [70]. IGF-1 could induce enhancement of type II collagen and reduction in MMP-13 in rat endplate chondrocytes, but this regulation is through different signaling pathways. The PI3K pathway mainly transduces the IGF-1 effect on type II collagen expression, while the extracellular signal-regulated kinase (ERK) pathway mediates the IGF-1 inhibitory effect on MMP-13 expression [71].

3.4. Proteases

SIRT1 (Sirtuin 1) is a nicotinamide adenosine dinucleotide (NAD)-dependent deacetylase that removes acetyl groups from various proteins. Its activity is negatively correlated with increased expression of MMP-13 mediated by an intermediate factor LEF1 in human primary chondrocytes [72]. This effect was confirmed in the SIRT1 knockout mouse models of OA that SIRT1 repressed LEF1 protein expression, reducing LEF1 transcriptional activity, sequentially lifting its inhibitory effects on downstream MMP-13 expression in the articular cartilage [73]. Another study further exhibited that increased SIRT1 prevents apoptosis and ECM degradation in resveratrol-treated OA chondrocytes via the Wnt/β-catenin signaling pathways [74]. At the same time, LEF1 is a key mediator of the Wnt/β-catenin signaling pathway, which interacts with β-catenin to regulate Wnt target gene expression. MMP-13 is a target protein downstream of the Wnt/β-catenin signaling pathway [73]. These results suggest SIRT1 may downregulate MMP-13 in OA via Wnt/β-Catenin/LEF1 pathway. High-temperature requirement A1 (HTRA1), a serine protease, is strongly expressed in both human OA cartilage and the articular cartilage in mouse models of OA [75]. Once HTRA1 degrades the pericellular matrix components, including fibronectin, matrilin3, collagen oligomeric matrix protein, biglycan, fibromodulin, and type VI collagen, the membrane of the chondrocyte is exposed to the type II collagen, activating the transmembrane discoidin domain-containing receptor 2 (DDR2), a cell surface collagen receptor. DDR2 induces the upregulation of MMP-13 in response to its cartilage-specific ligand, type II collagen, which results in further degradation of the interterritorial matrix [76].

3.5. Receptors

Low-density lipoprotein (LDL) receptor-related protein 1 (LRP1) is a type I transmembrane cell surface receptor that can internalize extracellular proteins. It has been demonstrated that LRP1 is the major endocytic receptor of MMP-13 in human chondrocytes through directly binding to MMP-13 via hemopexin domain, mediating its internalization for subsequent lysosomal degradation [77]. This was supported by experiments in which the addition of receptor-associated protein (a ligand-binding antagonist for the LDL receptor family) or gene silencing of LRP1 markedly inhibited the cellular uptake of proMMP-13 from culture media. Osteoclast-associated receptor (OSCAR), an immunoglobulin-like collagen-recognition receptor, was reported increased during OA pathogenesis in human and mouse articular cartilages [78]. It was demonstrated that the inhibition of OSCAR activity by OSCAR deletion or treatments with human OSCAR-Fc fusion protein attenuates OA development. OSCAR deficiency resulted in downregulated expression of the ECM-degrading enzymes, such as MMP-3, MMP-13, and ADAMTS5 (a disintegrin and metalloproteinase with thrombospondin motifs 5), and upregulation of aggrecan and type II collagen. These results collectively suggest that OSCAR is involved in OA pathogenesis in mice and indirectly associated with the expression of MMP-13. Integrins are cell surface receptors that can bind cartilage ECM proteins to regulate cell proliferation, differentiation, and matrix remodeling [79]. For instance, the matrix protein fibronectin fragment (FN-f) stimulates chondrocytes to produce MMP-13 through binding with $\alpha 5 \beta 1$ integrins [80]. An increase in the specific MMP-cleavage of collagen type II is observed with age, accompanied by a corresponding upregulation of MMP-13 due to the increased anaplastic lymphoma kinase (ALK) ratio of ALK1/ALK5 with age [81]. In chondrocytes from aged and OA cartilage, the ratio of TGF-β receptor ALK1/ALK5 increases, leading to downregulation of the TGF-β pathway and shift from matrix synthesis activity to catabolic MMP expression [82]. These results indicate that the partial reason for enhanced collagen type II degradation by MMP-13 may be attributed to the increased ratio of ALK1/ALK5 with age. The sex hormone estrogen plays a critical role in OA pathogenesis in women over 50 years old or after menopause due to reduced estrogen levels. Estrogen receptor (ER) expressed in joint tissue and chondrocytes directly regulates some target genes' transcripts via DNA binding. MMP-13 mRNA levels are significantly suppressed by 17-β-estradiol (E2) in the articular chondrocytes of female patients, indicating that estrogen acts via ER to inhibit the catabolic activity of MMP-13 [83].

3.6. Others

Leptin, a peptide hormone involved in maintaining insulin sensitivity and contributing to the sensation of satiety, is expressed at very high levels in obese individuals. It appears to be correlated to with OA by intervening the level of MMP-13 expression. Down-regulation of leptin mRNA translation via small interference RNA (siRNA) inhibits MMP-13 expression in cultured osteoarthritic chondrocytes [84].

Many other proteins, like adiponectin [85], nuclear protein-1 [86], and estrogen [87], have also been found to be amplified accompanied with increased expression of MMP-13 in OA chondrocytes. It should be noted that the mediators of MMP-13 are not limited to those mentioned above.

4. Epigenetic Regulation of MMP-13

The "NIH Roadmap Epigenomics Project" defined epigenetics as both heritable changes in gene activity and expression, and stable, long-term alterations in a cell's transcriptional potential that are not necessarily heritable [88]. The epigenetic regulation will not change the underlying DNA sequence, which is contrary to gene regulation by changes in the DNA sequence. Thus, epigenetic mechanisms regulate gene expression either by affecting gene transcription or by acting post-transcriptionally [89]. Although OA's specific mechanism is unclear, genetic changes are considered critical factors in its pathology. There is increasing evidence that gene expression can be regulated by epigenetic processes, including DNA methylation, histone modification, and non-coding RNAs (Figure 3), as outlined in the following sub-chapters.

4.1. DNA Methylation

DNA methylation involves adding a methyl group to the 5′ position of cytosine within a CpG dinucleotide to form 5-methylcytosine in the presence of DNA methyltransferase (DNMT) without changing the DNA sequence [90]. DNA methylation is associated with transcriptional repression and is accomplished by blocking the binding of transcription factors to gene promoters and by altering the chromatin structure through the recruitment of repressive chromatin remodeling complexes [91]. The demethylation of specific CpG dinucleotides within MMP-13 promoters has been shown to alter transcription factor binding and thereby increase MMP-13 transcription in OA cartilage [92].

DNA methylation involved in the MMP-13-driven OA process can directly target the MMP-13 promoter. For example, Roach et al. [93] first investigated the abnormal gene expression of clonal OA chondrocytes is associated with heritable epigenetic alterations in the DNA methylation pattern. They found the overall percentage of nonmethylated sites for MMP-13 were significantly increased in OA patients (20%) compared with controls (4%), but not all CpG sites were equally susceptible to demethylation. The authors identified that both the −134 and −110 sites in the MMP-13 promoter became demethylated during the OA process, even at the early stage. Another study further showed that methylation of the −110 bp CpG site, which resides within a hypoxia-inducible factor (HIF) consensus motif in the MMP-13 promoter, produced the most significant suppression of its transcriptional activities. Methylation of the −110 bp CpG site in the MMP-13 promoter inhibited its HIF-2α-driven transactivation and decreased HIF-2α binding to the MMP-13 proximal promoter by chromatin immunoprecipitation assays [92]. DNA methylation can also target the promoters of genes encoding MMP-13-mediated proteins, further activate the downstream signaling pathway, and eventually lead to chondrocyte hypertrophy and cartilage destruction [94]. RUNX2 promoter activity is increased by demethylation of specific CpG sites in the P1 promoter. Overexpression of RUNX2 significantly enhances MMP-13 promoter activity, independent of the MMP-13 promoter methylation status, which may result in high expression of its protein product and further promote the transcriptional activity of MMP-13 in OA [95].

4.2. Histone Modification

Histones are basic proteins that associate with DNA in the nucleus and help condense it into chromatin, which is composed of DNA-wrapped protein octamers. Histone modification can alter the chromatin conformation and influence the binding of transcription factors with the promoter region [96]. Acetylation/deacetylation and methylation/demethylation of histones are the primary modifications studied in OA [97]. Acetylation decreases the binding ability of histones with DNA, allowing the transcription factor's binding leading to the initiation of gene expression. On the contrary, deacetylation carried out by histone deacetylases (HDAC) encourages high-affinity binding between the DNA backbone and histones, resulting in preventing the binding of transcription factors [98].

HDAC expression promotes chondrocytes' catabolic activity, and several HDACs are upregulated in OA chondrocytes, including HDAC1, HDAC2, and HDAC7 [99]. Overexpression of HDAC1 and HDAC2 represses transcription of ECM genes, including ACAN and COL2A1, whereas HDAC7 induces transcription of the matrix-degrading enzyme MMP-13. Higashiyama et al. found that the enhanced HDAC7 promotes cartilage destruction in OA patients by inducing the expression of MMP-13. The knockdown of HDAC7 by siRNA in SW 1353 human chondrosarcoma cells induced by IL-1β leads to a decrease in the expression of MMP-13 [100]. In addition, HDAC3 has also been shown to inhibit the phosphorylation of extracellular ERK and the downstream target gene activity in chondrocytes [101]. Ablation of HDAC3 in chondrocytes increased the temporal and spatial activation of Erk1/2 by decreasing the dual-specific phosphatase 6 (Dusp6), resulting in increased Runx2 phosphorylation and MMP-13 activation as downstream effects of activated Erk pathway. It is likely that HDAC3 deletion is directly affecting Runx2 activity and histone acetylation of the MMP-13 gene, in addition to controlling Erk1/2 activity through Dusp6.

4.3. Non-Coding RNAs

Non-coding RNAs (ncRNA) are functional RNA molecules that produce transcripts functioning as structural, catalytic, or regulatory RNAs rather than being translated into proteins. Based on the length, ncRNAs are classified as short ncRNAs (<30 nucleotides) and long ncRNAs (lncRNAs, >200 nucleotides) [102]. Further, short ncRNAs mainly include three types-microRNAs (miRNAs), short interfering RNAs (siRNAs), and P-Element induced wimpy testis (PIWI)-interacting RNAs (piRNAs) [103]. These ncRNAs regulate gene expression at transcription, splicing, or translation levels. Recent advances in ncRNAs have revealed their importance in the pathogenesis of OA [104].

4.3.1. Micro RNA

miRNAs are endogenous, single-stranded non-coding RNA in cytoplasm, usually 20–23 base pairs in length. They are involved in the posttranscriptional regulation of gene expression through binding to target mRNAs via complementary base pairing between the miRNA and the "seed sequence" present in the 3'-untranslated region (3'-UTR) or the open reading frame (ORF) of the target mRNA [105]. The incomplete base pairing can regulate gene expression by translational suppression, mRNA cleavage, and deadenylation [106,107].

Previous studies have shown that more than 30 miRNAs expressed in human joint tissue are related to cartilage homeostasis and OA development [108]. Among the miRNAs, some direct negative regulators for the expression of MMP-13 have been investigated, including miR-9, miR-146a, miR-127-5p, miR-27b, miR-320, miR-411, and miR-148, which have a direct binding site in the 3'-untranslated region (3'-UTR) of MMP-13 mRNA. The miR-9 expression is repressed while the MMP-13 expression level is elevated in OA cartilage tissues compared with normal specimens, in which miR-9 inhibits the expression level of MMP-13, thus suppressing its inhibitory effects on COL2A1 and enhancing COL2A1 expression levels, which consequently antagonizes the pathogenesis of OA. [109]. The results are consistent with previous studies conducted by Gu et al. [110] and Song et al. [111]. The miR-146 expression is correlated to cartilage degradation measured by Mankin scale in OA patients. miR-146a is significantly higher at grade I OA and lower at grade II and III OA. Furthermore, the variation in the expression of miR-146a is inversely related to the expression level of MMP-13 at a similar cartilage grade, but the increasing cartilage degradation is in parallel with increased MMP13 mRNA. Therefore, the expression of miR-146a is significantly higher during the early stages of OA than during the later stages [112]. The miR-320, which is expressed during the late stages of chondrogenic differentiation, was also significantly downregulated in OA cartilage. miR-320 targets MMP-13 during chondrogenesis and in IL-1β-activated chondrocytes [113]. miR-127-5p is an important regulator of MMP-13 in human chondrocytes and may contribute to the development of OA [114]. Upregulation of MMP-13 expression by IL-1β was correlated with downregulation of miR-127-5p expression in human chondrocytes. miR-127-5p suppressed IL-1β-induced MMP-13 production and the activity of a reporter construct containing the 3'-UTR of human MMP-13 mRNA. In contrast, treatment with anti-miR-127-5p remarkably increased reporter activity and MMP-13 production. Therefore, miR-127-5p could function as a direct negative regulator of MMP-13 in the development of OA. Overexpression of miR-27b also suppressed the activity of a reporter construct containing the 3'-UTR of human MMP-13 mRNA and inhibited the IL-1β–induced expression of MMP-13 protein in chondrocytes [115]. MMP-13 has also been identified as a direct target gene of miR-411 in chondrocytes. Overexpression of miR-411 inhibited the MMP-13 expression and increased the expression of type II collagen and type IV collagen expression in chondrocytes, suggesting that miR-411 is a crucial regulator of MMP-13 in chondrocytes and may respond to the development of OA [116]. Similarly, miR-148a is downregulated in OA cartilage, while the overexpression of miR-148a increases ECM ingredients accompanied by decreased production of degrading enzymes, including MMP-13 in chondrocytes [117].

Moreover, several miRNAs that are downregulated in OA indirectly enhance the MMP-13 expression, including miR-27a, miR-29a, miR-140, miR-222, miR-488, miR-602, miR-608, miR-24, miR-148a, miR-222, and miR-125b-5p. It was first reported that both miR-27a and miR-140, as possible regulators of MMP-13 and IGFBP-5, are reduced in OA chondrocytes. miR-140 could act directly on decreasing IGFBP-5 expression, but miR-27a indirectly decreases both MMP-13 and IGFBP-5 [118]. Co-transfection of miR-29a and miR-140, which are significantly downregulated in OA, notably affected the MMP-13 and TIMP1 gene expression that regulates ECM. Although co-transfection of miR-29a and miR-140 did not show a synergistic effect on MMP-13 protein expression and type II collagen release, both of them can significantly suppress the protein abundance of MMP-13 and restore the type II collagen release in IL-1β treated chondrocytes. The mediating effect on ECM caused by miR-29a and miR-140 may be explained by the restoration of TIMP1 that is able to promote cell proliferation and has an anti-apoptotic function [119]. miR-222 was significantly downregulated in OA chondrocytes, and its overexpression suppressed apoptotic death by downregulating HDAC-4 and MMP-13 levels; the treatment of chondrocytes with the HDAC inhibitor suppressed MMP-13 protein level and apoptosis. Altogether, miR-222 regulates MMP-13 via targeting HDAC-4 in the pathogenesis OA [120]. miR-488, which is also downregulated in OA chondrocytes, plays a protective role in OA pathogenesis by decreasing cartilage degradation by targeting the zinc transporter SLC39A8/ZIP8) since Zn^{2+} is required for the catalytic activity of MMP-13 [121]. Expression of sonic hedgehog (SHH) was inversely correlated with the expression of miR-608 in damaged cartilage and IL-1β-stimulated chondrocytes. Overexpression of miR-602 or miR-608 inhibited SHH mRNA expression, and stimulation with SHH-protein upregulated the MMP-13 expression in OA chondrocytes. Hence, suppression of miR-602 and miR-608 may contribute to the enhanced expression of MMP-13 in OA via SHH [122]. miR-24 is identified as a negative regulator of p16INK4a, which is a consequence of inherent age-associated disorders and sufficient to induce the production of MMP-13 expressed in OA chondrocytes, suggesting the downregulation of miR-24 is consistent with the increased production of MMP-13 [123]. Additionally, miR-125b-5p acts as a negative co-regulator of inflammatory genes, including MMP-13, via targeting TRAF6/MAPKs/NF-κB pathway in human OA chondrocytes [124].

However, some other miRNAs, like miR-33a, miR-181b, miR-145, miR-16-5p, and miR-483, are positively correlated with the expression of MMP-13 in OA chondrocytes. The upregulation of these miRNAs indirectly leads to an increased level of MMP-13. For example, treatment of normal chondrocytes with miR-33a resulted in significantly reduced ABCA1 (ATP-binding cassette transporter A1) and ApoA1 (apolipoprotein A1) expression levels, which were accompanied by elevated levels of MMP-13, promoting the OA phenotype, but the effects were reversed by miR-33a inhibitor [125]. Similarly, the use of an inhibitor to alter miR-181b levels can reduce MMP-13 expression, while inducing type II collagen expression [126]. Overexpression of miR-145 in OA chondrocytes induced by IL-1β resulted in a significant downregulation of ACAN and COl2A1, and increased expression of MMP-13. This effect of miR-145 on impaired ECM in OA cartilage is through direct targeting of Smad3 protein, which is essential for chondrocyte homeostasis [127]. It is reported miR-16-5p may also facilitate catabolism in cartilaginous tissues under the influence of SMAD3 [128]. The expression of miR-483 was significantly upregulated in murine OA, which was negatively correlated with the expression of BMP-7 and TGF-β, but positively correlated with MMP-13 [129].

4.3.2. Small Interfering RNAs (siRNAs)

siRNAs are artificially synthesized 19–23 nucleotide long double-stranded RNA molecules that can be used to "interfere" with the translation of target protein by binding to and promoting the degradation of messenger RNA (mRNA) at specific sequences to block its expression [130].

siRNA of MMP-13 or ADAMTS5 has been tested in surgically induced mice OA model to evaluate their effects by the individual or combined intra-cellular injection compared with a control group (non-targeting siRNA). Significant improvement was observed in all three siRNA-treated groups compared to the control siRNA-injected group. The degree of OA progression of the combined group was less than that of the ADAMTS5 siRNA-only group, whereas the combined injection of MMP-13 and ADAMTS5 siRNA resulted in almost the same inhibitory effects as MMP-13 siRNA alone on cartilage degradation at the early phase of OA [131]. The inhibitory effect of the MMP-13 siRNA on OA is consistent with the results previously studied [132,133].

4.3.3. Long Non-Coding RNAs (lncRNAs)

lncRNAs are fundamental regulators of transcription, and function as a signal, decoy, scaffold, guide, enhancer RNAs, and short peptides to regulate transcription in response to various stimuli [134]. Many lncRNAs have been identified differentially expressed in OA patients vs. Normal [135]. Recent literature showed that several lncRNAs potentially play a role in OA associated with MMP-13.

A lncRNA, termed as cartilage injury-related lncRNA (lncRNA-CIR), was highly expressed in OA cartilage. In contrast, silencing of lncRNA-CIR was confirmed to promote the formation of collagen and aggrecan and reduce the expression of matrix-degrading enzymes, such as MMP-13 and ADAMTS5 [136]. Another long non-coding RNA, GAS5, plays a critical role in the regulation of miR-21 in OA [137]. GAS5 was identified as a direct target of miR-21, and the overexpression of GAS5 was subsequently found to promote OA pathogenesis by increasing MMP-13 expression levels [137]. The expression of lncRNA-UCA1 (urothelial cancer associated 1) was also found upregulated in the OA cartilage, and it is negatively correlated with the expression of miR-204-5p. Moreover,

MMP-13 was a direct target gene of miR-204-5p in the chondrocytes. The results indicated that LncRNA-UCA1 enhances MMP-13 expression by inhibiting miR-204-5p in human chondrocytes [138].

In addition, circular RNAs (circRNAs) belong to the family lncRNA that, unlike linear RNAs, are characterized by a covalently closed circular RNA structure lacking 5′ cap and 3′ poly-adenylated tails [139]. It has been reported that circRNAs function as miRNA 'sponges' that naturally sequester and competitively suppress miRNA activity to affect cell behavior [140]. In a study to identify circRNA expression and explore the function of chondrocyte extracellular matrix related circRNAs (circRNA-CER) in cartilage, five miRNA binding sites for circRNA-CER are identified, including miR-636, miR-665, miR-217, miR-646, and miR-136, which can match the sequence of the circRNA-CER 3′UTR. miR-136 fits the 3′UTR of MMP-13 to suppress its expression, and knockdown of circRNA-CER by siRNA (si-CRE) in OA chondrocytes induced decreased MMP-13 and increased COLOA1 and AGGRN. However, as a consequence of co-transfection of the miR-136 inhibitor and si-CER into chondrocytes, the repression of MMP-13 via circRNA-CER knockdown was reversed by the miR-136 inhibitor, and the effect regarding the high expression of COL2 and ACAN was also eliminated. The results demonstrated that circRNA-CER regulated MMP-13 expression by functioning as a competing endogenous RNA and participated in the process of chondrocyte ECM degradation [141].

5. Selective Inhibitors of MMP-13

Since MMP-13 plays a crucial role in OA, it has become a hot spot that researchers are paying attention to. We might be able to treat OA if we are able to detect or to synthesize a species that is able to block a specific step in the transcriptional regulation pathway of MMP-13, to inhibit its synthesis, or to combine with MMP-13 to inhibit its activity. Such substances are called MMP-13 inhibitors. For example, there are some natural compounds such as resveratrol [142], curcumin [143], epigallocatechin-3-gallate [144], showing protective effects against matrix degradation and inflammation in OA-affected chondrocytes by indirectly inhibiting the expression of MMP-13. However, these natural compounds still have potentially toxic effects on other human tissues because they do not work only to MMP-13. Here we introduce some selective MMP-13 inhibitors, which means the compounds bind exclusively to MMP-13 without acting on other substrates. They can be divided into two types: biologically synthesized inhibitors and chemically synthesized inhibitors.

5.1. Chemically Synthetic Inhibitors

MMPs have a conserved active site motif, where a tris(histidine)-bound zinc ion acts as the catalytic site for substrate hydrolysis. MMP inhibition can be achieved by chelating the active site zinc ion via Zn^{2+} binding groups (ZBGs), including hydroxamic acid, carboxylates, thiols, and phosphorous acid-based ligand. The hydroxamic acid functionality has traditionally been the ligand of choice for the most potent MMP inhibitors. A number of different hydroxamic acid-based MMP inhibitors have been reported showing efficacy in the mono-iodoacetate-induced model of joint degeneration in rats [145]. However, the clinical utility of broad-spectrum MMP inhibitors has been restricted by developing musculoskeletal syndrome (MSS) due to high structural similarity among the various MMPs [146].

5.1.1. Zinc-Binding Inhibitors

To avoid broad MMP inhibition owing to the high structural homology of the different MMPs and to reduce the off-target effects observed in clinical trials, researchers have developed MMP-13 inhibitors with superior selectivity profiles over traditional MMP inhibitors through binding deeply in the S1′ region of MMP-13 [147]. This kind of zinc-binding inhibitors generally contain not only a ZBG to chelate with catalytic Zn^{2+}, but also a P1′ fragment that can be accommodated in the S1′ subsite of the enzyme active site.

A series N-O-Isopropyl sulfonamido-based hydroxamates, in which different aryl substituents on the sulfonamidic portion are introduced, are synthesized and evaluated as MMP-13 inhibitors for potential therapeutic agents of OA [148]. Among these inhibitors, compound 5 exhibited a nanomolar inhibiting activity for MMP-13 (IC_{50} = 3.0 ± 0.2 nM) and was highly selective for this enzyme compared to other MMPs. This compound acted as a slow-binding inhibitor of MMP-13 and was demonstrated to be effective in an in vitro collagen assay and a cartilage degradation model. A series of carboxylic acid inhibitors of MMP-13 were also designed for the treatment of OA without significantly inhibiting the related MMP-1 or TNF-α converting enzyme (TACE) [149]. A compound 24f, optimized from carboxylic acid lead 9, was identified as a subnanomolar inhibitor of MMP-13 (IC_{50} value 0.5 nM and Ki of 0.19 nM) having no activity against MMP-1 or TACE (IC50 of >10,000 nM), and significantly reduced proteoglycan release following oral dosing at 30 mg/kg (75% inhibition) and 10 mg/kg (40% inhibition) in a rat model of MMP-13-induced cartilage degradation [149]. Recently, it has reported the discovery of series of pyrimidine-2-carboxamide-4-one-based MMP-13 zinc-binding inhibitors as exemplified by compound 35, which is characterized by having a triazolone as the zinc-binding moiety connected via a biphenyl spacer with a sulfonyl linkage to the P1′ group, quinazoline-2-carboxamide. The triazolone inhibitor 35 exhibited excellent potency (IC50 = 0.071 nM) and selectivity (greater than 170-fold) over other MMPs (MMP-1, 2, 3, 7, 8, 9, 10, 12, and 14), but slow oral availability in rat pharmacokinetic studies [150]. A novel series of fused pyrimidine compounds that possess a 1,2,4-triazol-3-yl group as a ZBG were developed. Among them, 31f exhibited excellent potency for MMP-13 (IC50 = 0.036 nM) and selectivities (greater than 1500-fold) over other MMPs (MMP-1, -2, -3, -7, -8, -9, -10, and -14) and was shown to protect bovine nasal cartilage explants against degradation induced by interleukin-1 and oncostatin M [151].

5.1.2. Non-Zinc Binding Inhibitors

Another class of MMP-13 inhibitors were produced not to bind to the catalytic zinc ion, but to burry themselves deeper in the S1′ pocket, occupying the specificity loop leading to inhibitors that combine high potency with appealing selectivity profiles. An advantage of non-zinc-binding MMP inhibitors is a potential reduction in non-specific, off-target metalloenzyme inhibition. A number of highly selective and potent MMP-13 inhibitors with a variety of structural scaffolds, including diphenyl ethers, biaryls (aryltetrazoliums, arylfurans, pyrazole-indoles), pyrimidines, and aryl/cycloalkyl-fused pyrimidines, have been explored [152].

Several groups with various structural classes have shown efficacious results and, at the same time, can overcome safety problems associated with MMP inhibitors developed so far for the potential treatment of OA. For example, some pyrido [3,4-d] pyrimidin-4-ones were discovered as orally active and specific MMP-13 inhibitors for the treatment of OA. Some derivatives, such as compound 10a, possessed favorable absorption, distribution, metabolism, and elimination and safety profiles. More significantly, 10a effectively prevented cartilage damage in rabbit animal models of OA without inducing musculoskeletal side effects when given at extremely high doses to rats [153]. A group of highly selective and orally bioavailable MMP-13 inhibitors has been identified based upon a (pyridin-4-yl)-2H-tetrazole scaffold. The desired compound 29b demonstrated potent inhibition of full length MMP-13 (K_i = 4.4 nM) and excellent oral bioavailability in the rat (F = 100%, 1 mg/kg dose) with low clearance (14 mL/min/kg, T1/2Eff = 2.8 h). It was also found to inhibit production of type II collagen neoepitope, a biomarker of cartilage degradation, and afforded cartilage protection in a preclinical rat OA model [154]. A non-zinc binding MMP-13 selective inhibitor (4-methyl-1-(S)-({5-[(3-oxo-3,4-dihydro-2H-benzo[1,4]oxazin-6-ylmethyl)carbamoyl]pyrazolo[1,5-a]pyrimidine-7-carbonyl}amino)indan-5-carboxylic acid) is distinguished for its remarkable durability and minimized systemic exposure by IA injection in knee joint of rats. It is able to attain high, sustained concentrations (≥2 μM for 8 weeks) and sustained efficacy (100% inhibition for 3 weeks) without gross changes in the joint or signs of MSS [155]. PF152 was shown to decrease human cartilage degradation ex vivo and reduce cartilage lesions with decreased type II collagen and aggrecan degradation in dogs with OA induced by partial medial meniscectomy [156]. However, additional preclinical testing of PF152 indicated significant nephrotoxicity due to the compound's accumulation in the kidneys mediated by human organic anion transporter 3. Thus, a follow-up analysis produced an optimized compound N-(4-Fluoro-3-methoxybenzyl)-6-(2-(((2S,5R)-5-(hydroxymethyl)-1,4-dioxan-2-yl)methyl)-2H-tetrazol-5-yl)-2-methylpyrimidine-4- carboxamide lacking the previously observed preclinical toxicology at comparable exposures [157].

Although all of these compounds showed very impressive selectivity profiles toward MMP-13, no such molecules have yet been approved for use in the clinic, as some concerns remain about poor solubility, permeability, biodistribution, metabolic stability, or bioavailability, and thus the search for new MMP-13 inhibitors continues [150].

5.2. Biologically Synthetic Inhibitor

Monoclonal antibody (mAb) therapy is one of the biological treatments aiming to slow structural progression, control inflammation, and relieve the pain of OA. Several kinds of mAbs, including anti-ADAMTS mAbs, anti-IL-1 mAbs, anti-NGF mAbs, and anti-VEGF mAbs, have been developed for the treatment of OA in experimental to clinical studies and show the potential to be disease-modifying anti-OA drugs (DMOADs) [158]. Due to the pivotal role of MMP-13 in the pathogenesis of OA, anti-MMP-13 mAbs is also a targeted therapeutic approach. An interesting study by Naito et al. demonstrated the development of a novel MMP-13 neutralizing antibody by immunization with a synthetic peptide, which selectively binds the active MMP-13 and is highly selective over other MMPs [159]. Despite the encouraging results using antibodies, the potency is also limited by the immunogenicity of functional sites, rapid evolvement of genetic alteration occurring at protein surfaces under pathological conditions, limited administration routes, difficulties of penetrating cartilage, and expense [158,160]. Therefore, the therapeutic potential of antibodies against MMM-13 for OA has yet to be realized.

So far, there are no clinical trials for both chemically and biologically synthetic inhibitors selective for MMP-13. These inhibitors are still under development to eliminate side effects that cause great harm. Hence, more research is needed to evaluate their safety and efficacy before administration to patients.

6. Conclusions

In this review, we discuss the recent advances made in understanding the role of MMP-13 in OA development and the therapeutic potential of MMP-13 inhibition in that condition. MMP-13 is regulated by multiple pathways, and some of the regulatory mechanisms are mutually causal. Even so, MMP-13 plays a pivotal role in cartilage destruction for. Therefore, elucidation of the biological processes provides a foundation with which to understand mechanisms of MMP-13 regulation in OA and potentially to refine the specificity of MMP-13 inhibition as a therapeutic strategy for OA. However, limited data are available on the role of MMP-13 inhibitors in the treatment of OA, and further research is needed to develop highly selective agents to avoid the side effects of non-selective MMP inhibitors. In the future, MMP-13 inhibitors may bring a breakthrough in the treatment of OA.

Author Contributions: Conceptualization, Q.H.; methodology, Q.H.; investigation, Q.H.; data curation, Q.H.; writing—original draft preparation, Q.H.; writing—review and editing, Q.H. and M.E.; visualization, Q.H.; supervision, M.E.; project administration, M.E. All authors have read and agreed to the published version of the manuscript.

Funding: This research received no external funding.

Institutional Review Board Statement: Not applicable.

Int. J. Mol. Sci. **2021**, *22*, 1742

Informed Consent Statement: Not applicable.

Data Availability Statement: Not applicable.

Conflicts of Interest: The authors declare no conflict of interest.

Abbreviations

ADAMTS5: a disintegrin and metalloproteinase with thrombospondin motifs 5; ALK: anaplastic lymphoma kinase; AP-1: activator protein 1. $3'$-UTR: $3'$-untranslated region; C/EBPb: CCAAT/enhancer-binding protein-b; cirRNAs: circular RNAs; circRNA-CER: chondrocyte extracellular matrix related circRNAs; COL2A1: Collagen Type II Alpha 1 Chain; DDR2: discoidin domain-containing receptor 2; DNMT: DNA methyltransferase; DMM: destabilization of the medial meniscus; Dusp6: dual-specific phosphatase 6, ECM: extracellular matrix; ELF3: E-74 like factor 3; ER: Estrogen receptor; FN-f: fibronectin fragment; LEF1: lymphoid enhancer-binding factor 1; ERK: extracellular signal-regulated kinase; HDAC: histone deacetylase; Hes1: hairy and enhancer of split-1; HIF-2α: hypoxia-inducible factor-2 alpha; IL-1β: interleukin-1 beta; IGF-1: Insulin growth factor-1; LDL: Low-density lipoprotein; LRP1: Low-density lipoprotein receptor-related protein 1; lncRNA-CIR: cartilage injury-related lncRNA; mAb: monoclonal antibody; MAPK: mitogen-activated protein kinase; miRNA: microRNA; MMP: matrix metalloproteinase; ncRNA: non-coding RNA; NF-κB: Nuclear factor kappa-light-chain-enhancer of activated B cells; NSAIDs: non-steroidal anti-inflammatory drugs; OA: osteoarthritis; ORF: open reading frame; OSCAR: Osteoclast-associated receptor; PBX3: pre-B-cell leukemia transcription factor; PI3K/AKT: phosphoinositide 3-kinase/protein kinase B; PTGS: post-transcriptional gene silencing; RUNX2: runt-related transcription factor 2; SHH: sonic hedgehog siRNAs: short interfering RNA; TACE: TNF-α converting enzyme; TIMP: tissue inhibitors of metalloproteinases; TNF-α: tumor necrosis factor-α; UCA1: urothelial cancer associated 1; ZBG: Zn^{2+} binding group.

References

1. Castrogiovanni, P.; Musumeci, G. Which is the best physical treatment for osteoarthritis? *J. Funct. Morphol. Kinesiol.* **2016**, *1*, 54–68. [CrossRef]
2. Litwic, A.; Edwards, M.H.; Dennison, E.M.; Cooper, C. Epidemiology and burden of osteoarthritis. *Br. Med. Bull.* **2013**, *105*, 185–199. [CrossRef]
3. James, S.L.; Abate, D.; Abate, K.H.; Abay, S.M.; Abbafati, C.; Abbasi, N.; Abbastabar, H.; Abd-Allah, F.; Abdela, J.; Abdelalim, A.; et al. Global, regional, and national incidence, prevalence, and years lived with disability for 354 Diseases and Injuries for 195 countries and territories, 1990-2017: A systematic analysis for the Global Burden of Disease Study 2017. *Lancet* **2018**. [CrossRef]
4. Wilder, F.V.; Hall, B.J.; Barrett, J.P.; Lemrow, N.B. History of acute knee injury and osteoarthritis of the knee: A prospective epidemiological assessment. The clearwater osteoarthritis study. *Osteoarthr. Cartil.* **2002**, *10*, 611–616. [CrossRef] [PubMed]
5. Niu, J.; Zhang, Y.Q.; Torner, J.; Nevitt, M.; Lewis, C.E.; Aliabadi, P.; Sack, B.; Clancy, M.; Sharma, L.; Felson, D.T. Is obesity a risk factor for progressive radiographic knee osteoarthritis? *Arthritis Care Res.* **2009**, *61*, 329–335. [CrossRef] [PubMed]
6. Palazzo, C.; Nguyen, C.; Lefevre-Colau, M.M.; Rannou, F.; Poiraudeau, S. Risk factors and burden of osteoarthritis. *Ann. Phys. Rehabil. Med.* **2016**, *59*, 134–138. [CrossRef]
7. Donell, S. Subchondral bone remodelling in osteoarthritis. *EFORT Open Rev.* **2019**, *4*, 221–229. [CrossRef]
8. Melrose, J.; Fuller, E.S.; Little, C.B. The biology of meniscal pathology in osteoarthritis and its contribution to joint disease: Beyond simple mechanics. *Connect. Tissue Res.* **2017**, *58*, 282–294. [CrossRef] [PubMed]
9. Belluzzi, E.; Stocco, E.; Pozzuoli, A.; Granzotto, M.; Porzionato, A.; Vettor, R.; De Caro, R.; Ruggieri, P.; Ramonda, R.; Rossato, M.; et al. Contribution of Infrapatellar Fat Pad and Synovial Membrane to Knee Osteoarthritis Pain. *Biomed Res. Int.* **2019**, *2019*. [CrossRef]
10. Zeng, N.; Yan, Z.P.; Chen, X.Y.; Ni, G.X. Infrapatellar fat pad and knee osteoarthritis. *Aging Dis.* **2020**, *11*, 1317–1328. [CrossRef] [PubMed]
11. Malemud, C.J. Biologic basis of osteoarthritis: State of the evidence. *Curr. Opin. Rheumatol.* **2015**, *27*, 289–294. [CrossRef] [PubMed]
12. Martel-Pelletier, J.; Barr, A.J.; Cicuttini, F.M.; Conaghan, P.G.; Cooper, C.; Goldring, M.B.; Goldring, S.R.; Jones, G.; Teichtahl, A.J.; Pelletier, J.P. Osteoarthritis. *Nat. Rev. Dis. Prim.* **2016**, *2*. [CrossRef] [PubMed]
13. Takaishi, H.; Kimura, T.; Dalal, S.; Okada, Y.; D'Armiento, J. Joint Diseases and Matrix Metalloproteinases: A Role for MMP-13. *Curr. Pharm. Biotechnol.* **2008**, *9*, 47–54. [CrossRef] [PubMed]
14. Goldring, M.B. The role of the chondrocyte in osteoarthritis. *Arthritis Rheum.* **2000**, *43*, 1916–1926. [CrossRef]
15. Man, G.S.; Mologhianu, G. Osteoarthritis pathogenesis—A complex process that involves the entire joint. *J. Med. Life* **2014**, *7*, 37–41. [PubMed]

16. Zhang, F.J.; Yu, W.B.; Luo, W.; Gao, S.G.; Li, Y.S.; Lei, G.H. Effect of osteopontin on TIMP-1 and TIMP-2 mRNA in chondrocytes of human knee osteoarthritis in vitro. *Exp. Ther. Med.* **2014**, *8*, 391–394. [CrossRef]
17. Mitchell, P.G.; Magna, H.A.; Reeves, L.M.; Lopresti-Morrow, L.L.; Yocum, S.A.; Rosner, P.J.; Geoghegan, K.F.; Hambor, J.E. Cloning, expression, and type II collagenolytic activity of matrix metalloproteinase-13 from human osteoarthritic cartilage. *J. Clin. Investing.* **1996**, *97*, 761–768. [CrossRef]
18. Mueller, M.B.; Tuan, R.S. Anabolic/Catabolic balance in pathogenesis of osteoarthritis: Identifying molecular targets. *PM R* **2011**, *3*, S3–S11. [CrossRef]
19. Di Rosa, M.; Castrogiovanni, P.; Musumeci, G. The synovium theory: Can exercise prevent knee osteoarthritis? The role of "mechanokines", a possible biological key. *J. Funct. Morphol. Kinesiol.* **2019**, *4*, 11. [CrossRef]
20. Castrogiovanni, P.; Di Rosa, M.; Ravalli, S.; Castorina, A.; Guglielmino, C.; Imbesi, R.; Vecchio, M.; Drago, F.; Szychlinska, M.A.; Musumeci, G. Moderate physical activity as a prevention method for knee osteoarthritis and the role of synoviocytes as biological key. *Int. J. Mol. Sci.* **2019**, *20*, 511. [CrossRef]
21. Chow, Y.Y.; Chin, K.Y. The Role of Inflammation in the Pathogenesis of Osteoarthritis. *Mediators Inflamm.* **2020**. [CrossRef]
22. Sinusas, K. Osteoarthritis: Diagnosis and treatment. *Am. Fam. Physician* **2012**, *85*, 49–56. [CrossRef]
23. Flood, J. The role of acetaminophen in the treatment of osteoarthritis. *Am. J. Manag. Care* **2010**, *16*, S48–S54. [PubMed]
24. Darwiche, H.; Barsoum, W.K.; Klika, A.; Krebs, V.E.; Molloy, R. Retrospective analysis of infection rate after early reoperation in total hip arthroplasty. *Proc. Clin. Orthop. Relat. Res.* **2010**, *468*, 2392–2396. [CrossRef]
25. Mahler, E.A.M.; Minten, M.J.M.; Leseman-Hoogenboom, M.M.; Poortmans, P.M.P.; Leer, J.W.H.; Boks, S.S.; Van Den Hoogen, F.H.J.; Den Broeder, A.A.; Van Den Ende, C.H.M. Effectiveness of low-dose radiation therapy on symptoms in patients with knee osteoarthritis: A randomised, double-blinded, sham-controlled trial. *Ann. Rheum. Dis.* **2019**, *78*, 83–90. [CrossRef]
26. Stevens, R.M.; Ervin, J.; Nezzer, J.; Nieves, Y.; Guedes, K.; Burges, R.; Hanson, P.D.; Campbell, J.N. Randomized, Double-Blind, Placebo-Controlled Trial of Intraarticular Trans-Capsaicin for Pain Associated with Osteoarthritis of the Knee. *Arthritis Rheumatol.* **2019**, *71*, 1524–1533. [CrossRef]
27. Kloppenburg, M.; Peterfy, C.; Haugen, I.K.; Kroon, F.; Chen, S.; Wang, L.; Liu, W.; Levy, G.; Fleischmann, R.M.; Berenbaum, F.; et al. Phase IIa, placebo-controlled, randomised study of lutikizumab, an anti-interleukin-1α and anti-interleukin-1β dual variable domain immunoglobulin, in patients with erosive hand osteoarthritis. *Ann. Rheum. Dis.* **2019**, *78*, 413–420. [CrossRef] [PubMed]
28. Jin, Y.; Smith, C.; Monteith, D.; Brown, R.; Camporeale, A.; McNearney, T.A.; Deeg, M.A.; Raddad, E.; Xiao, N.; de la Peña, A.; et al. CGRP blockade by galcanezumab was not associated with reductions in signs and symptoms of knee osteoarthritis in a randomized clinical trial. *Osteoarthr. Cartil.* **2018**, *26*, 1609–1618. [CrossRef]
29. Jo, C.H.; Lee, Y.G.; Shin, W.H.; Kim, H.; Chai, J.W.; Jeong, E.C.; Kim, J.E.; Shim, H.; Shin, J.S.; Shin, I.S.; et al. Intra-articular injection of mesenchymal stem cells for the treatment of osteoarthritis of the knee: A proof-of-concept clinical trial. *Stem Cells* **2014**, *32*, 1254–1266. [CrossRef] [PubMed]
30. Meheux, C.J.; McCulloch, P.C.; Lintner, D.M.; Varner, K.E.; Harris, J.D. Efficacy of Intra-articular Platelet-Rich Plasma Injections in Knee Osteoarthritis: A Systematic Review. *Arthrosc. J. Arthrosc. Relat. Surg.* **2016**, *32*, 495–505. [CrossRef] [PubMed]
31. Sabatini, M.; Lesur, C.; Thomas, M.; Chomel, A.; Anract, P.; De Nanteuil, G.; Pastoureau, P. Effect of inhibition of matrix metalloproteinases on cartilage loss in vitro and in a guinea pig model of osteoarthritis. *Arthritis Rheum.* **2005**, *52*, 171–180. [CrossRef] [PubMed]
32. Renkiewicz, R.; Qiu, L.; Lesch, C.; Sun, X.; Devalaraja, R.; Cody, T.; Kaldjian, E.; Welgus, H.; Baragi, V. Broad-spectrum matrix metalloproteinase inhibitor marimastat-induced musculoskeletal side effects in rats. *Arthritis Rheum.* **2003**, *48*, 1742–1749. [CrossRef]
33. Xie, X.W.; Wan, R.Z.; Liu, Z.P. Recent Research Advances in Selective Matrix Metalloproteinase-13 Inhibitors as Anti-Osteoarthritis Agents. *ChemMedChem.* **2017**, *12*, 1157–1168. [CrossRef]
34. Whittaker, M.; Floyd, C.D.; Brown, P.; Gearing, A.J.H. Design and Therapeutic Application of Matrix Metalloproteinase Inhibitors. *Chem. Rev.* **1999**, *99*, 2735–2776. [CrossRef] [PubMed]
35. Jacobsen, J.A.; Major Jourden, J.L.; Miller, M.T.; Cohen, S.M. To bind zinc or not to bind zinc: An examination of innovative approaches to improved metalloproteinase inhibition. *Biochim. Biophys. Acta (BBA) Mol. Cell Res.* **2010**, *1803*, 72–94. [CrossRef] [PubMed]
36. Dufour, A.; Sampson, N.S.; Zucker, S.; Cao, J. Role of the hemopexin domain of matrix metalloproteinases in cell migration. *J. Cell. Physiol.* **2008**, *217*, 643–651. [CrossRef] [PubMed]
37. Laronha, H.; Caldeira, J. Structure and Function of Human Matrix Metalloproteinases. *Cells* **2020**, *9*, 1076. [CrossRef]
38. MacColl, E.; Khalil, R.A. Matrix metalloproteinases as regulators of vein structure and function: Implications in chronic venous disease. *J. Pharmacol. Exp. Ther.* **2015**, *355*, 410–428. [CrossRef]
39. Aureli, L.; Gioia, M.; Cerbara, I.; Monaco, S.; Fasciglione, G.; Marini, S.; Ascenzi, P.; Topai, A.; Coletta, M. Structural Bases for Substrate and Inhibitor Recognition by Matrix Metalloproteinases. *Curr. Med. Chem.* **2008**, *15*, 2192–2222. [CrossRef]
40. Overall, C.M.; Kleifeld, O. Towards third generation matrix metalloproteinase inhibitors for cancer therapy. *Br. J. Cancer* **2006**, *94*, 941–946. [CrossRef] [PubMed]

41. Park, H.I.; Jin, Y.; Hurst, D.R.; Monroe, C.A.; Lee, S.; Schwartz, M.A.; Sang, Q.X.A. The Intermediate S1′ Pocket of the Endometase/Matrilysin-2 Active Site Revealed by Enzyme Inhibition Kinetic Studies, Protein Sequence Analyses, and Homology Modeling. *J. Biol. Chem.* **2003**, *278*, 51646–51653. [CrossRef] [PubMed]

42. Lovejoy, B.; Welch, A.R.; Carr, S.; Luong, C.; Broka, C.; Hendricks, R.T.; Campbell, J.A.; Walker, K.A.M.; Martin, R.; Van Wart, H.; et al. Crystal structures of MMP-1 and -13 reveal the structural basis for selectivity of collagenase inhibitors. *Nat. Struct. Biol.* **1999**, *6*, 217–221. [CrossRef] [PubMed]

43. Cui, N.; Hu, M.; Khalil, R.A. Biochemical and Biological Attributes of Matrix Metalloproteinases. *Prog. Mol. Biol. Transl. Sci.* **2017**, *147*, 1–73.

44. Van Wart, H.E.; Birkedal-Hansen, H. The cysteine switch: A principle of regulation of metalloproteinase activity with potential applicability to the entire matrix metalloproteinase gene family. *Proc. Natl. Acad. Sci. USA.* **1990**, *87*, 5578–5582. [CrossRef]

45. Nagase, H.; Visse, R.; Murphy, G. Structure and function of matrix metalloproteinases and TIMPs. *Cardiovasc. Res.* **2006**, *69*, 562–573. [CrossRef] [PubMed]

46. Knäuper, V.; Will, H.; López-Otin, C.; Smith, B.; Atkinson, S.J.; Stanton, H.; Hembry, R.M.; Murphy, G. Cellular mechanisms for human procollagenase-3 (MMP-13) activation. Evidence that MT1-MMP (MMP-14) and gelatinase A (MMP-2) are able to generate active enzyme. *J. Biol. Chem.* **1996**, *271*, 17124–17131. [CrossRef]

47. Zijlstrat, A.; Aimes, R.T.; Zhu, D.; Regazzoni, K.; Kupriyanova, T.; Seandel, M.; Deryugina, E.I.; Quigley, J.P. Collagenolysis-dependent angiogenesis mediated by matrix metalloproteinase-13 (collagenase-3). *J. Biol. Chem.* **2004**, *279*, 27633–27645. [CrossRef]

48. Rowan, A.D.; Litherland, G.J.; Hui, W.; Milner, J.M. Metalloproteases as potential therapeutic targets in arthritis treatment. *Expert Opin. Ther. Targets* **2008**, *12*, 1–18. [CrossRef] [PubMed]

49. Howes, J.M.; Bihan, D.; Slatter, D.A.; Hamaia, S.W.; Packman, L.C.; Knauper, V.; Visse, R.; Farndale, R.W. The recognition of collagen and triple-helical toolkit peptides by MMP-13: Sequence specificity for binding and cleavage. *J. Biol. Chem.* **2014**, *289*, 24091–24101. [CrossRef]

50. Little, C.B.; Barai, A.; Burkhardt, D.; Smith, S.M.; Fosang, A.J.; Werb, Z.; Shah, M.; Thompson, E.W. Matrix metalloproteinase 13-deficient mice are resistant to osteoarthritic cartilage erosion but not chondrocyte hypertrophy or osteophyte development. *Arthritis Rheum.* **2009**, *60*, 3723–3733. [CrossRef]

51. Neuhold, L.A.; Killar, L.; Zhao, W.; Sung, M.L.A.; Warner, L.; Kulik, J.; Turner, J.; Wu, W.; Billinghurst, C.; Meijers, T.; et al. Postnatal expression in hyaline cartilage of constitutively active human collagenase-3 (MMP-13) induces osteoarthritis in mice. *J. Clin. Invest.* **2001**, *107*, 35–44. [CrossRef] [PubMed]

52. Shiomi, T.; Lemaître, V.; D'Armiento, J.; Okada, Y. Matrix metalloproteinases, a disintegrin and metalloproteinases, and a disintegrin and metalloproteinases with thrombospondin motifs in non-neoplastic diseases: Review Article. *Pathol. Int.* **2010**, *60*, 477–496. [CrossRef] [PubMed]

53. Li, H.; Wang, D.; Yuan, Y.; Min, J. New insights on the MMP-13 regulatory network in the pathogenesis of early osteoarthritis. *Arthritis Res. Ther.* **2017**, *19*, 1–12. [CrossRef] [PubMed]

54. Wang, X.; Khalil, R.A. Matrix Metalloproteinases, Vascular Remodeling, and Vascular Disease. *Adv. Pharmacol.* **2018**, *81*, 241–330.

55. Troeberg, L.; Nagase, H. Analysis of TIMP expression and activity. *Methods Mol. Med.* **2007**, *135*, 251–267. [CrossRef]

56. Brew, K.; Dinakarpandian, D.; Nagase, H. Tissue inhibitors of metalloproteinases: Evolution, structure and function. *Biochim. Biophys. Acta* **2000**, *1477*, 267–283. [CrossRef]

57. Sahebjam, S.; Khokha, R.; Mort, J.S. Increased collagen and aggrecan degradation with age in the joints of Timp3-/-mice. *Arthritis Rheum.* **2007**, *56*, 905–909. [CrossRef] [PubMed]

58. Black, R.A.; Castner, B.; Slack, J.; Tocker, J.; Eisenman, J.; Jacobson, E.; Delaney, J.; Winters, D.; Hecht, R.; Bendele, A. A14 Injected Timp-3 protects cartilage in a rat meniscal tear model. *Osteoarthr. Cartil.* **2006**, *14*, S23–S24. [CrossRef]

59. Kevorkian, L.; Young, D.A.; Darrah, C.; Donell, S.T.; Shepstone, L.; Porter, S.; Brockbank, S.M.V.; Edwards, D.R.; Parker, A.E.; Clark, I.M. Expression profiling of metalloproteinases and their inhibitors in cartilage. *Arthritis Rheum.* **2004**, *50*, 131–141. [CrossRef]

60. Strickland, D.K.; Ashcom, J.D.; Williams, S.; Burgess, W.H.; Migliorini, M.; Scott Argraves, W. Sequence identity between the α2-macroglobulin receptor and low density lipoprotein receptor-related protein suggests that this molecule is a multifunctional receptor. *J. Biol. Chem.* **1990**, *265*, 17401–17404. [CrossRef]

61. Chen, D.; Kim, D.J.; Shen, J.; Zou, Z.; O'Keefe, R.J. Runx2 plays a central role in Osteoarthritis development. *J. Orthop. Transl.* **2020**, *23*, 132–139. [CrossRef]

62. Hirata, M.; Kugimiya, F.; Fukai, A.; Saito, T.; Yano, F.; Ikeda, T.; Mabuchi, A.; Sapkota, B.R.; Akune, T.; Nishida, N.; et al. C/EBPβ and RUNX2 cooperate to degrade cartilage with MMP-13 as the target and HIF-2α as the inducer in chondrocytes. *Hum. Mol. Genet.* **2012**, *21*, 1111–1123. [CrossRef]

63. Yun, K.; Im, S.H. Transcriptional regulation of MMP13 by Lef1 in chondrocytes. *Biochem. Biophys. Res. Commun.* **2007**, *364*, 1009–1014. [CrossRef] [PubMed]

64. Yun, K.; So, J.-S.; Jash, A.; Im, S.-H. Lymphoid Enhancer Binding Factor 1 Regulates Transcription through Gene Looping. *J. Immunol.* **2009**, *183*, 5129–5137. [CrossRef] [PubMed]

65. Grall, F.; Gu, X.; Tan, L.; Cho, J.Y.; Inan, M.S.; Pettit, A.R.; Thamrongsak, U.; Choy, B.K.; Manning, C.; Akbarali, Y.; et al. Responses to the proinflammatory cytokines interleukin-1 and tumor necrosis factor α in cells derived from rheumatoid synovium and other joint tissues involve nuclear factor κB-mediated induction of the Ets transcription factor ESE-1. *Arthritis Rheum.* **2003**, *48*, 1249–1260. [CrossRef]

66. Otero, M.; Plumb, D.A.; Tsuchimochi, K.; Dragomir, C.L.; Hashimoto, K.; Peng, H.; Olivotto, E.; Bevilacqua, M.; Tan, L.; Yang, Z.; et al. E74-like Factor 3 (ELF3) impacts on Matrix Metalloproteinase 13 (MMP13) transcriptional control in articular chondrocytes under proinflammatory stress. *J. Biol. Chem.* **2012**, *287*, 3559–3572. [CrossRef] [PubMed]

67. Sugita, S.; Hosaka, Y.; Okada, K.; Mori, D.; Yano, F.; Kobayashi, H.; Taniguchi, Y.; Mori, Y.; Okuma, T.; Chang, S.H.; et al. Transcription factor Hes1 modulates osteoarthritis development in cooperation with calcium/calmodulin-dependent protein kinase 2. *Proc. Natl. Acad. Sci. USA.* **2015**, *112*, 3080–3085. [CrossRef] [PubMed]

68. Pombo-Suarez, M.; Castaño-Oreja, M.T.; Calaza, M.; Gomez-Reino, J.; Gonzalez, A. Differential upregulation of the three transforming growth factor beta isoforms in human osteoarthritic cartilage. *Ann. Rheum. Dis.* **2009**, *68*, 568–571. [CrossRef] [PubMed]

69. Aref-Eshghi, E.; Liu, M.; Harper, P.E.; Doré, J.; Martin, G.; Furey, A.; Green, R.; Rahman, P.; Zhai, G. Overexpression of MMP13 in human osteoarthritic cartilage is associated with the SMAD-independent TGF-β signalling pathway. *Arthritis Res. Ther.* **2015**, *17*. [CrossRef] [PubMed]

70. Massicotte, F.; Aubry, I.; Martel-Pelletier, J.; Pelletier, J.P.; Fernandes, J.; Lajeunesse, D. Abnormal insulin-like growth factor 1 signaling in human osteoarthritic subchondral bone osteoblasts. *Arthritis Res. Ther.* **2006**, *8*. [CrossRef]

71. Zhang, M.; Zhou, Q.; Liang, Q.Q.; Li, C.G.; Holz, J.D.; Tang, D.; Sheu, T.J.; Li, T.F.; Shi, Q.; Wang, Y.J. IGF-1 regulation of type II collagen and MMP-13 expression in rat endplate chondrocytes via distinct signaling pathways. *Osteoarthr. Cartil.* **2009**, *17*, 100–106. [CrossRef]

72. Dvir-Ginzberg, M.; Gagarina, V.; Lee, E.J.; Booth, R.; Gabay, O.; Hall, D.J. Tumor necrosis factor α-mediated cleavage and inactivation of sirT1 in human osteoarthritic chondrocytes. *Arthritis Rheum.* **2011**, *63*, 2363–2373. [CrossRef]

73. Elayyan, J.; Lee, E.J.; Gabay, O.; Smith, C.A.; Qiq, O.; Reich, E.; Mobasheri, A.; Henrotin, Y.; Kimber, S.J.; Dvir-Ginzberg, M. LEF1-mediated MMP13 gene expression is repressed by SIRT1 in human chondrocytes. *FASEB J.* **2017**, *31*, 3116–3125. [CrossRef] [PubMed]

74. Liu, S.; Yang, H.; Hu, B.; Zhang, M. Sirt1 regulates apoptosis and extracellular matrix degradation in resveratrol-treated osteoarthritis chondrocytes via the wnt/β-catenin signaling pathways. *Exp. Ther. Med.* **2017**, *14*, 5057–5062. [CrossRef] [PubMed]

75. Polur, I.; Lee, P.L.; Servais, J.M.; Xu, L.; Li, Y. Role of HTRA1, a serine protease, in the progression of articular cartilage degeneration. *Histol. Histopathol.* **2010**, *25*, 599–608. [CrossRef] [PubMed]

76. Xu, L.; Servais, J.; Polur, I.; Kim, D.; Lee, P.L.; Chung, K.; Li, Y. Attenuation of osteoarthritis progression by reduction of discoidin domain receptor 2 in mice. *Arthritis Rheum.* **2010**, *62*, 2736–2744. [CrossRef] [PubMed]

77. Yamamoto, K.; Okano, H.; Miyagawa, W.; Visse, R.; Shitomi, Y.; Santamaria, S.; Dudhia, J.; Troeberg, L.; Strickland, D.K.; Hirohata, S.; et al. MMP-13 is constitutively produced in human chondrocytes and co-endocytosed with ADAMTS-5 and TIMP-3 by the endocytic receptor LRP1. *Matrix Biol.* **2016**, *56*, 57–73. [CrossRef]

78. Park, D.R.; Kim, J.; Kim, G.M.; Lee, H.; Kim, M.; Hwang, D.; Lee, H.; Kim, H.S.; Kim, W.; Park, M.C.; et al. Osteoclast-associated receptor blockade prevents articular cartilage destruction via chondrocyte apoptosis regulation. *Nat. Commun.* **2020**, *11*. [CrossRef] [PubMed]

79. Loeser, R.F. Integrins and chondrocyte-matrix interactions in articular cartilage. *Matrix Biol.* **2014**, *39*, 11–16. [CrossRef]

80. Forsyth, C.B.; Pulai, J.; Loeser, R.F. Fibronectin fragments and blocking antibodies to α2β1 and α5β1 integrins stimulate mitogen-activated protein kinase signaling and increase collagenase 3 (matrix metalloproteinase 13) production by human articular chondrocytes. *Arthritis Rheum.* **2002**, *46*, 2368–2376. [CrossRef]

81. Hui, W.; Young, D.A.; Rowan, A.D.; Xu, X.; Cawston, T.E.; Proctor, C.J. Oxidative changes and signalling pathways are pivotal in initiating age-related changes in articular cartilage. *Ann. Rheum. Dis.* **2016**, *75*, 449–458. [CrossRef] [PubMed]

82. Blaney Davidson, E.N.; Remst, D.F.G.; Vitters, E.L.; van Beuningen, H.M.; Blom, A.B.; Goumans, M.-J.; van den Berg, W.B.; van der Kraan, P.M. Increase in ALK1/ALK5 Ratio as a Cause for Elevated MMP-13 Expression in Osteoarthritis in Humans and Mice. *J. Immunol.* **2009**, *182*, 7937–7945. [CrossRef] [PubMed]

83. Wang, W.; Wang, L.; Xu, Z.; Yin, Y.; Su, J.; Niu, X.; Cao, X. Effects of estradiol on reduction of osteoarthritis in rabbits through effect on matrix metalloproteinase proteins. *Iran. J. Basic Med. Sci.* **2016**, *19*, 310–315. [CrossRef]

84. Iliopoulos, D.; Malizos, K.N.; Tsezou, A. Epigenetic regulation of leptin affects MMP-13 expression in osteoarthritic chondrocytes: Possible molecular target for osteoarthritis therapeutic intervention. *Ann. Rheum. Dis.* **2007**, *66*, 1616–1621. [CrossRef] [PubMed]

85. Francin, P.J.; Abot, A.; Guillaume, C.; Moulin, D.; Bianchi, A.; Gegout-Pottie, P.; Jouzeau, J.Y.; Mainard, D.; Presle, N. Association between adiponectin and cartilage degradation in human osteoarthritis. *Osteoarthr. Cartil.* **2014**, *22*, 519–526. [CrossRef] [PubMed]

86. Yammani, R.R.; Loeser, R.F. Brief report: Stress-inducible nuclear protein 1 regulates matrix metalloproteinase 13 expression in human articular chondrocytes. *Arthritis Rheumatol.* **2014**, *66*, 1266–1271. [CrossRef]

87. Liang, Y.; Duan, L.; Xiong, J.; Zhu, W.; Liu, Q.; Wang, D.; Liu, W.; Li, Z.; Wang, D. E2 regulates MMP-13 via targeting miR-140 in IL-1β-induced extracellular matrix degradation in human chondrocytes. *Arthritis Res. Ther.* **2016**, *18*. [CrossRef]

88. Romanoski, C.E.; Glass, C.K.; Stunnenberg, H.G.; Wilson, L.; Almouzni, G. Epigenomics: Roadmap for regulation. *Nature* **2015**, *518*, 314–316. [CrossRef]

89. Bird, A. Perceptions of epigenetics. *Nature* **2007**, *447*, 396–398. [CrossRef] [PubMed]
90. Lev Maor, G.; Yearim, A.; Ast, G. The alternative role of DNA methylation in splicing regulation. *Trends Genet.* **2015**, *31*, 274–280. [CrossRef] [PubMed]
91. Reynard, L.N.; Loughlin, J. Genetics and epigenetics of osteoarthritis. *Maturitas* **2012**, *71*, 200–204. [CrossRef] [PubMed]
92. Hashimoto, K.; Otero, M.; Imagawa, K.; De Andrés, M.C.; Coico, J.M.; Roach, H.I.; Oreffo, R.O.C.; Marcu, K.B.; Goldring, M.B. Regulated transcription of human matrix metalloproteinase 13 (MMP13) and interleukin-1β (IL1B) genes in chondrocytes depends on methylation of specific proximal promoter CpG sites. *J. Biol. Chem.* **2013**, *288*, 10061–10072. [CrossRef] [PubMed]
93. Roach, H.I.; Yamada, N.; Cheung, K.S.C.; Tilley, S.; Clarke, N.M.P.; Oreffo, R.O.C.; Kokubun, S.; Bronner, F. Association between the abnormal expression of matrix-degrading enzymes by human osteoarthritic chondrocytes and demethylation of specific CpG sites in the promoter regions. *Arthritis Rheum.* **2005**, *52*, 3110–3124. [CrossRef]
94. Cheung, K.S.C.; Hashimoto, K.; Yamada, N.; Roach, H.I. Expression of ADAMTS-4 by chondrocytes in the surface zone of human osteoarthritic cartilage is regulated by epigenetic DNA de-methylation. *Rheumatol. Int.* **2009**, *29*, 525–534. [CrossRef] [PubMed]
95. Takahashi, A.; de Andrés, M.C.; Hashimoto, K.; Itoi, E.; Otero, M.; Goldring, M.B.; Oreffo, R.O.C. DNA methylation of the RUNX2 P1 promoter mediates MMP13 transcription in chondrocytes. *Sci. Rep.* **2017**, *7*. [CrossRef]
96. Kouzarides, T. Chromatin Modifications and Their Function. *Cell* **2007**, *128*, 693–705. [CrossRef]
97. Khan, N.M.; Haqqi, T.M. Epigenetics in osteoarthritis: Potential of HDAC inhibitors as therapeutics. *Pharmacol. Res.* **2018**, *128*, 73–79. [CrossRef] [PubMed]
98. Clayton, A.L.; Hazzalin, C.A.; Mahadevan, L.C. Enhanced Histone Acetylation and Transcription: A Dynamic Perspective. *Mol. Cell* **2006**, *23*, 289–296. [CrossRef]
99. Hong, S.; Derfoul, A.; Pereira-Mouries, L.; Hall, D.J. A novel domain in histone deacetylase 1 and 2 mediates repression of cartilage-specific genes in human chondrocytes. *FASEB J.* **2009**, *23*, 3539–3552. [CrossRef] [PubMed]
100. Higashiyama, R.; Miyaki, S.; Yamashita, S.; Yoshitaka, T.; Lindman, G.; Ito, Y.; Sasho, T.; Takahashi, K.; Lotz, M.; Asahara, H. Correlation between MMP-13 and HDAC7 expression in human knee osteoarthritis. *Mod. Rheumatol.* **2010**, *20*, 11–17. [CrossRef]
101. Carpio, L.R.; Bradley, E.W.; Westendorf, J.J. Histone deacetylase 3 suppresses Erk phosphorylation and matrix metalloproteinase (Mmp)-13 activity in chondrocytes. *Connect. Tissue Res.* **2017**, *58*, 27–36. [CrossRef]
102. Ma, L.; Bajic, V.B.; Zhang, Z. On the classification of long non-coding RNAs. *RNA Biol.* **2013**, *10*, 924–933. [CrossRef] [PubMed]
103. Mattick, J.S.; Makunin, I.V. Non-coding RNA. *Hum. Mol. Genet.* **2006**, *15*, R17–R29. [CrossRef] [PubMed]
104. Barter, M.J.; Young, D.A. Epigenetic mechanisms and non-coding rnas in osteoarthritis. *Curr. Rheumatol. Rep.* **2013**, *15*. [CrossRef]
105. Sondag, G.R.; Haqqi, T.M. The Role of MicroRNAs and Their Targets in Osteoarthritis. *Curr. Rheumatol. Rep.* **2016**, *18*, 56. [CrossRef] [PubMed]
106. Bartel, D.P. MicroRNAs: Genomics, Biogenesis, Mechanism, and Function. *Cell* **2004**, *116*, 281–297. [CrossRef]
107. Eulalio, A.; Huntzinger, E.; Nishihara, T.; Rehwinkel, J.; Fauser, M.; Izaurralde, E. Deadenylation is a widespread effect of miRNA regulation. *RNA* **2009**, *15*, 21–32. [CrossRef] [PubMed]
108. Asahara, H. Current Status and Strategy of microRNA Research for Cartilage Development and Osteoarthritis Pathogenesis. *J. Bone Metab.* **2016**, *23*, 121. [CrossRef] [PubMed]
109. Zhang, H.; Song, B.; Pan, Z. Downregulation of microRNA-9 increases Matrix metalloproteinase-13 expression levels and facilitates osteoarthritis onset. *Mol. Med. Rep.* **2018**, *17*, 3708–3714. [CrossRef]
110. Gu, R.; Liu, N.; Luo, S.; Huang, W.; Zha, Z.; Yang, J. MicroRNA-9 regulates the development of knee osteoarthritis through the NF-kappaB1 pathway in chondrocytes. *Medicine* **2016**, *95*, e4315. [CrossRef]
111. Song, J.; Kim, D.; Chun, C.H.; Jin, E.J. MicroRNA-9 regulates survival of chondroblasts and cartilage integrity by targeting protogenin. *Cell Commun. Signal.* **2013**, *11*. [CrossRef] [PubMed]
112. Yamasaki, K.; Nakasa, T.; Miyaki, S.; Ishikawa, M.; Deie, M.; Adachi, N.; Yasunaga, Y.; Asahara, H.; Ochi, M. Expression of microRNA-146a in osteoarthritis cartilage. *Arthritis Rheum.* **2009**, *60*, 1035–1041. [CrossRef]
113. Meng, F.; Zhang, Z.; Chen, W.; Huang, G.; He, A.; Hou, C.; Long, Y.; Yang, Z.; Zhang, Z.; Liao, W. MicroRNA-320 regulates matrix metalloproteinase-13 expression in chondrogenesis and interleukin-1β-induced chondrocyte responses. *Osteoarthr. Cartil.* **2016**, *24*, 932–941. [CrossRef] [PubMed]
114. Park, S.J.; Cheon, E.J.; Lee, M.H.; Kim, H.A. MicroRNA-127-5p regulates matrix metalloproteinase 13 expression and interleukin-1β-induced catabolic effects in human chondrocytes. *Arthritis Rheum.* **2013**, *65*, 3141–3152. [CrossRef]
115. Akhtar, N.; Rasheed, Z.; Ramamurthy, S.; Anbazhagan, A.N.; Voss, F.R.; Haqqi, T.M. MicroRNA-27b regulates the expression of matrix metalloproteinase 13 in human osteoarthritis chondrocytes. *Arthritis Rheum.* **2010**, *62*, 1361–1371. [CrossRef]
116. Wang, G.; Zhang, Y.; Zhao, X.; Meng, C.; Ma, L.; Kong, Y. MicroRNA-411 inhibited matrix metalloproteinase 13 expression in human chondrocytes. *Am. J. Transl. Res.* **2015**, *7*, 2000–2006.
117. Vonk, L.A.; Kragten, A.H.M.; Dhert, W.J.A.; Saris, D.B.F.; Creemers, L.B. Overexpression of hsa-miR-148a promotes cartilage production and inhibits cartilage degradation by osteoarthritic chondrocytes. *Osteoarthr. Cartil.* **2014**, *22*, 145–153. [CrossRef] [PubMed]
118. Tardif, G.; Hum, D.; Pelletier, J.P.; Duval, N.; Martel-Pelletier, J. Regulation of the IGFBP-5 and MMP-13 genes by the microRNAs miR-140 and miR-27a in human osteoarthritic chondrocytes. *BMC Musculoskelet. Disord.* **2009**, *10*. [CrossRef] [PubMed]
119. Li, X.; Zhen, Z.; Tang, G.; Zheng, C.; Yang, G. MiR-29a and MiR-140 protect chondrocytes against the anti-proliferation and cell matrix signaling changes by IL-1β. *Mol. Cells* **2016**, *39*, 103–110. [CrossRef] [PubMed]

120. Song, J.; Jin, E.H.; Kim, D.; Kim, K.Y.; Chun, C.H.; Jin, E.J. MicroRNA-222 regulates MMP-13 via targeting HDAC-4 during osteoarthritis pathogenesis. *BBA Clin.* **2015**, *3*, 79–89. [CrossRef]
121. Song, J.; Kim, D.; Lee, C.H.; Lee, M.S.; Chun, C.H.; Jin, E.J. MicroRNA-488 regulates zinc transporter SLC39A8/ZIP8 during pathogenesis of osteoarthritis. *J. Biomed. Sci.* **2013**, *20*. [CrossRef]
122. Akhtar, N.; Makki, M.S.; Haqqi, T.M. MicroRNA-602 and microRNA-608 regulate sonic hedgehog expression via target sites in the coding region in human chondrocytes. *Arthritis Rheumatol.* **2015**, *67*, 423–434. [CrossRef] [PubMed]
123. Philipot, D.; Guérit, D.; Platano, D.; Chuchana, P.; Olivotto, E.; Espinoza, F.; Dorandeu, A.; Pers, Y.M.; Piette, J.; Borzi, R.M.; et al. P16INK4a and its regulator miR-24 link senescence and chondrocyte terminal differentiation-associated matrix remodeling in osteoarthritis. *Arthritis Res. Ther.* **2014**, *16*. [CrossRef] [PubMed]
124. Rasheed, Z.; Rasheed, N.; Abdulmonem, W.A.; Khan, M.I. MicroRNA-125b-5p regulates IL-1β induced inflammatory genes via targeting TRAF6-mediated MAPKs and NF-κB signaling in human osteoarthritic chondrocytes. *Sci. Rep.* **2019**, *9*. [CrossRef] [PubMed]
125. Kostopoulou, F.; Malizos, K.N.; Papathanasiou, I.; Tsezou, A. MicroRNA-33a regulates cholesterol synthesis and cholesterol efflux-related genes in osteoarthritic chondrocytes. *Arthritis Res. Ther.* **2015**, *17*. [CrossRef]
126. Song, J.; Lee, M.; Kim, D.; Han, J.; Chun, C.H.; Jin, E.J. MicroRNA-181b regulates articular chondrocytes differentiation and cartilage integrity. *Biochem. Biophys. Res. Commun.* **2013**, *431*, 210–214. [CrossRef] [PubMed]
127. Yang, B.; Kang, X.; Xing, Y.; Dou, C.; Kang, F.; Li, J.; Quan, Y.; Dong, S. Effect of microRNA-145 on IL-1β-induced cartilage degradation in human chondrocytes. *FEBS Lett.* **2014**, *588*, 2344–2352. [CrossRef] [PubMed]
128. Li, L.; Jia, J.; Liu, X.; Yang, S.; Ye, S.; Yang, W.; Zhang, Y. MicroRNA-16-5p Controls Development of Osteoarthritis by Targeting SMAD3 in Chondrocytes. *Curr. Pharm. Des.* **2015**, *21*, 5160–5167. [CrossRef] [PubMed]
129. Qi, Y.; Ma, N.; Yan, F.; Yu, Z.; Wu, G.; Qiao, Y.; Han, D.; Xiang, Y.; Li, F.; Wang, W.; et al. The expression of intronic miRNAs, miR-483 and miR-483*, and their host gene, Igf2, in murine osteoarthritis cartilage. *Int. J. Biol. Macromol.* **2013**, *61*, 43–49. [CrossRef]
130. McManus, M.T.; Sharp, P.A. Gene silencing in mammals by small interfering RNAs. *Nat. Rev. Genet.* **2002**, *3*, 737–747. [CrossRef] [PubMed]
131. Hoshi, H.; Akagi, R.; Yamaguchi, S.; Muramatsu, Y.; Akatsu, Y.; Yamamoto, Y.; Sasaki, T.; Takahashi, K.; Sasho, T. Effect of inhibiting MMP13 and ADAMTS5 by intra-articular injection of small interfering RNA in a surgically induced osteoarthritis model of mice. *Cell Tissue Res.* **2017**, *368*, 379–387. [CrossRef] [PubMed]
132. Akagi, R.; Sasho, T.; Saito, M.; Endo, J.; Yamaguchi, S.; Muramatsu, Y.; Mukoyama, S.; Akatsu, Y.; Katsuragi, J.; Fukawa, T.; et al. Effective knock down of matrix metalloproteinase-13 by an intra-articular injection of small interfering RNA (siRNA) in a murine surgically-induced osteoarthritis model. *J. Orthop. Res.* **2014**, *32*, 1175–1180. [CrossRef] [PubMed]
133. Hoshi, H.; Sasho, T.; Akagi, R.; Muramatsu, Y.; Mukoyama, S.; Akatsu, Y.; Fukawa, T.; Katsuragi, J.; Endo, J.; Yamamoto, Y. Effective knock down of MMP13 and ADAMTS5 by intra-articular injection of small interference RNA (siRNA) in a surgically induced osteoarthritis model of mice. *Osteoarthr. Cartil.* **2014**, *22*, S372–S373. [CrossRef]
134. Mercer, T.R.; Dinger, M.E.; Mattick, J.S. Long non-coding RNAs: Insights into functions. *Nat. Rev. Genet.* **2009**, *10*, 155–159. [CrossRef] [PubMed]
135. Fu, M.; Huang, G.; Zhang, Z.; Liu, J.; Zhang, Z.; Huang, Z.; Yu, B.; Meng, F. Expression profile of long noncoding RNAs in cartilage from knee osteoarthritis patients. *Osteoarthr. Cartil.* **2015**, *23*, 423–432. [CrossRef]
136. Liu, Q.; Zhang, X.; Dai, L.; Hu, X.; Zhu, J.; Li, L.; Zhou, C.; Ao, Y. Long noncoding RNA related to cartilage injury promotes chondrocyte extracellular matrix degradation in osteoarthritis. *Arthritis Rheumatol.* **2014**, *66*, 969–978. [CrossRef]
137. Song, J.; Ahn, C.; Chun, C.H.; Jin, E.J. A long non-coding RNA, GAS5, plays a critical role in the regulation of miR-21 during osteoarthritis. *J. Orthop. Res.* **2014**, *32*, 1628–1635. [CrossRef]
138. Wang, G.; Bu, X.; Zhang, Y.; Zhao, X.; Kong, Y.; Ma, L.; Niu, S.; Wu, B.; Meng, C. LncRNA-UCA1 enhances MMP-13 expression by inhibiting miR- 204-5p in human chondrocytes. *Oncotarget* **2017**, *8*, 91281–91290. [CrossRef]
139. Seda Yar Saglam, A.; Alp, E.; Ilke Onen, H. Circular RNAs and Its Biological Functions in Health and Disease. In *Gene Expression and Phenotypic Traits*; IntechOpen: London, UK, 2020. [CrossRef]
140. Hansen, T.B.; Jensen, T.I.; Clausen, B.H.; Bramsen, J.B.; Finsen, B.; Damgaard, C.K.; Kjems, J. Natural RNA circles function as efficient microRNA sponges. *Nature* **2013**, *495*, 384–388. [CrossRef]
141. Liu, Q.; Zhang, X.; Hu, X.; Dai, L.; Fu, X.; Zhang, J.; Ao, Y. Circular RNA Related to the Chondrocyte ECM Regulates MMP13 Expression by Functioning as a MiR-136 "Sponge" in Human Cartilage Degradation. *Sci. Rep.* **2016**, *6*. [CrossRef]
142. Gu, H.; Jiao, Y.; Yu, X.; Li, X.; Wang, W.; Ding, L.; Liu, L. Resveratrol inhibits the IL-1β-induced expression ofMMP-13 and IL-6 in human articular chondrocytes viaTLR4/MyD88-dependent and -independent signaling cascades. *Int. J. Mol. Med.* **2017**, *39*, 734–740. [CrossRef] [PubMed]
143. Yang, Q.; Wu, S.; Mao, X.; Wang, W.; Tai, H. Inhibition effect of curcumin on TNF-α and MMP-13 expression induced by advanced glycation end products in chondrocytes. *Pharmacology* **2013**, *91*, 77–85. [CrossRef]
144. Rasheed, Z.; Anbazhagan, A.N.; Akhtar, N.; Ramamurthy, S.; Voss, F.R.; Haqqi, T.M. Green tea polyphenol epigallocatechin-3-gallate inhibits advanced glycation end product-induced expression of tumor necrosis factor-α and matrix metalloproteinase-13 in human chondrocytes. *Arthritis Res. Ther.* **2009**, *11*. [CrossRef] [PubMed]

145. Janusz, M.J.; Hookfin, E.B.; Heitmeyer, S.A.; Woessner, J.F.; Freemont, A.J.; Hoyland, J.A.; Brown, K.K.; Hsieh, L.C.; Almstead, N.G.; De, B.; et al. Moderation of iodoacetate-induced experimental osteoarthritis in rats by matrix metalloproteinase inhibitors. *Osteoarthr. Cartil.* **2001**, *9*, 751–760. [CrossRef] [PubMed]

146. Fingleton, B. Matrix Metalloproteinases as Valid Clinical Target. *Curr. Pharm. Des.* **2006**, *13*, 333–346. [CrossRef] [PubMed]

147. Johnson, A.R.; Pavlovsky, A.G.; Ortwine, D.F.; Prior, F.; Man, C.F.; Bornemeier, D.A.; Banotai, C.A.; Mueller, W.T.; McConnell, P.; Yan, C.; et al. Discovery and characterization of a novel inhibitor of matrix metalloprotease-13 that reduces cartilage damage in vivo without joint fibroplasia side effects. *J. Biol. Chem.* **2007**, *282*, 27781–27791. [CrossRef]

148. Nuti, E.; Casalini, F.; Avramova, S.I.; Santamaria, S.; Cercignani, G.; Marinelli, L.; La Pietra, V.; Novellino, E.; Orlandini, E.; Nencetti, S.; et al. N-O-isopropyl sulfonamido-based hydroxamates: Design, synthesis and biological evaluation of selective matrix metalloproteinase-13 inhibitors as potential therapeutic agents for osteoarthritis. *J. Med. Chem.* **2009**, *52*, 4757–4773. [CrossRef]

149. Monovich, L.G.; Tommasi, R.A.; Fujimoto, R.A.; Blancuzzi, V.; Clark, K.; Cornell, W.D.; Doti, R.; Doughty, J.; Fang, J.; Farley, D.; et al. Discovery of potent, selective, and orally active carboxylic acid based inhibitors of matrix metalloproteinase-13. *J. Med. Chem.* **2009**, *52*, 3523–3538. [CrossRef] [PubMed]

150. Nara, H.; Sato, K.; Kaieda, A.; Oki, H.; Kuno, H.; Santou, T.; Kanzaki, N.; Terauchi, J.; Uchikawa, O.; Kori, M. Design, synthesis, and biological activity of novel, potent, and highly selective fused pyrimidine-2-carboxamide-4-one-based matrix metalloproteinase (MMP)-13 zinc-binding inhibitors. *Bioorg. Med. Chem.* **2016**, *24*, 6149–6165. [CrossRef]

151. Nara, H.; Kaieda, A.; Sato, K.; Naito, T.; Mototani, H.; Oki, H.; Yamamoto, Y.; Kuno, H.; Santou, T.; Kanzaki, N.; et al. Discovery of novel, highly potent, and selective matrix metalloproteinase (MMP)-13 inhibitors with a 1,2,4-triazol-3-yl moiety as a zinc binding group using a structure-based design approach. *J. Med. Chem.* **2017**, *60*, 608–626. [CrossRef] [PubMed]

152. De Savi, C.; Morley, A.D.; Ting, A.; Nash, I.; Karabelas, K.; Wood, C.M.; James, M.; Norris, S.J.; Karoutchi, G.; Rankine, N.; et al. Selective non zinc binding inhibitors of MMP13. *Bioorg. Med. Chem. Lett.* **2011**, *21*, 4215–4219. [CrossRef]

153. Jie, J.L.; Nahra, J.; Johnson, A.R.; Bunker, A.; O'Brien, P.; Yue, W.S.; Ortwine, D.F.; Man, C.F.; Baragi, V.; Kilgore, K.; et al. Quinazolinones and pyrido[3,4-d]pyrimidin-4-ones as orally active and specific matrix metalloproteinase-13 inhibitors for the treatment of osteoarthritis. *J. Med. Chem.* **2008**, *51*, 835–841. [CrossRef]

154. Schnute, M.E.; O'Brien, P.M.; Nahra, J.; Morris, M.; Howard Roark, W.; Hanau, C.E.; Ruminski, P.G.; Scholten, J.A.; Fletcher, T.R.; Hamper, B.C.; et al. Discovery of (pyridin-4-yl)-2H-tetrazole as a novel scaffold to identify highly selective matrix metalloproteinase-13 inhibitors for the treatment of osteoarthritis. *Bioorg. Med. Chem. Lett.* **2010**, *20*, 576–580. [CrossRef] [PubMed]

155. Gege, C.; Bao, B.; Bluhm, H.; Boer, J.; Gallagher, B.M.; Korniski, B.; Powers, T.S.; Steeneck, C.; Taveras, A.G.; Baragi, V.M. Discovery and evaluation of a non-Zn chelating, selective matrix metalloproteinase 13 (MMP-13) inhibitor for potential intra-articular treatment of osteoarthritis. *J. Med. Chem.* **2012**, *55*, 709–716. [CrossRef]

156. Settle, S.; Vickery, L.; Nemirovskiy, O.; Vidmar, T.; Bendele, A.; Messing, D.; Ruminski, P.; Schnute, M.; Sunyer, T. Cartilage degradation biomarkers predict efficacy of a novel, highly selective matrix metalloproteinase 13 inhibitor in a dog model of osteoarthritis: Confirmation by multivariate analysis that modulation of type II collagen and aggrecan degradation pepti. *Arthritis Rheum.* **2010**, *62*, 3006–3015. [CrossRef] [PubMed]

157. Ruminski, P.G.; Massa, M.; Strohbach, J.; Hanau, C.E.; Schmidt, M.; Scholten, J.A.; Fletcher, T.R.; Hamper, B.C.; Carroll, J.N.; Shieh, H.S.; et al. Discovery of N-(4-Fluoro-3-methoxybenzyl)-6-(2-(((2S,5R)-5-(hydroxymethyl)-1,4-dioxan-2-yl)methyl)-2H-tetrazol-5-yl)-2-methylpyrimidine-4-carboxamide. A Highly Selective and Orally Bioavailable Matrix Metalloproteinase-13 Inhibitor for the Potential Treat. *J. Med. Chem.* **2016**, *59*, 313–327. [CrossRef]

158. Zheng, S.; Hunter, D.J.; Xu, J.; Ding, C. Monoclonal antibodies for the treatment of osteoarthritis. *Expert Opin. Biol. Ther.* **2016**, *16*, 1529–1540. [CrossRef] [PubMed]

159. Naito, S.; Takahashi, T.; Onoda, J.; Yamauchi, A.; Kawai, T.; Kishino, J.; Yamane, S.; Fujii, I.; Fukui, N.; Numata, Y. Development of a neutralizing antibody specific for the active form of matrix metalloproteinase-13. *Biochemistry* **2012**, *51*, 8877–8884. [CrossRef]

160. Amar, S.; Fields, G.B. Potential clinical implications of recent matrix metalloproteinase inhibitor design strategies. *Expert Rev. Proteomics* **2015**, *12*, 445–447. [CrossRef]

MDPI

St. Alban-Anlage 66

4052 Basel

Switzerland

Tel. +41 61 683 77 34

Fax +41 61 302 89 18

www.mdpi.com

International Journal of Molecular Sciences Editorial Office

E-mail: ijms@mdpi.com

www.mdpi.com/journal/ijms

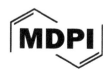